WS 200 FEL

EVIDENCE-BASED
PEDIATRICS

EVIDENCE-BASED
PEDIATRICS

William Feldman, MD, FRCPC

Professor Emeritus of Pediatrics

University of Toronto

Editor, Annals of the Royal College

of Physicians and Surgeons of Canada

Ottawa, Canada

2000

B.C. Decker Inc.

Hamilton • London • Saint Louis

B.C. Decker Inc.
4 Hughson Street South
P.O. Box 620, L.C.D. 1
Hamilton, Ontario L8N 3K7
Tel: 905-522-7017; 1-800-568-7281
Fax: 905-522-7839
E-mail: info@bcdecker.com
Website: http://www.bcdecker.com

00 01 02 03 / PC / 6 5 4 3 2 1

ISBN 1-55009-087-9

Printed in Canada

Sales and Distribution

United States
B.C. Decker Inc.
P.O. Box 785
Lewiston, NY USA
Tel: 905-522-7017/1-800-568-7281
Fax: 905-522-7839
e-mail: info@bcdecker.com

Canada
B.C. Decker Inc.
4 Hughson Street South
P.O. Box 620, L.C.D. 1
Hamilton, Ontario, Canada L8N 3K7
Tel: 905-522-7017; 1-800-568-7281
Fax: 905-522-7839
e-mail: info@bcdecker.com

Japan
Igaku-Shoin Ltd.
Foreign Publications Department
3-24-17 Hongo, Bunkyo-ku,
Tokyo 113-8719, Japan
Tel: 3 3817 5676
Fax: 3 3815 6776
e-mail: fmbook@ba2.so-net.or.jp

South America
Ernesto Reichmann, Distribuidora
De Livros Ltda.
Rua Coronel Marques
335-Tatuape, 03440-000
Sao Paulo-SP-Brazil
Tel/Fax: 011-218-2122

U.K., Europe, Scandinavia, Middle East
Blackwell Science Ltd.
Osney Mead
Oxford OX2 0EL
United Kingdom
Tel: 44-1865-206206
Fax: 44-1865-721205
e-mail: info@blackwell-science.com

Australia
Blackwell Science Asia Pty, Ltd.
54 University Street
Carlton, Victoria 3053
Australia
Tel: 03 9347 0300
Fax: 03 9349 3016
e-mail: info@blacksci.asia.com.au

South Korea
Seoul Medical Scientific Books Co.
C.P.O. Box 9794
Seoul 100-697
Seoul, Korea
Tel: 82-2925-5800
Fax: 82-2927-7283

Foreign Rights
John Scott & Co.
International Publishers' Agency
P.O. Box 878
Kimberton, PA 19442
Tel: 610-827-1640
Fax: 610-827-1671

Notice: The authors and publisher have made every effort to ensure that the patient care recommended herein, including choice of drugs and drug dosages, is in accord with the accepted standard and practice at the time of publication. However, since research and regulation constantly change clinical standards, the reader is urged to check the product information sheet included in the package of each drug, which includes recommended doses, warnings, and contraindications. This is particularly important with new or infrequently used drugs.

Contributors

Adelle Roberta Atkinson, RN, BSc, MD, FRCPC, FAAP
Fellow, Division of Immunology and
   Allergy
The Hospital for Sick Children
Toronto, Canada

Carol S. Camfield, MD, FRCPC
IWK Grace Health Centre
Professor of Pediatrics
Department of Pediatrics
Dalhousie University Medical School
Halifax, Canada

Peter R. Camfield, MD, FRCPC
IWK Grace Health Centre
Professor and Chair, Department of
   Pediatrics
Dalhousie University Medical School
Halifax, Canada

H. Dele Davies, MD, MSc, FRCPC
Director, Child Health Research Unit
Alberta Children's Hospital
Associate Professor
Departments of Pediatrics, Microbiology
   and Infectious Diseases and
   Community Health
University of Calgary
Calgary, Canada

Paul T. Dick, MDCM, MSc, FRCPC
Pediatrician, Division of Pediatric
   Medicine
The Hospital for Sick Children
Assistant Professor of Pediatrics
University of Toronto
Toronto, Canada

J.M. Dooley, MBBCh, FRCPC
Division of Pediatric Neurology
IWK-Grace Health Centre
Associate Professor, Department of
   Pediatrics
Dalhousie University
Halifax, Canada

Darcy L. Fehlings, MD, MSc, FRCPC
Hospital for Sick Children
Bloorview MacMillan Centre
Assistant Professor in Pediatrics
University of Toronto
Toronto, Canada

Brian M. Feldman, MD, MSc, FRCPC
Staff Rheumatologist
The Hospital for Sick Children
Clinical Chief, Arthritis Team
Bloorview MacMillan Centre
Assistant Professor
University of Toronto
Toronto, Canada

Mark E. Feldman, MD, FRCPC
Chief of Pediatrics
St. Joseph's Health Centre
Assistant Professor
University of Toronto
Toronto, Canada

William Feldman, MD, FRCPC
Professor Emeritus of Pediatrics
University of Toronto
Editor, Annals of the Royal College
   of Physicians and Surgeons of
   Canada
Ottawa, Canada

Norma Goggin, MBBCh, MRCP
Lecturer in Ambulatory Paediatrics,
    Department of Child Health
Royal Free and University College Medical
    School
University College London
Royal Free Hospital
London, United Kingdom

Ronald Gold, MD, MPH, FRCPC
Honorary Consultant
The Hospital for Sick Children
Professor Emeritus of Pediatrics
Faculty of Medicine
University of Toronto
Toronto, Canada

Eudice Goldberg, MD, FRCPC
Head, Division of Adolescent Medicine
The Hospital for Sick Children
Associate Professor of Pediatrics
Department of Pediatrics
Faculty of Medicine
University of Toronto
Toronto, Canada

K.E. Gordon, MD, MS, FRCPC
Division of Pediatric Neurology
IWK-Grace Health Centre
Associate Professor, Department of
    Pediatrics
Dalhousie University
Halifax, Canada

Saul Greenberg, MD, FRCPC
Staff Physician
The Hospital for Sick Children
Associate Professor
University of Toronto
Toronto, Canada

R. I. Hilliard, MD, EdD, FRCPC
Division of Pediatric Medicine
The Hospital for Sick Children
Professor of Pediatrics
University of Toronto
Toronto, Canada

Moshe Ipp, MBBCh, FRCPC, FAAP
The Hospital for Sick Children
Associate Professor
University of Toronto
Toronto, Canada

Sheila J. Jacobson, MBBCh
Division of Pediatric Medicine
The Hospital for Sick Children
Assistant Professor in Pediatrics
University of Toronto
Toronto, Canada

Debra K. Katzman, MD, FRCPC
Medical Director, The Eating Disorder
    Program
The Hospital for Sick Children
Associate Professor of Pediatrics
Department of Pediatrics
University of Toronto
Toronto, Ontario

Kevin B. Laupland, MD, FRCPC
Division of Infectious Diseases
Alberta Children's Hospital
Fellow, Infectious Diseases and Critical
    Care
University of Calgary
Calgary, Canada

Katherine A. Leonard, MD, FRCPC
Adolescent Health Service
North York General Hospital
Pediatric Department/Teen Clinic
Centenary Health Centre
North York, Canada

Brian W. McCrindle, MD, MPH, FRCPC
Staff Cardiologist
The Hospital for Sick Children
Associate Professor of Pediatrics
University of Toronto
Toronto, Canada

Golda Milo-Manson, MD, MHSc, FRCPC
Developmental Pediatrician
Bloorview-MacMillan Centre
The Hospital for Sick Children
North York General Hospital
Assistant Professor
University of Toronto
Toronto, Canada

Michael E.K. Moffatt, MSc, FRCPC
Health Sciences Centre
Professor and Head, Department of
    Pediatrics and Child Health
University of Manitoba
Winnipeg, Canada

Arne Ohlsson, MD, MSc, FRCPC
Director, Evidence Based Neonatal Care
    and Outcomes Research
Staff Neonatologist
Mount Sinai Hospital
Professor, Departments of Pediatrics,
    Obstetrics and Gynecology, and Public
    Health Sciences
University of Toronto
Toronto, Canada

Patricia C. Parkin, MD, FRCPC
Associate Professor
Department of Pediatrics
University of Toronto Faculty of Medicine
Head, Division of Pediatric Medicine
Hospital for Sick Children
Toronto, Canada

Hema Patel, MD, MSc, FRCPC
Ambulatory Care Pediatrician
The Montreal Children's Hospital
Assistant Professor in Pediatrics
McGill University
Montreal, Canada

Norman R. Saunders, MD, FRCPC
Associate Professor in Pediatrics
University of Toronto
Toronto, Canada

Vibhuti Shah, MD, MRCP(UK)
Department of Newborn and
    Developmental Pediatrics
Research Fellow in Neonatology
Sunnybrook and Women's College Health
    Sciences Centre
Toronto, Canada

Amir Shanon, MD, MPA
Director, Department of Medical
    Professionals
Ministry of Health
Tel Aviv, Israel

Michelle Kiran Shouldice, MSc, MD,
FRCPC
Section Head, Pediatric Outpatient
    Consultation
The Hospital for Sick Children
Assistant Professor
University of Toronto
Toronto, Canada

Michael B.H. Smith, MBBCh, FRCPC
Division Head in Pediatric Medicine
Physician Leader Acute and Chronic Care
IWK Grace Health Centre
Assistant Professor in Pediatrics
Dalhousie University
Halifax, Canada

Lynne J. Warda, MD, FRCPC
Pediatric Emergency Physician
Children's Hospital, Winnipeg
Medical Director, IMPACT—The Injury
    Prevention Centre of Children's
    Hospital, Winnipeg
Assistant Professor, Department of
    Pediatrics and Child Health
University of Manitoba
Winnipeg, Canada

This book is dedicated to infants, children, and adolescents, and to the physicians who care for them. The recipients and providers of health care all benefit when the care is evidence based.

Preface

Appropriate medical care for infants and children has three components. The first consists of the clinical skills of the practitioner to provide the preventive, diagnostic, and therapeutic interventions that are required to maintain health and to solve clinical problems. The second component is the practitioner's awareness of the need to ascertain the patients' and parents' knowledge of the nature of the problem and their values regarding how it should be solved. The third component, and by no means the least important, is the practitioner's determination that all interventions—preventive, diagnostic, therapeutic, and rehabilitative—should only be offered when the evidence that the intervention does more good than harm has been thoroughly reviewed.

The purpose of this book is to provide the physicians and nurses who care for infants and children with the best available evidence regarding the benefit/risk ratios underlying their interventions.

To quote those who have made the concept of "evidence-based medicine" recognized throughout the world: "...evidence-based medicine involves the integration of our clinical expertise, and our patients' values, with the best available research evidence."[1]

As the editor of *Evidence-Based Pediatrics*, I was faced with a number of challenges. The first was the choice of topics and problems to be included in the book. Because the likeliest readers are those engaged in the frontline provision of child health care, I decided that the emphasis would be on the most prevalent problems that pediatricians, family physicians, and nurses would face in day-to-day practice.

Although only a few rare conditions are discussed, the "red flags" that should alert the practitioner that a rare or serious condition may be causing the child's problems, are highlighted throughout the book.

The second challenge was the choice of authors. Having practiced as a primary care pediatrician, a subspecialist, and mainly as a general consultant pediatrician, I was aware that pediatricians in all three categories have valuable perspectives regarding child health care. I chose, therefore, not to select chapter writers on the basis of whether they were primary-care pediatricians, general consultants, or subspecialists, but rather on the basis of their clinical expertise and their knowledge and practice of evidence-based pediatrics. Thus, some of the authors are in busy primary care practices, some are hospital-based general consultants, and some are subspecialists.

Finally, the challenge of how to evaluate the quality of the evidence and the strength of the recommendations required careful consideration. I chose the system of evaluation of evidence used by the Canadian Task Force on the Periodic Health Examination.[2] A similar system has also been used by the U.S. Preventive Services Task Force.[3] In this system (Table 1), the highest quality (level I) of evidence is that obtained from properly conducted randomized controlled trials (RCTs), and the lowest level (level III) is that derived from opinions of authorities or expert committees, or from descriptive studies. An "A" recommendation, usually based on level I evidence, advises the practitioner to perform the intervention because the benefit/risk ratio is clearly high. A "C" recommendation advises the practitioner that the evidence either to use or not use a particular intervention is poor. An "E" recommendation advises that the intervention should not be used, either because the evidence is good that the maneuver is ineffective or is actually harmful. The "B" and "D" recommendations are based on "fair" evidence that the maneuver should (B) or should not (D) be performed.

This system of grading the evidence and recommendations was chosen because it has been widely used throughout North America for at least 20 years and appears to be well understood and accepted. In correspondence with a colleague, who practices and teaches Family Medicine, the system is described as having "real clinical utility as a way to summarize evidence. I know of no other that is better or more transparent." As he states, "In my discussions with practicing family doctors, they have often said that they really want the bottom line. What they mean is that at the community level, they need to know concisely and in a timely fashion (without having to search out the original studies) what they should do with the patient in the office. Having "A", "B", "C", etc. is helpful and straightforward."[4]

I hope the readers of this book will find the evidence and the recommendations concise, timely, helpful, and straightforward.

William Feldman, MD, FRCPC

QUALITY OF EVIDENCE

I: Evidence obtained from at least one properly randomized controlled trial.

II-1: Evidence obtained from well-designed controlled trials without randomization

II-2: Evidence obtained from well-designed cohort or case-control analytic studies, preferably from more than one center or research group.

II-3: Evidence obtained from comparisons between times or places with or without the intervention. Dramatic results in uncontrolled experiments (such as the results of treatment with penicillin in the 1940s) could also be included in this category.

III: Opinions of respected authorities, based on clinical experience, descriptive studies or reports of expert committees.

CLASSIFICATION OF RECOMMENDATIONS

A: There is *good* evidence to support the recommendation that the intervention be performed.

B: There is *fair* evidence to support the recommendation that the intervention be performed.

C: There is *poor* evidence regarding the value or harm of the intervention; recommendations may be made on other grounds.

D: There is *fair* evidence to support the recommendation that the intervention *not* be performed.

E: There is *good* evidence to support the recommendation that the intervention *not* be performed.

REFERENCES

1.   Sackett DL, Rosenberg WMC, Gray JAM, Haynes RB, Richardson WS. Evidence-based medicine: What it is and what it isn't. BMJ 1996;312:71–2.

2.   The Canadian Guide to Clinical Preventive Health Care. The Canadian Task Force on the Periodic Health Examination. Canada Communication Group Publishing, Ottawa, 1994.

3.   Guide to Clinical Preventive Services, Second Edition. Report of the U.S. Preventive Services Task Force, William and Wilkins Publishers, USA, 1996.

4.   McIsaac, Warren, MD. personal communication. May 1999.

Contents

CHAPTER 1

Problems of the Newborn: Prevention and Management

Vibhuti Shah, MD, MRCP

Arne Ohlsson, MD, MSc, FRCPC

The goals of evidence-based neonatal care are to decrease perinatal mortality and morbidity, improve long-term outcomes, and increase parents' and care providers' satisfaction.[1] An increasing number of health-care professionals with varying backgrounds and degrees of training are involved in the care of the critically ill preterm/term newborn as well as the healthy infant born at term. Thus, effective teamwork that includes the active participation of the parents is essential to optimize short- and long-term outcomes. This chapter focuses on effective interventions to prevent conditions commonly occurring in term infants who are born healthy. The reader is referred to systematic reviews in the Cochrane Library for evidence of effectiveness of interventions applied to the pregnant woman, the fetus, or the critically ill preterm/term newborn infant. The systematic reviews in the Cochrane Library are based on randomized controlled trials (RCTs) and are regularly updated.[2] Pediatric practitioners need to base their decisions on the best evidence available from such reviews and other sources of up-to-date information. In addition to knowledge about the most current evidence from the literature, health-care providers need to maintain a high level of technical skills related to their specialty. In our opinion, the provision of evidence-based health care is dependent on a number of additional provider skills/qualities including (1) active listening and communication, (2) empathy, (3) sensitivity to and respect of ethnic and cultural differences, (4) collection and analysis of relevant data and a timely response, (5) individualized care, (6) continuity of care, (7) appropriate consultation, and (8) flexibility — the ability to change practice, when appropriate.

PERINATAL STATISTICS, PERINATAL SURVEILLANCE, AND BENCHMARKING

In 1996, there were 364,732 births in Canada. In the same year, Canada ranked 14th in the world with regard to its infant mortality rate.[3] In the year 1996, out of 1,000 live births, 5 to 6 infants died before they reached 1 year of age, the total reaching approximately 2,000 infants.[3] To match the infant mortality rates of the countries with the lowest rates (Singapore, Japan, Finland, Sweden, Norway, Hong Kong), (3.9 to 4.0/1,000 live births), an additional 500 infants born in Canada in 1996 should have survived till the age of 1 year. An increase in the infant mortality rate in Canada in 1993 was likely due to an increased registration of infants weighing less than 500 g as live births.[4] The infant mortality rate was 5.8 in Australia and 6.1 per 1,000 live births in the United Kingdom in 1996.[3] A study has shown an increase in the preterm birth rate in Canada (from 6.3 percent in 1981–1983 to 6.8 percent in 1992–1994; a relative increase of 9 percent) related to increase in obstetric interventions, multiple pregnancies, and ultrasonographic dating of the pregnancy.[5] Maternal education, a modifiable aspect of socioeconomic status, has consistently been found to be inversely related to infant mortality.[6] A recent study from the province of Quebec in Canada confirms that fetal and infant mortality rates are higher among the offspring of mothers with less than 12 years of education, compared with mothers with at least 14 years of education, even after adjusting for maternal age, parity, marital status, and infant's gender.[7] If groups of all education levels had the same low rates as that of the higher-education group, the number of fetal and infant deaths would be reduced by approximately 20 percent.

Significant variations in survival rates exist among neonates admitted to different Canadian neonatal intensive care units.[8] "Benchmarking" techniques can be used to improve the care and outcomes in a unit with marked variance from the norm.[9]

Perinatal surveillance is a system of data collection, data analysis, and response. The Canadian Perinatal Surveillance System (CPSS) plans to collect and analyze data on all recognized pregnancies in Canada, regardless of their outcome — abortion, ectopic pregnancy, stillbirth, or live birth — and the data on the determinants of health during the first year of life. Such data collection and analysis will allow for benchmarking at a national, regional, or local level.[9] Standardized perinatal records carried by the pregnant woman would increase her feeling of having control over her antenatal care and also would facilitate data collection.[10,11]

ANTENATAL INTERVENTIONS TO IMPROVE PERINATAL OUTCOMES

The Cochrane Library is the best single source of reliable evidence on the effects of perinatal/neonatal health care.[2] It currently includes 149 full reviews and 24 protocols from the Pregnancy and Child Birth Review group and 73 reviews and 21 protocols from the Neonatal Review group.[2] As new reviews are added quarterly and old reviews are updated regularly, the Cochrane Library should be made available in the delivery/postpartum areas and consulted for the most up-to-date information. A new "obstetric wheel" that is an improvement on the existing obstetric calendar wheels has been developed.[12,13] It incorporates evidence-based information in an innovative way. It should facilitate prenatal care, education, and communication and foster realistic expectations about the likely timing of delivery.

RESUSCITATION

All health-care givers attending deliveries should be trained in neonatal resuscitation in accordance with the latest guidelines by the American Academy of Pediatrics (AAP) and the American Heart Association.[14]

EXAMINATION AT BIRTH

If at all possible, the examination of the newborn should take place in the presence of at least one of the parents so that any deviation from the norm can be discussed with the parents and any questions can be answered. Proper hand-washing prior to the examination is essential. The hips and the genital and anorectal areas should be examined last. Table 1–1 lists the chronological steps that will facilitate the physical examination of the newborn infant, cause minimal amount of stress, and reduce the risk of nosocomial infections. Admission and discharge examinations of the newborn should be done on two separate occasions.

VITAMIN K

To prevent hemorrhagic disease of the newborn, vitamin K_1 should be given as a single intramuscular dose of 1.0 mg within the first 6 hours after birth to all newborns with a birth weight >1,500 g; if the birth weight is <1,500 g, 0.5 mg should be given.[15] The pain response to an intramuscular injection of vitamin K_1 may be less, if given shortly after birth.[16]

OPHTHALMIA NEONATORUM

Ophthalmia neonatorum is defined as conjunctivitis with discharge occurring in the first month of life. Untreated, it can lead to blindness, especially if the infectious agent is *Neisseria gonorrhea*. Etiologic agents may be chemical (topical antimicrobial agents), bacterial, or rarely viral, such as herpes virus, molluscum contagiosum, and papilloma virus. Neonates present with redness of the conjunctiva, swelling of the eyelids, and purulent dis-

Table 1–1 History and Examination of the Newborn*

- Family, obstetric, and labor history

- Weight, length, head circumference (growth in relation to gestational age)

- Presence of any unusual facial features (facial nerve palsy) or external malformations/deformations. Normal eyes. Normal sucking reflex

- Head (fontanels, sutures, presence of cephalic hematoma, caput succedaneum, vacuum extraction or forceps marks), nostrils patent, palate intact, normally formed external ears

- Vital signs (pink in room air, normal breathing pattern [absence of flaring of nostrils, grunting, retractions, stridor], heart rate, perfusion, level of consciousness, tone, normal temperature)

- Skin (cyanosis, jaundice, rash, abrasion, petechiae, distribution of hair)

- Auscultation of chest and heart (air entry equal on both sides, heart sounds heard best to the left of the midline, regular heart rate, no murmur detected)

- Examination of the abdomen (shape, masses, size of liver/spleen)

- Normal umbilical cord with three vessels

- Presence of femoral pulses. Absence of inguinal masses

- Genitalia (descended testes, normal sized penis without hypospadias, ambiguous genitalia, hyperpigmentation of genitalia, vaginal secretions)

- Neurological: presence of neonatal reflexes (symmetric Moro reflex: no brachial plexus injury, presence of grasp reflex)

- Hips (dislocation: ultrasound examination for confirmation)

- Normal cry

- Spine (deep pinonidal sinus, hair-tuft: ultrasound examination to rule out/in spina bifida occulta)

- Anus (patency)

- Any concerns raised by family members or attending health-care workers to be addressed

*to be performed after birth and at discharge from hospital in the presence of a family member

charge. Gonococcal ophthalmia neonatorum tends to start earlier and be more severe than chlamydial infection. The efficacy of single-dose topical antimicrobial prophylaxis in preventing ophthalmia neonatorum has been established. Universal ocular prophylaxis, which is a routine practice in Canada and the United States, should be administered as soon as possible (within 1 hour) after birth.[17] One percent silver nitrate,[18] 0.5 percent erythromycin, or 1 percent tetracycline ointment[19-21] have comparable efficacy in preventing conjunctivitis caused by most bacterial pathogens, including penicillin-sensitive *Neisseria gonorrhea*. Although *Chlamydia trachomatis* is sensitive to erythromycin, tetracycline, and silver nitrate, the evidence supporting the efficacy of these agents has not been established.[22-23] Recent studies[24,25] evaluating the efficacy of 0.5 percent erythromycin, 1 percent silver nitrate, and 2.5 percent povidone-iodine as prophylactic agents demonstrated that the use of povidone-iodine was associated with fewer cases of ophthalmia neonatorum and was found to be more effective against chlamydial conjunctivitis as compared with the other two agents. The potential advantages of povidone-iodine include a broader antibacterial spectrum, and an antiviral spectrum, which includes herpes simplex and human immunodeficiency virus (HIV); it is less costly and can be prepared locally. Further studies are needed to assess its effectiveness and possible toxicity in ophthalmia neonatorum. The availability of effective ocular prophylaxis, however, does not diminish the importance of prenatal screening for and appropriate treatment of maternal gonococcal and chlamydial infections.

METABOLIC SCREENING

Guthrie developed newborn screening for inborn errors of metabolism, using dried blood samples on filter paper in the 1960s.[26] Since then screening for phenylketonuria (PKU) and congenital hypothyroidism (CH) has been recommended for all newborns prior to discharge from the nursery in the developed countries; screening for other disorders is highly variable. Phenylketonuria, a disorder of phenylalanine metabolism has an incidence of 1:10,000 to 1:25,000 births in North America.[27] Without treatment, affected individuals develop severe mental retardation, seizures, spasticity, eczema, and autistic-like behavior. Since the implementation of screening and early dietary interventions, these manifestations have rarely developed in children born after the mid-1960s.[28-32] The AAP and the American Academy of Family Physicians recommend screening of all newborns prior to discharge from the nursery and repeat screening at 1 to 2 weeks of age for infants discharged prior to 24 hours.[33] Similar recommendations have been published by the Canadian Task Force, except that repeat screening be performed at 2 to 7 days of age for infants discharged prior to 24 hours of age.[34] Premature infants and those with illnesses should be tested at or near 7 days of age. There is a growing concern that the practice of early discharge from the nursery may lead to a falsely negative screening result as the test is most reliable when performed at 24 to 48 hours of age, 24 hours after the first protein feed.[35]

Congenital hypothyroidism, also detected by newborn screening, has an incidence of 1:3,600 to 1:5,000.[36] Deficiency of the thyroid hormone leads to mental retardation, if not diagnosed early and treated. Most infants appear to be clinically normal until 3 months of age; therefore laboratory tests are the only reliable means of diagnosing CH. Treatment is simple and effective, with thyroid hormone replacement. Screening has been extremely successful in eradicating severe mental retardation resulting from CH. However, despite early diagnosis through screening, children with severe CH (ie, those with marked retardation of bone age and/or low circulating thyroxine [T4] before treatment) have lower IQ than children with less severe CH.[37] Recent studies suggest that this developmental gap may be closed with early treatment (within 2 weeks of birth), using a higher dose of levothyroxine.[38]

BREAST-FEEDING

There is compelling evidence that breast-feeding is the natural and normal way to provide optimal nutritional, immunologic, and emotional nurturing for the growth and development of infants.[39] Human milk is uniquely superior and species specific; all substitute feeding options differ markedly from it. The advantages of breast-feeding are listed in Table 1–2.[40-47] Despite being endorsed as the ideal method of infant feeding by all levels of government and many Canadian health professional associations, optimal initiation and duration rates have not been achieved in Canada. The Canadian Pediatric Society (CPS) recommends breast-feeding for the first 6 months of life.[48] Despite the recommendations, a 1990 survey revealed that approximately 80 percent of Canadian mothers chose to breast feed, but that only 30 percent continued to do so for at least 6 months.[49] Factors affecting feeding practices during the first 4 months include the perceived inadequacy of milk supply and/or the perceived hunger of the baby, difficulties encountered in the feeding process such as poor sucking, sore nipples, and breast infection, and mothers with low educational levels.[50] Mothers who chose to breast feed during the preconception period or in early pregnancy were more likely to

---

Table 1–2 Advantages of Breast-Feeding

- Provides ideal nutrition for infants and contributes to their healthy growth and development[40,41]

- Reduces incidence and severity of infectious disease, thereby lowering infant morbidity and mortality[42,43]

- Protects against allergies[44,45]

- Contributes to women's health by reducing the risk of breast and ovarian cancers, and by increasing the spacing between pregnancies[46,47]

- Provides social and economic benefits to the family and the nation

- Brings mother and baby together emotionally as well as physically, and helps to build a secure and loving relationship

---

breast feed longer than mothers who made their decision later.[51,52] Also, mothers with previous breast-feeding experience were noted to have high initiation and duration rates.[53]

Recently, breast-feeding difficulties have been compounded by a trend toward early discharge of newborns and mothers. Both the CPS[54] and AAP[55] have set standards for early discharge, which include breast-feeding criteria, and emphasize the need for an early follow-up visit for newborns discharged less than 48 hours after birth. Two of the best measures of breast-feeding adequacy include infant weight and elimination patterns.[56] Traditionally, physicians have been trained to accept a weight loss of 10 percent of birth weight as normal; however, by redefining excessive weight loss as 8 percent of birth weight, more at-risk infants could be targeted for early interventions. A newborn's elimination pattern is also a sensitive indicator of adequacy of milk intake. Usually, within a day or two after the initiation of breast-feeding, a newborn should be voiding urine six to eight times and passing more than four yellow, seedy "milk" stools per day.

There are few contraindications to breast-feeding, and these include maternal HIV infection, active tuberculosis, or drug abuse and galactosemia in the infant.[57,58] The use of a small number of maternal medications prohibits breast-feeding (eg, cytotoxic and immunosuppressive drugs and gold salts). Comprehensive tables of drugs that are safe or contraindicated are available to the physician for reference.[59]

In newborns, structural defects such as cleft lip and palate, and alterations in neurological functions such as in Down syndrome or hydrocephalus require special management to facilitate breast-feeding.[60]

In 1989, the World Health Organization (WHO) and the United Nations Children's Fund (UNICEF) jointly launched the "Baby-Friendly Hospital Initiative," which emphasized the creation of a hospital environment friendly to mothers and babies. This initiative was based on principals summarized in a joint statement issued by the two organizations in 1989 to support, protect, and promote breast-feeding.[61,62] A baby-friendly code of practice standards was drafted by the UNICEF and WHO (Table 1–3). To date, no hospital in Canada has been assigned as baby-friendly by the UNICEF, whereas in a less technologically developed country such as the Sultanate of Oman, all delivery units have been designated as "baby-friendly."[63]

In summary, optimizing breast-feeding outcomes begins in the perinatal period with effective breast-feeding education and screening for lactation risk factors. Early initiation of nursing, bedside instruction in the proper breast-feeding technique, rooming-in, and avoidance of pacifiers and unnecessary supplementation of breast-fed infants fosters successful breast-feeding during hospital stay. Early follow-up of infants after hospital discharge should be advocated to assess the effectiveness of breast-feeding.

Table 1–3 "Ten Steps to Successful Breast-Feeding"

1. Have a written breast-feeding policy that is routinely communicated to all health care staff.

2. Train all health-care staff in the skills necessary to implement this policy.

3. Inform all pregnant women about the benefits and management of breast-feeding.

4. Help mothers initiate breast feeding within 1 hour of birth.

5. Show mothers how to breast feed, and how to maintain lactation even if they are separated from their infants.

6. Give newborn infants no food or drink other than breast milk unless medically indicated.

7. Practice rooming-in: allow mothers and infants to stay together 24 hours a day.

8. Encourage breast-feeding on demand.

9. Give no artificial teats or pacifiers (also called dummies and soothers) to breast-feeding infants.

10. Foster the establishment of breast-feeding support groups and refer mothers to them on discharge from hospital or clinic.

With permission from World Health Organization/United Nations Children's Fund: Protecting, promoting and supporting breastfeeding: the special role of maternity services, a joint WHO/UNICEF statement. 1989. Geneva, Switerland.

CIRCUMCISION

The evidence for possible benefits and harms of circumcision is evenly balanced, therefore circumcision of newborns should not be routinely performed.[64] When parents are making a decision about circumcision, they should be advised of the present state of knowledge about its benefits and harms. Their decision may ultimately be based on personal, religious, or cultural factors.[64] If circumcision is performed adequate analgesia/anesthesia should be provided.[65]

EARLY DISCHARGE

Postpartum hospital stays have decreased markedly over the past two decades from 4.1 days to 2.6 days between 1970 and 1992 in the United States[66] and from 5.3 days in 1984 to 1985 to 3.0 days in 1994 to 1995 (including cesarean sections) in Canada.[67] Since 1992, the length of stay has further decreased, with many infants being discharged at 24 hours or less after vaginal birth, and at 72 hours or less after cesarean birth. Similar reductions have also been observed in other jurisdictions such as the United Kingdom, Australia, and Scandinavia.[68-71] This trend that began as a consumer-driven movement has now been generalized, without adequate study, to all low-risk newborns.[72] The theoretical advantages of shorter postpartum hospital stay are economic (eg, fewer hospital days), medical (eg, reduction in the number of iatrogenic events such as cross-infection), increased breast feeding,[73] psychosocial (eg, parental preference, facilitation of bonding and attachment, enhanced family interactions),[74] improved patient satisfaction,[73] and better postpartum adjustment.[61] The potential disadvantages are social (eg, other parental preference, fewer opportunities to teach breast-feeding and parental skills) and medical (inability or failure to detect medical problems that become apparent only after 24 to 72 hours of age). The AAP[47] and the CPS, in conjunction with the Society of Obstetricians and Gynecologists of Canada,[54] have published guidelines that list explicit criteria for discharge prior to 48 hours. Two reviews published recently concerning early newborn discharge conclude that the definitive study of early newborn discharge has not been done.[75,76] Both groups conclude that published research to date provides little information on the consequences of shorter hospital stays or varying postdischarge practices for the low-risk population. Most of these studies were applied under restricted circumstances or were too small to detect a clinically significant effect on important outcomes. No adequately designed studies have examined early discharge without additional postdischarge services. A recent Canadian study concluded that a decrease in the mean length of stay from 4.5 days to 2.7 days, without community follow-up, was associated with increased re-admission rate in the first 2 weeks of life.[77] The main reasons for re-admission were jaundice and dehydration. Thus, decisions regarding the timing of discharge of the newborn should be individualized and made by the practitioner on the basis of the "unique characteristics of each mother and newborn," the ability and confidence of the parents to care for the newborn, the support system at home, and the access to appropriate follow-up.

NEONATAL HYPERBILIRUBINEMIA

Between 25 and 50 percent of full-term and a higher percentage of preterm infants develop clinical jaundice. Jaundice results from accumulation in the skin of unconjugated (indirect) lipid-soluble bilirubin derived from the breakdown of heme-containing proteins in the reticuloendothelial system. In the liver, unconjugated bilirubin is converted to water-soluble conjugated (direct) bilirubin by glucuronyl transferase enzyme and excreted through the bile into intestines and out through the feces. Neontal hyperbilirubinemia (NHB) can be broadly categorized into two groups:

Physiologic Jaundice

1. In the term infant, jaundice usually appears by the 2nd or 3rd day of life, peaks between 102 and 136 mmol/L (6 to 8 mg/dL) by 3 days of age, with a maximum level of 204 mmol/L (12 mg/dL), and then declines.
2. In the preterm infant, the peak level may be 170 to 204 mmol/L (10 to 12 mg/dL) by the 5th day of life, with a maximum level of 255 mmol/L (15 mg/dL) without any specific abnormality of bilirubin metabolism.

Factors responsible for physiologic jaundice include increased red blood cell volume, decreased red blood cell survival, increased ineffective erythropoiesis and turnover of non hemoglobin heme proteins, increased enterohepatic circulation, and defective conjugation due to decreased activity of glucuronyl transferase in infants.

Pathologic or Nonphysiologic Jaundice

This type is characterized by the following:

1. Jaundice visible within the first 24 hours of life.
2. Hemolysis due to maternal isoimmunization, G-6-PD deficiency, spherocytosis, or other causes.
3. A rise in serum bilirubin of more than 8 to 9 mmol/L (0.5 mg/dL) per hour.
4. Signs of underlying illness in any infant (vomiting, lethargy, poor feeding, temperature instability).
5. Elevation of serum bilirubin requiring phototherapy.
6. Jaundice persisting after 8 days in a term infant or after 14 days in a preterm infant.

A bilirubin level that justifies consideration for phototherapy should mandate investigation of the cause of hyperbilirubinemia. Management should include pertinent history of mother, description of labor and delivery, physical examination, and infant's clinical course. Table 1–4 lists the initial and subsequent laboratory investigations that should be undertaken.

Table 1–4 Laboratory Investigation for Hyperbilirubinemia in Term Newborn Infants

Indicated (if bilirubin plasma/serum concentrations reach phototherapy levels)

- Total or unconjugated bilirubin concentration
- Conjugated bilirubin concentration
- Blood groups (mother and infant) with direct antibody test (Coombs' test)
- Hemoglobin and hematocrit

Optional (in specific clinical circumstances)

- Complete blood count including manual differential white cell count
- Blood smear for red cell morphology
- Reticulocyte count
- Glucose-6-phosphate dehydrogenase screen
- Serum/plasma electrolytes and albumin or protein concentrations

With permission from Fetus and Newborn Committee, CPS. Approach to management of hyperbilirubinemia in term newborn infants. Pediatr Child Health 1999; 161-4.

Treatment for jaundice includes adequate hydration, phototherapy, and exchange transfusion. The goal of treatment is to avoid bilirubin concentrations that may result in kernicterus. The effectiveness of phototherapy is related to the area of exposed skin and the radiant energy and wavelength of the light.[78-82] It causes bilirubin to be changed by structural photoisomerization into water-soluble lumirubin, which is excreted in the urine.[78] Double or triple phototherapy is recommended to optimize the exposed skin surface and, thus, the efficacy of phototherapy. Except the eyes, all areas of the body should be exposed to light. Exchange transfusion is performed when phototherapy fails to control the rising bilirubin levels.

In 1994, the AAP issued a "practice parameter" with the aim to assist pediatricians and other health-care providers in managing hyperbilirubinemia in a healthy term infant without risk factors.[83] The Fetus and Newborn Committee of the CPS has recently published guidelines that recommend lower levels of bilirubin at which to start phototherapy (Figure 1–1).[84]

The current practice of early discharge of neonates means that jaundice is often not present/recognized at the time of discharge.[85] Appropriate parental education regarding feeding, signs of dehydration, and jaundice must be implemented in those nurseries where early discharge of neonates is practiced. Testing for serum bilirubin concentrations must be available on an outpatient basis, with adequate follow-up in place.

Bhutani and colleagues developed a nomogram for healthy term and near-term infants by which an hour-specific total serum bilirubin before hospital discharge can predict which infant is at high (values ≥ 95th percentile), intermediate (values between the 40th and 95th percentiles) or low risk (below the 40th percentile) for developing clinically significant hyperbilirubinemia.[86] The intermediate zone was further divided into lower intermediate (between the 40th and 75th percentiles) and upper intermediate (between the 76th and 95th percentiles) zones. In their study, the likelihood ratio for developing clinically significant jaundice was increased 14-fold in the high-risk zone, 3.2-fold in the upper intermediate zone, 0.5-fold in the lower intermediate zone, and none in the low risk zone. Thus, in conjunction with the practice parameter, a universal predischarge total serum bilirubin measurement would facilitate targeted intervention and follow-up in a safe manner.

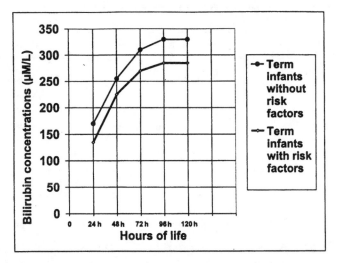

Figure 1–1 Guidelines for initiation of phototherapy for hyperbilirubinemia in term infants with and without risk factors. Some risk factors include gestional age younger than 37 weeks, birth weight less than 2500 g, hemolysis, jaundice at younger than 24 h of age, sepsis and the need for resuscitation at birth.

SUDDEN INFANT DEATH SYNDROME

Sudden infant death syndrome (SIDS) is defined as "sudden death of an infant under 1 year of age that remains unexplained after a thorough case investigation, including performance of a complete autopsy, examination of the death scene, and review of the clinical history." Sudden infant death syndrome is a leading cause of postneonatal infant mortality.[87] Various risk factors such as male infants, infants of unmarried women, increased parity, maternal smoking, low birth weight, and prematurity have been identified.[88] The CPS has issued a statement addressing strategies to reduce SIDS,[89] which has recently been updated.[90] The recommendations are summarized in Table 1–5. Sleeping on the stomach increases the risk of SIDS, and sleeping on the back or side reduces the risk. Exceptions to this recommendation include infants with Pierre Robin syndrome and infants with gastroesophageal reflux. Infants exposed to maternal smoking during pregnancy and postnatally have a higher risk of SIDS. Parents should therefore be advised to avoid smoking and exposing their infants to smoke. Overheating either from high room temperatures or wrapping should be avoided. The spe-

---

Table 1–5 Recommendations to Reduce the Risk of Sudden Infant Death Syndrome

- Normal, healthy infants should be placed on their back for sleep.

- Infants should be cared for in a smoke- and drug-free environment.

- Infants should be dressed and covered in a manner that will avoid overheating, even during illness.

- All women should be encouraged and helped to breast feed their babies.

- Firm flat bedding should be used for normal healthy infants, with sheets and light blankets as needed, but without products to maintain the sleeping position.

With permission from Canadian Foundation for the Study of Infant Deaths, the Canadian Institute of Child Health, the Canadian Paediatric Society, and Health Canada. Joint statement. Reducing the risk of sudden infant death syndrome in Canada. Pediatr Child Health 1999; 4: 223-6.

Table 1–6 Interventions in the Neonatal Period, the Quality of Evidence and Recommendations

Condition	Intervention	Quality of Evidence	Recommendation
Ophthalmia neonatorum	Universal ocular prophylaxis within one hour of birth with 1% silver nitrate solution, 0.5% erythromycin, 1% tetracycline ointment or 2.5% povidone-iodine solution	I, II-1, II-3	Good evidence to recommend ocular prophylaxis in newborns (A)
Hemorrhagic disease of the newborn	Prophylactic use of vitamin K at birth (1 mg by intramuscular route)	II-2, III	Good evidence to recommend prophylaxis (A)
Phenylketonuria (PKU) and congenital hypothyroidism (CH)	Newborn screening prior to discharge from the hospital. Infants discharged prior to 24 hours of age should have a repeat screening test between 2 and 7 days	II-2, II-3,III	Good evidence to ensure screening for PKU and CH (A)
Breast-feeding	Promote breast-feeding	II-2	Good evidence to counsel women regarding breast-feeding (A)
Sudden infant death syndrome	"Back to sleep" campaign	II-2, II-3, III	Good evidence to support "sleeping on the back" (A)

cific protective effect of breast-feeding against SIDS has not been proven; however it should be promoted because of its other well-documented benefits.[89]

LEVEL OF EVIDENCE

Table 1–6 outlines the quality of evidence and recommendations for interventions for different neonatal conditions.

Table 1–7 Websites that Provide Up-to-date Information Related to Perinatal/Neonatal Care

- American Academy of Pediatrics: http://www.aap.org

- British Association of Perinatal Medicine: http://www.bapm-London.org

- Canadian Pediatric Society: www.cps.ca

- Canadian Perinatal Surveillance System — Laboratory Center for Disease Control: http://www.hc-sc.gc.ca/hpb/lcdc/brch/reprod.html

- Cochrane Library (abstracts of Cochrane reviews): http:hiru.mcmaster.ca/cochrane/

- Cochrane Library (full Cochrane neonatal reviews): http://silk.nih.gov/silk/cochrane

- Society of Obstetricians and Gynecologists of Canada: http://www.medical.org

- The College of Family Physicians of Canada: http://www.cfpc.ca

INFORMATION AVAILABLE ON THE INTERNET

Table 1–7 lists websites of different organizations providing information on perinatal/neonatal care.

REFERENCES

1. Ohlsson A. Randomized controlled trials and systematic reviews: a foundation for evidence-based perinatal medicine. Acta Pediatr 1996;85:647-55.

2. The Cochrane Library. The Cochrane Library Issue 2. 1999. Update Software Ltd.

3. Guyer B, MacDorman MF, Martin JA, et al. Annual summary of vital statistics — 1997. Pediatrics 1998;102:1333-49.

4. Joseph KS, Kramer MS. Recent trends in Canadian infant mortality rates: effect of changes in registration of live newborns weighing less than 500 g. Can Med Assoc J 1996;155:1047-52.

5. Joseph KS, Kramer MS, Marcoux S, et al. Determinants of preterm birth rates in Canada from 1981 through 1983 and from 1992 through 1994. N Engl J Med 1998;339:1434-9.

6. Kramer MS. Determinants of low birth weight: methodological assessment and meta-analysis. Bull WHO 1987;65:663-737.

7. Chen J, Fair M, Wilkins R, Cyr M, Fetal and Infant Mortality Group of the Canadian Perinatal Surveillance System. Maternal education and fetal and infant mortality in Quebec. Health Rep Stat Can 1998;10:53-65.

8. Lee SK, Ohlsson A, Synnes AR, et al. Mortality variations and illness severity (SNAP-II) in Canadian NICUs [abstract]. Pediatr Res 1999;45:248A.

9. Mohr JJ, Mahoney CC, Nelson EC, et al. Improving health care, Part 3: Clinical benchmarking for best patient care. Quality Improvement 1996;22:599-616.

10. Elbourne D, Richardson M, Chalmers I, et al. The Newbury maternity care study: a randomized controlled trial to assess a policy of women holding their own obstetric records. Br J Obstet Gyn 1987;94:612-9.

11. Lacy B, Bartlett L, Ohlsson A. A standard perinatal care record in Canada: justification, acceptability and feasibility. J Soc Obstet Gyn Can 1998;20:557-65.

12. Grzybowski S, Nout R, Kirkham CM. Maternity care calendar wheel. Improved obstetric wheel developed in British Columbia. Can Fam Phys 1999;45:661-6.

13. Kirkham CM, Gryzbowski S. Maternity care guidelines checklist. To assist physicians in implementing CPGs. Can Fam Phys 1999;45:671-8.

14. Bloom RS, Cropley C, AHA/AAP Neonatal Resuscitation Program Steering Committee. Textbook of neonatal resuscitation. Elk Grove Village, Illinois: American Academy of Pediatrics, American Heart Association; 1994.

15. Fetus and Newborn Committee Canadian Pediatric Society, Committee on Child and Adolescent Health, College of Family Physicians of Canada. Routine administration of vitamin K to newborns. Pediatr Child Health Care 1997;2:429-31.

16. Bergqvist LL, Baumann P, Katz-Salamon M, et al. The stress of birth modifies the response to pain during the first hours after birth. [abstract] Pediatr Res 1999;45:350A.

17. Canadian Task Force on the Periodic Health Examination. Periodic health examination, 1992, update 4. Prophylaxis for gonococcal and chlamydial ophthalmia neonatorum. Can Med Assoc J 1992;147:1449-54.

18. Crede CSR. Die Verhutung der Augenentzundung der Neugeborenen. Arch Gyn 1881;18:367-70.

19. Lund RJ, Kibel MA, Knight GJ, van der Elst C. Prophylaxis against gonococcal ophthalmia neonatorum. A prospective study. S Afr Med J 1987;72:620-2.

20. Hammerschlag MR, Chandler JW, Alexander ER, et al. Erythromycin ointment for ocular prophylaxis of neonatal chlamydial infection. JAMA 1980;244:2291-3.

21. Bell TA, Sandstrom KI, Gravett MG, et al. Comparison of ophthalmic silver nitrate solution and erythromycin ointment for prevention of natally acquired *Chlamydia trachomatis*. Sex Trans Dis 1987;14:195-200.

22. Laga M, Plummer FA, Piot P, et al. Prophylaxis of gonococcal and chlamydial ophthalmia neonatorum. A comparison of silver nitrate and tetracycline. N Engl J Med 1988;318:653-57.

23. Hammerschlag MR, Cummings C, Roblin PM, et al. Efficacy of neonatal ocular prophylaxis for the prevention of chlamydial and gonococcal conjunctivitis. N Engl J Med 1989;320:769-72.

24. Isenberg SJ, Apt L, Yoshimori R, et al. Povidone-iodine for ophthalmia neonatorum prophylaxis. Am J Ophthalmol 1994;118:701-6.

25. Isenberg SJ, Apt L, Wood M. A controlled trial of povidone-iodine as prophylaxis against ophthalmia neonatorum. N Engl J Med 1995;332:562-6.

26. Guthrie R, Susi A. A simple phenylalanine method for detecting phenylketonuria in large populations of newborn infants. Pediatrics 1963;32:338-43.

27. Allen DB, Farrell PM. Newborn screening: principles and practice. Adv Pediatr 1996;43:231-70.

28. Berman PW, Waisman HA, Graham FK. Intelligence in treated phenylketonuric children: a developmental study. Child Develop 1966;37:731-47.

29. Hudson FP, Mordaunt VL, Leahy I. Evaluation of treatment begun in first three months of life in 184 cases of phenylketonuria. Arch Dis Child 1970;45:5-12.

30. Williamson ML, Koch R, Azen C, Chang C. Correlates of intelligence test results in treated phenylketonuric children. Pediatrics 1981;68:161-7.

31. Azen CG, Koch R, Friedman EG, et al. Intellectual development in 12-year old children treated for phenylketonuria. Am J Dis Child 1991;145:35-9.

32. Koch R, Yusin M, Fishler K. Successful adjustment to society by adults with phenylketonuria. J Inherited Metabolic Dis 1985;8:209-11.

33. U.S. Preventive Services Task Force. Guide to clinical preventive services: an assessment of the effectiveness of 169 interventions. Baltimore: Williams & Wilkins; 1989. p. 115-9.

34. Feldman W. Screening for phenylketonuria. In: Canadian Task Force on the Periodic Health Examination, editors. The Canadian Guide to Clinical Preventive Health Care. Ottawa: Minister of Public Works and Government Services Canada; 1994. p. 179-88.

35. Charles S, Prystowsky B. Early discharge, in the end: maternal abuse, child neglect, and physician harassment. Pediatrics 1995;96:746-7.

36. Committee on Genetics. Newborn screening fact sheets. Pediatrics 1996;98:467-72.

37. Glorieux J, Dussault J, Van Vliet G. Intellectual development at age 12 years of children with congenital hypothyroidism diagnosed by neonatal screening. J Pediatr 1992;121:581-4.

38. Van Vliet G. Neonatal hypothyroidism: treatment and outcome. Thyroid 1999;9:79-84.

39. Lawrence RA. Breastfeeding: a guide for the medical profession. St. Louis: Mosby; 1999.

40. Wang YS, Wu SY. The effect of exclusive breastfeeding on the development and incidence of infection in infants. J Human Lactation 1996;12:27-30.

41. Brandt KA, Andrews CM, Kvale J. Mother-infant interaction and breastfeeding outcome 6 weeks after birth. J Obstet Gyn Neonatal Nursing 1998;27:169-74.

42. Cushing AH, Samet JM, Lambert WE, et al. Breastfeeding reduces risk of respiratory illness in infants. Pediatrics 1998;147:863-70.

43. Railser J, Alexander C, O'Campo P. Breast-feeding and infant illness: a dose-response relationship? Am J Public Health 1999;89:25-30.

44. Lucas A, Brooke OG, Morley R, et al. Early diet of preterm infants and development of allergic or atopic disease: a randomized prospective study. Br Med J 1990;300:837-40.

45. Saarinen UM, Kajosaari M. Breastfeeding as prophylaxis against atopic disease: prospective follow-up study until 17 years old. Lancet 1995;346:1065-9.

46. Rosenblatt KA, Thomas DB. Prolonged lactation and endometerial cancer. WHO collaborative study of neoplasia and steroid contraceptives. Int J Epidemiol 1993;22:192-7.

47. Newcomb PA, Storer BE, Longnecker MP, et al. Lactation and a reduced risk of premenopausal breast cancer. N Engl J Med 1994;330:81-7.

48. Nutrition Committee, CPS. Meeting the iron needs of infants and young children: an update. Can Med Assoc J 1991;44:1451-4.

49. Health and Welfare Canada. Present patterns and trends in infant feeding in Canada. 1990. Ottawa: Ministry of Supply and Services, Canada.

50. Barber CM, Abernathy T, Steinmetz B, Charlebois J. Using a breastfeeding prevalence survey to identify a population for targeted programs. Can J Pub Health 1997;88:242-5.

51. Beaudry M, Aucoin-Larade L. Who breastfeeds in New Brunswick, when and why? Can J Pub Health 1989;80:166-72.

52. Mackey S, Fried PA. Infant breast and bottle feeding practices: some related factors and attitudes. Can J Pub Health 1981;72:312-8.

53. Agnew T, Gilmore J. Breastfeeding support. 1993. Ottawa: Health and Welfare Canada, Ministry of Supply and Services.

54. Fetus and Newborn Committee, CPS, Maternal Fetal Medicine and Clinical Practice Committees SOGC. Facilitating discharge home following a normal term birth. Pediatr Child Health Care 1996;1:165-9.

55. American Academy of Pediatrics Committee on Fetus and Newborn. Hospital stay for healthy term newborns. Pediatrics 1995;96:788-90.

56. Neifert MR. The optimization of breast-feeding in the perinatal period. Clin Perinatol 1998;25:303-26.

57. The Australian College of Pediatrics. Policy statement on breastfeeding. J Pediatr Child Health 1998;34:412-3.

58. American Academy of Pediatrics Work Group on Breastfeeding. Breastfeeding and use of human milk. Pediatrics 1997;100:1035-9.

59. American Academy of Pediatrics Committee on Drugs. The transfer of drugs and other chemicals into human milk. Pediatrics 1994;93:137-50.

60. Biancuzzo M. The compromised infant: impact on breastfeeding. In: Ledbetter M, editor. Breastfeeding the newborn: clinical strategies for the nurse. St.Louis, MO: Mosby Inc; 1999. p. 163-219.

61. Powers NG, Naylor AJ, Wester RA. Hospital policies: crucial to breastfeeding success. Semin Perinatol 1994;18:517-524.

62. World Health Organization/United Nations Children's Fund. Protecting, promoting and supporting breastfeeding: the special role of maternity services, a joint WHO/UNICEF statement. 1989. Geneva, Switzerland: WHO

63. Ohlsson, A. Report on perinatal/neonatal mortality, Sultanate of Oman: 1999. Muscat, Oman: Unicef/Ministry of Health Sultanate of Oman [in press].

64. Fetus and Newborn Committee, CPS. Neonatal circumcision revisited. Can Med Assoc J 1996;154:769-80.

65. American Academy of Pediatrics Task force on Circumcision. Circumcision policy statement. Pediatrics 1999;103:686-93.

66. Anonymous. Trends in length of stay for hospital deliveries — United States, 1970-1992. MMWR 1995;44:335–7.

67. Wen SW, Liu S, Marcoux S, Fowler D. Trends and variations in length of hospital stay for childbirth in Canada. Can Med Assoc J 1998;158:875-80.

68. Gee A. Transfer home — two aspects of transfer home of mother and baby. Midwives Chronicle 1984;97:8-9.

69. James ML, Hudson CN, Gebski VJ, et al. An evaluation of planned early postnatal transfer home with nursing support. Med J Austral 1987;127:434-8.

70. Waldenström U. Early discharge with domiciliary visits and hospital care: parents' experiences of two modes of post-partum care. Scand J Caring Sci 1987;1:51-8.

71. Waldenström U, Sundelin C, Lindmark G. Early and late discharge after hospital birth. Health of mother and infant in the postpartum period. Upsala J Med Sci 1987;92:301-14.

72. Annas GJ. Women and children first. N Engl J Med 1995;333:1647-51.

73. Carty EM, Bradley CF. A randomised, controlled evaluation of early postpartum hospital discharge. Birth 1990;17:199-204.

74. Waldenström U. Early and late discharge after hospital birth: father's involvement in infant care. Early Human Development 1988;17:19-28.

75. Britton JR, Britton HL, Beebe SA. Early discharge of the term newborn: a continued dilemma. Pediatrics 1994;94:291-5.

76. Braveman P, Egerter S, Pearl M, et al. Problems associated with early discharge of newborn infants. Early discharge of newborns and mothers: a critical review of the literature. Pediatrics 1995;96:716-26.

77. Lee KS, Perlman M, Ballantyne M, et al. Association between duration of neonatal hospital stay and readmision rate. J Pediatr 1995;127:758-66.

78. Vogl TP. Phototherapy of neonatal hyperbilirubinemia: bilirubin in unexposed areas of the skin. J Pediatr 1974;85:707-10.

79. Rubaltelli FF, Carli M. The effect of light on cutaneous bilirubin. Biol Neonate 1971;18:457-62.

80. Sisson TR, Kendall N, Shaw E, et al. Phototherapy of jaundice in the newborn infant: 2. Effect of various light intensities. J Pediatr 1972;81:35-8.

81. Anonymous. Importance of radiant flux in the treatment of hyperbilirubinemia: failure of overhead phototherapy units in intensive care units. Pediatrics 1976;57:505.

82. Warshaw JB, Gagliardi J, Patel A. A comparison of fluorescent and nonfluorescent light sources for phototherapy. Pediatrics 1980;65:795-8.

83. American Academy of Pediatrics PCfQIaSoH. Practice parameter. Management of hyperbilirubinemia in the healthy term newborn. Pediatrics 1994;94:558-65.

84. Fetus and Newborn Committee, CPS. Approach to management of hyperbilirubinemia in term newborn infants. Pediatr Child Health Care 1999;4:161-4.

85. Maisels MJ, Newman TB. Jaundice in full-term and near-term babies who leave the hospital within 36 hours. The pediatrician's nemesis. Clin Perinatol 1998;25:295-302.

86. Bhutani VK, Johnson L, Sivieri EM. Predictive ability of a predischarge hour-specific serum bilirubin for subsequent significant hyperbilirubinemia in healthy term and near-term neonates. Pediatrics 1999;103:6-14.

87. Willinger M, James LS, Catz C. Defining the sudden infant death syndrome (SIDS): deliberations of an expert panel convened by the National Institute of Child Health and Human Development. Pediatr Pathol 1991;11:677-84.

88. Millar WJ, Hill GB. Prevalence of and risk factors for sudden infant death syndrome in Canada. Can Med Assoc J 1993;149:629-35.

89. Injury Prevention Committee, CPS. Reducing the risk of sudden infant death. Pediatr Child Health Care 1996;1:63-7.

90. Canadian Foundation for the Study of Infant Deaths, the Canadian Institute of Child Health, the Canadian Pediatric Society, and Health Canada. Joint statement. Reducing the risk of sudden infant death syndrome in Canada. Pediatr Child Health Care 1999;4:223-6.

CHAPTER 2

Health Maintenance Visits: a Critical Review

Norman R. Saunders, MD, FRCPC
Michelle Shouldice, MSc, MD, FRCPC

The prime purpose of the pediatric health maintenance visit is to help children reach their full potential physically, developmentally, and emotionally. So vital is this aspect of medicine that the American Academy of Pediatrics (AAP) has long declared that preventive pediatrics is the core of quality medical care for children.[1]

Clearly, the goal of providing excellent preventive care is a noble one, but do our current practices in the periodic pediatric health examination serve to optimally achieve the intended aim? This chapter reviews the many important issues pertaining to screening methods, preventive health measures, and anticipatory guidance, which are integral to health maintenance visits in childhood. What primary care physicians have done in the past, are attempting to do currently, and, perhaps, should do will be critically examined using the available scientific evidence as a basis.

GENERAL CONSIDERATIONS

Historical Perspectives

Over the years, a significant shift in focus has occurred concerning the function and goals of the periodic health maintenance examination in childhood. Earlier priorities had centered mainly on the prompt detection of physical problems, and the composition of the well-child visit reflected this emphasis. In 1980, Reisinger reported that whereas the typical pediatric health maintenance visit was scheduled to last 15 minutes, it actually averaged 10.8 minutes in duration, and a seemingly inadequate amount of time was devoted to anticipatory guidance. For children under 6 months of age, an average of just 98 seconds was given to counseling, while the time spent on adolescent counseling averaged only 2.8 seconds.[2]

In the last two decades, there has been an increasing recognition of an expanded role for primary-care physicians, which includes not just treating physical disease but also the morbidity that is due to behavioral, developmental, and social problems.[3,4] In one recent report, the overwhelming majority of parents (98 percent) viewed their children as being in either good or excellent physical health, but 79 percent of parents wanted more information in at least one area of parenting and more than half (53 percent) desired help in at least 3 of 6 areas.[5] McCune and colleagues reported that 81 percent of parental questions during health maintenance visits concerned psychosocial issues.[6] Hickson and colleagues found that 70 percent of mothers were more concerned about some aspect of their parenting or their child's behavior than they were about the physical health of their child.[7] Cheng and colleagues found that although ensuring the physical health of their children was the most common goal for mothers during a well-child examination, 75 percent had as a goal ensuring the emotional health and behavioral well being of their child. Furthermore, these mothers viewed their physician as the main source of parenting information.[8]

In response to this expanded vision of child health, the practice of pediatrics has changed. The mean duration of child visits to primary-care providers has increased from 11.8 minutes in 1979 to 14.1 minutes in 1994 (p for trend $< .001$).[9] The frequency of counseling reported during well-child visits during the same period increased from 39.1 percent of visits in 1979 to 71 percent of visits in 1994 (*p* for trend <.001). Still, there is obvious room for improvement; in 1994, for example, only 2 percent of adolescents were counseled about smoking.

Accessibility, Coordination, and Continuity of Care

It is generally agreed that health supervision should be (1) a longitudinal process that promotes a partnership over time among the health professional, the child, and the family; (2) personalized to fit individual needs; (3) contextual, in that it views the child in the context of the family and community; and (4) complementary to the health-promotion and disease-prevention efforts of the family, school, community, and the media.[10] Although there is a clear recognition that 10 or 15 minutes in a face-to-face encounter is not the unit of importance,[11] there is consensus that children should have a medical home.[12] Fortunately, over 90 percent of children are described as having a usual source of care.[13] Significantly, however, poor children, especially if they have no Medicaid, are less likely to have a medical home. Children receiving routine care at community clinics were more likely to receive sick care at a different location than those children whose routine care occurred at physicians' offices (40 percent versus 4 percent *p*<.001) and also were more likely to identify an emergency department as their usual source of sick care (9 percent versus 2 percent *p*<.001).[13] The lack of Medicaid or other insurance is not the only problem. A growing body of literature suggests that being a member of a minority group can, in and of itself, constitute a barrier to access.[14] It is a source of concern that in 1997, in the United States, the infant mortality rate for African American children was 2.3 times greater than that of Caucasians (14.7 versus 6.1 deaths per 1,000 live births).[15]

Scheduling Visits

The ideal number of health maintenance visits for children has not been established. As not every family has identical needs, some flexibility in the scheduling of routine check-ups seems prudent. The Committee on Practice and Ambulatory Medicine of the AAP has recommended 10 preventive health visits in the first 24 months of life following neonatal discharge.[16] The Canadian Pediatric Society (CPS) suggests that well-baby visits be organized according to the immunization schedule with additional visits within the first month and also at 9 months of age.[17] Gilbert and colleagues could find no advantage in 10 scheduled well-baby visits, compared with only five for healthy, low-risk newborns.[18] No significant difference in the incidence of illness, prevalence of undetected abnormalities, physical development, developmental progress, maternal anxiety, and parental satisfaction could be found between the two groups. It is worth noting that in this study, the group with 10 scheduled visits ultimately averaged only 7.89 well-baby visits, whereas the five-visit group averaged 6.19 well-baby visits in the first 2 years[18] (Table 2–1).

A prenatal visit is often felt to be useful, particularly for first-time parents. Several objectives can be served by this meeting, particularly, promoting the physician-patient relation-

Table 2–1 Frequency of Health Maintenance Visits

Intervention	Quality of Evidence	Recommendation
5 to 6 well-baby visits for healthy low risk newborns	I	A
Office visit at 3 to 4 days of age for low risk newborns	II-3	B

ship, obtaining relevant information about the medical and social history of the family, providing information about several issues such as circumcision, breast feeding, and office routines. Collectively, these three objectives should promote a fourth, which is building parenting skills.[19] The format of the prenatal visit need not be rigid; it can vary from a telephone encounter to a brief office visit or even a more detailed counseling session. The merits of a prenatal visit have not been evaluated by controlled trials.

Because of the trend toward shorter postpartum hospitalization periods, the optimal time for scheduling the first office visit has changed. Early neonatal discharge increases the possibility of missing significant jaundice or dehydration and hypernatremia due to feeding difficulties. A number of referral centers have reported an increasing admission rate for neonates with these problems.[20,21] In a 1995 review of the topic, Braveman and colleagues concluded that published research provided little knowledge on the consequences of short neonatal hospital stays and advised caution in discharge planning.[22] It, therefore, would seem advisable to evaluate even low-risk newborns within a few days of initial discharge.

PREVENTIVE GUIDANCE

The effectiveness of preventive counseling in primary care is hard to qualify and, indeed, its value debatable. There are a remarkably limited number of conditions for which the efficacy of prevention has been clearly demonstrated with scientific rigor. Nonetheless, theoretical arguments exist for promoting disease and accident prevention as part of the periodic pediatric health maintenance examination. First, the primary-care physician is seen as a trustworthy source of reliable information. Thus, the doctor-patient relationship can be used to educate parents and to advocate practices that promote health and safety in children. Behaviors may be improved on by the combined efforts of counseling, widespread community education, and legislative change, all based on sound clinical research. As stated in the Canadian Guide to Clinical Preventive Health Care, "prevention does not take place in a vacuum. Clinical prevention must be seen in the broadest context of public health and healthy public policy."[23] Second, the scale of most studies may be too limited to demonstrate small but significant behavior changes due to preventive counseling. Even if a relatively small percentage of a population modify their actions in a favorable manner, the end result may be very significant, if the population concerned is large enough. Imagine, for example, the health impact of convincing only 3 percent of North Americans to quit smoking.

Accident prevention is a major component of anticipatory counseling and serves to illustrate many of the broader issues in preventive care. It is clearly recognized that accidents and injuries are an important cause of morbidity and mortality in children. In the United States, accidents represent the leading cause of death in childhood.[15] Between 1990 and 1992, approximately 1,500 Canadian children per year died of injuries. In Canada, injuries were the second leading cause of hospital admissions of children during the same period.[24] These numbers, of course, represent the most severe (and easiest to measure) sequelae of injuries in children and do not account for those treated in other settings.

A number of studies have attempted to determine the effectiveness of injury prevention counseling in pediatric primary care. The results of these investigations vary. Randomized controlled trials have demonstrated improvements in safety knowledge[25] and behavior with respect to home safety[25–27] and car seat use[25,28] after physician counseling. One study showed an increase in the use of socket covers but not cupboard guards (which are harder to install) after provision of free safety devices, in a group that received safety information.[29] Another showed a significant decrease in hot water temperature but not an increase in smoke detector use after burn prevention counseling.[30] However, other well-designed trials have demonstrated no improvement in home safety knowledge and practices[29] and car seat use[31] with counseling. In the majority of the literature supporting the effectiveness of counseling, advice was supplemented by written materials given to parents. Provision of free or low-cost safety devices did not consistently improve frequency of their use. The average time spent counseling was 20 minutes. No studies have demonstrated a difference in injury occurrence after physician counseling.

Despite recommendations by the AAP, the Canadian Task Force for the Periodic Health Exam, and the U.S. Preventive Services Task Force,[1,16,23,32] that injury prevention counseling be included in the routine health maintenance visit, a significant proportion of primary-care physicians do not appear to be fulfilling this role. It has been shown that even when physicians are aware that they are being evaluated, they provide little anticipatory guidance in the form of injury prevention counseling during well-child visits. For example, less than half the well-child visits in an urban pediatric clinic serving low-income families included injury prevention counseling, when studied by audiotaping.[33] In another study, only 20 percent of surveyed parents reported being advised about injury prevention during their children's check-ups.[34] An average of less than two injury topics were covered and the average time spent on the topic was 1 minute per visit. Interestingly, these parents cited pamphlets from doctor's offices and drug stores and media coverage as their most frequent sources of injury prevention information. These parents seemed aware of the importance of childhood accidents but not their most common causes.

In summary, counseling for injury prevention may result in an improvement in parental safety knowledge and, possibly, practices. The evidence to support the latter is not strong. Nonetheless, it seems prudent to include safety counseling in the health maintenance visit. The important issue of which are the most appropriate safety topics to cover and the optimal number per session remains uncertain. Furthermore, the most effective methods are still undetermined. For a more detailed discussion on injury prevention, see Chapter 14.

IMMUNIZATIONS

The topic of immunization is discussed in greater detail in Chapter 3. Briefly, it is hard to imagine a more successful or cost-effective health measure than routine immunization programs for children. For example, polio which once afflicted children in epidemic proportions has essentially vanished from North America. The 1985 Pan-American Health Organization goal of the hemispheric elimination of poliomyelitis was achieved by September, 1995.[35] In Canada, the number of diphtheria cases has been reduced from 9,000 annually in 1924 to just 2 to 5 per year, and tetanus mortality has not been reported since 1991.[35] Since the introduction of the *Haemophilus influenzae* type b vaccine in the 1980s, the incidence of invasive disease from this bacteria has fallen by more than 90 percent.[36] Similar success stories exist for measles, mumps, and rubella.[35] Furthermore, of all the life-saving interventions, scheduled pediatric immunization programs are among the most cost effective.[37] Routine vaccination programs for children not only save lives, but they also actually save more money than they cost. Thus, there is strong evidence to recommend current immunization practices. They are, and should remain, the cornerstones in the pediatric health maintenance visit.

DEVELOPMENTAL SCREENING

Developmental monitoring is recognized by physicians and parents as an essential component of health supervision. Developmental problems are common in childhood, with a quoted prevalence of between 8 and 16 percent.[38–42] Although parents have clearly identified developmental issues to be a major concern,[7] and developmental delay is a common problem, primary-care providers frequently omit developmental examinations during routine well-child visits. There may be many reasons for this. A commonly identified issue is the planned duration of the typical health supervision visit. Physicians may find standardized developmental screening tools too lengthy or cumbersome for routine use, when they are expected to also obtain an interim history, conduct a physical examination, address parental questions and concerns, administer appropriate immunizations, and provide anticipatory guidance. However, pediatricians and family practitioners who have frequent, ongoing, and regular contact with young children can play a critical role in the early identification of developmental problems.

The role of screening is to identify problems that do not manifest obvious signs and symptoms, to provide early treatment and thus avoid unnecessary morbidity. A screening test should have high sensitivity and few false negative results. Clinical judgment of developmental progress, based only on history and physical examination, has been shown to be very insensitive in determining the presence or absence of developmental delays. In one study, less than half the cases of mild mental retardation or significant behavior problems were identified this way.[43,44] Interestingly, familiarity with the patient through previous contact did not improve the intelligence quotient (IQ) estimate. These values were underestimated in chronically-ill children and overestimated in mental retardation. The problem of imprecise clinical diagnosis of scholastic problems seems to be a universal one. In the United Kingdom, where clinical impression is the widely used method of identification, only 45 to 55 percent of children with developmental problems have been identified before school entrance.[45,46] In Ireland, only 6 percent of children with learning difficulties were identified during preschool health supervision, although 98 percent of children were seen in well-child visits at 4 years of age.[39] In Sweden, a group of 6-year-old children were screened for neurodevelopmental and neuropsychiatric problems; 10 percent of these youngsters were identified as having such disorders. Significantly, just 15 percent of these had been previously diagnosed.[40]

A number of studies have evaluated the common developmental screening tests used to evaluate children. Currently, there is no test with sufficient evidence to justify its use. A number of studies have shown the Denver Developmental Screening Test—the most widely known, used, and studied of the available tests—to be insensitive for developmental delay.[47,48] Other standardized developmental tests, such as the Battelle Developmental Inventory and the Minnesota Child Developmental Inventory, appear to be highly sensitive screening tools.[47,48] However, as yet, these tests have not been adequately studied in the primary-care setting to recommend their use. It has been shown that parental concerns about speech and language, fine motor, behavior, and global developmental delays are highly predictive of developmental problems.[49–51]

The early identification of developmental problems has many potential benefits. It can result in the diagnosis of an underlying medical condition, which, in turn, can lead to necessary genetic counseling and prognostic information to the family. It can permit early therapeutic intervention. However, to truly justify mass developmental screening, the benefits of this earlier intervention should be clear. Currently, this is not the case. A number of studies have indicated that there has been little or no benefit to early intervention, and there may even be a possible morbidity associated with it.[52,53] These reports are part of an enormous body of literature regarding developmental delays, which, to date, has not provided the definitive answer about the value of early intervention. The problem has been a difficult area to study because of the large variety of developmental problems and their causes, the differences in children's individual personality traits, home environment, parenting, and culture, as well as the wide array of different treatment services available. In addition, many of the studies use IQ gains as the outcome measure rather than functional effect. Of note, there is a recent trend in the literature that suggests that early intervention is important and beneficial.[54–57] In particular, there is evidence to support developmental screening by primary-care providers for high-risk children. These include those at risk due to biomedical factors (prematurity, low birth weight, significant early medical illness or trauma, and family history of developmental delay, learning disability, social difficulties, or autism) and those sociologically disadvantaged (eg, poverty, teenaged parents) as well as those children whose parents are concerned about development (Table 2–2).

Table 2–2 Screening for Development

Intervention	Quality of Evidence	Recommendation
Clinical assessment of developmental stage	II-2	B
Denver Developmental Screening Test	II-1, II-3	C

PHYSICAL EXAMINATION

General Considerations

A complete physical examination has long been considered an essential component of the pediatric preventive health care visit.[16] However, most primary-care physicians schedule only 15 minutes for these appointments that should also include a developmental, nutritional, and behavioral history as well as appropriate anticipatory guidance and immunizations. It seems hard, therefore, to imagine that all these aspects of preventive pediatrics can be adequately provided, given the pragmatic realities of everyday practice. Realistically, therefore, the physical examination performed at a check-up must be focused, and efficient and emphasize anticipated age-related problems.

The initial postnursery physical examination should focus on how well the neonate has adapted to extrauterine life. As mentioned, early neonatal discharge creates a situation in which significant jaundice or dehydration due to inadequate intake must be promptly identified. At this first office visit, as throughout infancy, the physical examination should seek to identify subtle or late-presenting congenital abnormalities. Three percent of children are born with a structural defect that is serious enough to interfere with normal function.[58] Other conditions, such as developmental dysplasia of the hip or inherited deafness may not present until later in life. Thus, in total, it is estimated that 5 to 6 percent of children may be affected with a significant congenital defect, and the cumulative morbidity of these individually rare abnormalities accounts for almost a third of hospitalized children.[58]

During the toddler stage, much of a health maintenance visit tends to be devoted to developmental issues and behavioral concerns. Often, proportionally less time is spent on the detailed re-examination of a less-than-compliant child. Usually, most practitioners will accept some degree of compromise in the examination process at these visits. School-aged children are generally quite healthy, aside from the usual transient infectious diseases of childhood. Often, the physical examination needs to carefully address specific concerns such as recurrent abdominal pain, headaches, or minor knee problems. As for the adolescent, the examination tends to center upon the physiologic processes associated with puberty as well as specific concerns that often are related to acne, weight, sexuality, or the physical effects of experimentation with alcohol and/or drugs.

A number of the individual components of the physical examination recommended during health maintenance visits have been specifically analyzed. The following review seeks to highlight some of the main issues and controversies associated with these aspects of preventive care.

Height and Weight Measurement

Interpreted judiciously, a child's growth pattern can serve as a useful monitor of health. It is, therefore, a recommended part of a scheduled pediatric preventive health visit.[32] It is important to remember that cross-sectional growth charts are based on the height and weight measurements of many children at each age and may inadequately portray the acceptably normal variation in the growth of any given child. During infancy, percentile changes in length frequently occur as the child undergoes a physiologic shift from predominantly intrauterine influences to individual genetic growth potential.[59] The linear growth rate during the first 18 months of life shifts in two-thirds of normal infants with an equal number moving upwards and downwards.[60] Later on, during adolescence, the wide range in pubertal onset diminishes the reliability of the standard height chart. Between the opposite poles of childhood/infancy and adolescence, children do tend to follow a given growth percentile fairly closely and a falling-off in growth may well indicate an abnormal condition.

The main justification for monitoring height and weight is to identify growth failure. The term "failure to thrive" has been traditionally used in clinical pediatrics to describe children whose growth lags behind that of their peers. The phrase lacks precision and its designation does not constitute a diagnosis. A number of clinical patterns of growth failure have been recognized.[61] The majority of children who fail to thrive are found to have a normal head circumference and a weight that is reduced disproportionately to height. Undernutrition is usually the cause. Although a small percentage of these children will turn out to have intestinal malabsorption as the cause of their poor nutritional status, most cases result from problematic infant-parent interactions. Children whose head circumference, weight, and height are all proportionally reduced are more likely to suffer from hereditary or congenital disorders. Those patients with normal head circumference but whose weight and height are reduced in proportion tend to have constitutional short stature or, rarely, an endocrine disorder. In a population that is two standard deviations below the mean height for age, about 20 percent will have pathologic short stature, while the rest are equally divided between familial short stature and constitutional growth delay.[59] On the other hand, most children who are three standard deviations below the mean for height will have a pathologic cause for their shortness[59] (Table 2–3).

The issue of monitoring children's weight as a screening process for obesity is a complex one. Too many children and adults exceed the recommended guidelines for obesity. Estimates for the prevalence of obesity in children range from 5 to 25 percent.[62] About one-fifth of adolescents[63] and approximately one-third of adult Americans are estimated to be overweight.[64] Furthermore the incidence of obesity is thought to be increasing in all age groups.[62,64,65] Several studies have linked obesity to cardiovascular disease, hypertension, diabetes, and increased mortality, yet the exact etiologic role of obesity for these conditions is less certain.[23,32] What is of little doubt is the effect of obesity on quality of life. Because of the cultural bias against obesity, it is clear that obese children in North America suffer significant social and emotional difficulty.[66]

Generally speaking, a screening test is deemed worthwhile only if there exists an effective intervention that can be implemented when detection of the screened condition occurs. Using this criterion, screening for obesity is of questionable value. The long-term results of traditional weight reduction methods are disappointing.[23,32] Thus, there is little evidence to support screening for obesity as part of the pediatric health maintenance visit. Counseling about proper nutrition and sufficient exercise, however, is recommended on the grounds that it seems harmless and may provide an incentive for motivated individuals to reduce their weight and improve their lifestyles (Table 2–4).

Table 2–3 Height and Weight Measurement

Intervention	Quality of Evidence	Recommendation
Routine measurement of height, weight, and head circumference	II-2	B

Table 2–4 Screening for Obesity

Intervention	Quality of Evidence	Recommendation
Routine measurement of weight	II-2	C
Counseling about nutrition and exercise	I	C

Vision Screening

Vision screening and the ophthalmologic examination are recommended components of preventive pediatric care.[67,68] The eye examination should result in early detection of congenital anomalies and other eye abnormalities that threaten vision and in timely treatment to prevent vision loss. Missed visual problems, such as strabismus or unequal refractive error, can result in amblyopia and irreversible visual defects. The prevalence of visual defects in children is high. Undetected vision problems are estimated to occur in 5 to 10 percent of pre-school children with 2 to 5 percent displaying amblyopia and/or strabismus.[23] One study of inner-city school children found amblyopia present in 3.9 percent, strabismus in 3.1 percent, and refractive errors in 8.2 percent of the children.[69] By late adolescence, nearly 20 percent of the population has a refractive error, requiring the use of eyeglasses.[67]

It is generally agreed that the inspection of the external eye structures, conjunctiva, cornea, iris, and pupil should be considered an integral part of the physical examination of children of all ages. In the neonatal period and during early infancy, the red reflex should be checked to screen for opacities in the visual axis and for signs of posterior eye disease such as retinoblastoma. The corneal light reflex should be used to evaluate ocular misalignment. When a child becomes capable of cooperating, visual acuity should be tested. Extraocular muscle imbalance can be checked using the unilateral cover test.[67,68]

The sensitivity of the visual screening procedures is incompletely validated. These screening tests in children are considered imperfect, especially in the young.[68] Noncompliance, the time required for testing, and the inaccuracy of the testing methods were all cited as impediments to screening in one cross-sectional study, in which a third of 3- to 5-year-old children were not visually screened.[70] Screening using the Snellen letters is sensitive for refractive errors but not for the detection of amblyopia or strabismus.[71] The sensitivity of the unilateral cover test to detect strabismus in a primary-care setting is uncertain. DeBecker and colleagues found that a screening program comprising visual inspection and test of visual acuity had a negative predictive value of 98.7 percent.[72]

Although no randomized trial evaluating amblyopia screening is yet available, there is fair evidence that the early detection and treatment of amblyopia and strabismus improve the prognosis for normal vision. Once diagnosed, visual impairment resulting from a refractive problem is easily corrected with eyeglasses. However, there is no evidence to show benefit from screening older children for refractive error versus waiting till these patients complain about their vision. Furthermore, whether or not uncorrected refractive error adversely affects school performance is debatable. Still, screening children for visual problems, particularly in the neonatal period and at a preschool examination, seems reasonable. Feldman and colleagues found that visually screened preschoolers had fewer vision problems 1 year later than those who were not screened[73] (Table 2–5).

Hearing Screening

There is a growing consensus that screening for hearing defects should be universally done in the neonatal period.[74,75] Recent cohort studies have demonstrated the effectiveness of such programs in efficiently identifying significant hearing loss.[76–79] When such routine neonatal

Table 2–5 Vision Screening

Intervention	Quality of Evidence	Recommendation
Visual acuity testing	II-1	B

screening is unavailable, those infants with known risk factors for hearing deficit should have their hearing tested.

Significant hearing loss can still occur beyond the neonatal period. About 20 to 30 percent of children who subsequently display persistent hearing loss develop their impairment during childhood.[75] In spite of this, pediatric screening programs for hearing impairment appear to be of dubious value.[73] O'Mara and colleagues evaluated the results of screening 1,653 3- and 4-year-old Canadian children using pure-tone audiometry. Only 5 children (0.3 percent) were found to have a previously undiscovered problem. All were caused by persistent middle-ear effusions.[78A] Although, at any given time, 5 to 7 percent of children aged 5 to 8 years suffer a 25 dB hearing loss,[79] the great majority will have only a transient problem, usually related to middle-ear effusions. As a result, the usefulness of screening all school-aged children for hearing loss is diminished. Audiologic screening is recommended for children known to be at higher risk for hearing loss. Primary-care practitioners must maintain a vigilance for any sign or symptom of hearing difficulty, including apparent language or developmental delay. Clinicians are particularly well advised to heed parental concerns, as 70 percent of hearing impairment is first identified by parents. Furthermore, parental concern is felt to be of better predictive value than informal testing undertaken in the physician's office.[80]

No randomized controlled trials exist to confirm the effectiveness of early intervention for hearing impairment. Furthermore, for ethical reasons, such an investigation is unlikely to be performed. Recently, it has been demonstrated in a cohort comparison study that significantly better language development is associated with earlier detection and intervention (Table 2–6).

Blood Pressure

Incorporating routine blood pressure measurement into children's scheduled health visits allows the early detection of asymptomatic hypertension. Elevated blood pressure can be caused either by underlying disease, or it may be due to essential hypertension. About 66 percent of sustained hypertension in childhood appears caused by renal parenchymal or renovascular disease, 10 percent of hypertensive children have a nonrenal cause, and approximately 25 percent have primary or essential hypertension.[82] The prevalence of primary hypertension in the pediatric population increases with age.

The morbidity and mortality from cardiovascular disease is significantly greater in hypertensives compared with normotensives at all ages and in both sexes.[23] The risk of childhood hypertension is seldom immediate but adverse cardiac ventricular and hemodynamic changes have been demonstrated prior to the third decade of life.[23] The best predictor of

Table 2–6 Hearing Screening

Intervention	Quality of Evidence	Recommendation
Neonatal auditory brain stem response measurement	II-2	C
Pure tone audiometry	II-1, II-2	D

adult blood pressure is the blood pressure in childhood.[83] Elevated blood pressure in childhood correlates well with hypertension in early adulthood.[84] Thus, screening for hypertension at the time of the health maintenance visit is advised.[16]

The measurement of blood pressure requires standardization. Hypertension is defined as average systolic or diastolic blood pressure equal to or greater than the 95th percentile for age and sex, when measured on at least three separate occasions.[32] A proper-sized cuff is essential for accurate measurement; at least two-thirds of the upper arm should be covered by the cuff. The right arm is preferred both for consistency and comparison with standard tables.[32] Ideally, measurement should be taken with the patient seated and the cubital fossa at heart level after a period of 3 to 5 minutes' rest. Systolic blood pressure is determined by the onset of the "tapping" Korotkoff's sound. It is now recommended that the diastolic blood pressure be defined by the disappearance of Korotkoff's sounds rather than by the onset of muffling of sound.[32] For those children whose muffled sound can still be heard at 0 mm Hg, diastolic hypertension can be considered excluded (Table 2–7).

Screening for Developmental Dysplasia of the Hips

Developmental dysplasia of the hips (DDH) is a more complex entity than earlier appreciated. It encompasses a broad range of deformities that includes combinations of acetabular hypoplasia, maldirection, torsion, diminished articular cartilage, erosion of margins, and abnormalities of shape.[85] The exact incidence of DDH is uncertain. In general, about 1 percent of Caucasian neonates will have hip dysplasia and 0.1 percent will have dislocated hips, with females at four-fold risk.[86] The incidence is lower in African Americans and East Asian Americans and higher in aboriginal Americans. Other risk factors include breech presentation, torticollis, club feet, metatarsus adductus, positive family history, and being the first-born.[86] The natural history of hip dysplasia is incompletely understood. Some cases of dysplasia appear to resolve spontaneously,[87] while late presentation of dysplasia of previously normal hips also occurs.[88]

Screening for developmental dysplasia in the neonatal period and throughout early infancy is generally clinical. The two tests used are Barlow's and Ortolani's. Barlow's test is a provocative procedure, in which longitudinal pressure is exerted on an adducted hip to demonstrate abnormal movement between the femoral head and the acetabulum in a dysplastic joint. Ortolani's test is an abduction procedure, which detects dislocation.[86] The "clunk" that is heard in a positive test is due to reduction of the dislocated hip. It is not a "click," which is now felt to be of no clinical significance.[89] After infancy, Barlow's and Ortolani's tests become less reliable, and clinical detection depends on limited abduction of the hip, asymmetric skin folds (an insensitive finding present in about 30 percent of infants), and the presence of relative shortening of the femoral segment. Clinical screening is effective in detecting DDH,[90,91] but it is not perfect.[92] Not surprisingly, the skill of the examiner has been shown to significantly affect detection rates.[91]

Ultrasound examination of the hip has been shown to be a sensitive tool in confirming the diagnosis of DDH; it is both safe and reliable.[88,89,92,93] It is particularly useful in newborns and infants under 4 months of age and whose ossification centers are incomplete, which makes plain radiography unreliable. Ultrasonography also has been shown to be reliable in older children and has been recommended as the primary imaging technique in this age group as well.[94]

Table 2–7 Blood Pressure Measurement

Intervention	Quality of Evidence	Recommendation
Routine measurement of blood pressure	II-3	B

Abnormal hips, left untreated, usually will develop long-term complications, which include osteoarthritis and leg length discrepancies, which, in turn, produce pain, gait abnormalities, and reduced agility.[86] Hips that remain clinically unstable beyond the first few days of life need treatment. Early diagnosis permits a relatively simple treatment— dynamic splinting generally employing a Pavlik harness. Later diagnosis requires more extensive management—either closed reduction under general anesthetic followed by casting (for those 6 to 18 months of age) or surgical repair (for children diagnosed after 18 months). If the initial diagnosis of DDH is delayed beyond age 4 years in bilateral cases or beyond age 8 years in unilateral DDH, it is probably too late to attempt surgical repair.[86]

In brief, a large body of evidence supports the routine clinical screening of all newborns and infants for developmental dysplasia of the hips. Ultrasonography of the hips is useful in confirming the clinical diagnosis of DDH, but universal screening of all newborns is not recommended at this time, as it may be too sensitive and lead to unnecessary treatment.[85,88] To date, there has been no randomized controlled trial of hip screening comparing ultrasonography with clinical assessment (Table 2–8).

Scoliosis Screening

Scoliosis, defined as a lateral spinal curve of greater than 10°, is present in 2 to 3 percent of adolescents by the end of their growth, with 0.5 percent of teenagers developing a curve in excess of 20°.[95] Severe curves can produce restrictive pulmonary disease and increased mortality, but these curves are generally the result of severe early-onset scoliosis.[96] Back pain, lowered self-esteem, and cosmetic deformity have also been considered to be potential consequences of scoliosis. However, the magnitude of these adverse effects that result from milder forms of idiopathic scoliosis is uncertain and debated.[32]

Scoliosis is principally screened by upright visualization of the back and the Adams forward-bending test. The accuracy of the testing is dependent on the skill of the examiner and the size of the curve.[32] Trained public health nurses have been shown to identify all children with a Cobb angle of greater than 20°. For curves greater than 10°, a sensitivity of 73.9 percent and a specificity of 77.8 percent was obtained.[97]

The rationale for routine screening rests on the assumption that early diagnosis and treatment are effective. A major concern about scoliosis screening has been the paucity of evidence to support the contention that early initiation of therapy will prevent progression of the curve and thus avoid the complications of severe disease or surgery. Recently, a prospective study by the Scoliosis Research Society showed that bracing was superior to either observation alone or surface electrical stimulation in preventing an increase of at least 6° in the scoliotic curve.[98] A 1997 meta-analysis of the efficacy of nonoperative treatments for idiopathic scoliosis also concluded that bracing for 23 hours a day was effective in halting the progression of the curve.[99]

Should screening for idiopathic scoliosis remain part of the routine pediatric preventive examination? Although clinical methods of detection may be imperfect, the extent of morbidity uncertain, and the efficacy of treatment incompletely proven, it would still seem pru-

Table 2–8 Screening for Developmental Dysplasia of the Hips

Intervention	Quality of Evidence	Recommendation
Physical examination of the hips during the first year of life	II-1	B
Universal ultrasound screening	II-1	D

dent to include screening for scoliosis as part of the preadolescent and adolescent examinations (Table 2–9).

SCREENING LABORATORY TESTS

Urinalysis

Screening urinalyses have been a recommended part of pediatric preventive care for years.[100] However, the utility of routine urinalysis is questionable. Gutgesell found that 88.5 percent of asymptomatic patients with abnormal findings on an initial urinalysis had normal urine upon follow-up.[101] In a large Japanese screening program conducted over a 13-year period, only 0.017 percent of elementary students and just 0.015 percent of junior high school students were discovered to have renal disease.[102] Not surprisingly, Kaplan and colleagues concluded that the multiple screening dipstick urinalyses that had been recommended by the AAP were costly and should be discontinued, to be replaced by only a single urinalysis at school entry.[103] A number of guidelines now advise that routine periodic urine screening in children be discontinued, including the 1995 U.S. Preventive Service Task Force and the Canadian Task Force on the Periodic Health Examination.[23,32]

The purpose of urinary screening in pediatrics primarily has been to identify occult renal parenchymal disease or infection. The prevalence of asymptomatic bacteriuria in school-aged girls is 1.9 percent while school-aged boys have a lower prevalence of only .02 percent.[104] Current screening techniques usually involve either dipstick measurement of leukocyte esterase and urinary nitrites or microscopic urinalysis. The leukocyte esterase test serves as an indirect measure of degraded leukocytes presumed to be present due to infection. Nitrites are the metabolic byproducts of bacteria, specifically gram-negative organisms, and, hence, their presence indicates bacterial presence in the urine. Both tests are more effective if performed on concentrated morning urine. Although possessing a very high negative predictive value, the sensitivities and specificities of these methods are only around 80 percent, when compared with urine cultures,[105] which is about the same level of reliability as the microscopic examination of the urine.

Even when early diagnosis of asymptomatic bacteriuria is made and treatment promptly instituted, there is no demonstrated improvement in patient outcome. It seems that in most cases, asymptomatic bacteriuria is of little or no clinical significance, and those cases that do represent true infection are likely to become symptomatic, prompting appropriate treatment.

The value of screening urine for asymptomatic microscopic hematuria is also questionable. Around 5 percent of school-aged children show detectable blood on a single urine sample, of which more than half clear within 1 week. The annual incidence of new cases of hematuria in children 6 to 12 years of age is 0.4 percent.[106] Most of these are inconsequential. It is estimated that 75 percent are caused by either benign recurrent or benign persistent hematuria.[107] Dipstick testing for hematuria is extremely sensitive and very specific for detecting even tiny amounts of blood in the urine.[108] In fact, from a practical perspective, dipstick testing for blood may be too sensitive. A false-positive/transient hematuria rate of 88 percent has been reported.[101]

On the basis of available evidence, repeated screening urinalysis seems hard to justify as part of the routine health maintenance visit (Table 2–10).

Table 2–9 Screening for Scoliosis

Intervention	Quality of Evidence	Recommendation
Adams forward-bending test	II-2	B

Table 2–10 Urinalysis

Intervention	Quality of Evidence	Recommendation
Dipstick urinalysis in asymptomatic children, for detection of renal disease	II-2	D
Dipstick urinalysis in asymptomatic children, for detection of urinary infection	I, II-1	E

Anemia and Iron Deficiency

In the United States, the overall incidence of iron deficiency anemia (IDA) has fallen over the years to around 3 percent.[32] Due to the heterogeneity of society, much variability exists in this rate among subpopulations. Middle-class children rarely suffer from iron deficiency, and when they do, the problem is mild.[109] On the other hand, aboriginal people, immigrants, and low-income groups have a much higher incidence of anemia.[110] Although most cases of IDA seem unaccompanied by obvious clinical symptoms, an association has been reported between iron deficiency in early childhood and abnormal behavior and development.[32]

Testing hemoglobin concentration is the principal method of screening for anemia. It is reliable and sensitive for the diagnosis of actual anemia but will miss milder iron deficiency states that maintain normal hemoglobin levels.[111] Capillary sampling, which is often used in infants because of its convenience, is less accurate than venipuncture samples.[112] Other tests such as serum ferritin, serum iron binding capacity, or mean cell volume may be used to diagnose depletion of iron stores. Of these, serum ferritin is the most sensitive, when compared with the gold standard of bone marrow aspiration.[23,32]

What are the clinical effects of treating iron deficiency states in young children? The definitive answer to this critical question remains unclear. Low levels of both hemoglobin and iron stores can be easily normalized with oral iron therapy. The effect of iron supplementation on infant development is less certain. Some trials have been unable to demonstrate benefit, either in the short term or after months of treatment.[32] However, Idjradinata and Pollitt were able to show significant improvement in both intellectual and motor development.[113] Four months of oral iron therapy given to infants aged 12 to 18 months produced a 20-point improvement in the Bayley scales and a 14-point gain on motor scores. By comparison, the placebo-treated group showed no improvement. In reasonably nourished school-aged children and adolescents, oral iron treatment shows little clinical effect.[32]

Should children be routinely screened for iron deficiency anemia? Different organizations have produced differing recommendations. There is a consensus that high-risk infants should be screened before 1 year of age. The AAP suggests hemoglobin screening of all infants at around 9 months of age.[16] Most groups do not advocate routine testing of older children, although the AAP suggests screening menstruating adolescents. Regardless of whether or not children receive hemoglobin screening and blood film examination, it seems prudent for physicians and health-care professionals to promote breast-feeding and encourage an appropriate diet for infants and children. Please see Chapter 16 for a more detailed discussion.

Tuberculin Skin Testing

The intradermal skin test is the only practical tool for diagnosing tuberculosis in asymptomatic children.[114] Only the Mantoux test is now recommended for screening and diagnosis.[115] A dosage of five TU (tuberculin units) of purified protein derivative (PPD) is preferred, as the interpretation of this amount is the most standardized.[114] There is little difficulty interpreting clearly positive tests (> 15 mm of induration) or those that are definitely negative (< 5 mm induration), but intermediate reactions of 5 to 14 mm produce considerable inter-observer variability and create the potential for mislabeling.[23] Multiple puncture tests, such as the tine test, are considered inferior to the Mantoux test.[115]

False-negative Mantoux test results can occur. Malnutrition, certain viral illnesses (such as varicella, measles, and influenza), immunodeficiency states such as HIV infection, over-whelming tuberculosis, and very young age can all significantly reduce the size of induration at the test site. Approximately 10 percent of culture-proven tuberculosis cases are Mantoux test negative.[115] False-positive test results can also happen, either from prior bacille Calmette-Guérin (BCG) vaccination, nontuberculous mycobacteria infection or the booster effect caused by serial tuberculin testing. However, it is rare for these factors to create a true diagnostic dilemma.

Routine tuberculin skin testing of all children is no longer recommended.[23,114,115] In North America, regular assessment, including routine Mantoux skin testing, is recommended every 1 to 2 years for all children considered at increased risk for tuberculosis.[114,115] Children whose parents immigrated from endemic regions or who themselves reside in high prevalence areas should be considered for testing at 4 to 6 years and again at 11 to 16 years[114] (Table 2–11).

Screening for Hemoglobinopathies

There are 2,000 new cases of sickle cell disease diagnosed in the United States every year. This condition is easily and inexpensively diagnosed. Universal or targeted screening is currently performed in some states, although not included as a recommendation by the CPS or AAP. The rationale for early detection is the prevention of deaths from infections with encapsulated organisms by instituting penicillin prophylaxis and early, aggressive treatment of febrile illness. The risk of invasive infection with *Streptococcus pneumoniae* is 30 to 100 times greater in those with sickle cell disease, particularly young children. A cost-effectiveness analysis done in Alaska suggested that targeted screening would be the most cost-effective strategy for neonatal screening for sickle cell disease in areas of low prevalence and universal screening in areas where it is more common.[116] However, Shafer and colleagues suggest that targeted screening would have resulted in 58 undetected cases of sickle cell disease in non–African American infants and almost 7,000 patients with sickle cell trait not being identified.[117] The effectiveness of neonatal screening in preventing deaths or morbidity associated with sickle cell disease is not known.

Screening for Lead Toxicity

Elevated blood lead levels in children are associated with neurotoxicity and decreased intelligence quotient. The AAP, in a recent review of screening for elevated blood lead levels,[118] suggests that targeted screening be performed. Children considered at increased risk are those living in older houses or homes that are being renovated or in areas known to have higher prevalence of elevated blood lead levels, children with pica or iron deficiency and those from low-income families. The past recommendation for universal screening has been revised, due to a recent study suggesting that there is a decline in the prevalence of elevated blood lead levels[119] (Table 2–12).

Table 2–11 Tuberculin Skin Testing

Intervention	Quality of Evidence	Recommendation
Routine tuberculin skin testing of all children	II-2	E

Table 2–12 Screening for Lead Toxicity

Intervention	Quality of Evidence	Recommendation
Blood lead measurement in high-risk children	II-2	B

Conclusion

The routine health maintenance visit has become an established cornerstone of pediatric care. Its components of scheduled immunizations, anticipatory guidance, developmental assessment, screening history, physical examination, and selected investigations all have values of varying degrees. Collectively, they may result in a sum that is greater than the individual parts. Strong physician-family relationships can be created and maintained by this ongoing process, which may be hard to quantify but is very important to appreciate. It is because health maintenance visits are so important that researchers in primary pediatric care must strive to provide the best evidence for those components which clearly work and should be enhanced and those which can safely be deleted.

References

1. American Academy of Pediatrics, CoSoCH. Preventive child care. Standards of child care, 3rd ed. Evanston: AAP; 1977.

2. Reisinger KS, Bires JA. Anticipatory guidance in pediatric practice. Pediatrics 1980;66(6):889–92.

3. American Academy of Pediatrics CoPAocaFH. Pediatrics and the psychosocial aspects of child and family health. Pediatrics 1982;70:126–7.

4. American Academy of Pediatrics CoPAoCaFH. The pediatrician and the new morbidity. Pediatrics 1993;92:731–3.

5. Young K, Davis K, Schoen C, Parker S. Listening to parents: national survey of parents with young children. Arch Pediatr Adolesc Med 1998;152:255–62.

6. McCune Y, Richardson M, Powell J. Psychosocial health issues in pediatric practices: parents' knowledge and concerns. Pediatrics 1984;74:180–90.

7. Hickson G, Altemeler W, O'Connor S. Concerns of mothers seeking care in private pediatric offices: opportunities for expanding services. Pediatrics 1983;72:619–24.

8. Cheng T, Savageau J, DeWitt T. Expectations, goals and perceived effectiveness of child health supervision: a study of mothers in a pediatric practice. Clin Pediatr 1996;35:129–37.

9. Ferris T, Saglam D, Stafford R. Changes in the daily practice of primary care for children. Arch Pediatr Adolesc Med 1998;152:227–33.

10. Green M. Bright futures: guidelines for health supervision of infants, children, and adolescents. Arlington, VA: National Center for Education in Maternal and Child Health; 1994.

11. Palfrey J. Comprehensive child health: is it in the picture? Arch Pediatr Adolesc Med 1998;152:222–3.

12. American Academy of Pediatrics. The medical home. Policy reference guide of the American Academy of Pediatrics: a comprehensive guide to AAP policies issued through December 1996, 10th ed. Elk Grove Village, IL: American Academy of Pediatrics; 1997. p. 529.

13. St. Peter R, Newacheck P, Halfon N. Access to care for poor children: separate and unequal? JAMA 1992;267:2760–4.

14. Friedman E. Money isn't everything: nonfinancial barriers to access. JAMA 1994;271:1535–6.

15. Guyer B, MacDorman M, Martin J, et al. Annual summary of vital statistics-1997. Pediatrics 1998; 102:1333–49.

16. American Academy of Pediatrics CoPaAM. Recommendations for preventive pediatric health care. Pediatrics 1995;96:373–4.

17. Canadian Task Force on the Periodic Health Examination. Periodic health examination, 1990 update: well-baby care in the first two years of life. Can Med Assoc J 1990;143:867–72.

18. Gilbert J, Feldman W, Siegel L. How many well-baby visits are necessary in the first two years of life? Can Med Assoc J 1984;130:857–61.

19. American Academy of Pediatrics CoPAoCaFH. The prenatal visit. Pediatrics 1996;97:141–2.

20. Lee K, Perlman M, Ballantyne M, et al. Association between duration of neonatal hospital stay and readmission rate. J Pediatr 1995;127:758–66.

21. Cooper W, Atherton H, Kahana M, Kotagal U. Increased incidence of severe breast feeding malnutrition and hypernatremia in a metropolitan area. Pediatrics 1995;96:957–60.

22. Braveman P, Egerter S, Pearl M. Problems associated with early discharge of newborn infants. Early discharge of newborns and mothers: a critical review of the literature. Pediatrics 1995;96:716–26.

23. Canadian Task Force on the Periodic Health Examination. Canadian guide to clinical preventive health care. Ottawa: Canada Communications Group; 1994.

24. Health Canada. For the safety of Canadian children and youth. From injury data to preventive measures. Ottawa: Ministry of Public Works and Government Services, Canada; 1997.

25. Kelly B, Sein C, McCarthy P. Safety education in a pediatric primary care setting. Pediatrics 1987;79:818–24.

26. Clamp M, Kendrick D. A randomised controlled trial of general practitioner safety advice for families with children under 5 years. Br Med J 1998;316:1575–9.

27. Katcher M, Landry G, Shapiro MM. Liquid-crystal thermometer use in pediatric office counseling about tap water burn prevention. Pediatrics 1989;83:766–71.

28. Scherz R. Restraint systems for the prevention of injury to children in automobile accidents. Am J Public Health 1976;66:451–6.

29. Dershewitz R, Williamson J. Prevention of childhood household injuries: a controlled clinical trial. Am J Public Health 1977;67:1148–53.

30. Thomas K, Hassanein R, Christophersen E. Evaluation of group well-child care for improving burn prevention practices in the home. Pediatrics 1984;74:879–82.

31. Miller J, Pless B. Child automobile restraints: evaluation of health education. Pediatrics 1977;59:907–11.

32. U.S. Preventive Services Task Force. Guide to clinical preventive services: report of the U.S. Preventive Service Task Force, 2nd ed. Baltimore: Williams & Wilkins; 1996:p. 219–29.

33. Gielen A, McDonald E, Forrest C, et al. Injury prevention counseling in an urban pediatric clinic. Analysis of audiotaped visits. Arch Ped Adolesc Med 1997;151:146–51.

34. Hu X, Wesson D, Parkin P, Rootman I. Pediatric injuries: parental knowledge, attitudes and needs. Can J Public Health 1996;87:101–5.

35. Canadian Medical Association. Canadian immunization guide, 5th ed. Ottawa: CMA; 1998.

36. Immunization Monitoring Program—Active (IMPACT) of the Canadian Pediatric Society and the Laboratory Center for Disease Control. Recent trends in pediatric *Haemophilus influenzae* type b infection in Canada. Can Med Assoc J 1996;154:1041–7.

37. Tengs T, Adams M, Pliskin J, et al. Five hundred life-saving interventions and their cost-effectiveness. Risk Analysis 1995;15:369–90.

38. Boyle C, Decoufle P, Yeargin-Allsopp M. Prevalence and health impact of developmental disabilities in U.S. children. Pediatrics 1994;93:399–403.

39. Corrigan N, Stewart M, Scott M, Fee F. Predictive value of preschool surveillance in detecting learning difficulties. Arch Dis Child 1996;74:517–21.

40. Landgren M, Pettersson R, Kjellman B, Gillberg C. ADHD, DAMP and other neurodevelopmental/psychiatric disorders in 6-year-old children: epidemiology and comorbidity. Dev Med Child Neurol 1996;38:891–906.

41. Sanford M, Offord D, Boyle M, et al. Ontario child health study: social and school impairments in children aged 6 to 16 years. J Am Acad Child Adolesc Psych 1992;31:60–7.

42. Yeargin-Allsopp M, Murphy C, Oakley G, Sikes R. A multiple-source method for studying the prevalence of developmental disabilities in children: the Metropolitan Atlanta Developmental Disabilities Study. Pediatrics 1992;89:624–30.

43. Bierman JM, Connor A, Vaage M, et al. Pediatricians' assessment of intelligence of two year olds and their mental test scores. Pediatrics 1964;43:680–90.

44. Korsch B, Cobb K, Ashe B. Pediatricians' appraisals of patients' intelligence. Pediatrics 1961;29:990–5.

45. Dearlove J, Kearney D. How good is general practice developmental screening? Br Med J 1990;300:1177–80.

46. Dworkin P. Developmental screening: expecting the impossible? Pediatrics 1989;83:619–22.

47. Meisels S. Can developmental screening tests identify children who are developmentally at risk? Pediatrics 1989;83:578–85.

48. Glascoe F, Martin E, Humphrey S. A comparative review of developmental screening tests. Pediatrics 1990;86:547–54.

49. Cunningham R. Parents' concerns about children's development: prescreening techniques or screening test? Pediatrics 1997;100:901–2.

50. Glascoe F, Sandler H. Value of parents' estimates of children's developmental ages. J Pediatrics 1995;127:831–5.

51. Glascoe F, Dworkin P. The role of parents in the detection of developmental and behavioral problems. Pediatrics 1995;95:829–36.

52. Cadman D, Chambers L, Walter S. Evaluation of public health preschool child developmental screening: the process and outcome of a community program. Am J Public Health 1987;77:45–51.

53. Gittleman R, Reingold I. Children with reading disorders: 1. Efficacy of reading remediation. J Child Psychol Psychiatry 1983;23:167–91.

54. Fewell R, Glick M. Program evaluation findings of an intensive early intervention program. Am J Mental Retardation 1996;101:233–43.

55. Parush S, Hahn-Markowitz J. The efficacy of an early prevention program facilitated by occupational therapists: a follow up study. Am J Occu Ther 1997;51:247–51.

56. Berlin L, Brooks-Gunn J, McCarton C, McCormick M. The effectiveness of early intervention: examining risk factors and pathways to enhanced development. Prevent Med 1998;27:238–45.

57. Majnemer A. Benefits of early intervention for children with developmental disabilities. Semin Pediatr Neurol 1998;5:62–9.

58. Aase J. Dysmorphologic diagnosis for the pediatric practitioner. Pediatr Clin N Am 1992;39(1):135–56.

59. Mahoney CP. Evaluating the child with short stature. Pediatr Clin N Am 1987;34(4):825–49.

60. Smith DW, Truog W, Rogers JE, et al. Shifting linear growth during infancy: illustration of genetic factors in growth from fetal life through infancy. J Pediatr 1976;89:225–30.

61. Gahagan S, Holmes R. A stepwise approach to evaluation of undernutrition and failure to thrive. Pediatr Clin N Am 1998;45(1):169–87.

62. Dietz W. Childhood obesity: susceptibility, cause and management. J Pediatr 1983;103:676–86.

63. Centers for Disease Control and Prevention. Prevalence of overweight among adolescents— United States, 1988-1991. MMWR 1994;43:818–21.

64. Kuczmarski R, Flegal K, Campbell S. Increasing prevalence of overweight among U.S. adults. JAMA 1994;272:205–11.

65. Gortmaker SL, Dietz WH, Sobol AM, Wehler CA. Increasing pediatric obesity in the United States. Am J Dis Child 1987;141:535–40.

66. Wadden T, Stunkard A. Social and psychological consequences of obesity. Ann Intern Med 1985;103:1062–7.

67. American Academy of Pediatrics CoPaAM. Section on ophthalmology Eye examination and vision screening in infants, children and young adults. Pediatrics 1996;98:153–7.

68. Canadian Pediatric Society CPC. Vision screening in infants and children. Pediatr Child Health 1998;3:261–2.

69. Preslan M, Novak A. Baltimore vision screening project. Ophthalmology 1996;103:105–9.

70. Wasserman R, Croft C, Brotherton S. Pre-school vision screening in pediatric practice: a study from the Pediatric Research Group in Office Settings (PROS) Network. Pediatrics 1992;89:834–8.

71. Lieberman S, Cohen A, Stolzberg M, Ritty J. Validation of the New York State Optometric Association (NYSOA) vision screening battery. Am J Optom Physiol Opt 1985;62:165–8.

72. DeBecker I, MacPherson H, LaRoche G. Negative predictive value of a population-based preschool vision screening program. Ophthalmology 1992;99:998–1003.

73. Feldman W, Milner R, Sackett B, Gilbert S. Effects of preschool screening for vision and hearing on prevalence of vision and hearing problems 6-12 months later. Lancet 1980;2:1014–6.

74. American Academy of Pediatrics AAoPJcoIH. 1994 position statement. Pediatrics 1995;95:152–6.

75. National Institutes of Health. NIH consensus statement. Early identification of hearing impairment in infants and young children. 1993;11:1–24.

76. Mason J, Hermann K. Universal infant hearing screening by auditory brainstem response measurement. Pediatrics 1998;101:221–8.

77. Mehl A, Thomson V. Newborn hearing screening: the great omission. Pediatrics 1998;101:E4.

78. Vohr B, Carty L, Moore P, LeTourneau K. The Rhode Island Hearing Assessment Program: experience with statewide hearing screening (1993-1996). J Pediatr 1998;133:353–7.

78A. O'Mara LM, Issacs S, Chambers LW. Follow-up of participants in a preschool hearing screening program in child care centres. Can J Public Health 1992;83:373–8.

79. Cross A. Health screening in schools. Part I. J Pediatr 1985;107:487–94.

80. Bachmann KR, Arvedson JC. Early identification and intervention for children who are hearing impaired. Pediatr Rev 1998;19(5):155–65.

81. Yoshinaga-Itano C. Language of early- and later-identified children with hearing loss. Pediatrics 1998;102:1161–71.

82. Arar M, Hogg R, Arant B, Seikaly M. Etiology of sustained hypertension in children in the southwestern United States. Pediatric Nephrol 1994;8:186–9.

83. Gillman M, Ellison R. Childhood prevention of essential hypertension. Pediatr Clin N Am 1993;40(1):179–94.

84. Lauer R, Clarke W, Mahoney L, Witt J. Childhood predictors for high adult blood pressure. The Muscatine study. Pediatr Clin N Am 1993;40(1):23–40.

85. Wedge J. Hip joint acetabular dysplasia. J Pediatr Orthop 1997;17:141–2.

86. Novachek T. Developmental dysplasia of the hip. Pediatr Clin N Am 1996;43(4):829–48.

87. Castelein R, Sauter A, DeVleiger M, VanLinge B. Natural history of ultrasound hip abnormalities in clinically normal newborns. J Pediatr Orthop 1992;12:423–7.

88. Aronsson D, Goldberg M, King TJ, Roy D. Developmental dysplasia of the hip. Pediatrics 1994;94(2 Pt 1):201–8.

89. Bond C, Hennrikus W, DellaMaggiore E. Prospective evaluation of newborn soft tissue hip 'clicks' with ultrasound. J Pediatr Orthop 1997;17:199–201.

90. Darmonov A, Zagora S. Clinical screening for congenital dislocation of the hip. J Bone Joint Surg Am 1996;78:383–8.

91. Krikler S, Dwyer N. Comparison of results of two approaches to hip screening in infants. J Bone Joint Surg Br 1992;74:701–3.

92. Berman L, Klenerman L. Ultrasound screening for hip abnormalities: preliminary findings in 1001 neonates. Br Med J 1986;293:719–22.

93. Harcke H, Kujmar S. The role of ultrasound in the diagnosis and management of congenital dislocation and dysplasia of the hip. J Bone Joint Surg Am 1991;73:622–8.

94. Terjesen T, Runden T, Johnsen H. Ultrasound in the diagnosis of congenital dysplasia and dislocation of the hip joints in children older than two years. Clin Orthop 1991;262:159–69.

95. Renshaw T. Screening school children for scoliosis. Clin Orthop 1988;229:26–33.

96. Dickson R. Conservative treatment for idiopathic scoliosis. J Bone Joint Surg Br 1985;67:176–81.

97. Viviani G, Budgell L, Dok C, Tugwell P. Assessment of accuracy of the scoliosis school screening examination. Am J Public Health 1984;74:497–8.

98. Nachemson A, Peterson L. Effectiveness of treatment with a brace in girls who have adolescent idiopathic scoliosis. A prospective randomized controlled study based on data from the Brace Study of the Scoliosis Research Society. J Bone Joint Surg Am 1995;77:815–22.

99. Rowe D, Bernstein S, Riddick M, et al. A meta-analysis of the efficacy of non-operative treatments for idiopathic scoliosis. J Bone Joint Surg Am 1997;79:664–74.

100. American Academy of Pediatrics. Recommendations for preventive pediatric health care. Policy reference guide: a comprehensive guide to AAP policy statements published through December 1992, 6th ed. Elk Grove Village, IL: AAP; 1993. p. 608.

101. Gutgesell M. Practicality of screening urinalysis in asymptomatic children in a primary care setting. Pediatrics 1978;62:103–5.

102. Murakami M, Yamamoto H, Ueda Y, et al. Urinary screening of elementary and junior-high school children over a 13 year period in Tokyo. Pediatr Nephrol 1991;5:50–3.

103. Kaplan R, Springate J, Feld L. Screening dipstick urinalysis: a time to change. Pediatrics 1997;100:919–21.

104. Asymptomatic bacteriuria in schoolchildren in Newcastle upon Tyne. Arch Dis Child 1975;50:90–102.

105. Lohr J. Use of routine urinalysis in making a presumptive diagnosis of urinary tract infection in children. Pediatr Infect Dis J 1991;10:646–50.

106. Dodge W, West E, Smith E. Proteinuria and hematuria in school children: epidemiology and early natural history. J Pediatr 1976;88:327–47.

107. Norman M. An office approach to hematuria and proteinuria. Pediatr Clin N Am 1987;34(3):545–60.

108. Moore G, Robinson M. Do urine dipsticks reliably predict microhematuria? Ann Emerg Med 1988;17:257–60.

109. Yip R, Walsh K, Goldfarb M. Declining prevalence of anemia in childhood in a middle-class setting: a pediatric success story? Pediatrics 1987;80:330–4.

110. Centers for Disease Control. Pediatric nutrition surveillance system—United States, 1980-1991. MMWR 1992;41(SS-7):1–24.

111. Rybo E. Diagnosis of iron deficiency. Scand J Hematol Suppl 1985;43:5–39.

112. Thomas W, Collins T. Comparison of venipuncture blood counts with microcapillary measurements in screening for anemia in one-year-old infants. J Pediatr 1982;101:32–5.

113. Idjradinata P, Pollitt E. Reversal of developmental delays in iron-deficient anemia infants treated with iron. Lancet 1993;341:1–4.

114. American Academy of Pediatrics. Tuberculosis. In: Peter G, editor. Report of the Committee on Infectious Diseases, 24th ed. Elk Grove Village, IL: AAP; 1997. p. 541–62.

115. Canadian Pediatric Society IDaIC. Childhood tuberculosis: current concepts in diagnosis. Can J Pediatr 1994;1:97–100.

116. Gessner B, Teutsch S, Shaffer P. A cost-effectiveness evaluation of newborn hemoglobinopathy screening from the perspective of state health care systems. Early Human Dev 1996;45:257–75.

117. Shafer F, Lorey F, Cunningham G, et al. Newborn screening for sickle cell disease: 4 years of experience from California's newborn screening program. J Ped Hematol Oncol 1996;18:36–41.

118. American Academy of Pediatrics. Screening for elevated blood lead levels. American Academy of Pediatrics Committee on Environmental Health. Pediatrics 1998;101:1072–8.

119. Daniel K, Sedlis M, Polk L, et al. Childhood lead poisoning, New York City, 1988. MMWR 1990;39:1–7.

CHAPTER 3

Immunization

Ronald Gold, MD, MPH, FRCPC

———•———

Immunization prevents disease and saves lives. It is also one of the few health interventions that saves more money than it costs. Successful implementation of childhood immunization programs requires that both the health professionals involved in administering vaccines and parents be knowledgeable about the risks of the diseases and the benefits as well as the risks of the vaccines. In particular, it is extremely important that the true precautions and contraindications are understood.

The only absolute contraindications to immunization are as follows:[1,2]
- Anaphylaxis to a previous dose of vaccine
- Anaphylaxis to a constituent of a vaccine (eg, severe allergic reaction to influenza and yellow fever vaccines after eating eggs or allergy to neomycin in the case of inactivated polio vaccine[IPV] or mumps-measles-rubella [MMR] vaccine)
- Pregnancy, in the case of MMR
- Immunodeficiency, in the case of MMR

Precautions which may indicate deferral of immunization include the following:
- Recent administration of immunoglobulin, in the case of MMR (see[1,3] for details)
- Moderate or severe acute illness with or without fever

Conditions which are *not* contraindications to immunization are as follows:[1,2]
- Local reaction to previous dose of vaccine
- Mild acute illness with or without fever
- Convalescent phase of an acute minor illness
- Current antimicrobial therapy
- Recent exposure to infection
- Prematurity
- Personal or family history of allergy
- Family history of convulsions, sudden infant death syndrome (SIDS)
- Convulsion, hypotonic–hypo-responsive (HHR) episode, or high fever ($\geq 40.5°C$) within 48 hours or persistent inconsolable crying lasting ≥ 3 h after prior dose of diphtheria-pertussis-tetanus (DPT) vaccine
- Pregnancy, in the case of hepatitis B and influenza vaccines
- Diagnosis of multiple sclerosis, any other autoimmune disorder, or muscular dystrophy

Viral respiratory and gastrointestinal infections are very common in children less than 2 years of age. Studies have demonstrated that there is no increase in adverse events and no diminution of the immune responses if vaccination is performed while a child has a minor illness. Deferral of vaccination because of minor illness is all too common but should be avoided because children whose vaccinations are delayed have an increased probability of not being fully immunized.

Immunization Schedules

The Canadian schedule for routine immunization of children is given in Table 3–1.[1] The combined diphtheria, tetanus, acellular pertussis, inactivated polio and *Haemophilus influenzae* type b vaccine is now used in all Canadian provinces and territories. Differences exist

Table 3–1   Routine Immunization of Infants and Children in Canada

Age	DTaP	IPV	Hib	MMR	Td	HB
2 mo	X	X	X			X or
4 mo	X	X	X			
6 mo	X	X	X			
12 mo				X		
18 mo	X	X	X	X or		
4–6 y	X	X		X		
9–12 y						X
14–16 y					X	

DTaP = diphtheria, tetanus, acellular pertussis vaccine, usually combined with IPV and PRP-T. DTaP should be used for all doses, including completion of the series in those started with whole-cell pertussis vaccine; IPV = inactivated polio vaccine; Hib = *Haemophilus influenzae* type b conjugate vaccine: tetanus toxoid conjugate (PRP-T) used with combined DTaP-IPV in Canada; MMR = measles mumps rubella vaccine, first dose on or after first birthday, second dose either at 18 mo or at 4 to 6 y, depending on province; Td = adult tetanus, diphtheria vaccine with reduced dose of diphtheria toxoid for those ≥7 years of age; HB = hepatitis B vaccine: 3 doses at 0, 1, and 6 months either in infancy or in preadolescence, depending on province.

between jurisdictions regarding at what age the second dose of MMR and at which grade school–based hepatitis B vaccination should be administered. Information on schedules for children whose immunization did not begin in early infancy can be found in the Canadian Immunization Guide. The routine immunization schedules differ between the United States and Canada because (1) the combined vaccine is not yet available, (2) a sequential killed–live polio vaccine schedule is recommended, and (3) both hepatitis B and varicella vaccines are recommended for infants in the United States (Table 3–2).[4,5]

DIPHTHERIA

Epidemiology

Since 1983, less than five cases of diphtheria have been reported annually in Canada, almost all of which were in adults who had been either partially immunized or not immunized at all. Diphtheria is still a severe disease—the case fatality rate is 5 to 10 percent.

Diphtheria Toxoid

Diphtheria toxoid (D) is available in Canada and the United States, either separately or combined with one or more vaccines, including tetanus toxoid (T), acellular pertussis vaccine (aP), and (IPV). The combination recommended for routine immunization in Canada is D, T, aP, and IPV, DTaP-IPV, which is used to dissolve lyophilized *Haemophilus influenzae* type b vaccine (tetanus toxoid conjugate polyribose-phosphate, [PRP-T]). The resulting combination, DTaP-IPV/PRP-T, is administered as a single injection. The recommended vaccine in the United States is DTaP since combinations with IPV and/or Haemophilus b (Hib) vaccine are not yet licensed.[4]

For children over 7 years old and adults, a reduced amount of diphtheria toxoid is used (2 Lf units per dose rather than 12 to 25 Lf units) to minimize local reactions in persons who

Table 3–2 Routine Immunization of Infants and Children in the United States[*]

	Birth	1 mo	2 mo	4 mo	6 mo	12 mo	15 mo	18 mo	4–6 y	11–12 y	14–16 y
Hepatitis[1]	Hep B		Hep B			Hep B				Hep B	
Diphtheria, Tetanus, Pertussis[2]			DTaP	DTaP	DTaP		DTaP	DTaP	DTaP	Td	
H. influenzae type b[3]			Hib	Hib	Hib	Hib	Hib				
Polio[4]			IPV	IPV	Polio	Polio			Polio		
Measles, Mumps, Rubella[5]						MMR	MMR		MMR	MMR	
Varicella[6]						Var	Var			Var	

[*] modified from [4,5]

Vaccines are listed under recommended ages. Bars indicate the range of ages recommended for immunization. Shaded bars indicate vaccines to be given if previously recommended doses were missed or given earlier than minimum age.

1. Infants born to HbsAg–negative mothers should receive the 2nd dose of HBV vaccine at least 1 month after 1st dose. The 3rd dose should be given at least 4 months after the 1st dose and at least 2 months after the 2nd dose but not before 6 months of age.

2. DTaP (diphtheria and tetanus toxoids and acellular pertussis vaccine) is preferred vaccine for all doses, including completion of series in those that began with whole-cell DTP. The 4th dose of DTaP can be given as early as 12 months, provided 6 months have elapsed since the 3rd dose and if the child is unlikely to return at 15 to 18 months. Td is recommended at 11 to 12 months of age if at least 5 years have elapsed since the last dose of DTP, DTaP, or DT. Subsequent doses of Td should be given every 10 years.

3. Three Hib conjugate vaccines are licensed for infant use. Consult package insert for appropriate schedule.

4. Both inactivated (IPV) and oral (OPV) polio vaccines are licensed. The first two doses should be IPV to minimize the risk of vaccine-associated paralytic polio. The 3rd and 4th doses can be either IPV (for all IPV schedule) or OPV (for sequential IPV–OPV schedule). OPV is no longer recommended for the first two doses.

5. The 2nd dose of MMR is recommended at 4 to 6 years of age but may be given at any visit provided at least 4 weeks have elapsed since the administration of the 1st dose. The 1st dose should be given at or after 12 months of age.

6. Varicella vaccine is recommended at any visit on or after the first birthday for susceptible children, that is, those who lack a reliable history of chickenpox. Susceptible persons 13 years of age or older should receive two doses, given at least 4 weeks apart.

have previously been vaccinated.[6–8] The adult formulation is usually combined with Td or with Td and IPV (Td-IPV).

Adverse Events

The most common reaction caused by diphtheria toxoid is redness, swelling, pain, and tenderness at the site of the injection. The pain may cause babies to cry and be irritable. Local reactions are much more common in children and adults receiving boosters of the diphtheria toxoid than in infants receiving the first three doses.

Efficacy

Diphtheria toxoid prevents disease in most children and adults who are fully immunized. Those who do get diphtheria in spite of being fully vaccinated have a milder illness with fewer complications.

Evidence for the efficacy of diphtheria toxoid includes

- trials in school children in Toronto, which demonstrated a 75 percent reduction in the incidence of diphtheria in vaccinated compared to unvaccinated children;[9]
- the virtual disappearance of diphtheria cases in all countries in which immunization of infants and children is routine;[10–13]
- milder disease and fewer complications in fully immunized persons.[14]

Indirect evidence supporting the effectiveness of diphtheria toxoid is provided by the current experience in Russia, Ukraine, and other states of the former Soviet Union.[13] A marked decrease in the number of children being vaccinated was followed by epidemics of diphtheria; over 100,000 cases of diphtheria and more than 1,200 deaths occurred in Russia and Ukraine since 1990.[13]

Recommendations

There is good evidence to support the recommendation of routine immunization of all children with diphtheria toxoid, including one well-designed controlled trial without randomization, dramatic declines in disease incidence in all countries within a short period of introduction of mass immunization, and resurgence of epidemics when vaccination coverage declines (Table 3–3). The optimal schedule of boosters for adults remains to be determined.

TETANUS

Epidemiology

The frequency of tetanus has declined in all countries with successful immunization programs. Since 1985, there have been fewer than five cases per year in Canada. Most cases of tetanus now occur in persons over 60 years who have never been vaccinated.

Table 3–3 Summary of Quality of Evidence Supporting Use of DTaP-PV and Hib Vaccines

Immunizing Agent	Quality of Evidence	Recommendation
Diphtheria toxoid	II–1, II–3	A
Tetanus toxoid	I, II–3	A
Acellular pertussis vaccine	I, II–2	A
Inactivated polio vaccine	I, II–3	A
Hib vaccine	I, II–3	A

Tetanus Toxoid

Tetanus toxoid is supplied in Canada and the United States either by itself or combined with one or more other vaccines, including diphtheria toxoid, pertussis vaccine, and IPV. (See section above on "Diphtheria Toxoid" for description of combinations available in Canada.)

Adverse Events

Redness, swelling, pain, and tenderness at the site of injection are the most common reactions occurring after administration of tetanus toxoid.[15] The likelihood of local reactions increases with the number of doses given.[16] Severe local reactions after boosters occur in less than 2 percent of adults, primarily in those who have too many boosters, that is more than once every 10 years.[17]

Other reactions following tetanus vaccination include swollen lymph glands (especially those near the site of injection), fever, headache, and muscle aches.

Allergic reactions (usually hives) do occur but are rare.[18] As tetanus toxoid is usually given in combination with other vaccines, the exact factor causing a reaction may not be easy to identify. Severe allergic reactions are much less common in infants and young children than in adults.[19]

Adverse neurologic events have been reported following administration of tetanus toxoid. The frequency of neurologic reactions is estimated to be less than one per million doses of vaccine, making it impossible to determine whether the association is coincidental or causal.[20]

Efficacy

Routine immunization of U.S. soldiers during World War II resulted in a 30-fold reduction in the incidence of tetanus occurring after war wounds, compared with World War I.[21] Programs to prevent tetanus of newborns in the developing countries confirm that tetanus toxoid is extremely effective; in a double-blind controlled trial, no disease was seen in infants born to mothers who had received at least two doses of tetanus toxoid compared with a rate of 78 per 1,000 live births in control infants.[22] Tetanus is extremely rare in all countries with effective programs for vaccination of children.[23]

Recommendations

There is good evidence to support the recommendation of routine immunization of all children with tetanus toxoid including the reduced incidence of tetanus in U.S. military personnel in World War II compared with World War I;[21] the dramatic declines in incidence in all countries within a short period of introduction of mass immunization;[23] and randomized, double-blind controlled trials confirming the efficacy of tetanus toxoid in preventing neonatal tetanus in the developing countries (see Table 3–3).[22] The optimal schedule of boosters for adults remains to be determined.

PERTUSSIS

Epidemiology

Introduction of routine immunization with DPT in the 1940s resulted in a 90 percent decrease in reported cases of pertussis, from an average of 17,463 cases reported annually in the immediate prevaccine era to 4,900 cases per year for 1986 through 1995.[24] The actual number of cases is 10 to 15 times greater than the reported number because of incomplete reporting of the disease by physicians.[25]

The introduction of routine DPT vaccination was also followed by a significant change in the age distribution of pertussis. In the prevaccine era, the peak incidence of pertussis occurred in children 1 to 5 years of age and less than 15 percent of reported cases occurred in infants.[26] With routine vaccination, the peak incidence switched from young children to infants less than 1 year of age, among whom approximately 50 percent of reported cases occurred. Concurrently, there has been a significant increase in the proportion of cases occurring in adolescents and young adults.[27]

Approximately 85 percent of Canadian children have received 4 doses of DPT by 2 years of age and >90 percent have received 5 doses by 6 years of age.[24] However, disease continues to occur, along with epidemics every 3 to 5 years.[24,25] The lack of change in the interval between epidemics is strong evidence that routine vaccination, as presently practiced with a primary series of DPT at 2, 4, and 6 months followed by boosters at 18 months and at 4 to 6 years, has failed to interrupt the transmission of *Bordetella pertussis* in the population.[26]

Acellular Pertussis Vaccine

The new acellular pertussis vaccines consist of purified proteins extracted from the bacteria. The acellular vaccines differ in both the number and concentration of the following proteins purified from *B. pertussis:* pertussis toxoid (PT), filamentous hemagglutinin (FHA), pertactin (PRN, formerly designated 69 kD protein), and fimbriae (FIM) 2 and 3 (Table 3–4). The Canadian acellular pertussis vaccine contains PT, FHA, PRN, and both FIM 2 and FIM 3. It has completely replaced the use of whole-cell pertussis vaccine throughout Canada. The routine immunization schedule did not change with the replacement of whole-cell by acellular pertussis vaccine (see Table 3–1). The Canadian vaccine has not yet been licensed in the United States, where four acellular pertussis vaccines from other manufacturers are available.[4]

Adverse Events

The frequency of adverse effects after whole-cell and acellular pertussis vaccines are summarized in Table 3–5. These results were obtained from Canadian studies comparing whole-cell pertussis (DPT–IPV/PRP–T) with acellular pertussis combination vaccines (DTaP–IPV/PRP–T), given at 2, 4, and 6 months of age.[28] Both local and systemic adverse events were two to four times less common after acellular vaccine. The severity of reactions was also significantly less with acellular vaccine. Similar results have been obtained with all acellular pertussis vaccines.[29,30]

Severe allergic reactions such as anaphylaxis have been described after immunization with whole-cell pertussis vaccine. With both whole-cell and acellular pertussis vaccines that

Table 3–4   Components of *B. pertussis* Involved in Pathogenesis of Disease and Immunity

Pertussis proteins	*Role of pertussis proteins in*		
	Attachment to mucosa		*Immunity*
Pertussis toxin	++	++	++
Filamentous hemagglutinin	++	0	±
Pertactin	++	?	++
Fimbriae 2 and 3	++	0	++
Adenylate cyclase	0	++	?
Tracheal cytotoxin	0	±	?

++ = important ; ± = possibly important; 0 = not important; ? = importance unknown are currently available, the occurrence of anaphylaxis has been so rare that it is not possible to calculate the risk. Naturally, any child who has an allergic reaction of any kind after pertussis or any other vaccine should not receive the same vaccine again until the cause of the reaction has been identified by appropriate evaluation.

Other severe reactions that may occur after both whole-cell and acellular pertussis vaccines include prolonged crying, "collapse" reaction (also known as hypotonic–hypo-responsive episode), and convulsions. All these events are less frequent after immunization with acellular than with whole-cell pertussis vaccine.[31] About 1 in 100 infants have nonstop, inconsolable crying or screaming lasting more than 3 hours after administration of whole-cell vaccine, but this reduction is much less frequent after acellular pertussis vaccines. There is no evidence that prolonged crying is caused by a neurologic reaction, and recovery is complete.

Hypotonic–hypo-responsive episodes occur most often after the first dose of DPT and almost never after the fourth or fifth dose.[32] They occur about once in every 1,750 DPT injections. Symptoms begin within 12 hours of the injection and may last up to 1 day. The infant becomes pale, floppy, and less responsive than normal. The cause of HHE is unknown. Infants with HHE recover completely and can receive additional doses of pertussis vaccine without risk of recurrence of HHE.[33,34]

Any vaccine which can induce fever can precipitate febrile convulsions in susceptible children. The incidence of convulsions after whole-cell pertussis vaccination is between 1 in 1,700 vaccinations and 1 in 10,000 vaccinations.[35,36] Convulsions are more common after the third and fourth doses than after the first two doses. Febrile convulsions do not cause permanent brain damage and do not increase the risk of epilepsy or any other disorder of the brain.[37] Immunization is *not* associated with an increased incidence of afebrile convulsions.[38]

Table 3–5   Incidence of Adverse Events after Whole-Cell or Acellular Pertussis Combined Pentavalent Vaccines in Canadian Infants

	Incidence of Adverse Events (%)	
Adverse Event	*DPT-IPV/PRP-T**	*DTaP-IPV/PRP-T**
Local redness	33.3	10.7
Local swelling	31.1	10.0
Local tenderness	59.5	24.4
Fever — 38.0°C	61.8	17.7
Fever — 39.0°C	9.8	0.7
Fussiness	80.5	44.7
Crying	69.8	33.3
Drowziness	65.5	32.9
Anorexia	44.2	21.3
Vomiting	11.6	6.2
Diarrhea	11.9	8.2

*DPT-IPV/PRP-T, DtaP-IPV/PRP-T: whole-cell and acellular pertussis combined pentavalent vaccines (Pasteur Mérieux Connaught, Canada)

Febrile seizures, prolonged crying, and HHE have been observed following the administration of acellular pertussis vaccine.[31,39,40] The rates of such reactions appear to be lower with acellular than with whole-cell pertussis vaccine.[31] However, since none of the reactions that occurred after whole-cell vaccine are known to cause permanent brain damage, it is unlikely that damage will occur after administration of the acellular vaccine.

Many other conditions have been blamed on the pertussis vaccine. Such allegations are based on anecdotes rather than scientific studies. There are no valid scientific studies which demonstrate a causal link between pertussis vaccine and encephalopathy, brain damage, autism, infantile spasms, epilepsy, mental retardation, learning disorders, hyperactivity, SIDS, asthma, or atopic diseases.[1,41,42]

The only contraindication to administration of pertussis vaccine is an anaphylactic reaction to a previous dose.

Efficacy

Routine vaccination of infants and young children has resulted in a marked decline in the frequency of pertussis in every country with effective childhood vaccination programs. Conversely, discontinuation or declines in vaccine coverage have resulted in large epidemics in Japan, Sweden, the United Kingdom, and the newly independent states of the former Soviet Union.[43] When vaccine coverage rose again in Japan and England, the incidence of pertussis declined.[44]

Randomized, placebo-contolled studies in Sweden showed that the Canadian acellular vaccine protected 85 percent of infants against pertussis.[39,40] Similar results were obtained with other acellular pertussis vaccines.[45]

Products containing multiple pertussis antigens are more effective than those with PT alone or PT plus FHA against pertussis. The Canadian vaccine is also very effective against mild disease.[39,40] The results from recent efficacy trials have confirmed that there are antibody correlates of protection; vaccinated children with high antibody levels against PT, PRN, and FIM had a much lower secondary attack rate after household exposure to pertussis than did vaccinated children with low titers. The titer of antibody to FHA did not correlate with protection.[46,47]

Another very important finding of the recent studies is the demonstration that re-infection with pertussis is a common event because of waning immunity, which occurs not only in vaccinated individuals but also in those with prior pertussis infection.[27] Such re-infection may be asymptomatic, being detectable only by demonstrating a rise in antibodies to pertussis antigens but may also result in illness with cough.[48,49]

Because adverse reactions are so much less common with acellular than with whole-cell vaccine, it is possible to give boosters to adolescents and adults. It has become increasingly recognized that pertussis is very common in adolescents and young adults. In fact, the greatest rise in incidence of disease during the 1990s in North America occurred in persons 10 to 29 years of age. Approximately 15 to 25 percent of young adults presenting with cough of more than 7 days duration have pertussis.[50–52]

A single booster of either Td or Td-IPV combined with acellular pertussis vaccine has been shown to be safe and highly immunogenic in those between 10 and 60 years of age.[53,54] Such boosters may prolong the duration of protection against pertussis, thereby resulting in reduced transmission of B. pertussis in the population. If routine boosters do reduce the incidence of pertussis in adolescents and adults, infants under 6 months of age who have not yet completed the primary series would greatly benefit because of reduced risk of exposure to infection from siblings and parents.

Recommendations

There is good evidence to support the recommendation of routine immunization of all children with acellular pertussis vaccine, including two well-designed randomized, placebo-controlled trials[39,55] and one randomized controlled trial without placebo;[40] several case-control trials; epidemiologic evidence of dramatic declines in disease incidence in all countries within a short period of introduction of mass immunization and resurgence of epidemics when vaccination coverage declines (see Table 3–3). The optimal schedule of boosters for adolescents and adults remains to be determined.

POLIOMYELITIS

Epidemiology

Within 12 years after the introduction of IPV in 1955, the incidence of paralytic polio decreased by almost 99 percent in Canada, United States, and all other countries with successful polio vaccine programs using either IPV or oral polio vaccine (OPV). The global campaign to eradicate polio has been remarkably successful.[56] Indigenous transmission of wild polioviruses has been interrupted throughout the entire western hemisphere and the region was certified as polio free in 1994. Today, the remaining major foci of transmission of wild polioviruses are in Africa.[57] Because of the speed and extent of travel in all parts of the world, we must continue to immunize children until polioviruses have been eliminated worldwide.

Polio Vaccine

In Canada, an IPV–only schedule is used.[1] The change from OPV to IPV was based on the efficacy on an IPV–only schedule, the eradication of wild polio from the western hemisphere and declining risk of importation of wild polio viruses because of the success of the World Health Organization (WHO) polio eradication program in most parts of the world, and the desire to avoid the risk of vaccine-associated paralytic polio (VAPP) due to OPV.

Inactivated polio vaccine contains types 1, 2, and 3 wild-type polio viruses which have been killed with formalin. The viruses in IPV are grown in either human MRC-5 cells or Vero cells.

In Canada, IPV is supplied either by itself or in combination with the following vaccines: DTP-IPV, DTaP-IPV, DT-IPV, or Td-IPV. Both DPT/IPV and DTaP-IPV can be used to dissolve the lyophilized Hib vaccine so that all five vaccines can be administered as a single injection.

In the United States, either IPV-only or sequential IPV-OPV schedules are recommended by the American Academy of Pediatrics.[5] Oral polio vaccine consists of attenuated strains of live type 1, 2, and 3 polio viruses grown on monkey kidney cell cultures.

Adverse Events Associated with IPV

Other than minor pain and redness at the injection site, side effects with IPV are extremely rare. Current methods of production and testing before release of each batch of IPV ensure that there is no live polio virus in the vaccine.

In 1960, some batches of rhesus monkey kidney cells used to grow polio virus were discovered to be infected with a monkey virus called simian virus 40 (SV40). Live SV40 was subsequently found in some batches of both IPV and OPV, which had been used in many parts of the world. Vaccine production methods were altered in order to ensure that SV40 was not present in cells used to grow polio viruses. All polio vaccines, both IPV and OPV, used since 1963 have been free of SV40.

Simian virus 40 is a papovavirus, a group of viruses known to cause cancer in several species of animals. No differences in death rates from all causes or in cancer deaths have been detected among groups who had received vaccine containing SV40 compared with those given vaccine free of SV40.[58] A workshop on SV40 at the National Institutes of Health (NIH) concluded that there is no evidence of harm to humans as a result of exposure to SV40 in polio vaccines.[59]

Adverse Effects

Paralytic poliomyelitis following the use of monovalent type 3 OPV was first described in 1962.[60] Vaccine-associated paralytic polio also occurs with trivalent OPV. For immunocompetent infants receiving their first dose of OPV, the risk of VAPP is estimated to be 1 case per 750,000 children vaccinated.[61] The risk decreased nearly 20–fold with subsequent doses. There is also a risk of VAPP in household and community contacts of children vaccinated with OPV because the vaccine virus is excreted in the stool for several weeks. The risk in contacts is much lower than in vaccinated children. The risk of VAPP is more than 3,000-times higher in immunodeficient persons, especially those with agammaglobulinemia or hypogammaglobulinemia.[62] The risk of VAPP is eliminated entirely by an IPV-only schedule. The IPV-OPV sequential schedule is estimated to reduce the risk of VAPP by 95 percent.[63]

Efficacy

Field trials of the original IPV showed that it offered protection against paralytic polio in 55 percent of school children after one dose, 80 percent after two doses, 91 percent after three doses, and 96 percent after four doses.[64] Current vaccines are much more potent than the original Salk vaccine and have been shown to be 90 percent effective after just two doses.[65] Protection lasts for many years following vaccination with IPV.[66]

The experience in Sweden, Finland, the Netherlands, France, and some Canadian provinces (Ontario, Nova Scotia, Newfoundland) has demonstrated that paralytic polio can be eliminated by the use of IPV alone.[66–71] Even though the virus has been brought back into these countries many times over the past 50 years by travelers infected with polio, only three small outbreaks of paralytic polio have occurred. All cases involved small groups of people who had refused immunization for religious reasons. No disease occurred in those who had been vaccinated.[72]

The eradication of polio from the western hemisphere and many other parts of the world led to a change from OPV to IPV in all of Canada to avoid the very small risk of paralytic polio associated with OPV.

Recommendations

There is good evidence to support the recommendation of routine immunization of all children with IPV, including a large well–designed randomized, placebo–controlled trial in school children and strong epidemiologic evidence of elimination of paralytic polio and of eradication of indigenous transmission of wild polio viruses in all countries which have high vaccine coverage with IPV (see Table 3–3).

HAEMOPHILUS INFLUENZAE TYPE B (HIB)

Epidemiology

Before 1985, Hib was the most common cause of bacterial meningitis in children throughout the world. Every year, in Canada, about 1,500 cases of Hib meningitis occurred in children under 5 years of age and an equal number of other forms of invasive Hib disease. However, Hib infections have almost disappeared in countries such as Canada where Hib vaccine is part of the routine immunization schedule.[73–75]

HIB VACCINE

Haemophilus b vaccine is the purified capsular polysaccharide, PRP. Because the pure polysaccharide is not sufficiently immunogenic in infants, current vaccines are composed of the polysaccharide covalently bound to a protein carrier such as tetanus toxoid (PRP-T), diphtheria toxoid (PRP-D), a nontoxic form of diphtheria toxin produced by a mutant strain of *Corynebacterium diphtheriae* (PRP-CRM$_{97}$), or the outer membrane protein of group B

Meningococcus (PRP-OMP). The conjugated vaccines are safe and highly immunogenic in infants. The Hib vaccine currently used in Canada is PRP-T.

Adverse Events

Haemophilus b vaccines are extremely safe. When given as a separate injection, Hib conjugated vaccines cause local redness and pain in 5 to 15 percent of infants. Local reactions are milder and much less common than those seen after DPT vaccine. The addition of the Hib vaccine to DPT, DPT-IPV, DTaP or DTaP-IPV vaccines has no bearing on the frequency and severity of side effects.[28,76]

The only contraindication to Hib vaccine is the occurrence of a severe allergic reaction to a previous dose of the vaccine. Children who have such allergic reactions after vaccinations should be seen and evaluated by a physician to identify the cause of the reaction.

Efficacy

Antibodies against PRP that are induced by Hib vaccine protect children in two ways
- The vaccinated child is protected against invasion by Hib.[76,77]
- The vaccinated child is less likely to become a carrier of Hib, thereby reducing transmission of Hib in the population.[78,79]

The efficacy of Hib vaccines has been shown to be over 95 percent in randomized, placebo-controlled trials.[76,77] Active surveillance has demonstrated greater than 99 percent reduction in incidence in Scandinavia, United States, and Canada following introduction of routine immunization, regardless of which conjugate vaccine is used.[77] However, in certain native populations that have extremely high carriage rates and high incidence of disease, differences in efficacy between different conjugates have been observed.[80] For such populations, conjugates such as PRP–OMP, which induce antibodies after the first dose at 2 months of age, may be required.

Recommendations

There is good evidence to support the recommendation of routine immunization of all children with conjugated Hib vaccine, including many well-designed randomized, placebo–controlled trials, and epidemiologic evidence of dramatic declines in disease incidence in all countries within a short period of introduction of mass immunization (see Table 3–3).

MEASLES

Epidemiology

Before measles vaccine became available, almost everyone got measles by 18 years of age. An average of 350,000 cases occurred every year in Canada and there were 50 to 75 deaths, 5,000 hospital admissions, and 400 cases of encephalitis.

Since licensure of measles vaccine in 1963, there has been a dramatic decline in the annual number of cases in every country with routine immunization programs. In 1998, there were only 12 laboratory-confirmed cases of measles reported in Canada, a decline of >99.99 percent since the prevaccine era.[81]

The measles virus is highly contagious and is able to survive in small droplets in the air for at least several hours. This survival ability ensures airborne spread, which explains the high level of contagiousness of the virus.[82] The secondary attack rate among susceptible persons exposed at home to a child with measles is over 90 percent.[83]

Immunoglobulin Prophylaxis

Administration of immunoglobulin (Ig) after exposure can prevent or attenuate the severity of measles, if given less than 6 days after exposure to measles. Immunoglobulin is recommended, if the person exposed to measles is at increased risk of severe disease and/or complications of measles:

- An infant less than 12 months old
- A pregnant woman
- Those with problems involving the immune system.[1,84]

Measles Vaccine

Measles vaccine is a live, attenuated vaccine grown in chick embryo cells. Sorbitol and hydrolyzed gelatin are added to stabilize the lyophilized virus. Because exposure to sunlight or heat will kill the measles vaccine virus, it must be refrigerated at the proper temperature (5 to 8°C). If the vaccine virus dies before it is injected, it does not induce any protection. Improper storage is responsible for many vaccine failures.[85]

Adverse Events

Side effects after measles vaccine, whether given by itself or combined with mumps and rubella vaccine, are usually mild. When children are given a second dose of measles vaccine, no reactions occur in those who are immune as a result of the first dose.[86]

The most common side effect is fever. In a placebo-controlled, randomized, cross-over study in identical twins, about 2 percent had fever of ≥39.4°C occurring 8 to 10 days after vaccination and lasting 24 to 48 hours.[87] The fever may be high enough to cause seizures in children who are susceptible to febrile seizures. Rash occurs in about 2 percent of twins and lasts 1 to 2 days. The frequency of sides effects in the Finnish twin study are lower than the rates in almost all other studies because the twin study was one of the very few to include a placebo, thereby enabling more accurate assessment of events attributable to the vaccine.

The illness caused by the vaccine (fever and rash for 1 to 2 days in 2 percent of recipients)[87] is much less severe than the actual illness associated with measles (fever, rash, cough, and bronchitis lasting 7 to 10 days in 100 percent of cases).[88]

Severe adverse events after measles vaccine are rare. The risk of encephalitis after measles vaccine is less than one per one million doses, lower than the background incidence of encephalitis.[89] Measles itself, on the other hand, causes encephalitis in about 1 of every 1,000 cases. In countries where all children are vaccinated against measles, measles encephalitis has disappeared.[90] As subacute sclerosing panencephalitis (SSPE) has disappeared in countries with effective vaccine programs, it seems unlikely that the vaccine causes SSPE.[91] Transient thrombocytopenia during the month following vaccination with MMR occurs rarely.

Egg Allergy and Measles Vaccination

In the past, it was recommended that children who have allergic reactions after eating eggs should not be vaccinated with measles or mumps vaccines, unless skin testing was performed and a special vaccine schedule was used. However, review of all the studies about vaccinating children with egg allergy has shown that they can be safely vaccinated with measles and mumps vaccine without the need for special precautions.[92,93]

Measles is often very severe in persons with problems involving the immune system. Moreover, the original measles vaccine caused pneumonia in a few children with leukemia. Therefore, it is recommended that measles vaccine not be given to persons with severe disorders of the immune system. However, measles vaccine is recommended and has been shown to be safe for children with HIV infection or with AIDS.

Immunoglobulin (Ig) and other blood products may contain antibodies to the measles virus that will interfere with measles vaccine. Vaccination must be delayed for 3 to 11 months, depending on the type and dose of Ig or blood product used.

Efficacy

With a one-dose schedule, the incidence of measles was reduced by over 90 percent. However, measles is so highly contagious that school outbreaks would occur even though 85 to 90 percent of children were immune. Therefore, Canada has adopted a two-dose schedule whereby children are given one dose of measles vaccine in infancy and a second before starting school.[81] The purpose of the second dose is to ensure that the number of children who remain susceptible is less than 1 percent. A two-dose schedule is required if Canada is to achieve its national objective of measles eradication. Today, all Canadian provinces (except New Brunswick) have adopted a two-dose measles schedule. The introduction, in 1996 of the routine 2-dose schedule combined with school catch-up programs, has resulted in a dramatic fall in measles incidence; less than 20 cases were reported in 1998.[94]

Vaccine Failure

About 5 to 10 percent of infants fail to respond to the first dose of measles vaccine when administered on or soon after the first birthday.[95] The most important cause of failure is persistence of transplacentally acquired maternal antibodies against measles. If the titer of maternal antibodies at the time of immunization is great enough, the live vaccine virus is destroyed before it can induce an immune response.

Improper storage of measles vaccine is the second most important cause of vaccine failure. Because the vaccine virus must be alive when it is injected, it must be stored at 5 to 8°C at all times until just before it is used.

Recommendations

There is good evidence to support the recommendation of routine immunization of all children with two doses of measles vaccine, including many well-designed randomized trials in institutionalized populations,[96] epidemiologic evidence of dramatic declines in disease incidence in all countries within a short period of introduction of mass immunization,[81,97,98] eradication of indigenous measles in Cuba, the English-speaking islands of the Caribbean and Finland,[99,100] and rapid elimination of measles following introduction of the two-dose schedule (see Table 3–6).[81,100]

MUMPS

Epidemiology

Data from Canada, the United States, France, the United Kingdom, Sweden, and Finland show that the number of cases of mumps decreased by over 90 percent after mumps vaccine became available. Before mumps vaccination programs began, mumps was the most common cause of encephalitis in children. Mumps encephalitis has virtually disappeared from countries with effective vaccination programs.[90]

Table 3–6 Summary of Quality of Evidence Supporting Use of MMR Vaccine

Immunizing agent	Quality of Evidence	Recommendation
Measles vaccine	I, II–2, II–3	A
Mumps toxoid	I, II–2, II–3	A
Rubella vaccine	I, II–2, II–3	A

Mumps Vaccine

Mumps vaccine is a live attenuated virus vaccine produced in chick embryo cell cultures. After passing all tests for potency and safety, the virus is lyophilized. Trace amounts of neomycin remain in the vaccine. Mumps vaccine is most often combined with measles and rubella vaccines to produce MMR vaccine.

Because exposure to sunlight or heat will kill the mumps vaccine virus, it must be refrigerated at the proper temperature (5 to 8°C). Improper storage remains a problem and may be responsible for many of the vaccine failures.

Side effects of mumps vaccine

Side effects of the Jeryl Lynn strain of mumps vaccine have been rare. A few children develop swelling of the salivary glands 10 to 14 days after vaccination. Meningitis has been reported to occur at a rate of 1 case per 800,000 doses. No permanent brain damage has occurred after the rare cases of meningitis or encephalitis caused by mumps vaccine.

Mumps vaccine can be given, without any special precautions, to children with egg allergy (see section on "Measles Vaccine").

Efficacy

Over 90 percent of those vaccinated are protected against mumps. The vaccine provides the same protection, whether given separately or combined with measles and rubella vaccines.

Because fewer antibodies are induced by the vaccine than by the natural infection, there has been concern about the duration of protection after vaccination. Small outbreaks of mumps still occur, mainly in vaccinated teenagers and young adults (aged 13 to 25 years).[101] It has not been determined whether this vaccine failure is due to lack of response to the vaccine or to gradual loss of immunity. Introduction of a routine two-dose schedule of MMR vaccine should reduce the occurrence of such outbreaks.[100]

Recommendations

There is good evidence to support the recommendation of routine immunization of all children with two doses of mumps vaccine, including epidemiologic evidence of dramatic declines in disease incidence in all countries within a short period of introduction of mass immunization (see Table 3–6).

RUBELLA

Epidemiology

Prior to the introduction of rubella vaccine in 1969, outbreaks of rubella used to occur annually in North America with larger epidemics occurring about every 7 years. Approximately 85 percent of people developed rubella by 20 years of age; the remaining 15 percent of adults were therefore still susceptible to rubella. Of greatest concern were women of childbearing age because of the risk of congenital rubella syndrome (CRS).

If a pregnant woman is infected with rubella during the first 20 weeks of pregnancy, the probability of fetal infection is over 80 percent.[102] If infection occurs in the first 12 weeks of pregnancy, the baby is usually born with multiple handicaps; if infection occurs between 16 and 20 weeks, deafness is usually the only complication. Regardless of the timing of onset of infection, the infected fetus almost always sustains damage. Infection is fatal in about 20 percent of fetuses, and 10 percent of infected babies die of complications during the first year of life.

Rubella Vaccine

Rubella vaccine is a live, attenuated vaccine grown in human diploid cells (WI38 cells). After passing all tests for potency and safety, the virus is lyophilized. Rubella vaccine can be given alone, combined with measles vaccine (MR), or, most commonly, as measles, mumps, rubella vaccine (MMR). Although rubella vaccine is not as sensitive to light and heat as measles vaccine, it should be refrigerated at 5 to 8°C until it is used.

All women should have a blood test for immunity to rubella, preferably before their first pregnancy. If the blood lacks antibodies to rubella and the woman is not pregnant, she should be immunized with rubella vaccine or MMR. Women should not become pregnant for 3 months after vaccination to allow immunity to develop.

If the woman is already pregnant and tests reveal that she lacks antibodies, vaccination should be delayed until after delivery of the baby to avoid potential harm to the fetus. However, there have been no cases of CRS in over 1,000 infants born to women who were vaccinated in the first 2 months of pregnancy.[103]

Adverse Events

Infants rarely have any side effects after rubella vaccination.[104] The frequency and severity of side effects increase with age, as does severity of the disease. Following vaccination, a few people develop mild fever, sore throat, headache, a rash, and swollen glands, just like a mild case of rubella. Most of these reactions are probably due to measles vaccine rather than rubella or mumps vaccine; the frequency of reactions is the same in children receiving MMR or the plain measles vaccine.

The most significant side effect of the rubella vaccine is arthralgia, most often experienced by adult women. Following vaccination, about 25 percent of adult women have some joint pain compared with less than 1 percent of vaccinated children. The incidence of arthralgia is twice as high after natural infection than after vaccination. A recent randomized, placebo-controlled trial of rubella vaccination of susceptible women in the immediate postpartum period failed to confirm any increased risk of chronic arthritis associated with the vaccine.[105]

Transient thrombocytopenia during the month after rubella vaccination occurs rarely.[104] However, the incidence of thrombocytopenia is 10 times higher after natural infection than after vaccination.

Efficacy

The incidence of rubella and of congenital rubella syndrome have declined by over 99 percent in all countries with routine immunization programs.[106] Between 1994 and 1996, only three cases of congenital rubella syndrome were reported per year, one third of which were imported.[107]

Recommendations

There is good evidence to support the recommendation of routine immunization of all children with two doses of rubella vaccine, including epidemiologic evidence of dramatic declines in disease incidence in all countries within a short period of introduction of mass immunization (see Table 3–6).

HEPATITIS B

The incidence of infection with hepatitis B virus (HBV) displays very marked geographic variation. In Canada, the United States, and other developed countries, the prevalence of chronic carriage of hepatitis B surface antigen (HBsAg) is about 0.5 percent.[108] In China, Southeast Asia, and parts of Africa, chronic carrier rates are over 10 percent.

In Canada, the two most common means of spread are sexual activity and sharing of needles by users of injectable drugs.[109] The infection rate is highest among older teenagers and young adults. Infection of infants born to infected mothers still occurs, but the rate is decreasing.

Prevention of HBV infection with HBIg

Hepatitis B immunoglobulin (HBIg) prevents infection following exposure to HBV. For those exposed to HBV, HBIg is recommended in the following circumstances:
- Accidental needle-stick or other injury
- Sexual activity with an infected person
- An infant born to an infected mother

HB Vaccine

Hepatitis B vaccine consists of the protein that forms the outer coat of the virus particle, hepatitis B surface antigen (HbsAg). The vaccines currently used in Canada are prepared by recombinant gene technology.

Adverse Events

Pain and tenderness at the site of the injection occur after about 15 percent of vaccinations. The soreness is mild and lasts less than 24 hours.[110,111] Carefully controlled studies have found that other symptoms, such as fever, headache, muscle aches and pain, nausea, vomiting, loss of appetite, and fatigue occur at the same rates in persons who receive the vaccine as in those who are given a placebo.[111] No causal link between hepatitis B vaccination and chronic fatigue syndrome has been demonstrated.[112] Although there have been anecdotal reports associating administration of hepatitis B with onset or exacerbation of multiple sclerosis and a variety of other neurologic and connective tissue disorders, epidemiologic studies have failed to demonstrate any causal links.[113]

Allergic reactions are rare, occurring after only less than 1 percent of vaccinations. Such reactions may be caused by allergy to yeast proteins or to the preservative, thimerosal. Thimerosal is used as an antiseptic in many contact lens solutions. Persons who are allergic to contact lens solutions may have severe local reactions to HB vaccine.

Contraindications

The only reason not to give hepatitis B vaccination is anaphylaxis (hypersensitivity leading to respiratory distress) or any other severe allergic reaction to a previous dose of the vaccine.

Control of Hepatitis B through Vaccination

When HB vaccine first became available, it was recommended for persons at increased risk of infection with HBV, including the following:
- Health care workers and others at risk of infection because of frequent exposure to blood, as part of their occupation (eg, doctors, nurses, dentists)
- Persons with underlying diseases that require treatment with blood or blood products (eg, hemophilia and chronic kidney failure treated with dialysis)
- Infants whose mothers have chronic HBV infection
- Persons living with someone with chronic HBV infection
- Those travelling to areas with high rates of HBV infection

This approach of targeting high-risk groups has been very effective in reducing the number of infections in persons in the first three groups listed above. However, vaccination of high-risk groups has had little or no effect on the overall rate of HBV infections in Canada or the United States.[114]

To control HBV infection, medical authorities in both Canada and the United States now recommend immunization of all children.[2,112,115] Italy, New Zealand, and several Asian countries have already introduced routine vaccination of all infants. Because there is a lag of 15 to 30 years between infection with HBV and the development of chronic liver disease, several decades must pass before the benefits of routine immunization of children are seen.

The current strategy for prevention of HBV infection in Canada focuses on three groups:

1. Pregnant women who are tested for HbsAg so that newborns of such mothers can be protected as soon as possible with HBIg followed by vaccine
2. School-age children who are vaccinated prior to adolescence so that they are protected before becoming sexually active. School vaccination programs have been introduced in all provinces and territories
3. Persons at high risk of infection because of occupational exposure, or life-style or behavior

The decision to recommend vaccination of all children was based on these facts: the vaccine is safe, effective, and the vaccination program is affordable. It costs more to treat chronic liver disease caused by hepatitis B than to vaccinate all children.[116,117] In Canada, routine vaccination of school-age children rather than infants is recommended for the following reasons:[112]

- The rate of HBV infection is very low in children under 12 years of age but begins to rise rapidly after 15 years of age
- A product combining diphtheria, tetanus, pertussis, polio, and *Haemophilus b* vaccines with HB vaccine is not yet available; a 6-in-1 vaccine would be better for infants to minimize the number of injections they receive

The school vaccination programs in Canada have been very successful, reaching over 90 percent of eligible children with three doses of vaccine.[110,118] Infant vaccination programs may become routine once combination vaccines become available.

Overall, HB vaccine is very effective. Over 95 percent of those vaccinated develop antibodies and are protected against infection with HBV. Those who do become infected despite vaccination appear to be protected against developing chronic HBV infection. Studies in Taiwan have documented that the incidence of hepatocellular carcinoma caused by HBV is decreasing in those cohorts that had been vaccinated as infants.[119]

The duration of protection is not yet known. It does, however, last at least 10 years, and probably much longer. For now, booster doses of vaccine are not considered necessary.

Recommendations

There is good evidence to support the recommendation of routine immunization of all children with hepatitis B vaccine, including randomized, placebo-controlled trials,[120–122] epidemiologic evidence of declines in disease incidence in all countries within a short period of introduction of mass immunization,[123] and studies in Taiwan showing a decline among vaccinated cohorts of primary hepatocellular carcinoma (see Table 3–7).[119]

VARICELLA

Epidemiology

Varicella, or chickenpox, is a common infection of childhood; almost 85 percent of the Canadian population is infected by 12 years of age. Although chickenpox is usually a mild disease in children, it is a costly one. Parents generally stay home for an average of 3 days with their children who get chickenpox. The vaccine is cost effective compared with the wages lost by

Table 3–7 Summary of Quality of Evidence Supporting Use of Hepatitis B Vaccine

Immunizing Agent	Quality of Evidence	Recommendation
Hepatitis B vaccine	I, II–2, II–3	A

Table 3–8 Summary of Quality of Evidence Supporting Use of Varicella Vaccine

Immunizing Agent	Quality of Evidence	Recommendation
Varicella vaccine	I	A

parents and/or sick leave benefits incurred by them, the costs of doctor visits, and the management of the complications of chickenpox.[124,125]

Varicella Vaccine

A live attenuated vaccine was licensed in Canada in December, 1998. The vaccine currently licensed in the United States and Canada is unstable unless stored in a freezer at −15°C, which may create problems in the distribution of the vaccine.

In healthy children, the vaccine is very safe and immunogenic. Seroconversion occurs in over 97 percent of children less than 12 years of age after one dose. The vaccine is less immunogenic in adolescents and adults; two doses, administered 1 month apart, are recommended for susceptible persons over 12 years of age. The vaccine prevents chickenpox in over 80 percent of recipients.[126] Disease is mild in those who are infected in spite of vaccination. Very mild symptoms, such as low-grade fever and rash around the injection site, develop in less than 10 percent of normal children and adults. Chickenpox does occur in vaccinated persons due to the vaccine strain, but the rate is significantly lower than that following infection with wild virus.[126]

To date, neither the duration of protection nor the need for boosters is known. Studies in Japan suggest that immunity lasts many years.[127,128]

Recommended Use of Varicella Vaccine

Recommendations for the use of varicella vaccine in Canada have been issued by the National Advisory Committee on Immunization (NACI) and are the same as in the United States. Universal vaccination is recommended for all children after the first birthday. It can be given concurrently with MMR vaccine. A combined MMR-varicella vaccine is under investigation but not yet available. Varicella vaccination is also recommended for adolescents and adults who have no history of chickenpox. It is unlikely that routine serologic testing for susceptibility would be cost effective in those without a definite history of chickenpox.

Recommendations

There is good evidence from randomized controlled trials that varicella vaccine is effective in preventing chickenpox and in reducing the incidence of zoster in children, adolescents and adults (Table 3–8). Routine immunization of all children, adolescents and adults without evidence of prior infection is recommended.

References

1. National Advisory Committee on Immunization. Canadian Immunization Guide, 4th ed. Ottawa: Health Canada; 1998.p.215.

2. Committee on Infectious Diseases. 1997 Red Book, 24th ed. Elk Grove Village, IL: American Academy of Pediatrics; 1997.p.26–35.

3. Committee on Infectious Diseases. 1997 Red Book, 24th ed. Elk Grove Village, IL: American Academy of Pediatrics; 1997.p.23.

4. Committee on Infectious Diseases. Recommended childhood immunization schedule—United States, January-December 1999. Pediatrics 1999;103:182–5.

5. Committee on Infectious Diseases. Poliomyelitis prevention: revised recommendations for use of inactivated and live oral polio virus vaccines. Pediatrics 1999;103:171–2.

6. Simonsen O, Klaerke M, Klaerke A, et al. Revaccination of adults against diphtheria. II: Combined diphtheria and tetanus revaccination with different doses of diphtheria toxoid 20 years after primary vaccination. Acta Pathol Microbiol Immunol Scand [C] 1986; 94:219–25.

7. Blennow M, Granstrom M, Strandell A. Adverse reactions after diphtheria-tetanus booster in 10-year-old schoolchildren in relation to the type of vaccine given for the primary vaccination. Vaccine 1994;12:427–30.

8. Aggerbeck H, Wantzin J, Heron I. Booster vaccination against diphtheria and tetanus in man. Comparison of three different vaccine formulations—III. Vaccine 1996;14:1265-72.

9. McKinnon N, Ross M, Defries R. Reduction of diphtheria in 36,000 Toronto school children as a result of an immunization campaign. Canad J Publ Hlth 1931;22:217–23.

10. Munford R, Ory H, Brooks G, et al. Diphtheria deaths in the United States, 1959-1970. JAMA 1974;229:1890–3.

11. Griffith A. The role of immunization in the control of diphtheria. Develop Biol Standard 1979; 43:3-13.

12. Dixon J. Diphtheria in North America. J Hyg Camb 1984; 93:419–32.

13. Hardy I, Dittmann S, Sutter R. Current situation and control strategies for resurgence of diphtheria in newly independent states of the former Soviet Union. Lancet 1996; 347:1739–44.

14. Naiditch MJ, Bower AG. Diphtheria. A study of 1433 cases observed during a ten-year period at Los Angeles County Hospital. Am J Med 1954;17:229–45.

15. Mackko MB. Comparison of the morbidity of tetanus toxoid boosters with tetanus-diphtheria toxoid boosters. Ann Emerg Med 1985;14:33–5.

16. Sisk CW, Lewis CE. Reactions to tetanus-diphtheria toxoid (adult). Arch Environ Health 1965;11:34–6.

17. Edsall G, Elliott MW, Peebles TC, et al. Excessive use of tetanus toxoid boosters. JAMA 1967;202:17–9.

18. Smith RE, Wolnisty C. Allergic reactions to tetanus, diphtheria, influenza and poliomyelitis immunization. Ann Allergy 1962;20:809–13.

19. Jacobs RL, Lowe RS, Lanier BQ. Adverse reactions to tetanus toxoid. JAMA 1982;247:40–2.

20. Vaccine Safety Committee. Diphtheria and tetanus toxoids. Adverse events associated with childhood vaccines: evidence bearing on causality. In Stratton KR, Howe CJ, Johnston RB editors. Research strategies for assessing adverse effects associated with vaccines. Washington, DC: National Academy Press; 1994. p.67–117.

21. Long AP, Sartwell PE. Tetanus in the U.S. Army in World War II. Bull US Army Med Dept 1947;7:371–85.

22. Newell KW, Duenas Lehman A, LeBlanc DR, et al. The use of tetanus toxoid for the prevention of tetanus neonatorum. Final report of a double-blind controlled field trial. Bull World Hlth Org 1966;35:863–71.

23. Izurieta HS, Sutter RW, Strebel PM, et al. Tetanus surveillance–United States, 1995-1997. Morb Mortal Wkly Rep 1998;47 (SS2):1-13.

24. Laboratory Center for Disease Control. Canadian national report on immunization, 1997. Paediatr Child Health 1998;3 (Suppl B):20–1B.

25. Halperin S, Bortolussi R, MacLean D, et al. Persistence of pertussis in an immunized population: results of the Nova Scotia Enhanced Pertussis Surveillance Program. J Pediatr 1989; 115:686–93.

26. Fine P, Clarkson J. Distribution of immunity to pertussis in the population of England and Wales. J Hyg 1984; 92:21–6.

27. Edwards K. Pertussis in older children and adults. Adv Pediatr Infect Dis 1998;13:59–77.

28. Mills E, Gold R, Thipphawong J, et al. Safety and immunogenicity of a combined five–component pertussis-diphtheria-tetanus-inactivated poliomyelitis-Haemophilus b conjugate vaccine administered to infants at two, four and six months of age. Vaccine 1998;16:576–85.

29. Edwards D, Meade B, Decker M, et al. Comparison of 13 acellular pertussis vaccines: overview and serologic response. Pediatrics 1995; 96(Suppl):548–57.

30. Decker M, Edwards K, Steinhoff M, et al. Comparison of 13 acellular pertussis vaccines: adverse reactions. Pediatrics 1995; 96(Suppl):557–66.

31. McDermott C, Grimsrud K, Waters J. Acellular pertussis vaccine and whole-cell pertussis vaccine: a comparison of reported selected adverse events [abstract]. 3rd Canadian National Immunization Conference,Calgary AB, December 2-6, 1998. 1998.p.67–8.

32. Gold R, Scheifele D, Halperin S, et al. Hypotonic-hypo-responsive episodes in children hospitalized at 10 Canadian pediatric tertiary-care centers, 1991-1994. Can Comm Dis Rep 1997; 23:73–7.

33. Miller E. Collapse reactions after whole-cell pertussis vaccination. Pertussis remains a bigger risk than collapse after vaccination. Br Med J 1998; 316:876–80.

34. Vermeer-de Bondt PE, Labadie J, Rumke HC. Rate of recurrent collapse after vaccination with whole-cell pertussis vaccine: follow up study. Br Med J 1998; 316:902–3.

35. Cody CL, Baraff LJ, Cherry JD, et al. Nature and rates of adverse reactions associated with DTP and DT immunizations in infants and children. Pediatrics 1981;68:650–60.

36. Griffin M, Ray W, Mortimer E, et al. Risk of seizures and encephalopathy after immunization with diphtheria-tetanus-pertussis vaccine. JAMA 1990;263:1641–5.

37. Baraff L, Shields W, Beckwith L, et al. Infants and children with convulsions and hypotonic-hypo-responsive episodes following diphtheria-tetanus-pertussis immunization: follow-up evaluation. J Pediatr 1988;81:789–94.

38. Hirtz DG, Nelson KB, Ellenberg JH. Seizures following childhood immunizations. J Pediatr 1983;102:14–8.

39. Gustafsson L, Hallander H, Olin P, et al. A controlled trial of a two-component acellular, a five-component acellular, and a whole-cell pertussis vaccine. N Eng J Med 1996; 334:349–55.

40. Olin P, Rasmussen F, Gustafsson L, et al. Randomized controlled trial of two-component, three-component, and five-component acellular pertussis vaccines compared with whole-cell pertussis vaccine. Lancet 1997;350:1569–77.

41. Howson C, Fineberg H. The ricochet of magic bullets: summary of the Institute of Medicine report. Adverse effects of pertussis and rubella vaccines. Pediatrics 1992; 89:318–24.

42. National Advisory Committee on Immunization. Canadian Immunization Guide. Ottawa: Health and Welfare Canada, 4th ed; 1993.p.160.

43. Gangarosa E, Galazka A, Wolfe C, et al. Impact of anti-vaccine movements on pertussis control: the untold story. Lancet 1998; 351:356–61.

44. Cherry JD. The epidemiology of pertussis and pertussis immunization in the United Kingdom and the United States: a comparative study. Curr Probl Pediatr 1984;14:1–77.

45. Plotkin S, Cadoz M. The acellular pertussis vaccine trials: an interpretation. Pediatr Infect Dis J 1997;16:508–17.

46. Storsaeter J, Hallander H, Gustafsson L, et al. Levels of anti-pertussis antibodies related to protection after household exposure to *Bordetella pertussis*. Vaccine 1998;16:1907–16.

47. Cherry J, Gornbein J, Heininger H, et al. A search for serologic correlates of immunity to *Bordetella pertussis* cough illnesses. Vaccine 1998;16:1901–6.

48. Jenkinson D. Duration of effectiveness of pertussis vaccine: evidence from a 10-year community study. Br Med J 1988;296:612–4.

49. He Q, Viljanen M, Nikkari S, et al. Outcomes of *Bordetella pertussis* infection in different age groups of an immunized population. J Infect Dis 1994;170:873–7.

50. Robertson P, Goldberg H, Jarvie B, et al. *Bordetella pertussis* infection: a cause of persistent cough in adults. Med J Australia 1097;146:522–5.

51. Mink C, Cherry J, Christenson P, et al. A search for *B. pertussis* infection in university students. Clin Infect Dis 1992;14:464–71.

52. Mink C, Sirota N, Nugent S. Outbreak of pertussis in a fully immunized adolescent and adult population. Arch Pediatr Adolesc Med 1994;148:153–7.

53. Begue P, Stagnara J, Vie-Le-Sage F, et al. Immunogenicity and reactogenicity of a booster dose of diphtheria, tetanus, acellular pertussis and inactivated poliomyelitis vaccines given concurrently with Haemophilus type b conjugate vaccine or as pentavalent vaccine. Pediatr Infect Dis J 1997;16:787–94.

54. Tran Minh N, Edelman K, He Q, et al. Antibody and cell-mediated immune responses to booster immunization with a new acellular pertussis vaccine in school children. Vaccine 1998;16:1604–10.

55. Greco D, Salmaso S, Mastrantonio T, et al. A controlled trial of two acellular vaccines and one whole-cell vaccine against pertussis. N Eng J Med 1996;334:341–8.

56. Centers for Disease Control. Progress toward global eradication of poliomyelitis, 1997. MMWR 1998;47:414–9.

57. Centers for Disease Control. Progress toward poliomyelitis eradication— West Africa, 1997—September 1998. MMWR 1998;47:882–6.

58. Strickler H, Rosenberg PS, Devesa SS, et al. Contamination of polio virus vaccines with simian virus 40 (1955-1963) and subsequent cancer rates. JAMA 1998; 279:292-5.

59. Brown F, Lewis AM. Simian Virus 40 (SV40): a possible human polyomavirus. Dev Biol Stand 1998;94:247–69.

60. Terry L. The association of cases of poliomyelitis with the use of type 3 oral poliomyelitis vaccines. Washington, DC: US Department of Health, Education and Welfare; 1962.

61. Strebel P, Sutter R, Cochi S, et al. Epidemiology of poliomyelitis in the United States one decade after the last reported case of indigenous wild virus—associated disease. Clin Infect Dis 1992;14:568–79.

62. Sutter RW, Prevost DR. Vaccine-associated paralytic poliomyelitis among immunodeficient persons. Infect Med 1994;11:426, 429–30, 435–8.

63. Centers for Disease Control and Prevention. Poliomyelitis prevention in the United States. Introduction of a sequential schedule of inactivated polio virus vaccine followed by oral polio virus vaccine. Morb Mortal Wkly Rep 1997;46(RR3):1–25.

64. Francis TJ, Korns R, Voight R, et al. An evaluation of the 1954 poliomyelitis trials [summary report]. Am J Publ Hlth 1955; 45:vol 5, Part 2.

65. Faden H, Modlin J, Thomas M, et al. Comparative evaluation of immunization with live attenuated and enhanced potency inactivated trivalent polio virus vaccines in childhood: systemic and local immune responses. J Infect Dis 1990;162:1291–7.

66. Plotkin S. IPV for the United States. Pediatr Infect Dis J 1995;14:835–9.

67. Bôttiger M. Long-term immunity following vaccination with killed polio virus vaccine in Sweden, a country with no circulating polio virus. Rev Infect Dis 1984;6(suppl 2):S548–51.

68. Lapinleimu K. Elimination of poliomyelitis in Finland. Rev Infect Dis 1984;6(suppl 2):S457–60.

69. Hofman B. Poliomyelitis in the Netherlands before and after vaccination with inactivated poliovaccine. J Hyg 1967;65:547–57.

70. Malvy DJ, Drucker J. Elimination of poliomyelitis in France: epidemiology and vaccine status. Publ Hlth Rev 1993;21:99–106.

71. Varughese PV, Carter AO, Acres SE, et al. Eradication of indigenous poliomyelitis in Canada: impact of immunization strategies. Can J Publ Hlth 1989:80:363–8.

72. Oostvogel PM, van Wijngaarden JK, van der Avoort HG, et al. Poliomyelitis outbreak in an unvaccinated community in the Netherlands, 1992-93. Lancet 1994;344:665–70.

73. IMPACT. Recent trends in pediatric *Haemophilus influenzae* type b infections in Canada. Can Med Assoc J 1996; 154:1041–7.

74. Grewal S, Scheifele D. *Haemophilus influenzae* type b at 11 pediatric centers, 1996-1997. Can Commun Dis Rep 1998;24:105–8.

75. Gold R, Scheifele D, Barreto L, et al. Safety and immunogenicity of *Haemophilus influenzae* vaccine (tetanus toxoid conjugate) administered concurrently or combined with diphtheria and tetanus toxoids, pertussis vaccine, and inactivated poliomyelitis vaccine to healthy infants at two, four, and six months of age. Pediatr Infect Dis J 1994;13:348–55.

76. Peltola H, Aavitsland P, Hansen K, et al. Perspective: a five-country analysis of the impact of four different *Haemophilus influenzae* type b conjugates and vaccination strategies in Scandinavia. J Infect Dis 1999;179:223–9.

77. Fritzell B, Plotkin S. Efficacy and safety of a *Haemophilus influenzae* type b capsular polysaccharide–tetanus conjugate vaccine. J Pediatr 1992;121:355–62.

78. Takela AK, Eskola J, Leinonen M, et al. Reduction of oropharyngeal carriage of *Haemophilus influenzae* type b (Hib) in children immunized with a Hib conjugate vaccine. J Infect Dis 1991;164:982–6.

79. Murphy TV, Pastor P, Medley F, et al. Decreased *Haemophilus* colonization in children vaccinated with *Haemophilus influenzae* type b conjugate vaccine. J Pediatr 1993;122:517–23.

80. Galil K, Sungleton R, Levine O, et al. Reemergence of invasive *Haemophilus influenzae* type b disease in a well-vaccinated population in remote Alaska. J Infect Dis 1999; 179:101–6.

81. Laboratory Center for Disease Control. Update on the elimination of measles in Canada, 1998. Can Comm Dis Rep 1998;25:41–2.

82. Bloch AB, Orenstein WA, Ewing WM, et al. Measles outbreak in a pediatric practice: airborne transmission in an office setting. Pediatrics 1985;75:676–83.

83. Hope-Simpson RE. Infectiousness of communicable diseases in the household. Lancet 1952; 2:549–54.

84. Committee on Infectious Diseases. 1997 Red Book, 24th ed. Elk Grove Village, IL: American Academy of Pediatrics; 1997.p.347.

85. Hayden GE. Measles vaccine failure. A survey of causes and means of prevention. Clin Pediatr 1979;18:155–67.

86. Chen RT, Moses JM, Markowitz LE, et al. Adverse events following measles-mumps-rubella and measles vaccine in college students. Vaccine 1991;9:297–9.

87. Peltola H, Heinonen O. Frequency of true adverse reactions to measles-mumps-rubella vaccine. Lancet 1986;i:939–42.

88. Robbins FC. Measles: clinical features. Pathogenesis, pathology and complications. Am J Dis Child 1962;103:266–73.

89. Stratton KR, Howe CJ, Johnston RB Jr. Adverse events associated with childhood vaccines other than pertussis and rubella. Summary of a report from the Institute of Medicine. JAMA 1994; 271:1602–5.

90. Koskiniemi M, Vaheri A. Effect of measles, mumps, rubella vaccination of pattern of encephalitis in children. Lancet 1989;i:31–4.

91. Redd SC, Markowitz LE, Katz SL. Measles vaccine. In: Plotkin SA, Orenstein WA, editors. Vaccines 3rd ed. Philadelphia: WB Saunders; 1999.p.246–7.

92. National Advisory Committee on Immunization. Egg allergy and MMR vaccine: new recommendations from the National Advisory Committee on Immunization. Paediatr Child Health 1996;1:200–1.

93. Beck SA, Williams LW, Shirrell A, et al. Egg hypersensitivity and measles-mumps-rubella vaccine administration. Pediatrics 1991;88:913–7.

94. Laboratory Centre for Disease Control. Vaccine-preventable diseases [summary]. Update: Vaccine Preventable Disease 1998;6:45.

95. Markowitz L, Orenstein W. Measles vaccines. Pediatr Clin N Am 1990;37:603–25.

96. Krugman S, Giles JP, Jacobs AM, et al. Studies with a further attenuated live measles-virus vaccine. Pediatrics 1963;31:919–28.

97. Centers for Disease Control and Prevention. Measles—1996, and the interruption of indigenous transmission. Morb Mortal Wkly Rep 1997;46:242–6.

98. Gay N, Ramsay M, Cohen B, et al. The epidemiology of measles in England and Wales since the 1994 vaccination campaign. Commun Dis Rep CDR Rev 1997;7:R17–21.

99. de Quadros CA, Olivé JM, Hersh BS, et al. Measles elimination in the Americas: evolving strategies. JAMA 1996;275:224–9.

100. Peltola H, Heinonen O, Valle M, et al. The elimination of indigenous measles, mumps, and rubella from Finland by a 12 year two-dose vaccination program. N Eng J Med 1994; 331:1397–402.

101. Cheek J, Baron R, Atlas H, et al. Mumps outbreak in a highly vaccinated school population. Arch Pediatr Adolesc Med 1995; 149:774–8.

102. Plotkin SA. Rubella vaccine. In: Plotkin SA, Orenstein WA, editors. Vaccines 3rd ed. Philadelphia; WB Saunders; 1999.p.409–40.

103. Centers for Disease Control. Rubella vaccination during pregnancy. MMWR 1987;36:457–61.

104. Howson C, Fineberg HV. Adverse events following pertussis and rubella vaccines. Summary of a report of the Institute of Medicine. JAMA 1992;267:392–6.

105. Tingle A, Mitchell L, Grace M, et al. Randomized double-blind placebo-controlled study of adverse effects of rubella immunization in seronegative women. Lancet 1997;349:1277–81.

106. Preblud SR, Serdula MK, Frank JA, et al. Rubella vaccination in the United States: A 10-year review. Epidemiol Rev 1980;2:171–94.

107. Centers for Disease Control and Prevention. Rubella and congenital rubella syndrome, United States, 1994-1997. Morb Mortal Wkly Rep 1997;46:350–4.

108. Kane M. Epidemiology of hepatitis B infection in North America. Vaccine 1995; 13(Suppl 1): S16–7.

109. Working Group on Hepatitis B. Report of the Hepatitis B Working Group. Can Dis Wkly Rep 1994;20:105–12.

110. Dobson S, Scheifele D, Bell A. Assessment of a universal, school-based hepatitis B vaccination program. JAMA 1995; 274:1209–13.

111. Stevens C, Taylor P, Rubenstein P, et al. Safety of hepatitis B vaccine. N Eng J Med 1985; 312:375–6.

112. Report of the working group on the possible relationship between hepatitis B vaccination and the chronic fatigue syndrome. Can Med Assoc J 1993;149(3):314–9.

113. Marshall E. A shadow falls on hepatitis B vaccination effort. Science 1998;281:630–1.

114. Alter M, Hadler S, Margolis H, et al. The changing epidemiology of hepatitis B in the United States: need for alternative vaccination strategies. JAMA 1990;263:1218–22.

115. National Advisory Committee on Immunization. Statement on universal immunization against hepatitis B. Can Dis Wkly Rep 1991;17:165–71.

116. Bloom B, Hellman A, Fendrick A, et al. A reappraisal of hepatitis B virus vaccination strategies using cost-effectiveness analysis. Ann Intern Med 1993;118:298–306.

117. Edmunds W, Medley G, Nikes D. Cost-effectiveness of hepatitis B virus immunization. JAMA 1982;97:362–6.

118. Bell A. Universal hepatitis B immunization: the British Columbia experience. Vaccine 1995; 13(Suppl 1):S77–81.

119. Lee C-L, Ko Y-C. Hepatitis B vaccination and hepatocellular carcinoma in Taiwan. Pediatrics 1997;99:351–3.

120. Szmuness W, Stevens CE, Harley EJ, et al. Hepatitis B vaccine: demonstration of efficacy in a controlled trial in a high risk population in the U.S. N Eng J Med 1980;303:833–41.

121. Francis DP, Hadler SC, Thompson SE, et al. Prevention of hepatitis B with vaccine. Report of the Centers for Disease Control multi-center efficacy trial among homosexual men. Ann Int Med 1982;97:362–6.

122. Beasley RP, Hwang LY, Lee GC, et al. Prevention of perinatally transmitted hepatitis B virus with hepatitis B immune globulin and hepatitis B vaccine. Lancet 1983;2:1099–102.

123. Mahoney F, Woodruff B, Erben J, et al. Evaluation of a hepatitis B immunization program on the prevalence of hepatitis B virus infection. J Infect Dis 1993;167:203–7.

124. Lieu T, Black S, Rieser N, et al. The cost of childhood chickenpox: parents' perspective. Pediatr Infect Dis J 1993;13:173–7.

125. Huse D, Meissner H, Lacey M, et al. Childhood vaccination against chickenpox: an analysis of benefits and costs. J Pediatr 1994; 124:869–74.

126. Gershon AA, LaRussa PS. Varicella vaccine. Pediatr Infect Dis J 1998;17:248–9.

127. Asana Y, Suga S, Yoshikawa T, et al. Twenty-year follow-up of protective immunity of the Oka strain live varicella vaccine. Pediatrics 1994;94:524–6.

128. Johnson C, Stancin T, Fattlar D, et al. A long-term prospective study of varicella vaccine in healthy children. Pediatrics 1997;100:761–6.

CHAPTER 4

Nutrition Problems in Childhood

R.I. Hilliard, MD, EdD, FRCPC

Although the nutritional status of children has generally improved through this century, nutritional problems still occur in the western world and even more in the developing world. There are still children who are undernourished or malnourished as well as children who are obese. Much of our management of children with nutritional problems is based on experience, assumptions, or presuppositions and not always on good clinical trials.

This chapter will review the common pediatric nutritional problems including children who are failing to thrive, specific nutritional deficiencies (particularly iron and vitamin D deficiencies), and vegetarianism.

FAILURE TO THRIVE

Failure to thrive (FTT) has been well presented in many texts and review articles.[1-8] The condition has been defined as when a child, usually an infant less than 3 years of age, fails to gain weight according to accepted standards, and there is no obvious medical cause for this. As such, FTT is a clinical feature, like anemia, but not a specific diagnosis.[9] The causes of FTT are frequently divided into organic and nonorganic, although this may be misleading as, frequently, there are both organic and psychosocial causes for the condition. However, to many health professionals working with child abuse and neglect, FTT is often linked with child neglect, but such is not always the case. To some parents, FTT means failure to be a good parent, and that is also not always the case.

There are many reasons why some children are smaller than others, and being small is not exactly the same as failing to thrive (Table 4–1).

Some children are small but healthy. They may be small because their parents are of a small build, others because they are from an ethnic group where all children tend to be smaller than North American or European children. Some children may have constitutional growth delay. This is more frequently an explanation for children who are short in mid-childhood or before puberty. These children have always been short and have a delayed bone age, within the normal variation, a delayed puberty and growth spurt, but a normal eventual adult size. Although this diagnosis is applied to children who are short, the growth delay may be seen at an earlier age, and some children as young as 2 years of age may fit this description.

Table 4–1 The Small Child

Healthy Children	Medical Illness (Pathology)	Non-organic FTT	Mixed
• Familial • Ethnic • Constitutional growth delay	• Primordial syndromes • Endocrine disorder: rare • Chronic illness • Lack of caloric intake	• Interaction between child and parent – *accidental* – *neglectful* – *deliberate*	• Medical illness • Psychosocial factors

Some children are small because they have a chronic medical illness. Some children have an inherent genetic disease, such as a chromosomal abnormality, or intrauterine growth retardation associated with maternal illness, infections, or drugs. The term primordial is used rather than genetic so as to not confuse the diagnosis with children born of small parents. Most children with a serious chronic illness will also be small. Children with hypopituitarism, hypothyroidism, or excess glucocorticoids will be small, but these endocrine causes of FTT are rare.

Finally, children may be small because of nonorganic or psychosocial factors.[10–12] There may be factors in the child, in the parents, or in the interaction between parent and child such that the child is not given enough food to eat or does not eat well enough to grow normally.[13–16] These occurrences are often accidental or due to neglect on the part of the parents and, fortunately, only rarely deliberate. Sometimes, there are risk factors in the parents: young inexperienced parents, poverty, psychiatric illness such as depression, alcohol/drug abuse, or unemployment. Sometimes, the children are described as picky eaters, who have to be forced to eat.

The reasons for the small size can sometimes be determined by the weight, the height, or both. Children who are genetically small or have a primordial syndrome will usually be both short and underweight, with the weight being proportional to their height. In children with a chronic illness or nonorganic FTT, the weight is usually more affected than the height. In children with an endocrine disorder, there is usually more effect on their height than their weight. As an exception to these generalizations, children who have a chronic renal disease and are often treated with corticosteroids are usually short rather than underweight.

Failure to thrive can also be considered when children do not reach their maximum growth potential. Considered this way, the causes of FTT include (1) inadequate intake of food and calories; (2) vomiting of what the child takes in; (3) inadequate digestion, absorption, and assimilation; (4) failure to use the nutrition and calories; (5) overuse of calories in association with a chronic infection, inflammation, or malignancy; and (6) loss of nutrition and calories through chronic diarrhea or renal losses of sugar or protein. The most common reason for a child not to gain weight appropriately is inadequate intake of food and calories. Here also, there are different reasons: (1) children who do not eat enough because there is not enough food available or they are not offered enough food; (2) children who cannot eat because of neuromotor abnormalities such as cerebral palsy; (3) children who are anorexic and are not interested in eating because they suffer from a chronic illness or depression; or (4) children who are able to eat but will not eat because of a behavioral problem. Therefore, even though the most common reason for a child not to gain weight appropriately is inadequate intake of food and calories, it takes a careful history, physical examination and observation of a child's eating to sort out the exact cause for the poor intake.

Most reference textbooks list the situations where physicians and families are concerned about the child's poor growth. This is usually based on the appropriate use of growth charts. In using growth charts, it is important to record as many different measurements as possible and, when necessary, to correct for any premature births. Generally, a child is considered to be failing to thrive if (1) the weight is much less than the third percentile; (2) the growth velocity is less than the third percentile, that is, as the child grows, the weight crosses 2 major percentile lines; (3) the weight is less than 80% of the expected weight for that age and height or ideal body weight; or (4) the weight is less than the fifth percentile on a weight-for-height chart. There are two caveats to these generalizations. First, in the first 6 months, infants' weights change from the birth weight, which is determined more by maternal health and intrauterine factors, to the percentile according to the child's genetic background. Children may progress up or down on a growth chart as they approach their genetic potential. Secondly, most growth charts are based on the United States or United Kingdom growth studies, and these charts may not hold true for children from other parts of the world.

Interestingly, there are growth charts for children with specific conditions such as Down syndrome or Turner's syndrome but few charts for children from Asia or Africa.

Laboratory Investigations

Most texts and references provide a long list of laboratory tests that should be done for children who are failing to thrive. These are often based on practice and anecdotal experience but with few clinical studies to suggest what laboratory tests are needed. More recently, it is recognized that the diagnostic yield of unfocused investigations is negligible.[17] A careful, complete, and problem-focused history and physical examination can usually diagnose the reason for a child's poor weight gain.[18] In a retrospective investigation of 185 patients hospitalized for FTT, only 1.4 percent of laboratory studies were of diagnostic assistance, and even then, the diagnosis already had been strongly indicated by findings on history and physical examination. In most cases, the diagnosis can be made following a thorough history complete with an assessment of the psychosocial features of the family, a full physical examination, and observation of the child's eating.[19,20] Some simple laboratory tests might be indicated. When children do not take in enough calories to gain weight normally, there may also be a poor intake of specific nutrients, such as iron. Much can be learned by watching what and how parents feed their child. It is also helpful to have a parent make a 3-day record of everything a child eats. A dietician can then calculate whether this is adequate in calories, proteins, and the essential vitamins and minerals.

Management

The management of a child who is failing to thrive will depend on the severity and cause of the child's FTT. In the case of healthy children, it is most important to reassure the family that their child is well. For most cases of organic FTT, the diagnosis is made through a complete and problem-oriented history and physical examination, but appropriate laboratory tests should be ordered to confirm the suspected cause for the child's FTT.

The management of children who are truly underweight usually involves encouraging higher-calorie meals, more appropriate foods, and more structure to meal times.[21] Many families that are concerned about their child not eating will spend a lot of time to coax, cajole, or even force their child to eat. Some severely malnourished infants are anorectic and will not acquire an appetite until partial nutritional recovery occurs. It is usually recommended that children be given 150 percent of the average daily caloric requirement for the ideal weight. Physicians may provide nutritional advice on their own, but it is frequently more effective if the physician works with a team, which might include a nurse, dietician, social worker, psychiatrist, and community health worker. Most programs have booklets containing advice to parents. Table 4–2 provides a sample text of such booklets.[22]

Despite appropriate medical and dietary management and psychosocial support, many children with nonorganic FTT continue to be small, have cognitive and school-related problems, or other behavioral problems.[23–33]

What evidence is there that this overall approach to investigating and managing children with FTT is the best? Most studies in the literature are descriptive studies and may be strongly influenced by bias in selecting their study population.

Hospital or Ambulatory Management

There are very few randomized controlled trials (RCTs) in managing children with FTT because of the difficulties of setting up such trials. Most of the studies of children who are failing to thrive are descriptive and are influenced by bias and the inclusion/exclusion criteria of the population being studied. Traditionally, authors have defined FTT as organic if a specific organic disease is diagnosed or as nonorganic if the cause is thought to be environmental or due to relationship issues with parents or caregivers. These, however, are all influ-

Table 4–2 Helping Your Child to Gain Weight

Calories

In most cases, children do not gain weight because they just do not take in enough food, enough good nutritious calories. You cannot force children to eat more, but you can make sure to offer food high in calories.

No medication has been found to stimulate children's appetite with the resulting weight gain on a long-term basis.
- Children should develop a routine of three meals and three snacks per day.
- Children should be offered high-caloric foods. Fats are generally higher in calories than carbohydrates or proteins; therefore, add cream, butter, margarine, or oil to their foods.
- For infants on formula feedings, the formula can be concentrated by adding less water;
- Restrict juices, which have very few calories, especially diluted juice.
- Use meats or alternatives such as cheese or soy products.
- Use supplemental foods, such as Caloreen®, Pediasure®, Boost®, Polycose®.
- Give vitamins/iron supplements.

Feeding Routines

Children need to develop a routine for feedings and meal times. Children do not like to sit still, but they should be encouraged to sit in a high chair or at the table for meal times.
- Maintain a routine of three meals/three snacks a day with family.
- Watch for signs that the child is full.
- Never force or bribe a child to eat.
- Offer only small amounts of food and fluids at a time.
- Serve meals with a variety of tastes, colors, and textures.
- Make meal times enjoyable.
- Do not hurry along meals.
- Ignore food throwing at first.
- Do not hover expectantly while a child eats.
- Encourage independence.
- Let toddlers pick food from the serving plate.

Food Refusal

Occasionally, children refuse to take any food, turning their face away, refusing to open their mouths when food is offered, or spitting out any food given to them. *You just cannot force children to eat more, but you can make sure you offer foods high in calories.*
- The meals should be well prepared, appetizing, and have the kind of food the child likes.
- Meal times should be fun times for the whole family.
- Children should sit down to a meal in a high chair or a chair at the table.
- Children should be offered three meals and three snacks a day, and not offered food at other times.
- If a child doesn't eat in a given time, for example, 20 or 30 minutes, then the food should be put away.
- If a child refuses to open the mouth, then put the food down and turn away and do not give any attention.
- Extra milk or a snack can be taken along for children when on a trip or shopping, but stop for a proper rest.

Parental Support
- Help parents understand their feelings about their child.
- Help parents cope with some of the behaviors of their child that they find difficult.
- Direct parents to agencies, support groups, and community resources, which may be helpful for the family.
- Help with specific psychiatric problems in the family, such as depression.
- Occasionally, refer to a child protection agency, if needed.

enced by the particular patients who are being studied, such as the referral bias of a particular clinic. Schmitt, for example, reviewed patients in an outpatient setting and reported that 70 percent of the cases were nonorganic FTT, and of these, 50 percent were neglectful, 19 percent accidental, <1 percent poverty related, and < 1 percent deliberate starvation.[34]

Many authors would recommend a period of observation and hospital admission prior to embarking on a protocol of investigations. It has been suggested that a child with nonorganic FTT will gain weight well in hospital; thus, if the child gains weight in hospital, this is almost diagnostic of nonorganic FTT.[35,36] Goldbloom stated that few of these children can be managed successfully and with quick effect at home, and hospital admission can offer several advantages.[2] In these times of decreasing numbers of hospital beds and shorter lengths of stay, what is the evidence that hospitalization will aid in the diagnosis of nonorganic FTT?

The opposite is, in fact, the case. Berwick reviewed the records of 122 infants between the ages of 1 and 25 months who were hospitalized for FTT without a diagnosis.[20] By the end of the hospital stay, one-third of the patients still did not have a diagnosis. Each patient had received an average of 40 laboratory tests and radiographic examinations, but only 0.8 percent of all tests showed an abnormality that contributed to a diagnosis. Further, children who have FTT of either organic or nonorganic etiology could gain or lose weight during hospitalization. In the case of children with an organic illness, more attention is paid to their illness and their food intake, so it is not surprising that they also may gain weight in hospital. At the same time, in the case of children with nonorganic FTT, if the problem is the parent-child interaction and the parents' inability to read the cues from their child, admitting a child to hospital just transfers some of the problems from the home to a hospital room. Bithoney also demonstrated that children with both organic and nonorganic FTT can gain weight when treated by a specialized multidisciplinary team consisting of a pediatrician, child psychiatrist, social worker, nutritionist, and nurse clinician.[37]

Multidisciplinary Team Approach

Most papers on the management of FTT are descriptive or uncontrolled studies. For example, Peterson and colleagues described a team approach to managing FTT.[38] The authors described an FTT team at the Children's Hospital Medical Center in Boston that included a developmental pediatrician, a pediatrician with expertise in gastroenterology/clinical nutrition, a pediatric nurse practitioner, a dietician, a psychiatrist or psychologist, a social worker, and a physical therapist. They felt their team was effective, but this is a descriptive rather than a comparative or controlled study.

Similarly, Bithoney reported on children referred to and managed in a growth-and-nutrition clinic.[37] The study population included 64 (74 percent) of children with nonorganic FTT and 22 (26 percent) with an organic cause. They did more tests than are usually recommended for children with FTT, probably as this was a research project: hemoglobin, urinalysis, urine culture, stool for pH, reducing substances and occult blood, serum lead levels, sweat test, electrolytes, blood urea, and other tests as deemed appropriate. The nonorganic (NFTT) and the organic (OFTT) groups were comparable for age, race, and degree of malnutrition, although those in the OFTT group tended to belong to poorer sections of population (not statistically significant). The patients were managed with advice from their multidisciplinary team, with concrete individualized therapies including psychosocial support, medical care, and hypercaloric diets. Children in both groups grew extremely well. The growth quotients for both groups were comparable: OFTT 1.81 ± 0.37, NFTT 1.67 ± 0.56. They concluded that the multidisciplinary team consisting of a pediatrician, child psychiatrist, nutritionist, nurse clinician, and social worker may be successful in managing children with FTT (both OFTT and NFTT).

Bithoney and colleagues reported on the effectiveness of a multidisciplinary team approach on weight gain in children with nonorganic FTT.[39] This was a study of 160 children who were felt to have FTT because either the weight or height was less than the fifth percentile or the growth velocity was less than the fifth percentile. The children did not have a specific medical or organic illness to explain the FTT. The major outcome was the growth quotient, a comparison of the rate of growth of the child during the study period compared with the normal rate of growth during that time at the child's age. They compared children who were seen in the multidisciplinary growth-nutrition clinic with children who were seen in more traditional primary-care clinic staffed by pediatricians and pediatric residents. They followed up the children over a 6-month period and felt that there was a significant difference in the growth quotients (GQ) of the children in the two clinics: growth-nutrition clinic mean GQ 1.75 ± 0.39; primary-care clinic GQ 1.18 ± 0.42. A GQ of 1.0 would mean that the child continued to grow parallel to the growth chart, with no improvement in the FTT. This was not an RCT, but the authors did not feel there were any demographic differences in the patients of the two clinics that would explain the differences. They concluded that the use of a multidisciplinary team offers special advantages in the rapid correction of undernutrition in children with non-organic FTT.

Home Interventions

Many centers dealing with children who are failing to thrive have tried to incorporate a home intervention, making use of community or public health nurses, or lay home visitors. There is the opinion that a professional or trained lay person visiting in the home would be better able to see the problems with feedings and meal times in the home than a doctor or nurse interviewing the parents in the office or clinic. Also, the home visitor who visits the family regularly would be better able to advise a family about good nutrition and good feeding practices.

Black and colleagues reported on an RCT that studied the efficacy of a home-based intervention on the growth and development of children with nonorganic FTT.[40] Many management regimes recommend liaison with community health-care workers or trained lay home visitors. All the children in this study received services in a multidisciplinary growth-and nutrition-clinic. This study included 130 children in a pediatric primary-care clinic who were less than 25 months of age and whose weight was less than the fifth percentile. There was no history suggesting a chronic illness. Most parents were single African-American mothers on public assistance. Some children were randomly allocated to a home intervention group or to a control group that received only the clinic visits. Under the supervision of a community health nurse, a trained home visitor made weekly visits for a year. Children in both groups showed significant improvements in weight-for-age and weight-for-height. Children in the home-intervention group demonstrated better receptive language over time and more child-oriented home environments. Children in both groups showed improved cognitive development, with more improvement in the younger children. There were no long-term assessments of the children after the home intervention had been discontinued. Their findings support a cautious optimism regarding home intervention provided by trained lay home visitors during the first year of life. Early home intervention can promote a nurturant home environment effectively and can reduce the developmental delays often experienced by infants with NOFTT in low-income, urban families. The researchers reviewed these same children at age 4 years, or 1 year after the home intervention ended. There were persistent positive effects on the children in the home-intervention group, on motor development among all children, and on cognitive development and behavior during play among children of mothers who reported low levels of negative activity. The study would support the use of home intervention for cognitive and behavioral development, but not necessarily for physical growth.[41]

Wright and colleagues in Newcastle upon Tyne, England, reported on an RCT of a home health visitor in addition to the standard care provided by a pediatrician, dietician, and social worker in a primary-care practice.[42] Twenty of the 38 primary-care teams were randomly allocated to take part in the intervention, while the remaining 18 primary-care teams constituted controls. There were no significant differences between the children in the intervention group and the control group. In the families who consented to home visits, children in the intervention group were significantly heavier and taller and were reported to have better appetites than children in the control group, although both groups were equally satisfied with the services they had received. When the children were weighed at follow-up, 76 percent in the intervention group had recovered from their FTT compared with 55 percent in the control group. They concluded that in FTT, health visitor intervention, with limited specialist support, can significantly improve growth compared with conventional management.

Perhaps more important than treating children with FTT are efforts through physicians or community health programs to try and prevent FTT. Casey reported on a randomized trial using home visits to decrease the incidence of FTT in a group of preterm infants with low birth weight, who were at risk for poor weight gain.[43] In a multicenter trial, they studied 914 preterm infants with low birth weights, who were born at eight different university centers. This was a prospective RCT with 330 children in an Infant Health and Development Program (IHDP) and 512 controls. In the program, families had visits by a trained lay home visitor weekly during the first year and then biweekly visits for years 2 and 3. The families also attended a child development center 5 days a week with their children from age 1 year up until they were 3 years of age. In the study, the outcome measurements included height, weight, body mass index (BMI), general health ratings, child behavior checklist, and a measure (Stanford-Binet) of intellectual ability. The incidence of FTT did not differ in the treatment group (20 percent) and the control group (22 percent). There were no significant differences in the mean IQ of children with or without FTT in the treatment group compared with the control group. However, after controlling for other factors, treatment group membership and compliance with IHDP significantly contributed to the 36 mos. IQ. In this randomized prospective trial, the intervention of home visits did not change the incidence of FTT or the 3-year outcomes, but after controlling for multiple independent variables, marked effects on 3-year IQ were noted. These beneficial effects were most pronounced in families who were most compliant with the intervention. A summary of the evidence for the interventions for FTT is provided in Table 4–3.

OBESITY

Overnutrition or obesity is a common problem in children but also a problem which most physicians feel inadequate to manage; this is because childhood obesity is difficult to treat, and most view obesity as a social problem, blaming parents and families for their inability to control their child's eating. In research on childhood obesity, most definitions of obesity are based on BMI (weight in kg/height in m²) and the triceps skinfold thickness. However, most physicians in practice dealing with children do not have calipers to measure skinfolds,

Table 4–3 Levels of Evidence and Recommendations for Interventions for Failure to Thrive

Condition	Intervention	Level of Evidence	Recommendation
Failure to thrive	• Laboratory / diagnostic protocols	III	C
	• Hospitalization	III	C
	• Multidisciplinary team approach	II-1	B
	• Home visitors	I	B

and few have experience with BMIs for children. Thus, for defining obesity, most practitioners use a weight >120 percent of the expected weight for age and height; by body appearance, this is due to excess fat rather than large frames and muscle mass.[44] Obesity is seen in 7[45] to 43 percent[46] of children in Canada. In the United States, it has been estimated that 10 to 25 percent of children are obese.[47-49] The incidence of pediatric obesity is increasing despite national efforts to promote weight reduction.[50] Obesity occurs when a child's intake of calories is greater than the calories required for the basal metabolic rate, for growth, and for energy for the child's activities. In most cases, children overeat and take in more calories than they need, but obesity can also occur in inactive or sedentary children, especially children with neuromuscular disease that limits their physical activity. Childhood obesity has both genetic and environmental components. It appears to be associated with parental obesity, lower socioeconomic class, family patterns of activity and inactivity, and television viewing, the last probably related to both inactivity and increased consumption of food.[51] Studies with adoptees, siblings, cousins, and dizygotic and monozygotic twins suggest that genetics also plays a part in the development of obesity.[52] It is generally believed that obesity is probably due to an interaction of both genetics and environment.[53,54]

Obesity is rarely seen—that is, in fewer than 5 percent of obese children—due to syndromes that affect growth and metabolism, specifically Prader-Willi syndrome (hypotonia, hypogonadism, developmental disability), Alström-Hallgren syndrome, Carpenter's syndrome, hypothyroidism, hypopituitary syndrome, Laurence-Moon-Biedl sydrome, Cushing's syndrome (hypercortisolism), hyperinsulinism (Beckwith-Weidemann syndrome), pseudohypoparathyroidism, and rarely disorders involving the appetite center of the hypothalamus because of infection, trauma, or neoplasms.[52] This chapter can not deal with all these rare endocrine disorders which are more completely dealt with in other references.[44] In general these disorders are associated with short stature, a delayed bone age that reflects impaired skeletal maturation or other dysmorphic features. Primary obesity generally is associated with increased height, advanced bone age and early pubertal development.

Tests for Diagnosing a Child with Obesity

Although there are rare specific endocrinal causes for obesity, a protocol of diagnostic tests is rarely indicated. Most of the above rare causes of obesity are usually associated with short stature. If the obese child is appropriate for height or taller, the physician can be almost certain that tests are not indicated. If the child is short or has developmental or cognitive delay, a history of hypotonia or feeding problems in early infancy, or undescended testes or small external genitalia, the genetic tests for Prader-Willi syndrome should be ordered to detect the deletion of the long arm of chromosome 15. If the child has other congenital anomalies or dysmorphic features, a genetics consultation may be requested. If the child has headaches associated with nausea or vomiting, a computed tomographic (CT) or magnetic resonance imaging (MRI) scan to assess the hypothalamus or pituitary fossa may be indicated. But, in general, despite parents' beliefs that their child does not eat excessively, if the child is healthy with an appropriate height, tests are not indicated.

Parents often report that the overweight child eats less but gains weight more easily than other children and expect that the metabolic rate must therefore be altered. There is no evidence that obese children are more energy efficient; rather, they probably eat more than is reported and probably are less active.[44] If there is any doubt, a calorimetry measurement of resting basal metabolic rate may be ordered.

Effective Management of Obesity in Children

At present, there is insufficient knowledge to effectively prevent or treat most cases of obesity in children. The main methods of treating childhood obesity are modification of diet, exercise, and child-oriented or family-based behavior modification programs.[55-57] There are major problems with most studies of treatment approaches; they have tended to use very small samples, many have used no control groups, or an inappropriate one, and the follow-up time has rarely been sufficient to evaluate the long-term success of the treatment.

Most physicians will encourage the obese child, with the family's support, to eat less and especially less high-fat foods that are high in calories. It is often helpful for the child and parents to make a record of *everything* the child eats, keeping in mind that children, especially obese children, often under-report what they eat. Parents, and the children themselves, are often surprised at how much the children actually eat. The physician may offer simple advice such as no second helpings, smaller portions at meal times, no or low calorie snacks, and no snacks after supper. The child should be encouraged to eat foods that are low in fats and simple sugars, such as skim or 1 percent milk instead of homo milk, baked or boiled potatoes instead of fried potatoes, fruit, celery, or carrots sticks as snacks instead of cookies, cakes, or ice cream. The fat intake of children and adolescents in North America accounts for more than 35 percent of daily caloric intake, and fat in the diet is more easily converted into fat in its storage form as compared with carbohydrates.[44] Highly restricted diets, drugs, and surgical procedures should be limited to the rare pediatric patient who has a morbid complication of obesity for which rapid weight reduction is essential.

The obese child should be encouraged to participate in regular physical activity suited to the child's interests and level of physical fitness and stamina, such as walking, bicycling, swimming, or more active sports such as soccer, hockey, jogging, gymnastics, or dance.[58] However, physical activity alone, without alterations in the diet, has not been shown to lead to weight reduction in children. Many physicians will also encourage less television time to increase physical activity and diminish exposure to the effect of television to promote eating.

In the case of infants who are fed by their parents, the parents must be motivated to reduce the infant's caloric intake. But, as children grow older, they must themselves want to lose excess weight or even to maintain their weight as they grow taller, and they must be supported in this by their parents.

Although physicians may offer good advice, the success rate in treating obesity in children is particularly poor unless the child is highly motivated and supported by the parents.[59] Obese adults lose a relatively small amount of their excess weight in most treatment programs and do not maintain these weight losses.[60] Long-term studies of weight-reduced children have shown that similarly 80 to 90 percent of children return to their previous weight percentiles.[61,62] Weight loss and weight control interventions in children and adolescents have been disappointing. Therapy for unselected patients is not only of limited value but is not likely to be cost effective.[63] Dramatic short-term weight loss has been demonstrated, although maintenance after weight loss is generally poor. Family-based interventions using a combination of behavioral techniques, long-term dietary modification, and changes in lifestyle activities produced decreases in percent overweight up to about 25 percent at 1 year, 14 percent at 5 years, and 7 percent at 10-year follow-up in select samples of obese 5- to 12-year-olds. Additionally, involving parents in the treatment process, particularly simultaneous treatment of an obese parent, has produced better results than interventions focusing on the child alone.

The more drastic methods of fat reduction, such as surgery, pharmacotherapy, and the use of gastric balloons, are not appropriate for children, and very low caloric diets may impair their growth.[64]

Evidence for Obesity in Childhood Resulting in Obesity in Adulthood, with Atherosclerosis, Hypertension, and Diabetes Mellitus

There are certain stages in children when obesity is more common: infancy and the pre-adolescent period. There are conflicting reports of the correlation between obesity in infants and children and adult obesity, but in general, the probability of an obese child becoming an obese adult decreases with increasing time intervals but increases with greater degree of childhood obesity, higher age of the obese child, and greater numbers of obese family members.[65-67] In most samples, only 25 to 50 percent of obese children and adolescents become obese adults, with the more severely obese and the preadolescent being at higher risk for being obese as adults.[44]

Is the obese child at risk of becoming an obese adult with hypertension, coronary artery disease, and diabetes mellitus? Reports suggest that, relative to thinner children, obese children have elevated blood pressures, and elevated total cholesterol, high levels of low-density lipoprotein (LDL) cholesterol, and decreased levels of high-density lipoprotein (HDL) cholesterol.[68-70]

Longitudinal studies that relate childhood obesity to adult morbidity and mortality are rare. In a 33 to 40-year follow-up of persons from Hagerstown, Maryland, the mean levels of adult fasting blood sugar, systolic and diastolic pressures, and adult prevalence of diabetes mellitus and cardiovascular disease were greatest in the highest childhood weight category, at age 9 to 13 years, although the differences were not statistically significant.[44] Relative weight status in childhood was not significantly associated with adult serum total cholesterol or beta-lipoprotein levels. In a 40-year follow-up of obese Swedish children, overall mortality, cardiovascular disease, and digestive diseases occurred significantly earlier than in the nonobese Swedish reference population.[71]

The lack of good studies indicating the effectiveness of treating childhood obesity led the Canadian Task Force on the Periodic Health Examination to conclude that there is insufficient evidence for short-term or long-term benefits from screening for or treatment of childhood obesity to recommend for or against such screening.[64]

There is insufficient evidence to include the measurement of height and weight in the periodic health examination of children or to exclude it. Physicians should continue to measure height and weight, recognizing that diagnosing childhood obesity may have little effect on adult obesity.[72-75] Diagnosing obesity may, in fact, lead to anxiety or poor self-esteem in children, and dietary restrictions may have adverse effects.[76]

There is insufficient evidence to include, or to exclude, family-based nutrition and exercise education and behavior modification in the treatment of childhood obesity.[77-82] Weight loss is maintained in only a few children, and the high cost of these programs, lack of availability, and the high motivation of the families involved in the study may limit generalization of the results. These programs are not readily applicable to primary-care pediatrics.

There is insufficient evidence to include, or to exclude, exercise programs in the routine treatment of obese children.[83-86]

There is fair evidence to recommend against very-low-caloric diets for preadolescents.[85,87] There is insufficient evidence to recommend for or against exercise programs or intensive family-based programs for most obese children.

This review would suggest that better controlled studies in the prevention and treatment of obesity with longer follow-up are needed. In the meantime, practicing physicians will continue to do what they have been trained to do, that is, monitor a child's height and weight on a growth chart, observe for risk factors for obesity, and offer advice and suggestions to families and children on an individual basis. We recognize that our widely held beliefs about the need to recognize and prevent obesity in children lack the evidence to support or to reject our present practices. A summary of interventions for childhood obesity is given in Table 4–4.

SPECIFIC NUTRITIONAL DEFICIENCIES: VITAMIN D

Vitamin D or cholecalciferol is a steroid compound found in animals and is important for calcium homeostasis, the absorption of calcium from the gastrointestinal tract, bone for-

Table 4–4 A Summary of Interventions for Childhood Obesity

Condition	Intervention	Level of Evidence	Recommendation
Obesity in Children	• Routine laboratory/diagnostic tests	III	D
	• Screening for obesity	II - 2	C
	• Dietary/physical activity management	I / II-2	C
	• Predictors for illness / complications in adults	III	C

mation, the deposition of calcium into bone, and the prevention of rickets. Vitamin D is also produced by the action of ultraviolet light on the cells in the dermis. The liver converts cholecalciferol to 25-hydroxycholecalciferol and this is further converted by the kidney to 1,25-diOH-D$_3$. There is some vitamin D$_2$ (ergocalciferol) found in vegetable sources. Vitamin D is fat soluble, and a deficiency of vitamin D may occur with a fat malabsorption syndrome. With a deficiency of vitamin D, rickets develops resulting in hypocalcemia and poor bone formation and growth. Because of the past experience with rickets, vitamin D is added to most milk in North America, and the prevalence of rickets has dramatically decreased.

Because human breast milk is low in vitamin D, the American Academy of Pediatrics (APP) and the Canadian Pediatric Society (CPS) have recommended that breast-fed infants receive vitamin D supplements, 400 IU/day until the diet provides a sufficient source of vitamin D.[88,89] This is double the estimated requirement for full-term infants. The requirement for dietary vitamin D may depend on many factors including exposure to sunlight, but it is still prudent to recommend 400 IU/day.[90] Vitamin D deficiency rickets is still seen in the developed countries, but it tends to be seen in dark-skinned infants, who are exclusively breast fed with no vitamin D supplementation and have had little or no exposure to sunlight.[91] In North America, this frequently involves immigrant children, who may be kept indoors during the winter. Adequate exposure to sunlight for white infants is 30 minutes per week if only in a diaper or 2 hours per week if fully clothed.

Breast-feeding proponents, however, have argued that even in northern countries, there is adequate vitamin D and calcium in most breast milk in healthy mothers who are eating a normal diet and that a broad general recommendation of vitamin D supplements for breast-fed infants is not necessary. According to La Leche League International, the world's recognized authority on breast-feeding, "rickets has rarely been found in fully breast-fed infants. This is true even in northern climates where there is less exposure to sunlight, which activates the formation of vitamin D. Research has shown that human milk contains adequate vitamin D for at least the first 6 months of life. Concerns are sometimes raised about the breast-fed baby's need for specific nutrients such as vitamin D because this nutrient is available in small quantities in human milk. If just a small patch of your baby's skin is exposed to sunlight for just a few minutes each day, this will provide plenty of vitamin D for most babies. If you live in a severe climate and go without any exposure to sunlight for months, or if you wear clothing that protects the skin from all sunlight, your baby may need a vitamin D supplement."[92]

Three factors influence the vitamin D status of an infant: (1) the newborn's vitamin D status at birth dependent on the mother's vitamin D status, (2) vitamin D intake, and (3) effective exposure to sunlight. Breast-fed infants of mothers who took vitamin D supplements had higher levels of vitamin D, but not as high as infants who were given a vitamin D supplement.[93] Children who are adequately exposed to sunlight may not need any vitamin

D supplements.[94] Women who do not consume milk or other foods fortified with vitamin D or have little exposure to sunlight are at risk of not providing their infants with adequate vitamin D prior to birth and through breast-feeding.

There is extensive literature, but there are no good controlled studies to answer the question, What is the evidence that vitamin D supplements should be given to all breast-fed infants?

1. Vitamin D deficiency rickets does occur, but it tends to occur in young infants who were not given any vitamin D supplements and were of low birth weight, dark skinned and/or kept out of the sunshine during the winter months of least sunshine, and breast fed by mothers who did not take any vitamin D supplements.[95-97]
2. If mothers take vitamin D supplements during pregnancy, their newborn infants are at a lower risk for developing biochemical or clinical rickets.[98-100] If breast-feeding mothers take vitamin D supplements, the risk of their infants developing rickets is reduced.
3. Some of the studies used to make recommendations about vitamin D are based on biochemical evidence of vitamin D deficiency: low serum 25-hydroxy-vitamin D, elevated alkaline phosphatase, or low serum phosphorus, but not necessarily clinical or radiologic evidence of rickets.[101]
4. The recommendations that commercial milk be supplemented with vitamin D in northern countries appears appropriate, given the reduction in nutritional rickets through this century.
5. Whether all breast-fed infants in northern countries or only at-risk infants, that is, dark-skinned infants who are covered or kept indoors during the winter, should receive a daily supplement of 400 IU of vitamin D still is debated, and there are no studies yet to resolve this issue. A summary of interventions for vitamin D deficient rickets is given in Table 4–5.

VEGETARIANISM

In the 1990s, there has been a dramatic increase in the popularity of vegetarian diets. Approximately 5 percent of Americans consider themselves vegetarians.[102-105] Many parents with these eating preferences feed their children vegetarian diets.[106,107] Certain cultural and ethnic groups have a long history of vegetarian diets and have remained in good health. Some families in North America and Europe follow a vegetarian diet to avoid atherosclerosis and high cholesterol associated with the intake of meat products, or for philosophical, spiritual, or ecological reasons; they may be at risk of developing deficiencies of vitamins and minerals. A vegetarian diet, if properly selected, can meet all the nutritional requirement of a growing child. But for some vegetarian families, their diet simply involves taking out meat and meat products; and therefore, many health professionals remain concerned about the adequacy of vegetarian diets. A vegetarian is usually defined as someone who does not eat animal flesh but may eat eggs (ovovegetarians) or dairy products (lactovegetarians). Some vegetarians aspire to being pure vegetarians, or vegans, and exclude all food of animal ori-

Table 4–5 A Summary of Interventions for Vitamin D Deficient Rickets

Condition	Intervention	Level of Evidence	Recommendation
Vitamin D deficient rickets	Vitamin D supplementation for breast-fed infants	III	B (high risk) C (low risk)
	Vitamin D fortification of milk and commercial foods	II-3	A

Table 4–6 A Summary of Interventions for Vegetarianism

Condition	Intervention	Level of Evidence	Recommendation
Vegetarian Diets	• Calcium and vitamin supplements for pregnant and lactating mothers	III	B
	• Vitamin supplements for breast-fed infants of vegetarian mothers	III	B
	• Nutritional counseling for vegetarian families	III	B

gin.[108] Some parents who choose alternative food habits for their children also have unconventional health-care beliefs or practices, including questioning the need for vaccinations, reliance on homeopathy, and avoiding western medicine. There are studies and case reports of mothers who are vegan and almost solely breast feed their infants, who may develop iron deficiency, vitamin D deficiency rickets, or vitamin B_{12} deficiency.[109-112] These infants are potentially at the greatest risk for other deficiency states. Older children are at risk as well because vegetarian diets also tend to be bulky and high in fiber, which limits caloric intake. The APP and the CPS recommend vitamin and iron supplements to breast-feeding vegetarian mothers and to vegetarian infants and children, as well as consultation with a dietician or nutritionist to ensure the adequacy of their infants' food intake and to assess the need for nutritional supplements. There are, however, few controlled trials of children from vegetarian families. A summary of interventions for vegetarianism is provided in Table 4–6.

CONCLUSION

For most physicians, the management of nutritional problems in infants and children is based on experience, common sense, and traditional medical treatment derived from descriptive studies. But families today are asking questions and challenging traditional management, and there is a need for real evidence and controlled clinical trials to resolve some of these important issues.

REFERENCES

1. Berwick D. Non-organic failure-to-thrive. Pediatr Rev 1980;1:265–70.

2. Goldbloom RB. Failure to thrive. Pediatr Clin N Am 1982;29:151–66.

3. Skuse DH. Non-organic failure to thrive: a reappraisal. Arch Dis Child. 1985;60:173–8.

4. Goldbloom RB. Growth failure in infancy. Pediatr Rev 1987;9:57–61.

5. Frank DA, Zeisel SH. Failure to thrive. Pediatr Clin N Am. 1988;35:1187–206.

6. Bithoney WG, Dubowitz H, Egan H. Failure to thrive/growth deficiency. Pediatr Rev 1992;13:453–60.

7. Bennett S. Failure to thrive. Pediatr Child Health 1996;1:206–10.

8. Zenel JA. Failure to thrive:a general pediatrician's perspective. Pediatr Rev 1997;18:371–8.

9. Wilcox WD, Nieburg P, Miller DS. Failure to thrive: a continuing problem of definition. Clin Pediatr 1989;28:391–4.

10. Oates RK. Non-organic failure to thrive. Austral J Pediatr 1984;20:95–100.

11. Oates RK. Child abuse and non-organic failure to thrive: similarities and differences in the parents. Austral J Pediatr. 1984;20:177–80.

12. Drotar D, Eckerle D. The family environment in nonorganic failure to thrive: a controlled study. J Pediatr Psychol 1989;14:245–57.

13. Altemeier WA, O'Connor SM, Sherrod KB, Vietze PM. Prospective study of antecedents for nonorganic failure to thrive. J Pediatr 1985;106:360–5.

14. Powell GF, Low JF, Speers MA. Behavior as a diagnostic aid in failure to thrive. Develop Behav Pediatr 1987;8:18–24.

15. Stier DM, Leventhal JM, Berg AT, et al. Are children born to young mothers at increased risk of maltreatment? Pediatrics 1993;91:642–8.

16. McCann JB, Stein A, Fairburn CG, Dunger DB. Eating habits and attitudes of mothers of children with non-organic failure to thrive. Arch Dis Child. 1994;70:234–6.

17. Glaser HH, Haegarty MC, Bullard DM Jr, et al. Physical and psychological development of children with early failure to thrive. J Pediatr 1968;73:690–8.

18. Gahagan S, Holmes R. A stepwise approach to evaluation of undernutrition and failure to thrive. Pediatr Clin N Am 1998;45:169–87.

19. Sills RH. Failure to thrive: the role of clinical and laboratory evaluation. Am J Dis Child. 1978;132:967–9.

20. Berwick DM, Levy JC, Kleinerman R. Failure to thrive: diagnostic yield of hospitalization. Arch Dis Child. 1982;57:347–51.

21. Maggioni A, Lifshitz F. Nutritional management of failure to thrive. Pediatr Clin N Am. 1995;42:79–810.

22. Finney JW. Preventing common feeding problems in infants and young children. Pediatr Clin N Am. 1986;33:775–88.

23. Elmer E, Gregg S, Ellison P. Late results of the failure to thrive syndrome. Clin Pediatr 1969;8:584–9.

24. Hutton IW, Oates RK. Non-organic failure to thrive: a long-term follow-up. Pediatrics 1977;59:73–7.

25. Oates RK, Peacock A, Forrest D. Development in children following abuse and nonorganic failure to thrive. Am J Dis Child 1984;138:764–7.

26. Oates RK, Peacock A, Forrest D. Long-term effects of nonorganic failure to thrive. Pediatrics 1985;75:36–40.

27. Ellerstein NS, Ostrov BE. Growth patterns in children hospitalized because of caloric-deprivation failure to thrive. Am J Dis Child 1985;139:164–6.

28. Bithoney WG, McJunkin J, Michalek J, et al. The effect of a multidisciplinary team approach on weight gain in nonorganic failure-to-thrive children. Develop Behav Pediatr 1991;12:254–8.

29. Drotar D, Sturm M. Personality development, problem solving, and behavior problems among preschool children with early histories of non-organic failure-to-thrive: a controlled study. Develop Behav Pediatr 1992;13:266–73.

30. Heffer RW, Kelley ML. Nonorganic failure to thrive: developmental outcomes and psychosocial assessment and intervention issues. Res Develop Disabilities. 1994;15:247–68.

31. Brown JL, Pollitt E. Malnutrition, poverty and intellectual development. Sci Am 1996;274:38–43

32. Wilensky DS, Ginsberg G, Altman M, et al. A community based study of failure to thrive in Israel. Arch Dis Child 1996;72:145–8.

33. Schmitt BD, Mauro RD. Nonorganic failure to thrive: an outpatient approach. Child Abuse and Neglect 1989;13:235–48.

34. Rosenn DW, Loeb LS, Jura MB. Differentiation of organic from nonorganic failure to thrive syndrome in infancy. Pediatrics 1980;66:698–704.

35. Singer L. Long-term hospitalization of nonorganic failure-to-thrive infants: patient characteristics and hospital course. Develop Behav Pediatr 1987;8:25–31.

36. Bithoney WG, McJunkin J, Michalek J, et al. Prospective evaluation of weight gain in both nonorganic and organic failure-to-thrive children: an outpatient trial of a multidisciplinary team intervention strategy. Develop Behav Pediatr 1989;10:27–31.

37. Bithoney WG, et al. The effect of a multidisciplinary team approach on weight gain in nonorganic failure-to-thrive children. Develop Behav Pediatr 1991;12:254–8.

38. Peterson KE, Washington J, Rathbun JM. Team management of failure to thrive. J Am Dietetic Assoc 1984;84:810–5.

39. Black MM, et al. A randomized clinical trial of home intervention for children with failure to thrive. Pediatrics 1995;95:807–14.

40. Hutcheson JJ, Black MM, Talley M, et al. Risk status and home intervention among children with failure-to-thrive: follow-up at age 4. J Pediatr Psychol 1997;22:651–68.

41. Wright CM, Callum J, Birks E, Jarvis S. Effect of community-based management in failure to thrive: randomised controlled trial. Br Med J 1998;317:571–4.

42. Casey PH, et al. A multifaceted intervention for infants with failure to thrive. A prospective study. Arch Pediatr Adolesc Med 1994;148:1071–7.

43. Deitz WH, Robinson TN. Assessment and treatment of childhood obesity. Pediatr Rev 1993;14:337–43.

44. King AJC, Robertson AS, Warren WK. Summary report: Canada Health Attitudes and Behaviors Survey: 9, 12 and 15 year olds, 1984-1985, Social Program Evaluation Group. Kingston, Ontario: Queens University;1985. p. 29.

45. Stephens T, Craig CL. The well-being of Canadians: the 1988 Campbells Survey on Well-Being in Canada. Ottawa, Ontario: Canadian Fitness and Lifestyle Research Institute;1990. p. 34, 74.

46. Paige DM. Obesity in childhood and adolescence: special problems in diagnosis and treatment. Postgrad Med 1986;79: p. 233–45.

47. Foreyt JP. Issues in the assessment and treatment of obesity. J Consult Clin Psychol 1987;55:677–84.

48. Rosenbaum M, Leibel RL. Obesity in childhood. Pediatr Rev 1989;11:43–55.

49. Schonfeld-Warden N, Warden CH. Pediatric obesity:an overview of etiology and treatment. Pediatr Clin N Am. 1997;44:339–61.

50. Kimm SY, Obarzanek E, Barton BR, et al. Race, socioeconomic status, and obesity in 9- to 10-year old girls: the NHLBI Growth and Health Study. Ann Epidemiol 1996;6:263–5.

51. Stunkard AJH, Sorensen TIA, Hanis C, et al. An adoption study of human obesity. N Engl J Med 1986;314:193–8.

52. Brook CGD, Huntley RMC, Slack J. Influence of heredity and environment in determination of skinfold thickness in children. Br Med J 1975;2:719–21.

53. Brjeson M. The etiology of obesity in children: a study of 101 twin pairs. Acta Paediatr Scand 1976;65:270–87.

54. Epstein LH, Wing RR, Valoski A. Childhood obesity. Pediatr Clin N Am 1985;32:363–79.

55. Mahan LK. Family-focused behavioral approach to weight control in children. Pediatr Clin N Am 1987;34:983–6.

56. Rocchini AP. Adolescent obesity and hypertension. Pediatr Clin N Am 1993;40:81–92.

57. Epstein LH, Coleman KJ, Myers MD. Exercise in treating obesity in children and adolescents. Med Sc Sports Exercise 1996;28:428–35.

58. Committee on Nutrition. Nutritional aspects of obesity in infancy and childhood. Pediatrics 1981;68:880–3.

59. Wing RR, Jeffery RJ. Outpatient treatments of obesity: a comparison of methodology and results. Int J Obesity 1979;3:261–79.

60. Loyd JK, Wolff OH. Childhood obesity: a long-term study of height and weight. Br Med J 1961;2:145–8.

61. Kleinman RE. Pediatric nutrition handbook, 4th edition. Committee on Nutrition. Elk Grove Village, IL: American Academy of Pediatrics;1998. p. 444.

62. Dietz WH. Prevention of childhood obesity. Pediatr Clin N Am 1986;33:823–33.

63. Goldbloom R, for Canadian Task Force on the Periodic Health Examination, 1994 update: 1. Obesity in childhood. Can Med Assoc J 1994;150:871–9.

64. Garn SM. Continuities and changes in fatness from infancy through adulthood. Curr Prob Pediatr 1985;15:1–47.

65. Nieto FJ, Szklo M, Comstock GW. Childhood weight and growth rate as predictors of adult mortality. Am J Epidemiol 1992;136:201–13.

66. Serdula MK, Ivery D, Coates RJ, et al. Do obese children become obese adults: a review of the literature. Prevent Med 1993;22:167–77.

67. Merritt RJ. Obesity. Curr Prob Pediatr 1982;12:1–58.

68. Berenson GS. Cardiovascular risk factors in children: the early natural history of atherosclerosis and essential hypertension. New York, NY Oxford University Press;1980.

69. Leung AK, Robson WLM. Childhood obesity. Postgrad Med 1990;87:123–33.

70. Mossberg HO. Forty-year follow-up of overweight children. Lancet 1989;2:491–3.

71. Johnston FE. Health implications of childhood obesity. Ann Intern Med 1985;103:1069–72.

72. Burns TL, Moll PP, Lauer RM. The relation between ponderosity and coronary risk factors in children and their relatives: the Muscatine Ponderosity Family Study. Am J Epidemiol 1989;129:973–87.

73. Abraham S, Collins G, Nordsieck M. Relationship of childhood weight status to morbidity in adults. Pub Health Rep 1971;86:273–84.

74. Must A, Jacques PF, Dallal GE, et al. Long-term morbidity and mortality of overweight adolescents: a follow-up of the Harvard growth study of 1922 to 1935. N Engl J Med 1992;327:1350–5.

75. Mallick MJ. Health hazards of obesity and weight control in children: a review of the literature. Am J Pub Health 1983;73:78-82.

76. Epstein LH, Wing RR, Woodall K, et al. Effects of family-based behavioural treatment on obese 5-8 year old children. Behav Ther 1985;16:205–12.

77. Epstein LH, Valoski A, Koeske R, et al. Family-based behavioral weight control in obese young children. J Am Diet Assoc 1986;86:481–4.

78. Israel AC, Stolmaker L, Sharp JP, et al. An evaluation of two methods of parental involvement in treating obese children. Behav Ther 1984;15:266–72.

79. Kirschenbaum DS, Harris ES, Tomarken AJ. Effects of parental involvement in behavioral weight loss therapy for preadolescents. Behav Ther 1984;15:485-500.

80. Epstein LH, Wing RR, Koeske R, et al. Long-term effects of family-based treatment of childhood obesity. J Consult Clin Psychol 1987;55:91–5.

81. Epstein LH, Valoski A, Wing RR, et al. Ten-year follow-up of behavioral, family-based treatment for obese children. J Am Med Assoc 1990;264:2519–23.

82. Ballew C, Liu K, Levinson S, Stamler J. Comparison of three weight-for-height indices in blood pressure studies in children. Am J Epidemiol 1990;131:532–7.

83. Ward DS, Bar-Or O. Role of the physician and physical education teacher in the treatment of obesity at school. Pediatrician 1986;13:44-51.

84. Ginsberg-Fellner F, Knittle JL. Weight reduction in young obese children. 1. Effects on adipose tissue cellularity and metabolism. Pediatr Res 1981;15:1381–9.

85. Epstein LH, Wing RR, Penner B, et al. Effect of diet and controlled exercise on weight loss in obese children. J Pediatr 1985;107:358–361.

86. Committee on Nutrition. Nutritional aspects of obesity in infancy and childhood. Pediatrics 1981;68:880–3.

87. Pediatric nutrition handbook, 4th edition. Committee on Nutrition. American Academy of Pediatrics. Elk Grove Village, IL, U.S.A. 1998

88. Nutrition for healthy term infants. Statement of the Joint Working Group. Ottawa Ontario: Canadian Pediatric Society, Dietitians of Canada, and Health Canada; Ministry of Public Works and Government Services, Ottawa, Canada 1998.

89. Specker BL, Ho ML, Oestreich A, et al. Prospective study of vitamin D supplementation and rickets in China. J Pediatr 1992;120:733–9.

90. Binet A, Kooh SW. Persistence of vitamin D deficiency rickets in Toronto in the 1990s. Can J Pub Health 1996;87:227–30.

91. La Leche League International. Website http://www.lalecheleague.org

92. Rothberg AD, Pettifor JM, Cohen DF, et al. Maternal-infant vitamin D relationships during breast-feeding. J Pediatr 1982;101:500–3.

93. Greer FR, Marshall S. Bone mineral content, serum vitamin D metabolite concentrations, and ultraviolet B light exposure in infants fed human milk with and without vitamin D_2 supplements. J Pediatr 1989;114:204–12.

94. Mughal MZ, Salama H, Greenaway T, et al. Lesson of the week: florid rickets associated with prolonged breast feeding without vitamin D supplementation. Br Med J 1999;318:39–40.

95. Pugliese MT, Blumberg DL, Hludzinski J, Kay S. Nutritional rickets in suburbia. J Am Coll Nutr 1998;17 637–41.

96. Davies PS, Bates CJ, Cole TJ, et al. Vitamin D: seasonal and regional differences in preschool children in Great Britain. Eur J Clin Nutr 1999;53:195–8.

97. Devlin EE, Salle BL, Glorieux FH, et al. Vitamin D supplementation during pregnancy: effect on neonatal calcium homeostasis. J Pediatr 1986;109:328–34.

98. Mallett E, Guigi B, Brunelle P, et al. Vitamin D supplementation in pregnancy: a controlled trial of two methods. Obstet Gyn 1986;68:300–4.

99. Ala-Houhala M, Koskinen T, Terho A, et al. Maternal compared with infant vitamin D supplementation. Arch Dis Child 1986;61:1159-63.

100. Mimouni F, Campaigne B, Neylan M, Tsang RC. Bone mineralization in the first year of life in infants fed human milk, cow-milk formula, or soy-based formula. J Pediatr 1993;122:348–54.

101. Sanders TAB, Reddy S. Vegetarian diets and children. Am J Clin Nutr 1994;59(Suppl):S1176–81.

102. Sanders TAB. Vegetarian diets and children. Pediatr Clin N Am 1995;42:955–65.

103. Jacobs C, Dwyer JT. Vegetarian children: appropriate and inappropriate diets. Am J Clin Nutr 1988;43(Suppl):811–8.

104. Dwyer JT. Nutritional consequences of vegetarianism. Ann Rev Nutr 1991;11:61-91.

105. Campbell M, Lofters WS, Gibbs WN. Rastafarianism and the vegan syndrome. Br Med J 1982;285:1617–8.

106. Sklar R. Nutritional vitmin B_{12} deficiency in a breast-fed infant of a vegan-diet mother. Clin Pediatr 1986;25:219–21.

107. Kuhne T, Bubl R, Baumgartner R. Maternal vegan diet causing a serious infantile neurological disorder due to vitamin B_{12} deficiency. Eur J Pediatr 1991;150:205–8.

108. Specter BL. Nutritonal concerns of lactating women consuming vegetarian diets. Am J Clin Nutr 1994;59(Suppl):1182S–86.

109. Von Schenck U, Bender-Gotze C, Koletzko B. Persistency of neurological damage induced by dietary vitamin B_{12} deficiency in infancy. Arch Dis Child 1998;72:137–9.

110. Oski FA. Iron deficiency facts and fallacies. Pediatr Clin N Am 1985;32:493–7.

111. Reeves JD. Iron supplementation in infancy. Pediatr Rev 1986;8:177–84.

112. Oski FA. Iron deficiency in infancy and childhood. N Engl J Med 1993;329:190–3.

CHAPTER 5

Acute Rhinitis and Pharyngitis

Michael B.H. Smith, MBBCh, FRCPC

Infections of the upper respiratory tract are a common experience for children throughout the world. A preschool child can have six to eight infections a year, or more (up to twelve) if they attend daycare.[1] Acute rhinitis and pharyngitis are the commonest types of respiratory infection and may prompt a visit to a primary care provider when symptoms do not resolve. The common cold is not usually a diagnostic problem but the treatment can be problematic. There are numerous nonprescription remedies that provide only modest benefits. Conversely, pharyngitis presents more of a diagnostic problem, but the treatment is effective and efficient. In both conditions, antibiotics are often prescribed unnecessarily, contributing to the increasing problem of bacterial resistance. The purpose of this review is to cover the pediatric management of these two prevalent conditions.

COMMON COLD

Disease overview

The common cold is caused by a wide variety of viruses (Table 5–1). There are about 100 antigenically different types of rhinovirus that are responsible for more than 30 percent of colds in adults. It is presumed that approximately the same proportion affects children. Other types of viruses causing colds include coronavirus, respiratory syncytial virus, and parainfluenza virus.[2]

Although most viral respiratory infections in children are clinically trivial, progression to lower respiratory illness can produce significant illness. In the developing nations, acute respiratory tract infections (ARTI) are a common cause of death in infants, especially in Central America, Africa, South America, and Asia.[3] In the developed nations, illness from ARTI is much less severe. Children in day-care face a significant risk and are more likely to be hospitalised and to endure more complications from viral ARTI than those looked after at home.[4]

There is a persisting misconception that respiratory viruses are transmitted directly through droplets from sneezing or coughing. However, the most effective spread occurs by the direct inoculation of infected secretions from the hands to the eyes or nasal mucosa. This fact led to the institution of an effective and inexpensive method of prevention: handwashing.[5] Re-infection is common with most of the respiratory viruses and usually results in less severe disease.

Clinical Features and Diagnosis

The common cold is a self-limited, inflammatory viral respiratory illness that affects primarily the nose and paranasal sinuses. Due to the universal experience of this illness, diagnosis is seldom difficult. The syndrome usually begins with nasal irritation, followed by a scratchy throat, sneezing, and profuse nasal discharge. A low-grade fever often accompanies this illness, but occasionally the temperature can reach 39°C. The nasal congestion and fever often interfere with eating and sleeping, especially in infants. Symptoms usually last from 4 to 7 days. A persistent nasal discharge without systemic symptoms usually turns out to be allergic rhinitis or chronic sinusitis. A unilateral nasal discharge suggests a nasal foreign body.

Table 5–1 Viruses That Cause Common Cold

Category	Agents	Type or Subtype
Common cause	Rhinovirus	1 to 100+
	Parainfluenza virus	1 to 4
	Respiratory syncytial virus	2
	Coronavirus	Numerous
Occasional causes	Adenovirus	~31
	Enterovirus	Coxsackie A (1 to 24), Coxsackie B (1 to 6), Echovirus (1 to 34)
	Influenza virus	A,B,C
	Reovirus	1 to 3
	Mycoplasma pneumoniae	
Rare causes	*Coccidioides immitis*	
	Histoplasma capsulatum	
	Bordetella pertussis	
	Chlamydia psittaci	
	Varicella virus	
	Rubeola virus	
	Epstein-Barr virus	
	Herpes simplex virus	

With permission from Spector SL. The common cold: current therapy and natural history. J Allergy Clin Immunol 1995;95:1133–8.

Current Management of the Common Cold

As there is no cure for the common cold, treatment is aimed at amelioration of symptoms. Treatment options available include over-the-counter (OTC) medications, nonpharmaceutical treatments, and home remedies. Few of these have been examined in well-designed studies. In addition, many of the trials have been performed predominantly in adults. Compared with children, adults have larger respiratory airways that are presumably more amenable to improvement in airway diameter and secretion clearance. Over-the-counter medications are the predominant choice of treatment for common cold in childhood. Several factors may contribute to the selection of a particular treatment by parents. Among the most prominent of these is pharmaceutical advertising, which is highly successful in persuading parents that medications must be bought for the treatment of every symptom. Parents are naturally very susceptible to this advertising because of their desire to help their child. Kogan found that more than half of all mothers surveyed in a nationally representative sample had given their 3-year-old children an OTC medication in the previous 30 days—usually acetaminophen or cough/cold medications.[6]

Several studies have highlighted the problem of inappropriate treatment of the common cold either by antibiotic prescriptions or incorrect medications.[7-10] Some families mistakenly believe that medications, either prescription or OTC, cure the viruses that cause an infection.[11] With some exceptions (see discussion below), medications are not recommended and may actually worsen the illness in the child by causing side effects, delaying the diagnosis, or causing further problems with the disease process. Physicians and pharmacists need to take the initiative to inquire about these medications to understand why the patients use them. Misconceptions need to be corrected and advice provided on the proper choice and use of any medication for the common cold. Further areas of research will need to address these issues.

Nondrug Therapy: Inhalation Therapy

Breathing in steam or warm mist has long been known to provide a measure of comfort for those suffering from nasal and sinus congestion. The physical benefit probably stems from the liquefaction of respiratory secretions, which enables more effective removal by either coughing or nose blowing. Additionally, warm, moist air is soothing to an irritated respiratory epithelium. Aromatics have also been added to steam to provide a sensation of relief, although these have not been examined scientifically. Menthol tablets create a subjective sense of nasal decongestion but have not been shown to change nasal airflow when measured objectively[12] (level I).

Studies on the effect of steam inhalation on the common cold have shown conflicting results. Two early studies lend support to the hypothesis that nasal hyperthermia reduced the symptoms of the common cold. The effects of steam inhalation on nasal patency and on nasal symptoms in 62 patients with the common cold were studied in a double-blind, randomized, placebo-controlled clinical trial[13] (level I). Treatment consisted of two 20-minute sessions, during which one patient group inhaled saturated, hot (42 to 44°C) air through the nose. This was compared with a control group which received inhalations of room air (20 to 24°C) for similar time periods. During the week following treatment, the subjective response was recorded by each patient on a daily symptom score card. Nasal patency was determined before treatment, the following day, and 1 week later by measuring peak nasal expiratory and inspiratory airflow. Steam inhalation resulted in the alleviation of cold symptoms and increased nasal patency in a significantly higher percentage of patients in the actively treated group than in the placebo-treated group. In the second study, 87 subjects with simple colds breathed warm, humidified air at 43°C for 20 minutes per day and were compared with 84 subjects breathing air at 30°C [14] (level I). Patients recorded their symptoms, and observers recorded symptoms and signs, weight of nasal secretions, isolation of virus, and antibody responses in volunteers. Patients treated with the warm air had roughly half the score for symptoms of those treated at 30°C. The study concluded that nasal hyperthermia will provide immediate relief of symptoms and improve the course of the common cold.

Two more recent trials have attempted to examine the effect of inhaling warm, humidified air. The first of these was a randomized double-blind trial performed on 68 volunteers with naturally occurring colds[15] (level I). The first part of the study indicated that in-vivo rhinovirus was greatly inhibited if exposed to temperatures higher than 43°C for 60 minutes. In the second part of the study, 32 individuals received a 1-hour treatment with steam (43°C) and were compared with 36 who received room air (20 to 24°C). A 7-day follow-up revealed no difference in symptom scores or objective scores of nasal airflow. A second trial was performed on 20 volunteers who were experimentally infected with rhinovirus[16] (level II-1). Eight participants received two 30-minute treatments of (42 to 44°C) steam at 1 and 2 days after inoculation. Six received a similar regime of room temperature vapor (22 to 23°C). The outcomes were assessed over the following 4 days. There was no difference in rhinovirus titers in nasal washings and no difference in symptom scores. The authors commented on the low power of this trial and its inability to detect symptom improvement. Certainly, the steam had no antiviral effect.

These studies (none of which included children) provide conflicting evidence for the effects of inhaled steam for the relief of nasal congestion (recommendation C). It should be noted that the steam was delivered by a specially designed ultrasonic heater that directs moist air to the nares, using a mask device. The practical issue of safely delivering this treatment to children will need to be addressed (Table 5–4).

Pharmacotherapy

The fact that there are so many widely differing therapies for the common cold suggests that none really work very well. Many parents understandably want to ease these minor but irritating symptoms in their children and often turn to OTC medications for help. Antihistamines, decongestants, cough suppressants or expectorants, analgesics, and various combinations of these are available. The breadth of choice is all the more striking, given the limited scientific information demonstrating their effectiveness.[17] Commonly used cough and cold medications can be divided into the following groups: antihistamines, decongestants, cough medications, ipratropium, combination products, analgesics/nonsteroidal anti-inflammatory drugs, zinc gluconate, antibiotics, antiviral therapies, and vitamin C. Antipyretics (reviewed in detail in another chapter) are often combined with many of the cold medications.

Antihistamines

Antihistamines exert their effects via their anticholinergic activity designed to dry up the respiratory secretions. The anticholinergic effect is often weak, given the dosages used in most OTC preparations. The antihistamine effect is also probably minimal due to the lack of histamine released during a viral nasopharyngitis.[18] The most common groups of antihistamines include the ethanolamines (diphenhydramine and dimenhydrinate) alkylamines (chlorpheniramine and brompheniramine), and the piperidines (terfenadine and astemizole). In certain circumstances, such as in a child with allergic rhinitis, antihistamines may be effective in relieving some of the symptoms. In therapeutic doses, some antihistamines act as a sedative. Many parents wrongly attribute this to a relief of symptoms. Paradoxically, use of these medications may occasionally result in overstimulation in children.

The literature has not supported the use of antihistamines for the common cold in children. In one systematic review of OTC cold medications, there was no evidence for antihistamines causing clinical improvement in children.[17] There was evidence for a beneficial effect brought about by chlorpheniramine in adolescents and adults. In addition, a few first-generation antihistamines have recently been found to be useful in the common cold in adults. Doxylamine succinate[19] (level I), clemastine fumarate[20,21] (level I), and chlorpheniramine maleate[22] (level I) all reduce rhinorrhea, sneezing, and volume of nasal secretion. Terfenadine has not been found to reduce symptoms, possibly because of its relative lack of anticholinergic activity.[18] Recently, the efficacy of brompheniramine maleate was tested in a randomized, controlled trial of volunteers with experimental rhinovirus colds[23] (level I). Brompheniramine (12 mg) or placebo was administered for 4 days after the onset of symptoms. During the first 3 days of treatment, nasal secretion weights, rhinorrhea scores, sneeze counts, sneeze severity scores, and cough counts were lower in subjects receiving brompheniramine than in controls. Treatment with brompheniramine was associated with adverse effects such as somnolence and confusion in a small number of subjects. Overall, it was concluded that brompheniramine was efficacious treatment for the sneezing, rhinorrhea, and cough associated with rhinovirus colds.

A recent systematic review examined whether studies on antihistamines showed clinically significant relief from the symptoms of the common cold in adults and children.[24] Three out of five studies reporting on sneezing found a statistically significant improvement in the antihistamine group; similarly, 3 of 7 studies reporting on nasal discharge found a statistically significant improvement with therapy. No study reported improvement in total symptom score at the significance level of $p=.05$. The validity of the studies was weakened by several flaws, such as inattention to clinical significance and functional impact, inappropriate use of statistical tests, and poorly described methodology. The authors of this review concluded that the medical literature offered little support for the use of antihistamines in the treatment of the common cold.

In summary, there is some evidence that antihistamines reduce nasal symptoms of the common cold in adolescents and adults, although the clinical significance of this benefit is questionable (recommendation C). There may be some benefit if there is a history of accompanying allergic disease. Younger children do not appear to respond to these medications (recommendation E) (see Table 5–4).

Decongestants (Alpha-Adrenergic Agents)

These sympathomimetic substances produce a physiologic response similar to that of the catecholamines. Decongestants either directly stimulate the alpha and beta adrenergic receptors or release endogenous noradrenaline from presynaptic nerve terminals. The main beneficial action of these medications is the vasoconstriction of the nasal mucosa, which reduces edema and therefore improves nasal airflow and reduces sinus congestion. These medications are found in bronchodilators, stimulants, and appetite suppressants as well as cough and cold medications. In a systematic review of OTC cold medications, there was no evidence for decongestants causing clinical improvement in the common cold in children.[17]

Oral alpha-adrenergic agents. Ephedrine and pseudoephedrine have a rapid onset of action, reaching a peak at 1 to 2 hours after ingestion. They can produce hypertension and tachycardia, which are more often a problem in adults than children.[25] Signs and symptoms of toxicity in the pediatric age group include headache, nausea, vomiting, diaphoresis, agitation, psychosis, hypertension, seizures, tremulousness, and rhabdomyolysis.[25] Phenylpropanolamine is another sympathomimetic compound with a similar action and side-effect profile to ephedrine and pseudoephedrine. This substance is used in combination with analgesics, antihistamines, anticholinergic, and antitussive medications. The major problem caused by it is hypertension, especially when it is taken in combination with caffeine.[26] Norephedrine has also been shown to be mildly effective.[27] Side effects (particularly, CNS overstimulation and hypertension) have been reported both in therapeutic doses and in excessive ingestion.

Topical alpha-adrenergic agents. The imidazolines (oxymetazoline, naphazoline, tetrahydrozoline, and xylometazoline) are used as topical agents for their vasoconstrictive action. Studies have reached different conclusions regarding their effectiveness: (level II-2),[28] (level I).[29,30] The imidazolines are used in sinusitis, allergic rhinitis, colds, and ocular irritations. In short-term use, topical vasoconstrictors are promptly effective, although when used continuously (especially over 3 to 4 days), they can result in rebound nasal congestion and thus prolong the cold. As a result, these medications are not recommended for use in children (recommendation D). Signs of clinical toxicity cover a wide range of symptoms from lethargy, somnolence, pallor, and cool extremities to miosis, bradycardia, hypotension, loss of consciousness, and respiratory depression.[31]

The evidence would suggest that these medications are effective in adolescents and adults, but the side effects may be significant in certain individuals (recommendation C) (see Table 5–4).

Cough Suppressants/Expectorants

Dextromethorphan is one of the most commonly used antitussive medications. It acts in a similar manner to codeine by suppressing the cough center in the medulla oblongata. Both codeine and dextromethorphan are frequently used for their antitussive effects, despite evidence to the contrary[32] (level I). Although generally considered safe, dextromethorphan has been shown to cause CNS side effects, including hyperexcitability, increased muscle tone, and ataxia.

Expectorants reduce the viscosity of the secretion to promote more effective expectoration. Guaifenesin is the most widely used of these medications. In one clinical trial, young adults with a cold perceived a minor reduction in the quantity of sputum after using this medication[33] (level I) (recommendation D). In some formulations, this substance is combined with a cough suppressant, which makes little sense. There is no evidence, therefore, that dextromethorphan and guaifenesin are effective in relieving cold symptoms in children (recommendation E) (see Table 5–4).

Ipratropium

Ipratropium is a parasympatholytic medication with a highly topical action. It has been used successfully as a bronchodilator in asthma. One randomized trial looked at the effectiveness of intranasal ipratropium bromide (IB) for the treatment of symptoms of the common cold[34] (level I). Four hundred and eleven university students were randomized to either IB nasal spray, a nasal spray of salt solution, or no treatment. The treatments were self-administered three or four times daily for 4 days. Recipients of IB had 26 percent less nasal discharge, 31 percent less rhinorrhea and less sneezing on days 2 and 4. The medication was well tolerated but was associated with higher rates of blood-tinged mucus and nasal dryness than the control spray. Patient assessments of the overall effectiveness of treatment were more favorable for IB than for the control spray. The study concluded that intranasal IB provides specific relief of rhinorrhea and sneezing associated with the common cold.

In another study, three doses of IB nasal spray were compared with the vehicle alone and with no treatment, for the relief of rhinorrhea in patients with naturally acquired colds[35] (level I). Rhinorrhea severity was measured by determination of nasal discharge weights and a subjective symptom scale. Compared with either the vehicle or no treatment, IB nasal spray produced a significant decrease in the severity of rhinorrhea. A dose of 84 micrograms (two sprays of a 0.06 percent solution) in each nostril was more efficacious than a dose of 42 micrograms per nostril and only marginally less efficacious than a dose of 168 micrograms per nostril. The dose of 84 micrograms per nostril also was associated with fewer adverse events than the higher dose. None of the adverse events related to intranasal IB therapy were of a serious nature. This study indicates the pharmacologic benefits of differing doses of this medication. The study concluded that the use of IB nasal spray appears to be an effective and safe approach to relieving rhinorrhea associated with the common cold.

Ipratropium bromide seems to be a promising therapy in alleviating rhinorrhea (recommendation B). Side effects may be a problem for some individuals. As the evidence is drawn from adult studies, it remains to be seen whether this treatment is effective in children (see Table 5–4).

Combination Products

Drug combinations are the most common form of treatment for simple viral upper respiratory infections and possess the theoretical advantage of treating the various symptoms that accompany a cold. However, this treatment is less desirable pharmacologically because of the fixed amounts and ratios of each of the component drugs. This makes it less than ideal for children with differing ages and weights. One systematic review identified a probable reduction in symptoms with a decongestant and antihistamine preparation in adolescents and adults.[17] Benefits included a reduction in nasal symptoms (decrease in congestion, postnasal drip, and rhinorrhea) as well as less cough and fewer ear symptoms. The inclusion of analgesics (acetaminophen or ibuprofen) in the preparation relieved headaches and generalized discomfort.

In a more recent trial on preschool children, an antihistamine-decongestant combination was compared with a placebo in temporarily relieving symptoms of upper respiratory tract infection (URI)[36] (level I). Preschool children with a cold were randomly assigned to receive brompheniramine maleate–phenylpropanolamine hydrochloride (ADC) or placebo, as needed for respiratory symptoms. Two hours after each dose of study medication, changes in the child's nasal discharge, nasal congestion, cough, and sleep status were assessed by means of a standardized questionnaire. There were no statistically significant differences in symptom improvement between the ADC and the placebo groups. However, the proportion of children still asleep 2 hours after receiving ADC was significantly higher than the proportion receiving placebo. Results were unchanged after control for the correlated nature of repeated responses, age, symptom duration, use of acetaminophen, time that the medication was given, and parental desire for medication. The study concluded that ADC was equivalent to the placebo in providing temporary relief of URI symptoms in preschool children. However, ADC did have significantly greater sedative effects than did the placebo.

There seems to be no evidence, therefore, that these medications are of benefit in preschool children, who arguably have the greatest need for symptom relief. Sedation may be a beneficial side effect, for both parents and child, but is not an acceptable reason to recommend this as a therapy (recommendation E). Combination products may provide benefit in older children, adolescents, and adults (recommendation B) (see Table 5–4).

Antipyretics, Analgesics, and Nonsteroidal Anti-inflammatory Drugs

The fever which commonly accompanies viral upper respiratory infections generates considerable anxiety in parents, leading them to seek medical attention early and frequently.[37,38] Many families aggressively treat even a mild elevation of temperature (37 to 37.8°C) with antipyretics, a level which includes the normal range. There has been considerable debate whether pharmacologic reduction of fever is beneficial or hazardous to the host.[39] Fever is a reliable sign of illness, and reduction may mask the onset of a more serious disease. High fever may also be a useful mechanism for fighting bacterial infections. On the other hand, an elevated temperature is uncomfortable, and adverse events such as seizures, confusion, or dehydration are more likely. Common OTC medications used for fever are acetaminophen, acetylsalicylic acid, naproxen, and ibuprofen. Due to the association between aspirin and Reye's syndrome, acetaminophen has virtually replaced all OTC analgesic preparations. Acetaminophen can be found in a variety of forms, either on its own or combined with a variety of substances, in cough and cold preparations. In a recent report, the use of aspirin and acetaminophen was associated with suppression of serum-neutralizing antibody response and increased nasal symptoms and signs in the common cold, compared with ibuprofen or placebo.[40] Naproxen sodium has been thought to increase nasal symptoms and virus shedding and decrease serum neutralising antibody response in patients infected with the rhinovirus. However, in a study of adults with experimental rhinovirus colds, naproxen treatment did not alter virus shedding or antibody responses[41] (level I). The medication had a beneficial effect on headache, mylagia, and cough. Overall, the consistent benefit from these medications seemed to be analgesia (recommendation B) (see Table 5–4).

Zinc Gluconate

There is suggestive evidence from the laboratory that zinc gluconate may be effective in the treatment of the common cold. Despite this evidence, there continues to be controversy regarding its effectiveness. Initially, it was thought to be effective,[42] but subsequent trials failed to confirm this when placebos were used (level I).[43–46] Two more recent trials demonstrated efficacy in adults (level I).[47,48]

A recent randomized, placebo-controlled study examined 249 students in grades 1 through 12[49] (level I). Ten milligram zinc gluconate glycine lozenges were given either five or six times a day. The time to resolution of the symptoms was based on daily symptom scores for cough, headache, hoarseness, muscle ache, nasal congestion, nasal drainage, scratchy throat, sore throat, and sneezing. The study showed that time to resolution of all cold symptoms did not differ significantly between students receiving zinc and those receiving placebo. In addition, more students in the zinc group reported adverse effects such as bad taste, nausea, oral discomfort, and diarrhea. In this community-based trial, zinc lozenges were thus not effective in treating cold symptoms in children and adolescents (recommendation E). Overall, the published evidence demonstrates conflicting results with regard to the use of zinc in adults (recommendation C) (see Table 5–4).

Antibiotics

A well-designed study from Switzerland found co-amoxiclav to be beneficial in 20 percent of adults with the common cold whose nasopharyngeal secretions contained *Haemophilus influenzae*, *Moraxella catarrhalis* or *Streptococcus pneumoniae*[50] (level I). It is not clear how this information can be used in practice, as patients would have to wait for cultures, by which time the major symptoms of the cold would have passed. The benefit to those with positive cultures appears marginal, and the risks of excessive antibiotic use are too high to recommend its routine use (recommendation D) (see Table 5–4).

Antiviral therapy

Antiviral drugs for respiratory viruses generally bind to hydrophobic pockets in the virion capsid and inhibit virion attachment or uncoating. The main difficulties in the development of effective antiviral drugs for the common cold include the wide variety of viruses, mutant strains, and the development of resistance. Several studies have treated rhinovirus colds with no appreciable benefit[51,52] (level I). In Hayden's trial, intranasal pirodavir was assessed in a randomized, double-blind manner. Adults with laboratory-documented rhinovirus colds were randomly assigned to intranasal sprays of pirodavir or placebo six times daily for 5 days. In this study, no significant differences in the resolution of respiratory symptoms were apparent between the treatment and control groups. The median duration of illness was 7 days in each group. Reduced frequencies of rhinovirus shedding were observed in the pirodavir group on days 3 and 5, but not after the cessation of treatment on day 7. No pirodavir-resistant viruses were recovered from treated individuals. The pirodavir group had higher rates of nasal dryness, blood in mucus, or unpleasant taste on several study days. In summary, intranasal sprays of pirodavir were associated with significant antiviral effects but no clinical benefit in treating naturally occurring rhinovirus colds. Other antiviral agents have been tried similarly with successful reduction of the viral load but, again, with little clinical benefit.

Interferon prevents viral invasion of the nasal mucosa. As with many common cold therapies, the results have been conflicting. Interferon alpha 2 has been tested in two studies. In both these studies, a nasal spray was administered once daily for 7 days when cold symptoms appeared in another family member. A decrease in colds due to rhinovirus as well as a decrease in all respiratory illnesses was observed.[53,54] This short-term prophylaxis of colds was not confirmed in another study.[55] Combination therapy with interferon alpha 2b, ipratropium bromide, and oral naproxen reduced cold symptoms (rhinorrhea, cough, malaise, and sore throat) effectively in a small study of adults[56] (level II-2). Overall, there has been no clear effective antiviral therapy for colds in adults (recommendation D). At the current time, there is no evidence supporting the use of antiviral medication in children for the prevention or treatment of the common cold (see Table 5–4).

Vitamin C

Vitamin C has long been felt to play both a preventive and therapeutic role in the common cold. There have been many studies of varying quality which have attempted to determine this issue. A recent review of 30 trials by the acute respiratory infection group of the Cochrane Collaboration has provided a useful contribution to this debate.[57] In this review, which was undertaken using strict criteria, the authors found that regular high-dose vitamin C had no important effect on the incidence of the common cold. However, there was a modest benefit in the treatment of the common cold by reducing its duration. The magnitude of this effect was a reduction of symptoms by 8 to 9 percent, or about a half symptom day per episode. The studies reviewed included both adult and children. The authors concluded that prophylaxis should be discouraged but that higher-dose therapy (>8 g/day) should be studied for its therapeutic benefit.

This is likely to be a topic of debate for many years. Further studies examining the therapy in high doses may reveal whether there is value in using this medication for the common cold. It is not currently recommended for use in children or adults (recommendation C) (see Table 5–4).

PHARYNGITIS

Disease Overview

Group A beta-hemolytic streptococci (GABHS) are the most common bacterial cause for acute pharyngitis. Establishing the diagnosis of GABHS is particularly important because of the acute morbidity of the illness as well as the potentially severe nonsuppurative sequelae (acute rheumatic fever and acute glomerulonephritis). The bacteria are spread by person-to-person contact with infected nasal or oral secretions. Transmission is more common in crowded environments, such as schools or dormitories.

Clinical Features and Diagnosis

For the majority of children with a sore throat, diagnosis focuses on either a viral cause or GABHS pharyngitis. Pharyngitis caused by a virus requires no treatment. If the patient has respiratory difficulty, then pharyngeal or peritonsillar abscess or tonsillar hypertrophy from Epstein-Barr virus infection needs to be considered. Buccal or gingival inflammation, vesicles on the posterior pharynx, or diffuse cervical or posterior lymphadenopathy imply a viral cause. Scarlet fever is distinguished by a fine sandpaper-like rash seen in children older than 3 years. It is seen about 24 hours after the development of the illness, beginning on the chest and spreading all over, with accentuation in the flexural creases. The redness fades in several days and the skin begins to desquamate as in the case of a sunburn downwards from the face extending out to the peripheries.

Children with GABHS infection present with sudden onset of a sore throat, painful swallowing, and fever (Table 5–2). These symptoms may also be accompanied by headache, nausea and vomiting, and abdominal pain. Examination shows tonsillopharyngeal erythema with or without exudate, a red swollen uvula, petechiae on the palate and large, tender, anterior cervical lymph nodes. The papillae on the tongue may be red and swollen giving the "strawberry tongue" appearance. Younger children may have a more prolonged course of GABHS with chronic low grade fever, generalized lymphadenopathy and coryza with crusting below the nares with little or no pharyngitis. This condition is known as streptococcosis.

Scoring Systems

The clinical diagnosis of GABHS infection is difficult as many of the clinical features are also associated with other forms of pharyngitis or viral illnesses. Several attempts have been made to establish a predictive score for GABHS infection by incorporating clinical and epidemiologic features.[59–61] One study looked specifically at the clinical features to determine whether these can suggest GABHS infection.[62] In 192 children presenting with acute pharyngitis, 89 percent had GABHS isolated by throat culture. Using otoscopic magnification, the pharynx was examined for the presence of nine clinical features. Children with GABHS pharyngitis were more likely to have one out of the following six features: (1)pharyngeal erythema, (2)palatal enanthem, (3)uvular erythema, (4)uvular edema, (5)tonsillar erythema, and

---

Table 5–2 Features Suggestive of GABHS Pharyngitis

Clinical findings	Sudden onset of sore throat
	Fever
	Headache
	Marked inflammation of the pharynx and tonsils
	Tonsillar hypertrophy
	Patchy discrete exudate
	Tender enlarged cervical lymph nodes
	Nausea, vomiting, abdominal pain
	Absence of coryza, cough, conjunctivitis, or diarrhea
Epidemiological findings	5 to 15 years
	Winter and early spring
	Exposure to others with infection

With permission from Gerber MA. Diagnosis of group A streptococcal pharyngitis. Pediatr Ann 1998;27:269–73.

(6)tonsillar exudate. The combinations of two or three of these findings produced a positive predictive value of greater than 90 percent. However, these combinations were never present in more than 30 to 40 percent of the patients studied.

In a recent study, a score based on clinical symptoms and signs was developed to identify, in general practice, GABHS infection in patients presenting with a new upper respiratory tract infection.[61] The score ranged in value from 0 to 4. A total of 521 patients (with ages ranging from 3 to 76 years) were studied. The management and outcome of patients using the clinical score was compared with those of patients receiving the usual physician care. The sensitivity of the score for identifying GABHS infection was 83.1 percent, compared with 69.4 percent for usual physician care; the specificity values of the two approaches were similar. Among patients aged 3 to 14 years, the sensitivity of the score approach was higher than that of usual physician care (96.9 percent versus 70.6 percent). The authors calculated that if the score were implemented, the proportion of patients receiving initial antibiotic prescriptions would have been reduced by 48 percent compared with usual physician prescribing, without any increase in the use of throat culture. They concluded that an age-appropriate sore throat score identified GABHS infection in children and adults better than the usual care by family physicians. It had the additional benefit of significantly reducing unnecessary prescription of antibiotics (Recommendation B) (Table 5–5).

Throat Culture

Throat swab culture on sheep blood agar plate remains the gold standard for the diagnosis of GABHS infection.[63,64] Unfortunately, this method is not without potential problems. Firstly, the swab must pass over both the tonsils and the posterior pharyngeal wall.[65] If this is not done correctly, the swab will often be negative. Secondly, negative results can also be obtained if the patient has been on antibiotics prior to obtaining the sample. Thirdly, the length of incubation is important, as 24 to 48 hours of incubation will identify more streptococci than that of 18 to 24 hours.[66] Fourthly, the number of colonies of growth, anaerobic versus aerobic incubation, and the bacitracin disc to identify GABHS are also important determinants of microbiological yield.[58,66,67]

Rapid Antigen Detection Kits

Rapid diagnosis of GABHS pharyngitis results in significant advantages. The spread of the illness can be checked and the morbidity of the illness reduced.[58,68,69] Most of the rapid antigen detection tests have an excellent specificity of around 95 percent when compared with sheep blood agar plates. This means that positive results can usually be trusted. However, as the sensitivity is often less than the specificity (around 80 to 90 percent), negative results cannot always be trusted. It has been recommended, therefore, that a negative antigen detection test be confirmed with a throat culture[70,71] (Recommendation A) (see Table 5–5).

Recently, newer antigen detection kits have been developed using enzyme immunoassay techniques, which have more sharply defined endpoints and an increased sensitivity. The most recent tests are optical immunoassay (OIA) and chemiluminescent DNA probes.[72–74] One trial compared the accuracy of an OIA for the rapid diagnosis of group A streptococcal pharyngitis with the gold standard blood agar plate (BAP) culture.[74] The trial took place in six pediatricians' offices in two cities. Over 2,000 patients with acute pharyngitis participated in it. In each office, the OIA was more sensitive than the BAP culture, with overall sensitivities of the OIA and BAP culture of 84 percent and 78 percent, respectively, while the specificities were 93 percent and 99 percent, respectively. The results of this office-based investigation suggest that, with adequately trained personnel, negative OIA test results need not always be routinely confirmed with BAP cultures. A 1998 decision analysis similarly concluded that confirmatory cultures do not have to be performed with the newer rapid diagnostic testing.[75]

Repeat diagnostic testing after therapy is not indicated for routine patients.[76] A significant number of them will demonstrate streptococcal carriage, which often results in additional antibiotic therapy. In addition, up to 25 percent of household contacts will harbor GABHS. As with carriers, it is not necessary to treat these individuals, unless they become symptomatic. It is only necessary to investigate and treat other asymptomatic individuals if there is an increased likelihood of nonsuppurative complications or if there is an outbreak of GABHS in a crowded community such as a school, day care, or long term care institution.

Treatment of GABHS Infection

The main benefits of correct treatment are the prevention of rheumatic fever and the relief of discomfort. Moreover, appropriate treatment will shorten the course of the illness, decrease the spread through the child's community, and reduce the likelihood of both suppurative and nonsuppurative complications.[77] Which treatment is most appropriate will depend on several factors such as clinical efficacy, likelihood of adherence, potential side effects, and cost to the patient. No medication or regimen provides 100 percent removal of GABHS from the pharynx. The various antibiotic treatment alternatives include penicillin, macrolides, cephalosporins, and others. Certain antibiotics should not be used. These treatment options are discussed below.

Penicillin

Penicillin is arguably the safest and most well known of all the antibiotics and is the standard choice in the treatment of GABHS pharyngitis. The only exception to this is for those individuals with penicillin allergy. It can be given either orally or intramuscularly with equal effectiveness. It has a very narrow spectrum of activity, and there have been no documented cases of resistance. However, oral penicillin fails to remove GABHS from the pharynx in 15 percent of those treated.[78] The reasons for this are unclear, although some have proposed that it may be due to poor compliance, inclusion of carriers in clinical trials, suboptimal doses, low penicillin concentration, or presence of beta-lactamase bacteria in the pharynx.[79]

The first-line therapy is oral penicillin V (phenoxymethyl penicillin) in the dose of 250 mg two or three times daily[77,80,81] (level III); or 25 to 30 mg/kg/day divided into two or three doses not exceeding 750 mg/day[82] (level III). Adolescents and adults probably need 500 mg three times daily[80] (level III). It is very important to remind patients to take the entire 10-day course, even though they will likely feel better in the first few days of treatment. This will improve the chance of GABHS eradication and prevent rheumatic fever. An injection of intramuscular penicillin G (Benzathine penicillin) can also be given in place of the 10-day course of the oral preparation. This is recommended when compliance is likely to be low or in cases of possible rheumatic fever. The injection is painful and should be given into a large muscle mass. The pain can be reduced by warming the injected solution or by using preparations that include procaine penicillin. The recommended dose is 600,000 Units IM (<27 kg) or 1.2 million Units (>27 kg).

Amoxicillin is often used in place of penicillin because of convenience or familiarity.[83] However, treatment with this broader-spectrum antibiotic is unnecessary and may increase antibiotic resistance.[84] One recent trial examined the use of this antibiotic as a once-daily therapy[85] (level I). One hundred and fifty children were randomly assigned to once-daily amoxicillin or three times daily penicillin V for 10 days. There was no significant difference in the clinical or bacteriologic outcome. Amoxicillin also requires a completed 10-day course of therapy.

The major problem with penicillin therapy, as noted above, is the potential for allergic reactions. These are rare and occur more often in adults than in children. Penicillin reaction can produce urticaria, angioneurotic edema, serum sickness, or, rarely, anaphylaxis. Many children are diagnosed with penicillin allergy due to the appearance of a rash during a previous antibiotic treatment. Although this rash may be due, in fact, to a viral agent, it is often mislabeled as an allergic reaction. Thus, many physicians opt to treat with a nonpenicillin antibiotic.

Even though there is little level I evidence for the use of penicillin as a first-line therapy, most would argue that the long experience with this medication, its safety profile, and lack of bacterial resistance, have proved it to be the drug of choice in GABHS pharyngitis (recommendation A) (Table 5–6).

Macrolides

The macrolide group of antibiotics provide an acceptable alternative to penicillin in the allergic patient.[86,87] Although rare in North America, there are some areas of the world where there is streptococcal resistance to macrolides[88]The major problems with the older versions of these drugs have been the gastrointestinal side effects such as abdominal discomfort. The most commonly prescribed macrolides are erythromycin estolate (20 to 40 mg/kg/day in two to four divided doses) or erythromycin ethylsuccinate (40 mg/kg/day in two to four divided doses)[79,82] (level III). Both these medications require a 10-day course. The newer macrolides are much better tolerated, being well absorbed orally and resulting in fewer gastrointestinal effects. Clarithromycin (15 mg/kg/day in two divided doses) can be given on a full or empty stomach but requires a 10-day course[89] (level I);[90,82,79] (level III). Azithromycin (12 mg/kg/day once daily, maximum 500 mg/day) must be given on an empty stomach but need only be given for 5 days.[91] (level I);[79] (level III). Both these newer medications compare favorably with oral penicillin in the treatment of GABHS pharyngitis.

There is good evidence that the newer macrolides provide an equivalent, though expensive, alternative to penicillin in patients with GABHS pharyngitis (recommendation A) (Table 5–6).

Cephalosporins

Cephalosporins are effective in a variety of infections including GABHS pharyngitis. Broad-spectrum cephalosporins (such as cefaclor, cefixime, cefprozil. cefuroxime axetil, cefpodoxime proxetil) should not be used as they provide a broader coverage than necessary. Antibiotics with a narrower spectrum (for example, cefadroxil or cephalexin) are preferable and require a 10-day course for the eradication of GABHS. It should be noted that approximately 20 percent of penicillin-allergic individuals are also allergic to cephalosporins.

Some reports have concluded that a 10-day course of an oral cephalosporin is superior to penicillin in the eradication of GABHS from the pharynx. In one study, a 10-day course of ceftibuten oral suspension was compared to penicillin V in children (aged between 3 and 18 years) who were treated for pharyngitis and scarlet fever[92] (level I). Overall clinical success at the primary end point of treatment was achieved in 97 percent of ceftibuten-treated patients versus 89 percent of penicillin V-treated patients. Streptococci elimination after 5 to 7 days of therapy was achieved in 91 percent of ceftibuten-treated patients versus 80 percent of penicillin V-treated patients. No patient developed rheumatic fever or nephritis. These data suggest that once-daily ceftibuten is as safe as and more effective than penicillin V three times daily for the treatment of GABHS pharyngitis.

In a similar study that compared cefuroxime axetil with penicillin V suspension, GABHS was eradicated from 94 percent of the cefuroxime patients and 84.1 percent of the penicillin-treated patients[93] (level I). In this study, cefuroxime axetil suspension given twice daily resulted in significantly greater bacteriologic and clinical efficacy than that of penicillin V suspension given three times daily to pediatric patients presenting with acute pharyngitis and a positive throat culture for GABHS. Another study reported similar results with cefpodoxime proxetil with greater eradication of *Streptococcus pyogenes* when compared with penicillin[94] (level I).

Results of these studies have been cited as evidence to encourage use of this class of antibiotics. However, most oral cephalosporins are still very expensive, and the broader versions may promote resistance. Currently, it would appear that these medications are not needed for the majority of patients but are an excellent alternative to penicillin. (Recommendation A) (see Table 5–6).

Additional Antibiotic Treatment

Clindamycin is useful in a few selected circumstances. It may be used as an alternative to penicillin in allergic individuals. Clindamycin (20 to 30 mg/kg/day in two to four doses for 10 days) can also be used in individuals with repeated culture-positive GABHS pharyngitis, especially if they fail to respond to penicillin[95] (level III) (Recommendation B) (see Table 5–6).

Certain antibiotics should not be used in treating GABHS pharyngitis as the bacterium has a high rate of resistance to tetracyclines, and sulphonamides do not eradicate GABHS from the pharynx. In addition, sulfadiazine does not prevent rheumatic fever. Chloramphenicol has unpredictable efficacy and is associated with more severe side effects.

Short Course Therapy

As has been noted, one of the major drawbacks of the oral penicillins, older macrolides and many of the cephalosporins is the 10-day duration of therapy. Many patients will discontinue treatment once they begin to feel better, which is often after 2 or 3 days. A shorter course of treatment thus has obvious advantages. There are a number of options available (Table 5–3)[79] (level III)). The choice of these options has to be balanced against both the greater cost and the problems associated with broader spectrum agents.

Current Management of Pharyngitis

Several studies have attempted to ascertain prevailing physician practice in the management of pharyngitis. In 1993, Schwartz found that only 44 percent of pediatricians used the currently recommended approach (defined as culture alone, or as a backup to a negative rapid test).[96] Hofer assessed pediatrician knowledge of and management strategies for GABHS pharyngitis.[83] This study surveyed 1,000 pediatricians chosen randomly from the membership of the American Academy of Pediatrics. The survey included questions relating to two

Table 5–3 Short-Course Therapy for GABHS Pharyngitis

Regimen	Dose and Duration
Benzathine penicillin	600,000 U IM injection (<27 kg) 1.2 million U IM injection (>27kg) once only
Cefadroxil	30 mg/kg/day po twice a day for 5 days
Cefuroxime axetil	20 mg/kg/day po twice a day for 4 to 5 days
Cefpodoxime proxetil	10 mg/kg/day po twice a day for 5 days
Azithromycin	12 mg/kg/day po once a day for 5 days

With permission from Dajani AS. Current therapy of group A streptococcal pharyngitis. Pediatr Ann 1998;27:277–80.

Table 5–4 Summary of Therapy: Common Cold

Intervention	Age Group	Level of Evidence	Recommendation
Steam inhalation therapy	Adults	Level I to II-1	C No evidence for children
Antihistamines	Children Adolescents and adults	Level I Level I	E C
Decongestants	Children Adolescents and adults	Level I to II-2 Level I to II-2	D C
Cough suppressants and expectorants	Children Adolescents and adults	Level I Level I	E D
Ipratropium nasal spray	Adolescents and adults	Level I	B No evidence for children
Combination products	Children Adolescents and adults	Level I Level I	E B
Antipyretics/ analgesics	Adolescents and adults	Level I	B No evidence for children
Zinc	Children Adolescents and adults	Level I Level I	E C
Antibiotics	Adults	Level I	D No evidence for children
Antivirals	Adults	Level I	D No evidence for children
Vitamin C	All ages	Level I	C

clinical scenarios, respondent demographics, and knowledge of streptococcal pharyngitis. Of the 510 respondents, antigen detection tests (ADTs) were used by 64 percent and throat cultures by 85 percent. Strategies for diagnosing streptococcal pharyngitis were throat culture alone (38 percent), considering positive ADTs definitive and using throat culture when ADTs are negative (42 percent), ADT alone (13 percent), ADT and throat culture for all patients with pharyngitis (5 percent), and no tests performed for GABHS (2 percent). Thirty-one percent usually or always were treated with antibiotics before test results were available. Only 29 percent of these "early treaters" always discontinued antibiotics when tests did not confirm the presence of group A streptococci. The drug of choice for treatment was penicillin (73 percent); another 26 percent preferred a derivative of penicillin, particularly amoxicillin. Follow-up throat culture was obtained by 51 percent of pediatricians after treatment

Table 5–5 Summary of Diagnostic Maneuvers: Streptococcal Pharyngitis

Diagnostic Maneuver	Level of Evidence	Recommendation
Scoring systems	Level II-2 to III	B
Rapid antigen detection systems	Level II-1	A, to use initially with backup culture, if negative. Newer tests may not require this.

Table 5–6 Summary of Therapy: Streptococcal Pharyngitis

Intervention	Level of Evidence	Recommendation
Penicillins	Level I to III	A
Macrolides	Level I to III	A, as an alternative to penicillin
Cephalosporins	Level I	A, as an alternative to penicillin
Clindamycin	Level III	B, for repeated culture positive pharyngitis

of recurrent streptococcal pharyngitis. The study concluded that most pediatricians managed acute GABHS pharyngitis appropriately, but 15 to 20 percent used diagnostic or treatment strategies that were not recommended. There was lack of a consensus about the management of recurrent GABHS pharyngitis and chronic carriage of GABHS.

A similar conclusion was found in a survey of Canadian family doctors, where the majority of physicians did not follow the recommendation to take a throat culture and wait for culture results before prescribing an antibiotic.[97] Another recent trial demonstrated that psychosocial factors play an important role in prescribing antibiotics even though symptom resolution was the same irrespective of the treatment.[98] This study found that antibiotic prescribing increased patients' desire to visit the doctor again. These studies suggest that the pressure on physicians to prescribe antibiotics results in frequent, inappropriate prescribing.

CONCLUSION

Colds and sore throats are frequently experienced by children and adolescents, affecting their sleep, and school and extracurricular activities. Although the common cold presents no diagnostic problems, treatment so far is, at best, only mildly effective. Additionally, the evidence would suggest that for preschool children, by far the most commonly affected, there is no effective treatment. For older children and, more convincingly, for adolescents, antihistamines, antihistamine-decongestant combinations, and ipratropium nasal spray will provide a measure of relief for some of the symptoms. The treatment of bacterial pharyngitis is straightforward, provided the diagnosis is made in an accurate fashion and there is appropriate follow-up. Currently, rapid throat antigen testing should be carried out first, followed by cultures if the initial testing is negative. The newer rapid tests may render the follow-up culture obsolete. Penicillin (or a macrolide, if allergic) still remains the best antibiotic for GABHS pharyngitis.

REFERENCES

1. Dingle JH, Badger GF, Jordan WS. Illness in the home: a study of 25,000 illnesses in a group of Cleveland families. Cleveland: Press of Western Reserve University; 1964.

2. Spector SL. The common cold: current therapy and natural history. J Allergy Clin Immunol 1995;95:1133–8.

3. Hemming VG. Viral respiratory diseases in children: classification, etiology, epidemiology and risk factors. J Pediatr 1994;124(Suppl 5):S13–6.

4. Glezen WP. Viral respiratory infections. Pediatr Ann 1991;20:407–12.

5. Smith MBH. Transmission and therapy of common respiratory viruses. Curr Opin Infect Dis 1995;8:209–12.

6. Kogan MD, Pappas G, Yu SM, Kotelchuck M. Over-the-counter medication use among US preschool age children. JAMA 1994;272:1025–30.

7. English JA, Bauman KA. Evidence-based management of upper respiratory infection in a family practice teaching clinic. Fam Med 1997;29:38–41.

8. Mainous AG III, Hueston WJ, Clark JR. Antibiotics and upper respiratory infection: do some folks think there is a cure for the common cold [see comments]. J Fam Pract 1996;42:357–61.

9. Mainous AG III, Hueston WJ, Love MM. Antibiotics for colds in children: who are the high prescribers? Arch Pediatr Adolesc Med 1998;152:349–52.

10. Pennie RA. Prospective study of antibiotic prescribing in children. Can Med Assoc J 1998;44:1850–5.

11. Smith MBH, Kogan MD. Over-the-counter medication use and toxicity in children. In: Kacew S, Lambert GH, editors. Environmental toxicology and pharmacology of human development. Washington DC: Taylor and Francis; 1997:175–86.

12. Eccles R, Jawad MS, Morris S. The effects of oral administration of menthol on nasal resistance to airflow and nasal sensation of airflow in subjects suffering from nasal congestion associated with the common cold. J Pharm Pharmacol 1990;42:652–4.

13. Ophir D, Elad Y. Effects of steam inhalation on nasal patency and nasal symptoms in patients with the common cold. Am J Otolaryngol 1987;8:149–53.

14. Tyrrell D, Barrow I, Arthur J. Local hyperthermia benefits natural and experimental common colds [published erratum appears in BMJ 1989;299(6699):600]. BMJ 1989;298:1280–3.

15. Forstall GJ, Macknin ML, Yen-Lieberman B, Medendorp SV. Effect of inhaling heated vapour on symptoms of the common cold. JAMA 1994;271:1109–11.

16. Hendley JO, Abott RD, Beasley PP, Gwaltney JM Jr. Effect of inhalation of hot humidified air on experimental rhinovirus infection. J Am Med Assoc 1994;271:1112–3.

17. Smith MB, Feldman W. Over-the-counter cold medications. A critical review of clinical trials between 1950 and 1991 [see comments]. JAMA 1993;269:2258–63.

18. Gaffey MJ, Kaiser DL, Hayden FG. Ineffectiveness of oral terfenadine in natural colds: evidence against histamine as a mediator of common cold symptoms. Pediatr Infect Dis 1988;7:223–8.

19. Eccles R, Cauwenberge PV, Tetzloff W, Borum P. A clinical study to evaluate the efficacy of the antihistamine doxylamine succinate in the relief of runny nose and sneezing associated with upper respiratory infection. J Pharm Pharmacol 1995;47:990–3.

20. Gwaltney JM Jr, Park J, Paul RA, et al. Randomized controlled trial of clemastine fumarate for treatment of experimental rhinovirus colds. Clin Infect Dis 1996;22:656–62.

21. Turner RB, Sperber SJ, Sorrentino JV, et al. Effectiveness of clemastine fumarate for treatment of rhinorrhea and sneezing associated with the common cold. Clin Infect Dis 1997;25:824-30.

22. Howard JC Jr, Kantner TR, Lilienfield LS, et al. Effectiveness of antihistamines in the symptomatic management of the common cold. JAMA 1979;242:2414–7.

23. Gwaltney JM Jr, Druce HM. Efficacy of brompheniramine maleate for the treatment of rhinovirus colds. Clin Infect Dis 1997;25:1188–94.

24. Luks D, Anderson MR. Antihistamines and the common cold. A review and critique of the literature. J Gen Intern Med 1996;11:240–4.

25. Cetaruk EW, Aaron CK. Hazards of nonprescription medications. Emer Med Clin N Am 1994;12:483–510.

26. Brown NJ, Ryder D, Branch RA. A pharmacodynamic interaction between caffeine and phenyl-propanolamine. Clin Pharmacol Therapeutics 1991;50:363–71.

27. Gronborg H, Winther B, Brofeldt S, et al. Effects of oral norephedrine on common cold symptoms. Rhinology 1983;21:3–12.

28. Winther B, Brofeldt S, Borum P, et al. Lack of effect on nasal discharge from a vasoconstrictor spray in the common cold. Euro J Res Dis 1983;64S:447–8.

29. Akerlund A, Klint T, Olen L, Rundcrantz H. Nasal decongestant effect of oxymetalazoline in the common cold: an objective dose-response study in 106 patients. J Laryngol Otol 1989;103:743–6.

30. Hamilton LH. Effect of xylometazoline nasal spray on nasal conductance in subjects with coryza. J Otolaryngol 1981;10:109–16.

31. Liebelt EL, Shannon M. Small doses, big problems: a selected review of highly toxic common medications. Pediatr Emer Care 1993;9:292–7.

32. Taylor JA, Novack AH, Almquist JR, Rogers JE. Efficacy of cough suppressants in children. J Pediatr 1993;122:799–802.

33. Kuhn JJ, Hendley JO, Adams KF, et al. Antitussive effect of guaifenesin in young adults with natural colds. Objective and subjective assessment. Chest 1982;82:713–8.

34. Hayden FG, Diamond L, Wood PB, et al. Effectiveness and safety of intranasal ipratropium bromide in common colds. A randomized, double-blind, placebo-controlled trial [see comments]. Ann Intern Med 1996;125:89–97.

35. Diamond L, Dockhorn RJ, Grossman J, et al. A dose-response study of the efficacy and safety of ipratropium bromide nasal spray in the treatment of the common cold. J Allergy Clin Immunol 1995;95:1139–46.

36. Clemens CJ, Taylor JA, Almquist JR, et al. Is an antihistamine-decongestant combination effective in temporarily relieving symptoms of the common cold in preschool children? [see comments]. J Pediatr 1997;130:463–6.

37. Schmitt BD. Fever phobia. Am J Dis Child 1980;134:176–81.

38. Kramer MS, Naimark L, LeDuc DG. Parental fever phobia and its correlates. Pediatr 1985;75:1110.

39. Drwal-Klein LA, Phelps SJ. Antipyretic therapy in the febrile child. Clin Pharm 1992;11:1005–21.

40. Graham NM, Burrell CJ, Douglas RM, et al. Adverse effects of aspirin, acetaminophen, and ibuprofen on immune function, viral shedding, and clinical status in rhinovirus-infected volunteers. J Infect Dis 1990;162:1277–82.

41. Sperber SJ, Hendley JO, Hayden FG, et al. Effects of naproxen on experimental rhinovirus colds. Ann Int Med 1992;117:37–41.

42. Eby GA, Davis DR, Halcomb WW. Reduction in duration of common colds by zinc gluconate lozenges in a double-blind study. Antimicrob Agents Chemother 1984;25:20–4.

43. Smith DS, Helzner EC, Nuttall CEJ, et al. Failure of zinc gluconate in the treatment of acute upper respiratory infection. Antimicrob Agents Chemother 1989;33:646–8.

44. Farr BM, Conner EM, Betts FR, et al. Two randomized controlled trials of zinc gluconate lozenge therapy of experimentally induced rhinovirus colds. Antimicrob Agents Chemother 1987;31:1183–7.

45. Farr BM, Gwaltney JM Jr. The problems of taste in placebo matching: an evaluation of zinc gluconate for the common cold. J Chronic Dis 1987;40:875–9.

46. Weismann K, Jakobsen JP, Weismann JE, et al. Zinc gluconate lozenges for common cold. A double-blind clinical trial. Dan Med Bull 1990;37:279–81.

47. Godfrey JC, Conant Sloan B, Smith DS, et al. Zinc gluconate and the common cold: a controlled clinical study. J Int Med Res 1992;20:234–46.

48. Mossad SB, Macknin M, Medendorp SV, et al. Zinc gluconate lozenges for treating the common cold: a randomized, double-blind, placebo-controlled study. Ann Intern Med 1996;125:81–8.

49. Macknin ML, Piedmonte M, Calendine C, et al. Zinc gluconate lozenges for treating the common cold in children: a randomized controlled trial [see comments]. JAMA 1998; 279:1962-7.

50. Kaiser DL, Lew D, Hirschel B, et al. Effects of antibiotic treatment in the subset of common cold patients who have bacteria in nasopharyngeal secretions. Lancet 1996;347:1507–10

51. Al-Nakib W, Higgins PG, Barrow GI, et al. Suppression of colds in human volunteers challenged with rhinovirus by a new synthetic drug (R61837). Antimicrob Agents Chemother 1989;33:522–5.

52. Hayden FG, Hipskind GJ, Woerner DH, et al. Intranasal pirodavir (R77,975) treatment of rhinovirus colds. Antimicrob Agents Chemother 1995;39:290–4.

53. Hayden FG, Albrecht JK, Kaiser DL, Gwaltney JM Jr. Prevention of natural colds by contact prophylaxis with intranasal alpha 2-interferon. N Engl J Med 1986;314:71–5.

54. Douglas RM, Moore BW, Miles HB, et al. Prophylactic efficacy of intranasal alpha 2-interferon against rhinovirus infections in the family setting. N Engl J Med 1986;314:65–70.

55. Monto AS, Schwartz SA, Albrecht JK. Ineffectiveness of postexposure prophylaxis of rhinovirus infection with low-dose intranasal alpha 2b interferon in families. Antimicrob Agents Chemother 1989;33:387–90.

56. Gwaltney JMJ Jr. Combined antiviral and antimediator treatment of rhinovirus colds. J Infect Dis 1992;166:776–82.

57. Douglas RM, Chalker EB, Treacy B. Vitamin C for the common cold (Cochrane Review). In: The Cochrane Library. Issue 4, 1998. Oxford, UK: Update Software.

58. Gerber MA. Diagnosis of group A streptococcal pharyngitis. Pediatr Ann 1998;27:269-73.

59. Breese BB. A simple scorecard for the tentative diagnosis of streptococcal pharyngitis. Am J Dis Child 1977;131:514–7.

60. Wald ER, Green MD, Schwartz B, Barbadora K. A streptococcal score card revisited. Pediatr Emer Care 1998;14:109–11.

61. McIsaac WJ, White D, Tannenbaum D, Low DE. A clinical score to reduce unnecessary antibiotic use in patients with sore throat. Can Med Assoc J 1998;158:75–83.

62. Schwartz RH, Gerber MA, McKay K. Pharyngeal findings of group A streptococcal pharyngitis. Arch Pediatr Adolesc Med 1998;152:927–8.

63. Gerber MA. Diagnosis of group A beta-hemolytic streptococcal pharyngitis. Use of antigen detection tests. Diag Microbiol Infect Dis 1986;4:5S–15.

64. Breese BB. Streptococcal pharyngitis and scarlet fever. Am J Dis Child 1978;132:612–6.

65. Brien JH, Bass JW. Streptococcal pharyngitis: optimal site for throat culture. J Pediatr 1985;106: 781–3.

66. Kellogg JA. Suitability of throat culture procedures for detection of group A streptococci and as reference standards for evaluation of streptococcal antigen detection kits. J Clin Microbiol 1990;28:165–9.

67. Roddey OF Jr, Clegg HW, Martin ES, et al. Comparison of throat culture methods for the recovery of group A streptococci in a pediatric office setting. JAMA 1995;274:1863–5.

68. Lieu TA, Fleisher GR, Schwartz JS. Clinical evaluation of a latex agglutination test for streptococcal pharyngitis: performance and impact on treatment rates. Pediatr Infect Dis J 1988;7:847–54.

69. Randolph MF, Gerber MA, DeMeo KK, et al. Effect of antibiotic therapy on the clinical course of streptococcal pharyngitis. J Pediatr 1985;106:870–5.

70. Gerber MA, Randolph MF, Chanatry J, et al. Antigen detection test for streptococcal pharyngitis: evaluation of sensitivity with respect to true infections. J Pediatr 1986;108:654–8.

71. Gerber MA. Culturing of throat swabs: end of an era? [editorial]. J Pediatr 1985;107:85–8.

72. Schlager TA, Hayden GA, Woods WA, et al. Optical immunoassay for rapid detection of group A beta-hemolytic streptococci. Should culture be replaced? Arch Pediatr Adolesc Med 1996;150:245–8.

73. Fries SM. Diagnosis of group A streptococcal pharyngitis in a private clinic: comparative evaluation of an optical immunoassay method and culture. J Pediatr 1995;126:933–6.

74. Gerber MA, Tanz RR, Kabat W, et al. Optical immunoassay test for group A beta-hemolytic streptococcal pharyngitis. An office-based, multicenter investigation [see comments]. JAMA 1997;277:899–903.

75. Webb KH. Does culture confirmation of high-sensitivity rapid streptococcal tests make sense? A medical decision analysis. Pediatrics 1998;101:2.

76. Gerber MA. Treatment failures and carriers: perception or problems? Pediatr Infect Dis J 1994;13:576–9.

77. Gerber MA, Markowitz M. Management of streptococcal pharyngitis reconsidered. Pediatr Infect Dis 1985;4:518–26.

78. Markowitz M, Gerber MA, Kaplan EL. Treatment of streptococcal pharyngotonsillitis: reports of penicillin's demise are premature. J Pediatr 1993;123:679–85.

79. Dajani AS. Current therapy of group A streptococcal pharyngitis. Pediatr Ann 1998;27:277–80.

80. Dajani AS, Taubert K, Ferrieri P, et al. Treatment of acute streptococcal pharyngitis and prevention of rheumatic fever: a statement for health professionals. Committee on Rheumatic Fever, Endocarditis, and Kawasaki Disease of the Council on Cardiovascular Disease in the Young, the American Heart Association. Pediatrics 1995;96:758–64.

81. Bass JW. Antibiotic management of group A streptococcal pharyngotonsillitis. Pediatr Infect Dis 1991;10:S43–9.

82. Marinac BL, Smith JL. Formulary. In: Dipchand AI, editor. The HSC handbook of pediatrics. Toronto: Mosby; 1997.p.557–633.

83. Hofer C, Binns HJ, Tanz RR. Strategies for managing group A streptococcal pharyngitis. A survey of board-certified pediatricians. Arch Pediatr Adolesc Med 1997;151:824–9.

84. Schwartz B, Marcy M, Phillips WR, et al. Pharyngitis—principles of judicious use of antimicrobial agents. Pediatr 1998;101:171–4.

85. Feder HM, Gerber MA, Randolph MF, et al. Once-daily therapy for streptococcal pharyngitis with amoxicillin. Pediatr 1999;103:47–51.

86. Breese BB, Disney FA, Talpey W, et al. Streptococcal infections in children. Comparison of the therapeutic effectiveness of erythromycin administered twice daily with erythromycin, penicillin phenoxymethyl, and clindamycin administered three times daily. Am J Dis Child 1974;128:457–60.

87. Derrick CW, Dillon HC. Erythromycin therapy for streptococcal pharyngitis. Am J Dis Child 1976;130:175–8.

88. Seppala H, Nissinen A, Jarvinen H, et al. Resistance to erythromycin in group A streptococci. New Eng J Med 1992;326:292–7.

89. Still JG, Hubbard WC, Poole JM, et al. Comparison of clarithromycin and penicillin VK suspensions in the treatment of children with streptococcal pharyngitis and review of currently available alternative antibiotic therapies [see comments]. Pediatr Infect Dis J 1993;12:S134–41.

90. Schrock CG. Clarithromycin vs. penicillin in the treatment of streptococcal pharyngitis. J Fam Pract 1992;35:622–6.

91. Hooton TM. A comparison of azithromycin and penicillin V for the treatment of streptococcal pharyngitis. Am J Med 1991;91:23S–30.

92. Pichichero ME, McLinn SE, Gooch WM III, et al. Ceftibuten vs. penicillin V in group A beta-hemolytic streptococcal pharyngitis. Members of the Ceftibuten Pharyngitis International Study Group. Pediatr Infect Dis J 1995;14:S102–7.

93. Gooch WM III, McLinn SE, Aronovitz GH, et al. Efficacy of cefuroxime axetil suspension compared with that of penicillin V suspension in children with group A streptococcal pharyngitis. Antimicrob Agents Chemother 1993;37:159–63.

94. Dajani AS, Kessler SL, Mendelson R, et al. Cefpodoxime proxetil vs. penicillin V in pediatric streptococcal pharyngitis/tonsillitis. Pediatr Infect Dis J 1993;12:275–9.

95. Bisno AL, Gerber MA, Gwaltney JM Jr, et al. Diagnosis and management of group A streptococcal pharyngitis: a practice guideline. Infectious Diseases Society of America [see comments]. Clin Infect Dis 1997;25:574–83.

96. Schwartz B, Fries S, Fitzgibbon AM, et al. Pediatricians' diagnostic approach to pharyngitis and impact of CLIA 1988 on office diagnostic tests. JAMA 1994;271:234–8.

97. McIsaac WJ, Goel V. Sore throat management practices of Canadian family physicians. Fam Pract 1997;14:34–9.

98. Little P, Williamson I, Warner G, et al. Open randomised trial of prescribing strategies in managing sore throat. Br Med J 1997;314:722–7.

CHAPTER 6

Otitis Media

Moshe Ipp, MBBCh, FRCPC, FAAP

The need to optimize the diagnosis and management of otitis media in children, on the basis of available evidence, has become crucial for several vitally important reasons. The continued emergence of bacteria resistant to antibiotics has become a worldwide problem, and the unnecessary and frequent prescribing of antibiotics for otitis media in children is considered to have contributed to the spread of antibiotic resistance. Otitis media is the dominant reason for the use of antibiotics in children, and the condition is being diagnosed more frequently now than ever before.[1,2] Data from the United States show that between 1975 and 1990, the number of physician visits due to otitis media increased from 9.9 million to 24.5 million visits[2] and that 2 to 4 billion dollars are spent each year in the medical and surgical management of pediatric otitis media.[3] Otitis media is frequently overdiagnosed or misdiagnosed, and it has been estimated that, on average, children receive more than a month of antibiotic therapy for otitis media in each of the first 2 years of life.[4] For all these reasons and primarily to improve the quality of care, to provide optimal standards for the management of otitis media, and to set meaningful clinical practice guidelines, the current evidence in the literature regarding the management of otitis media must be critically evaluated.

DIAGNOSIS

Definitions

The term "otitis media" encompasses a number of clinical conditions, each called by a variety of names. The diagnosis is based on the clinician's skill and knowledge of the criteria necessary to categorize middle-ear disease in its various forms. The importance of distinguishing the different forms of otitis media leads to a management strategy that supports the use of antibiotics in the children who need them and prevents the use in those for whom antibiotics would not be beneficial.

- *Acute otitis media* (AOM) is an inflammation of the middle ear that presents with a rapid onset of signs and symptoms. The Agency for Health Care Policy and Research (AHCPR) in the United States has defined AOM as fluid in the middle ear, accompanied by signs or symptoms of acute local or systemic illness.[5]
- *Otitis media with effusion* (OME), previously known as serous otitis media, has been defined as the presence of fluid in the middle ear, without signs and symptoms of an ear infection, and may arise following AOM or may occur spontaneously.[5]
- *Recurrent AOM* is defined as at least three episodes of AOM in a period of 6 months or four episodes in 12 months.
- *Acute otitis media with otorrhea* includes the presence of discharge (usually purulent) from the middle ear.

Acute Otitis Media

It is important to make an accurate diagnosis before treating AOM; and this may be difficult, especially in young infants, in whom crying, irritability, and lack of cooperation make otoscopic and pneumatoscopic examinations very difficult. It must be emphasized that because the frequency and severity of symptoms of otitis media vary so widely, the clinician cannot rely on history alone nor on visual inspection of the tympanic membrane alone to make the diagnosis of AOM. It has been estimated that even the best combination of signs and symptoms can only predict AOM correctly in ~70 percent of cases.[6] Some of the errors that can lead to the misdiagnosis of AOM include attempting to make the diagnosis without removing ear wax to properly visualize the tympanic membrane, a mistaken belief that a red membrane with normal mobility or the absence of a light reflex alone establishes the diagnosis of AOM, inadequate lighting (a halogen lamp rather than an incandescent bulb is mandatory), using a wrong-sized speculum (which prevents adequate penetration into the external auditory canal), and not ensuring proper restraint of the child (parent's lap is preferable and less traumatic for the child) or providing proper instructions prior to the examination.[7]

The problem with the clinical criteria used to diagnose AOM is that it is difficult to validate or standardize those criteria that are needed for an accurate diagnosis. In one survey of clinical diagnostic standards for AOM, 18 different criteria were used in 26 publications, and 147 different sets of diagnostic criteria were given by 165 practicing pediatricians.[8] The diagnosis of otitis media requires visualization of the tympanic membrane for position, color, translucency, and assessment of mobility by pneumatic otoscopy.[9,10] Pneumatic otoscopy is a two-step procedure. In the first instance, the physician inspects the ear canal and ear drum visually, removing any obstructing cerumen or debris. In the second step, a seal is created in the ear canal, using a flanged ear speculum, and then very slight positive and then negative pressure is applied while watching the movement of the tympanic membrane. The clinician should be aware that only a slight pressure is required to move the ear drum. The sensitivity of pneumatoscopy has been found to be 85 to 90 percent with a specificity of 70 to 79 percent.[9] Combining the position (bulging), color (red), and mobility of the tympanic membrane (impaired) results in >83 percent predictive value for middle-ear effusion when compared with the findings at myringotomy.[11] A mnemonic that is useful to ensure adequacy of examination for the diagnosis of otitis media has recently been published.[12] The components of this examination include *Color*, *Other* conditions (air-fluid level, bullae, atrophic areas, retraction pockets), *Mobility*, *Position*, *Lighting* (halogen, fully charged), *Entire* surface (anterior, superior, inferior etc.), *Translucency*, *External* auditory canal and *Seal* (COMPLETES).

Although earache is the most significant symptom predicting AOM, it may also occur in the absence of AOM, indicating that it is not a specific symptom of AOM; therefore, medication for AOM should not be prescribed on the basis of earache alone.[6] Furthermore, signs and symptoms such as fever, irritability, lethargy, anorexia, vomiting, diarrhea, tugging of the ear, and tympanic membrane erythema may accompany AOM but are not specific enough to make a diagnosis of AOM.[6,13,14] In Weiss' literature review of signs and symptoms of AOM, upper respiratory tract infection symptoms were present in 94 percent of cases, fever in 55 percent, and earache in 47 percent.[15]

In summary, it is clear that making the diagnosis of AOM is not an easy matter. Although the reality of practice by many primary care physicians is simple otoscopy without pneumatic insufflation, it cannot reliably detect the presence of middle-ear fluid and therefore is not sufficiently accurate in diagnosing AOM.[16] The diagnosis of AOM requires both signs and symptoms of acute local or systemic illness and a bulging eardrum, confirmed by reduced tympanic membrane mobility, which indicate fluid (pus) in the middle ear.

Otitis Media with Effusion

The clinical diagnosis of OME is based on the asymptomatic presence of fluid in the middle ear, verified by pneumatoscopy and confirmed by tympanometry.[5] The positive predictive value for middle-ear effusion of a flat tympanogram (ie, likelihood of an effusion being present, if the tympanogram is abnormal) has been found to be between 49 and 99 percent.[17] Problems have arisen, however, with the application of tympanogram findings to clinical practice because of the categorization of tympanograms and the absence of data that would allow calculation of true sensitivity, specificity, and negative predictive values.

MICROBIOLOGY

The appropriate treatment of otitis media depends on the knowledge of the etiologic agents, the natural history of spontaneous resolution, and the emerging patterns of microbial resistance. Understanding this is crucial for the clinician, since AOM is associated with a high incidence of actual and perceived unresponsiveness to therapy, relapse, recurrence, and chronicity despite the availability of effective antibiotics.

Etiologic Agents

Viral Causes

Although AOM is generally considered to be a bacterial disease, the role of viruses has become more important recently because of the implications of secondary prevention of AOM by vaccination[18,19] and the concept of withholding antibiotics[2] in the treatment of non-bacterial disease.

A viral upper respiratory tract infection is a frequent antecedent of AOM, and viral agents are considered to be solely responsible for one-third of cases of AOM,[10] which presumably do not require treatment with antibiotics. Acute otitis media has been documented in 20 to 50 percent of hospitalized patients with laboratory-confirmed respiratory viral infections,[20] in which respiratory syncytial virus, rhinovirus, adenovirus, and influenza virus have been the most frequently isolated. Infection with influenza virus alone, which is preventable by vaccination,[18] may result in AOM in 10 to 50 percent of cases.

In patients with AOM, the presence of a virus in the middle-ear fluid may be important for other reasons, since it is now thought that viruses may interfere with the bacteriologic and clinical responses to antibiotics and may be responsible for the persistence of symptoms in some patients. This occurs more frequently in patients with combined bacteria and viruses in the middle ear rather than in those with bacteria or viruses alone.[21]

Bacterial Causes

A bacterial pathogen is isolated from the middle-ear fluid in approximately 66 percent of children with AOM. This is based on results from cultures of the middle-ear fluid obtained by tympanocentesis or needle aspiration; with the exception of *Moraxella catarrhalis*, the cultures have been consistent over the past 40 years.[10] The three most common bacteria identified are *Streptococcus pneumoniae*, which accounts for 20 to 40 percent, nontypable *Haemophilus influenzae*, which accounts for 10 to 20 percent, and *M. catarrhalis*, which accounts for 5 to 15 percent of AOM. Group A *Streptococcus* and *Staphylococcus aureus* are much less common causes of AOM and account for only 2 to 3 percent of AOM.[20,22,23] These bacterial causes of AOM are indistinguishable by clinical signs, but disease due to *Pneumococcus* is more likely to be severe and less likely to remit spontaneously than disease due to *H. influenzae* and *M. catarrhalis*.[24]

Natural History and Spontaneous Resolution of Otitis Media

There appears to be a high rate of spontaneous bacterial resolution of AOM (Table 6–1), but the rate differs depending on the infecting organism.[24] The importance of this information is that it may ultimately affect management strategies in terms of antibiotic choices and whether or not to use antibiotics. The spontaneous resolution data have been estimated from placebo-treated children with AOM (see Table 6–1), in whom those episodes caused by

Table 6–1   Spontaneous Resolution of AOM by Etiologic Agent*

Organism	Spontaneous Resolution Rate (%)
S. pneumoniae	19
H. influenzae	48
M. catarrhalis	75
Virus	100

*Data from [23–25]

S. pneumoniae resolved spontaneously in 19 percent of cases, and in those caused by *H. influenzae*, they resolved spontaneously in 48 percent of cases.[25,26] Although data from placebo-controlled trials are not available for children with AOM caused by *M. catarrhalis*, amoxicillin-treated, beta-lactamase–positive *M. catarrhalis* (which is resistant to amoxicillin) resolved spontaneously in 75 percent of cases.[26]

From a clinical standpoint, the spontaneous resolution rate of AOM has been shown to be in excess of 80 percent.[27–29] In two recent well-designed clinical trials, spontaneous resolution of AOM occurred in 86 percent and 92 percent, respectively, of placebo-treated children (level I).[27,28] This favorable natural history of AOM has also been demonstrated in a meta-analysis of 5,400 children enrolled in 33 randomized controlled trials, in which 81 percent of untreated children had spontaneous resolution of their AOM (level l).[29] Further support for spontaneous resolution comes from data showing excellent (93 percent) concordance between bacteriologic and clinical success[30] and is consistent with the belief that many children improve clinically without antibiotic treatment. Despite the cumulative evidence from randomized controlled trials indicating that the majority of AOM resolves spontaneously without treatment, it is still considered that antibiotic therapy has a significant, though modest, effect on the primary control of AOM[29,31] and remains the standard of care for the treatment of AOM in North America.[2] It is estimated that seven children need antibiotic treatment in order to facilitate resolution in one.[29]

Antibiotic Resistance

An alarming increase of resistant strains among the three main bacteria causing otitis media has occurred over the last 20 years. For *H. influenzae* and *M. catarrhalis*, the percentage of beta-lactamase producing isolates has increased dramatically to 30 percent and 90 percent respectively,[32] producing profound resistance to the aminopenicillins.

Unlike the resistance seen with *H. influenzae* and *M. catarrhalis*, drug-resistant *S. pneumoniae* (DRSP) develops through alterations in penicillin-binding proteins.[33] *S. pneumoniae* may be divided into susceptible strains, with a minimal inhibitory concentration (MIC) <0.1 µg/mL and nonsusceptible strains (PNSP) with MIC ≥0.1 µg/mL. The subgroup among the nonsusceptible strains with MIC ≥2 µg/mL are considered resistant (PRSP)[34]. Older terminology refers to nonsusceptible strains as resistant strains; those with MIC between 0.1 and 2 µg/mL are termed intermediate level resistance and strains with MIC ≥2 µg/mL are seen to demonstrate high level resistance. The frequency of DRSP varies considerably, ranging from 10 to 30 percent in the United States to 40 to 70 percent in Spain, Hungary, South Africa, France, and some Asian countries.[22] Canada is experiencing a period of rapid increase in the prevalence of DRSP as has previously occurred in the United States and other countries. In 1993 to 1994, 7 percent of clinical isolates from community and hospital laboratories in Toronto were PNSP.[35] In 1994 to 1995, 11.7 percent of isolates obtained from 39 laboratories across Canada were PNSP, of which 3.3 percent were PRSP.[36] Risk factors for carriage of or disease with DRSP (see Table 6–2) include recent hospitalization, recent beta lactam antibiotic therapy, young age, and day-care attendance.[37,38]

There are indications that if unnecessary antibiotic use can be curtailed, both the individual patient and the community will benefit. In 1974, in Japan, 62 percent of all isolates of group A *Streptococcus* were resistant to macrolides, which accounted for 22 percent of all antibiotic use in that country. By 1988, less than 2 percent of isolates were resistant to erythromycin, which coincided with a decreased use of macrolides to 8 percent of all antibiotics used.[39] Similarly, antibiotic resistance in Spain[40] and in Iceland[41] have shown a correlation between those regions with the lowest antibiotic use and those with the lowest rate of penicillin resistant *S. pneumoniae*. This reduction in the spread of resistant bacteria appears to be controlled by the judicious use of antibiotics.

MANAGEMENT

General Considerations.

Physicians cannot usually determine clinically whether or not their patients with AOM will have spontaneous resolution of their illness and whether the very young infants will have adverse outcomes if untreated. Therefore, antibiotic therapy remains the current North American standard of care for AOM, even though the treatment effect is small.[2] Pooled data from four randomized controlled trials (RCT) in a single meta-analysis showed that antibiotics had a 14 percent increase in clinical cures over placebo or no antibiotic (level I).[29] The criteria used for clinical cure included complete resolution of all presenting clinical signs and symptoms, exclusive of asymptomatic middle-ear effusion. The management of AOM thus still focuses on the choice of appropriate antibiotics, but a serious trend towards developing alternative strategies for some patients is rapidly evolving because of the increasing concern felt by physicians regarding the overuse of antibiotics. A reasonable evolving strategy to the management of AOM can be based on the age of the child at presentation (similar to the age format used to manage other pediatric conditions such as fever). The dividing line is 2 years of age, as those under 2 years are considered to be more vulnerable and at higher risk for persistence and recurrence of AOM,[30,42,43] and should be managed differently from those older than 2 years of age.

Management in Children Under 2 Years of Age.

A conventional 10-day course of appropriate antibiotics remains the standard of care for children under 2 years of age.[2,44] It is considered by some that longer therapy may result in a limited short-term but no long-term advantage.[45] Shorter therapy may result in more treatment failures in this age group.[2,3,43,46] Most children will respond to antibiotics with significant resolution of acute signs within 48 to 72 hours. If the signs and symptoms are worse at any time or if there is no improvement by 72 hours, the child should be re-examined to determine if there is a need for an alternative treatment strategy or if another antibiotic should be pre-

---

Table 6–2 Children at Risk for Drug-Resistant *S.Pneumonia* (DRSP)

- Less than 18 to 24 months old

- Day-care attendance

- Antibiotics in previous 1 month

- Recent hospitalization

scribed. Once the child responds to therapy, the question of when a follow-up visit should be scheduled to assess the resolution of middle-ear fluid remains controversial. A visit at 10 to 14 days has been the standard practice to determine if the AOM has resolved or not.[47] A recent study, however, has challenged this timing by showing that parents' assessments were as accurate as those of physicians in determining whether the child's infection had resolved at 14 days or not[42] (level II, recommendation B) and only those children at high risk for AOM such as infants less than 15 months of age and those with a family history of recurrent AOM and those children with parents who feel the infection is not resolved required immediate post-treatment follow-up. Some experts suggest that it might be reasonable to re-examine the child's ears 8-12 weeks after the onset of the AOM to identify those children who might have persistent OME that may require further intervention.[47]

Management In Children Over 2 Years of Age.

The main thrust of new and alternative approaches to the management of AOM are now being directed toward defining a group of children considered at low risk for serious sequelae (see Table 6–3) and who can be treated with a short course of antibiotics[48–50] (level I, recommendation A), or, at least initially, can be treated with symptomatic therapy and possibly either delay or avoid the use of antibiotics altogether.[31] Low-risk children (see Table 6–3) are defined as those over 2 years of age, who do not present with severe pain, are not sick or toxic, do not have an ear discharge, have no underlying disease, are not immunocompromised, do not have a history of recurrent or chronic otitis media, and for whom good follow-up care is available.[2] While 10 days of antibiotic therapy is the current North American standard of care for AOM, children often fail to complete the course of treatment anyway reflecting more realistically the actual practices of parents in the real world.[51] Prescribing shorter courses of antibiotics for treatment of AOM can be costsaving and exert less selective pressure that would favor the emergence of resistant organisms.

Short Course Treatment

A recent meta-analysis of randomized controlled trials comparing short-course treatment with traditional treatment for AOM has suggested that 5 days of antibiotic treatment is effective for uncomplicated AOM[52] (level I, recommendation A). Until further data are available, short-course treatment should be restricted to children older than 2 years of age, since younger children appear to be at increased risk for treatment failure, even with conventional dosing.[2,3,43,46] The treatment should also exclude those children with underlying medical conditions, those with chronic or recurrent otitis media, and those with draining ears; none of these were included in the trials evaluated.

Table 6–3   Children with AOM Considered at Low Risk for Serious Sequelae

- Older than 2 years of age
- Mild and/or unilateral AOM
- Normal host (no immune deficiency, chronic disease)
- No otorrhea
- No toxicity or severe pain
- No history of chronic or recurrent otitis media
- Availability of good follow-up

Delayed Treatment with Antibiotics

In the Netherlands and some other European countries, the standard of care for treating AOM in children over 2 years of age is to delay treatment with antibiotics for up to three days and only to introduce antibiotics if there are continued symptoms.[49,53] In a Dutch randomized controlled trial with treatment and no treatment groups (but which was not placebo-controlled and was not properly blinded), it was found that antibiotic therapy and myringotomy were unnecessary in most cases of AOM and should be reserved for those with an irregular course, suppurative complications, and persistent discharge (level I, recommendation C).[54] There have been no controlled studies which have investigated whether the guidelines from the Netherlands result in worse outcome or complications when compared with North American guidelines but van Buchem reported results of an audit of this conservative management of AOM, consisting of nose drops and analgesics alone without antibiotics, noting that only 2.7% of 4,860 children had continued symptoms of pain or fever requiring treatment.[55]

Selecting an Antibiotic

The best approach for selecting an antibiotic for treating AOM should be based not simply on which agent to use but on whether it is to be used for first-line, second-line, or prophylactic therapy. First-line antibiotics are used for initial empiric treatment of uncomplicated AOM. Second-line agents are indicated for initial treatment failures. Recommended drugs for treating otitis media are listed in Table 6–4 .

First-Line Treatment

Aminopenicillins (Amoxicillin, Pivampicillin) remain the recommended first-line drug of choice for the treatment of uncomplicated AOM (level III, recommendation B).[56–58] Aminopenicillins are safe, well tolerated, have a proven and enduring track record, and are effective against the main organisms causing AOM.[59] It is not surprising why aminopenicillins are so effective in the treatment of uncomplicated AOM when the microbiological data and other factors are taken into account. It has been estimated that of 100 children presenting with AOM, only 10 will have resistant organisms (beta-lactamase-producing or penicillin-binding) that will be unresponsive to an aminopenicillin.[60] There is no therapeutic benefit to initial empiric treatment with second-line agents. A disturbing recent trend is the use of expensive, broad-spectrum agents for the treatment of AOM, and it is this aggressive approach that reflects the unrealistic expectations on the part of practitioners.[46]

Second-Line Treatment

Factors that must be considered when a child does not respond to initial therapy for AOM include poor compliance, inadequate dosing, vomiting, and the most important new development, failure or persistence of AOM due to the presence of a resistant organism.[61] Viral pathogens or copathogens in the middle ear may be another contributing factor to account for persistent AOM.[21] Since the cause of the failed initial treatment is usually not apparent, the choice of a second-line antibiotic is empirical and is often based on the experience of selected antibiotic use by each individual physician.[62] Differences in terms of clinical efficacy, if present, among the various antibiotics used as second-line treatment have been considered by some authorities to be too small to be detected.[63] All the antibiotics listed (see Table 6–4) have activity against the common bacterial pathogens causing otitis media, although variations favoring one antibiotic over another do exist. These include drug safety, patient compliance (eg, frequency and duration of administration, taste, cost), and drug efficacy (eg, resistance to certain organisms and pharmacokinetics manifest, in part, by the drug's ability to achieve satisfactory concentrations in middle-ear fluid).

Table 6–4 Antibiotics for Acute Otitis Media and Dosage Schedules

First-Line Choices		
Aminopenicillin (Amoxil, Pondocillin)	40 mg/kg/d	tid or bid
Second-Line Choices		
Aminopenicillins		
Amoxicillin (Amoxil)	80 to 90 mg/kg/d	tid or bid
Amoxicillin/Clavulanate (Clavulin)	40 to 90 mg/kg/d	tid (4:1 formulation) or bid (7:1 formulation)
Cephalosporins		
Second generation		
Cefaclor (Ceclor)	40 mg/kg/d	tid or bid
Cefuroxime (Ceftin)	30 to 40 mg/kg/d	bid
Third generation		
Cefprozil (Cefzil)	30 mg/kg/d	bid
Cefixime (Suprax)	8 mg/kg/d	od or bid
Ceftriaxone (Rocephin)	50 mg/kg/d	Daily x IM (1 to 3 doses)
Macrolide/Azalide		
Azithromycin (Zithromax)	10 mg/kg/d on day 1 5 mg/kg/d on days 2 to 5	od
Clarithromycin (Biaxin)	15 mg/kg/d	bid
Other		
Erythromycin-sulfisoxazole (Pediazole)	40 mg/kg/d erythromycin	tid
Trimethoprim-sulfamethoxazole (Bactrim, Septra)	8-12 mg/kg day trimethoprim	bid
Clindamycin (Dalacin)	15 mg/kg/d	tid or qid

Although amoxicillin is not commonly regarded as a second-line drug, when it is administered in high doses (80 to 90 mg/kg/day) its concentration in middle-ear fluid reaches levels high enough (2 to <9 µg/mL) to be effective against most strains of PNSP (MIC 0.1 to 1.0 µg/mL) and approximately one third of PRSP (MIC >1.0 µg/mL) isolates.[64] Amoxicillin has also been shown to have a greater time above the MIC than any other oral antibiotic.[65,66] This makes high-dose amoxicillin the only oral agent that appears to have a high enough therapeutic index to provide consistent activity against fully resistant DRSP (with MIC up to ~4µg/mL). When amoxicillin is combined with a low dose of clavulanic acid, it also becomes effective against beta-lactamase–producing organisms. A fixed formulation of a new 7:1 amoxicillin:clavulanate ratio is now available in Canada, and a 14:1 formulation of amoxicillin:clavulanate is currently under investigation. The initial data on gastrointestinal side effects show no increase with the new high-dose amoxicillin/clavulanate combination, where the total daily dose of clavulanate is not to exceed 10 mg/kg/day.[64,67] Cefuroxime axetil (Ceftin) is also effective against both DRSP and beta-lactamase-producing *H. influenzae*. However, the bacterial failure rates of cefuroxime increase markedly once *S. pneumoniae* resistance surpasses the mid-intermediate range (MIC >0.5 µg/mL).[58,68] Cefprozil (Cefzil) has *S. pneumoniae* activity that is less than that of amoxicillin and, like the macrolides, appears to be less clinically effective against *H. influenzae* and *M. catarrhalis*.[69–71] On the basis of these data, macrolides and cefprozil are relatively poor choices for second-line therapy of otitis media. Cefaclor (Ceclor), another commonly used cephalosporin, although effective against *H. influenzae* and *M. catarrhalis* is substantially less effective than amoxicillin against pneumococci.[68] Trimethoprim/sulfamethoxazole, which has been used in the past as both first- and second-line agent, is no longer considered an effective form of therapy for AOM.[72] *S. pneumoniae* resistance to trimethoprim/sulfamethoxazole occurs in ~ 25 percent of isolates and tends to be at a high level when it occurs.[66]

Intramuscular ceftriaxone, given as a single dose or three daily doses, has also been shown to be effective in the treatment of AOM,[73–75] but should be reserved for severe infections, for those situations where compliance with a 10-day oral regimen is unlikely, or when there is vomiting or diarrhea precluding the use of oral medication.

Clindamycin is another agent that is effective against DRSP, but it is not effective against *H. influenzae* or *M. catarrhalis*[76,77] and should only be used in culture-confirmed cases of *S. pneumoniae* disease.

Special Circumstances

Some circumstances may warrant initial treatment of AOM with agents known to have better activity against resistant organisms. When AOM is accompanied by purulent conjunctivitis, termed "otitis conjunctivitis syndrome," beta-lactamase–producing *H. influenzae* is often the causative organism, and a second-line agent would be a preferable choice for initial treatment.[78] Children who are toxic or have immunodeficiencies or known exposure to resistant *S. pneumoniae* (for example, those recently hospitalized) may be candidates for initial treatment with a second-line agent.

Treatment of Otitis Media with Effusion

The U.S. Agency for Health Care Policy and Research (AHCPR) has defined a patient with OME as a child between 1 and 3 years of age, with effusion present 6 weeks after an episode of otitis media but with no apparent symptoms and no underlying medical condition.[5] The treatment of such a child with OME is based on the current knowledge of the natural history of OME and its prevalence, which may vary according to the study being reported. There is no scientific evidence that has documented the frequency of OME but it has been estimated by the National Center for Health Statistics in the United States that 25 to 35 percent of cases of "otitis media" are represented by OME[79]. Two studies have helped clarify our understanding of the natural history of OME. In the first study, which looked at a large sample size of 1,439 Dutch children with OME, approximately 60 percent recovered within 3 months, without intervention[80] and in the second 2-year U.S study, 80 percent of 103 children aged 2 to 6 years with OME, cleared without treatment within 2 months.[81] On the basis of these data, an expert panel of the AHCPR has concluded that in the majority of cases of OME, antibiotics can be avoided while the OME is allowed to resolve spontaneously (level III).[5]

There are, however, three meta-analyses of published trials of antibiotic therapy for OME that have shown a small but statistically significant effect of short-term resolution.[5,82,83] Of greater importance, however, is that there was no significant difference in the incidence of OME when assessed 1 month after treatment was completed, whether placebo or antibiotic was used. This finding has led many experts to recommend that initial treatment of middle-ear effusion (OME) in the absence of AOM should not be treated with antibiotics at all (level III).[5]

Surgical intervention with bilateral myringotomy and insertion of tubes should *not* be performed for initial management of OME but is recommended for those otherwise healthy children in whom bilateral effusion has been documented to persist for 3 months or longer and which is accompanied by significant hearing loss (defined as 20 decibels hearing threshold level or worse in the better hearing ear)[5].

Prevention of Recurrent Acute Otitis Media

Antibiotics

The use of prophylactic antibiotics has been shown, in a meta-analysis of nine trials involving the evaluation of 958 patients, to be successful in reducing the number of episodes of

Table 6–5 Evolving New Strategies for the Management of Otitis Media

Condition	Intervention	Level of Evidence	Recommendation
1. AOM <2 y of age	Antibiotics for 10 days	I	A
a. No antibiotic last 1 month	a. amoxicillin (standard dose)*	I	A
b. Antibiotic last 1 month or treatment failure after 3 days	b. amoxicillin (high dose)† or amoxicillin/clavulanate (standard dose)‡ or amoxicillin/clavulanate (high dose)§ or cefuroxime axetil// (Choice of antibiotic based on local/regional prevalence of DRSP)	III	B
2. AOM >2 y of age uncomplicated, low risk (see Table 6–3)	a. Standard of care in North America amoxicillin (short course,# standard dose*)	I	A
	b. Standard of care in some European countries • Withhold or delay antibiotic treatment for 2 to 3 days. • Observation and analgesia, provided good follow-up available. • If persistent pain, treat as in 2a.	I	C
3. AOM >2 y of age Antibiotic last 1 month	Same as 1b (Choice of antibiotic based on local/regional prevalence of DRSP)	III	B
4. AOM any age Treatment failure Day 3	Amoxicillin/clavulanate (standard or high dose) or cefuroxime axetil// or ceftriaxone IM** or clindamycin†† (Choice of antibiotic based on local/regional prevalence of DRSP)	III	B
5. Recurrent AOM (see text for definition)	a. Prophylactic antiobiotics: effective, but benefits must be weighed against risks of producing antibiotic resistance	I	A
	b. Placement of tympanostomy tubes	I	A
	c. Others:		
	eliminate pacifier, eliminate	II-2	B
	smoking, sleep supine, reduce day	II-2	C
	care, encourage breast feeding,	II-2	B
	vaccination (influenza,	II-2	B
	pneumococcus).	I	B
6. OME			
a. ≤3 months duration	a. Antibiotics	III	D
	b. Tubes	III	D
	c. Decongestants, antihistamines	I	E
b. 4 to 6 months (bilateral, with >20 db hearing loss)	Consider placement of tympanostomy tubes	I	A

*amoxicillin 40 mg/kg/day tid

†amoxicillin 80 to 90 mg/kg/day bid

‡amoxicillin 40 mg/kg/day with clavulanate—standard 4:1 formula containing 250 mg amoxicillin and 62.5 mg clavulanate/5 mL administered bid or tid (or new 7:1 formula bid, containing 400 mg amoxicillin and 57 mg clavulanate/5 mL).

§amoxicillin 80 to 90 mg/kg/day with clavulanate 6.4 ~ 10 mg/kg/day (new 7:1 ratio) bid

//cefuroxime axetil 30mg/kg/day bid

#short course defined as 5-7 days

**ceftriaxone for 50 mg/kg/d daily for 3 days

††clindamycin 15mg/kg/d qid. (not effective against *Haemophilus influenzae, Moraxella catarrhalis*)

AOM in those children who have been shown to have a history of recurrent infections (level I, recommendation A).[83] Despite evidence from good RCTs this recommendation must be revised under the present circumstances of increasing antibiotic resistance. It must be emphasized that the decrease in the frequency of recurrent episodes of AOM is small, and any benefit of daily antibiotic prophylactic therapy must be weighed against its risk of contributing to the rise of resistant organisms. It has been estimated that to prevent a single occurrence of AOM with prophylactic antibiotics, it would require the treatment of 1 child for 9 months or the treatment of 9 children for 1 month.[46] The Centers for Disease Control and Prevention in the United States have raised concerns about the prolonged and continuous use of antibiotic prophylaxis contributing to the increasing incidence of bacterial resistance,[84] and there is now evidence that antibiotic prophylaxis specifically increases the likelihood of nasopharyngeal colonization with resistant *S. pneumoniae* and with beta-lactamase–producing organisms in middle-ear effusions.[85–87] It is for these reasons that it has been recommended that antibiotic prophylaxis for AOM be avoided, whenever possible (level III, recommendation B).[2]

Environmental Manipulation

There are certain environmental factors that can be altered to provide more protection for vulnerable infants and children who suffer from recurrent AOM. These include a smoke-free home environment, where second-hand smoke has been implicated in the occurrence of AOM (level II-2, recommendation B).[88] In addition, sleeping in the supine position has been shown not only to prevent sudden infant death syndrome but also to be protective against the development of otitis media (level II-2, recommendation C).[89] Discouraging the use of pacifiers may also help to reduce the incidence of AOM (level II-2, recommendation B).[90] Reducing day-care attendance would most definitely be advantageous (level II-2).[88] There are those who contend that it is the size of the day-care group (less than six children is associated with a reduced risk), not the day care itself that is responsible for the predisposition to recurrent AOM.[91,92] The discussion of the prevention of otitis media would not be complete without mention of the protective effect of breast feeding (4 months or longer), which has been shown to decrease the frequency of AOM in longitudinal studies (level II-2, recommendation B).[93,94]

Immunization

S. pneumoniae (Pneumococcal) Vaccine The importance of *S. pneumoniae* infections in infants and children with otitis media and the rapidly emerging antimicrobial resistance to this organism emphasizes the need for urgent prophylaxis by means of vaccination. Due to an inadequate immunologic response to polysaccharide antigens in young children, the currently available and effective 23-valent polysaccharide pneumococcal vaccine is recommended for children over 2 years who have chronic cardiovascular disease, chronic pulmonary disease, diabetes, or sickle cell hemoglobinopathy. The pneumococcal vaccine has not been shown to decrease the overall incidence of AOM in a randomized controlled trial, although it did reduce vaccine-type pneumococcal AOM (level I, recommendation B).[95] Given the high prevalence of AOM in children under 2 years of age, a conjugated pneumococcal vaccine similar to that produced against *H. influenzae b* and used successfully in early infancy would be beneficial in this population. Several manufacturers have developed conjugated vaccines against pneumococci that contain either meningococcal outer membrane protein complex (OMPC) or a nontoxic variant of diphtheria (CRM_{197}) as carrier proteins and have been shown to be immunogenic in infants.[19,96] In a recent study, a heptavalent pneumococcal vaccine has been shown to be highly effective in preventing invasive disease in young children.[19] Its effectiveness in preventing AOM has not been assessed.

Influenza Virus Vaccine There is now evidence that otherwise healthy children predisposed to otitis media might benefit from influenza vaccination. Studies in Finland[97] and

North Carolina[98] have demonstrated a decreased incidence of AOM in children in day-care centers who had received killed influenza virus vaccines. In a recent North American study, healthy children vaccinated with a new intranasal, live attenuated, cold-adapted influenza-virus vaccine, were shown to have a 35 percent reduction in the incidence of otitis media (level I, recommendation B).[18] Since the occurrence of otitis media was a secondary outcome in this study, further otitis media–specific RCTs are required before a strong recommendation can be made to use the live attenuated influenza vaccine to prevent AOM, when it becomes commercially available. In this era of increasing antibiotic resistance associated with excessive antibiotic exposure, universal influenza vaccination of children may become an increasingly important strategy to diminish febrile illnesses and particularly otitis media, for which antibiotics may be needed.

Surgery

Three trials have demonstrated that myringotomy and tympanostomy tubes are effective for the prevention of recurrent AOM in otitis-prone children (level I, recommended A).[87,99,100] A contrary opinion has been expressed in a utilization review in which it has been suggested that approximately one-quarter of procedures for placement of tympanostomy tubes were performed for inappropriate indications.[101] There are still those who consider the insertion of tympanostomy tubes to be a valuable procedure in children with severe and recurrent disease who have failed adequate medical therapy.[102,103] Adenoidectomy is another procedure that has been shown in one trial to be effective for prevention of AOM, but is best warranted on an individual basis according to the investigators (level I, recommendation B).[104]

Management of OME

Surgery

Investigators have shown that myringotomy and tube placement provides more effusion-free time and better hearing than either myringotomy alone or no surgery in children with chronic OME (level I, recommendation A).[105,106] The benefits of tube placement in selected children with OME appear to outweigh the risks and concerns of surgery which include the risks of anesthesia, early loss of the tubes into the ear canal or into the middle ear, scarring of the tympanic membrane, permanent perforations, and cholesteatomas.[47]

Other Adjunctive Therapies

The use of decongestants, antihistamines, and corticosteroids have theoretical benefits for the treatment of OME by reducing mucosal edema and promoting patency of the Eustachian tubes; however, no obvious benefit of this adjunctive therapy has been demonstrated in the treatment of OME.[107,108] In two large-scale clinical trials in infants and children in Pittsburgh, decongestants and antihistamines were shown to be ineffective (level I, recommendation E).[109,110]

Children receiving corticosteroid therapy in addition to antibiotics immediately following initial treatment, have shown a reduction in the incidence of middle-ear effusion, but this effect was transient with no appreciable difference in outcome within weeks to months of concluding the treatment.[111] Thus, none of these agents are indicated.

THE OTITIS PRONE CHILD

The term "otitis prone" was first described in 1975 and defined as six or more episodes of otitis media before the age of six years.[112] Some authorities now believe that a better definition would include the total time spent with middle-ear disease rather than just the number of episodes. Certainly, children who experience their first episode of AOM early in life, particularly if this occurs before 6 months of age, are more likely to have recurrent episodes compared with children who have their first episode later.[113,114] It is not clear if a child who has an early occurrence of AOM is predisposed to recurrence or whether the first episode alters the middle ear or the child's immune system, thus increasing susceptibility to further episodes of AOM. Factors other than age that are risk factors for the development of AOM include winter, lower socioeconomic class, male gender, native American ethnicity, and allergy.

CONCLUSION

Otitis media is extremely common in childhood and is frequently overdiagnosed or misdiagnosed. Physicians can improve their quality of clinical care by distinguishing AOM from OME, by using appropriate otoscopic instruments, and by using validated clinical criteria to make an accurate diagnosis. The judicious use of antibiotics is imperative at this time of increasing bacterial resistance, and the selection of children at low risk for complications may help diminish the use of antibiotics to treat this benign condition.

REFERENCES

1. McCaig LF, Hughes JM. Trends in antimicrobial drug prescribing among office-based physicians in the United States. JAMA 1995;273:214–9.

2. Dowell S, Marcy M, Phillips W, et al. Otitis media—principles of judicious use of antimicrobial agents. Pediatrics 1998;101:165–71.

3. Berman S, Roark R, Luckey D. Theoretical cost effectiveness of management options for children with persisting middle ear effusions. Pediatrics 1994;93:353–63.

4. Paradise JL, Rockette HE, Colborn K, et al. Otitis media in 2253 Pittsburgh - area infants: prevalence and risk factors during the first two years of life. Pediatrics 1997;99:318–33.

5. Stool SE, Berg AO, Berman S, et al. Otitis media with effusion in young children. Clinical practice guidelines. Agency for Health Care Policy and Research; 1994.Vol. 94 - 0622.

6. Kontiokari T, Koivunen P, Niemelä M, et al. Symptoms of acute otitis media. Pediatric Infect Dis 1998;17:676–9.

7. Schwartz RH. A practical approach to the otitis prone child. Contemp Pediatrics 1987;4:30–54.

8. Hayden GF. Acute suppurative otitis media in children. Diversity of clinical diagnostic criteria. Clin Pediatr 1981;20:99–104.

9. Kaleida P, Stool SE. Assessment of otoscopists' accuracy regarding middle-ear effusion. Am J Dis Child 1992;146:433–5.

10. Klein JO. Otitis media. Clin Infect Dis 1994;19:823–33.

11. Karma P, Sipila M, Kayaja M, et al. Pneumatic otoscopy and otitis media: the value of different tympanic membrane findings and their combinations. In: Lim DJ, Bluestone CD, Klein JO, et al, editors. Recent advances in otitis media: proceedings of the Fifth International Symposium. Burlington, Ontario, Canada; 1993.p.41–5.

12. Kaleida PH. The COMPLETES exam for otitis. Contemp Pediatrics 1997;14:93–101.

13. Ingvarsson L. Acute otalgia in children—findings and diagnosis. Acta Paediatr Scand 1982;71:705–10.

14. Niemelä M, Uhari M, Jounio-Ervasti K. Lack of specific symptomatology in children with acute otitis media. Pediatr Infect Dis J 1994;13:765–8.

15. Weiss J, Yates G, Quinn L. Acute otitis media: making an accurate diagnosis. Am Fam Phys 1996;53:1200–6.

16. Stool SE, Berg AO. Managing otitis media with effusion in young children. Can J Pediatr 1995.2.379–87.

17. Babonis TR, Weir MR, Kelly PC. Impedance tympanometry and acoustic reflectometry at myringotomy. Pediatrics 1991;87:475–80.

18. Belshe R, Mendelman P, Treanor J, et al. The efficacy of live attenuated, cold-adapted, trivalent, intranasal influenza virus vaccine in children. N Eng J Med 1998;338:1405–12.

19. Black S, Shinefield H, Ray P, et al. Efficacy of heptavalent conjugate pneumococcal vaccine (Wyeth Lederle) in 37,000 infants and children: results of the Northern California Kaiser Permanente Efficacy Trial. 38th ICAAC, San Diego, California; September 24–7, 1998.

20. Ruuskanen O, Heikkinen T. Otitis media: etiology and diagnosis. Pediatr Infect Dis J 1994;13:S23–6.

21. Chonmaitree T, Owen M, Patel H, et al. Effect of viral respiratory tract infection on outcome of acute otitis media. J Pediatr 1992;120:856–62.

22. Barnett E, Klein J. The problem of resistant bacteria for the management of acute otitis media. Pediatr Clin North am 1995;42:509–17.

23. Bluestone CD, Stephenson JS, Martin LM. Ten-year review of otitis media pathogens. Pediatr Infect Dis J 1992;11:S7–11.

24. McCracken GH. Considerations in selecting an antibiotic for treatment of acute otitis media. Pediatr Infect Dis J 1994;13:1054–7.

25. Howie VM. Eradication of bacterial pathogens from middle ear infections. Clin Infect Dis 1991;14:209–10.

26. Klein JO. Microbiologic efficacy of antibacterial drugs for acute otitis media. Pediatr Infect Dis J 1993;12:973–5.

27. Burke P, Bain J, Robinson D, et al. Acute red ear in children: controlled trial of non-antibiotic treatment in general practice. Br Med J 1991;303:558–62.

28. Kaleida PH, Casselbrant ML, Rockette HE, et al. Amoxicillin or myringotomy or both for acute otitis media: results of a randomized clinical trial. Pediatrics 1991;87:466–74.

29. Rosenfeld RM, Vertrees JE, Carr J, et al. Clinical efficacy of antimicrobial drugs for acute otitis media: meta-analysis of 5,400 children from thirty–three randomized trials. J Pediatr 1994;124:355–67.

30. Carlin S, Marchant C, Shurin P, et al. Host factors and early therapeutic response in acute otitis media 1991;118:178–84.

31. Del Mar C, Glasziou P, Hayem M. Are antibiotics indicated as initial treatment for children with acute otitis media? A meta-analysis. Br Med J 1997;314:1526–9.

32. Jacoby GA. Prevalence and resistance mechanisms of common bacterial respiratory pathogens. Clin Infect Dis 1994;18:951–7.

33. Friedland IR, Klugman KP. Antibiotic-resistant pneumococcal disease in South African children. Am J Dis Child 1992;146:920–3.

34. National Committee for Clinical Laboratory Standards. Performance standards for antimicrobial susceptibility testing. National Committee for Clinical Laboratory Standards, Villanova, Pennsylvania, 1997.

35. Simor A, Rachlis A, Louie L, et al. Emergence of penicillin-resistant *Streptococcus pneumoniae* in southern Ontario, 1993-94. Can J Infect Dis 1995;6:157–60.

36. Simor A, Louie M. The Canadian Bacterial Surveillance Network, Low DE. Canadian national survey of prevalence of antimicrobial resistance among clinical isolates of *Streptococcus pneumoniae*. Antimicrob Agents Chemother 1996;40:2190–3.

37. Dowell S, Schwartz B. Resistant pneumococci: protecting patients through judicious use of antibiotics. Am Fam Physician 1997;55:1647–54.

38. Committee on Infectious Diseases. American Academy of Pediatrics. Therapy for children with invasive pneumococcal infections. Pediatrics 1997;99:289–98.

39. Fugita K, Murono K, Yoshikawa Mi, et al. Decline of erythromycin resistance of group A streptococci in Japan. Pediatr Infect Dis J 1994;13:1075–8.

40. Baquero F, Martinez-Beltran J, Loza E. A review of antibiotic resistance patterns of *Streptococcus pneumoniae* in Europe. J Antimicrob Chemother 1991;28:31–8.

41. Arason V, Kristinsson K, Sigurdsson J, et al. Do antimicrobials increase the carriage rate of penicillin resistant pneumococci in children? Cross-sectional prevalence study. Br Med J 1996;313:387–91.

42. Hathaway TJ, Katz HP, Dershewitz RA, et al. Acute otitis media: who needs post-treatment follow-up? Pediatrics 1994;1994:143–7.

43. Cohen R, Levy C, Boucherat M, et al. A multicenter, randomized, double-blind trial of 5 versus 10 days of antibiotic therapy for acute otitis media in young children. J Peds 1998;133:634–9.

44. Paradise JL. Short-course antimicrobial treatment for acute otitis media. JAMA 1997;278:1640–2.

45. Mandel EM, Casselbrandt ML, Rockette HE, et al. Efficacy of 20 versus 10 day antimicrobial treatment for acute otitis media. Pediatrics 1995;96:5–13.

46. Rosenfeld RM. What to expect from medical treatment of otitis media. Pediatr Infect Dis J 1995;14:731–8.

47. Klein JO, Bluestone CD. Management of otitis media in the era of managed care. Adv Pediatric Infect Dis 1997;12:351–86.

48. Conrad D. Should acute otitis media ever be treated with antibiotics? Pediatr Ann 1998;27:66–74.

49. Culpepper L, Froom J. Routine antimicrobial treatment of acute otitis media: is it necessary? JAMA 1997;278:1643–5.

50. Majeed A, Harris T. Acute otitis media in children: fewer children should be treated with antibiotics. Br Med J 1997;315:321–2.

51. Charney E, Bynum R, Eldredge D, et al. How well do patients take oral penicillin? A collaborative study in private practice. Pediatrics 1967;40:188–95.

52. Kozyrskyj AL, Hildes-Ripstein GE, Longstaffe SE, et al. Treatment of acute otitis media with a shortened course of antibiotics. A meta-analysis. JAMA 1998;279:1736–42.

53. Grol R, Thomas S, Roberts R. Development and implementation of guidelines for family practice: lessons from the Netherlands. J Fam Pract 1995;40:435–9.

54. van Buchem FL, Dunk JHM, van'T Hof MA. Therapy of acute otitis media: myringotomy, antibiotics, or neither? Lancet 1981;ii:883–7.

55. van Buchem FL, Peeters M, van 'T Hof MA. Acute otitis media: a new treatment strategy. Br Med J 1985;290:1033–7.

56. Dowell S. Meeting of Centers for Disease Control Therapeutic Working Group on Drug Resistant *Streptococcus pneumoniae* in Otitis Media, Atlanta, GA, March 20-21, 1997.

57. Drugs for treatment of acute otitis media in children. Med Letter Drugs Ther 1994;36:19-21.

58. Poole MD. Implications of drug-resistant *Streptococcus pneumoniae* for otitis media. Ped Infect Dis J 1998;17:953–6.

59. Neu HC. Diagnosis and treatment: drugs five years later: amoxicillin. Ann Intern Med 1979;90:356–60.

60. Berman S. Otitis media in children. N Engl J Med 1995;332:1560–5.

61. Pichichero ME, Pichichero CL. Persistent acute otitis media: 1. Causative pathogens. Pediatr Infect Dis J 1995;14:178–83.

62. McCracken GH. Treatment of acute otitis media in an era of increasing microbial resistance. Pediatr Infect Dis J 1998;17:576–9.

63. Marchant CD, Carlin SA, Johnson CE, et al. Measuring the comparative efficacy of antibacterial agents for acute otitis media: The "Pollyanna phenomenon." Pediatr 1992;110:72–7.

64. Seikel K, Shelton S, McCracken GH. Middle ear fluid concentrations of amoxicillin after large dosages in children with acute otitis media. Pediatr Infect Dis J 1997;16:710–1.

65. Drusano G, Craig W. Relevance of pharmacokinetics and pharmacodynamics in the selection of antibiotics for respiratory tract infections. J Chemother 1997;3:38–44.

66. Craig W, Andes D. Pharmacokinetics and pharmacodynamics of antibiotics in otitis media. Pediatr Infect Dis J 1996;15:255–9.

67. Canafax D, Yuan Z, Chonmaitree T, et al. Amoxicillin middle ear fluid penetration and pharmacokimetics in children with acute otitis media. Pediatr Infect Dis J 1998;17:149–56.

68. Dagan R, Abramson O, Leibovitz E, et al. Impaired bacteriologic response to oral cephalosporins in acute otitis media caused by pneumococci with intermediate resistance to penicllin. Pediatr Infect Dis J 1996;15:980–5.

69. Pichichero ME, McLinn S, Aronovitz G, et al. Cefprozil treatment of persistent and recurrent acute otitis media. Pediatr Infect Dis J 1997;16:471–8.

70. Jones RN. Ceftibuten: a review of antimicrobial activity, spectrum and other microbiologic features. Pediatr Infect Dis J 1995;14:S77–83.

71. Doern G, Brueggemeann A, Pierce G, et al. Antibiotic resistance among clinical isolates of *Haemophilus influenzae* in the United States in 1994 and 1995 and detection of beta-lactamase-positive strains resistant to amoxicillin-clavulanate: results of a national multicenter surveillance study. Antimicrob Agents Chemother 1997;41:292–7.

72. Dowell SF, Butler JC, Giebink GS, et al. Acute otitis media: management and surveillance in an era of pneumococcal resistance—a report from the Drug-resistant *Streptococcus pneumoniae* Therapeutic Working Group. Pediatr Infect Dis J 1999;18:1–9.

73. Green SM, Rothrock SG. Single-dose intramuscular ceftriaxone for acute otitis media in children. Pediatrics 1993;1993:23–30.

74. Gehanno P, Berche P, N'Guyen L, et al. Resolution of clinical failure in acute otitis media confirmed by in vivo bacterial eradication: efficacy and safety of ceftriaxone injected once daily, for 3 days [abstract LM-45]. In: American Society for Microbiology, Abstracts of the 37th International Conference on Antimicrobial Agents and Chemotherapy, Toronto, September 28 - October 1, 1997.

75. Leibovitz E, Piglansky L, Raiz S. Bacteriologic efficacy of 3-day intramuscular ceftriaxone in non-responsive acute otitis media [abstract K-105]. In: American Society for Microbiology, 37th International Conference on Antimicrobial Agents and Chemotherapy, Toronto, Ontario, September 28 - October 1, 1997.

76. Nelson CT, Mason EO, Kaplan SL. Activity of oral antibiotics in middle ear and sinus infections caused by penicillin-resistant *Streptococcus pneumoniae:* implications for treatment. Pediatr Infect Dis J 1994;13:585–9.

77. Cetron M, Breiman R, Jorgensen J. Multi-site population-based surveillance for drug-resistant *Streptococcus pneumoniae* (DRSP) [abstract C-283], 97th General Meeting of the American Society for Microbiology, Miami Beach, FL, 1997. Washington, DC: American Society for Microbiology.

78. Bodor F. Systemic antibiotics for the treatment of the conjunctivitis–otitis media syndrome. Pediatr Infect Dis J 1989;8:287–90.

79. Schappert SM. Office visits for otitis media: United States, 1975-90. Advance Data from Vital and Health Statistics of the Centers for Disease Control/National Center for Health Statistics, U.S. Department of Health and Human Services, No. 214, 1992.

80. Zelhuis G, Straatman H, Rach G, et al. Analysis and presentation of data on the natural course of otitis media with effusion in children. Int J Epidemiol 1990;19:1037–44.

81. Casselbrandt M, Brostoff L, Cantekin E, et al. Otitis media with effusion in preschool children. Laryngoscope 1985;95:428–36.

82. Rosenfeld RM, Post JC. Meta-analysis of antibiotics for the treatment of otitis media with effusion. Otolaryngol Head Neck Surg 1992;106:378–86.

83. Williams RL, Chalmers TC, Stange KC, et al. Use of antibiotics in preventing recurrent acute otitis media and in treating otitis media with effusion. A meta-analytic attempt to resolve the brouhaha. JAMA 1993;270:1344–51.

84. Centers for Disease Control and Prevention. Drug-resistant *Streptococcus pneumoniae*: Kentucky and Tennessee, 1993. MMWR Morb Mortal Wkly Rep 1994;43:21–3.

85. Reichler MR, Allphin AA, Breiman RF, et al. The spread of multiple resistant *Streptococcus pneumoniae* at a day care center in Ohio. J Infect Dis 1992;166:1346–53.

86. Brook I, Gober A. Prophylaxis with amoxicillin or sulfisoxazole for otitis media: effect on the recovery of penicillin-resistant bacteria from children. Clin Infect Dis 1996;22:143–5.

87. Casselbrandt M, Kaleida P, Rockette H, et al. Efficacy of antimicrobial prophylaxis and of tympanostomy tube insertion for prevention of recurrent acute otitis media: results of a randomized clinical trial. Pediatr Infect Dis J 1992;11:278–86.

88. Klein JO. Lessons from recent studies on the epidemiology of otitis media. Pediatr Infect Dis J 1994;13:1031–4.

89. Gannon M, Haggard M, Golding J. Sleeping position: a new environmental risk factor for otitis media? In: Abstracts of the Sixth International Symposium on Recent Advances in Otitis Media, Fort Lauderdale, FL, June 4-8, 1995.

90. Niemelä M, Uhari M, Möttönen M. A pacifier increases risk of recurrent acute otitis media in day care centers. Pediatrics 1995;96:884–8.

91. Louhiala PJ, Jaakkola N, Ruotsalainen R, et al. Form of day care and respiratory infections in children. Am J Public Health 1995;85:1109–12.

92. Marx J, Osguthorpe JD, Parsons G. Day care and the incidence of otitis media in young children. Otolaryngol Head Neck Surg 1995;112:695–9.

93. Aniansson G, Alm B, Andersson B, et al. A prospective cohort study on breast-feeding and otitis media in Swedish infants. Pediatr Infect Dis J 1994;13:183–8.

94. Duncan B, Ey J, Holberg CJ, et al. Exclusive breast-feeding for at least four months protects against otitis media. Pediatrics 1993;91:867–72.

95. Sloyer JJ, Ploussard J, Howie VM. Efficacy of pneumococcal polysaccharide vaccine in preventing acute otitis media in infants in Huntsville, Alabama. Rev Infect Dis 1981;3:S119–23.

96. Ahman H, Kayhty H, Lehtonen H, et al. *Streptococcus pneumoniae* capsular polysaccharide–diphtheria toxoid conjugate vaccine is immuogenic in early infancy and able to induce immunologic memory. Pediatr Infect Dis J 1998;17:211–6.

97. Heikkinen T, Ruuskanen O, Waris M, et al. Influenza vaccination in the prevention of acute otitis media in children. Am J Dis Child 1991;145:445–8.

98. Clements D, Langdon I, Bland C. Influenza A vaccine decreases the incidence of otitis media in 6 to 30-month-old children in day care. Arch Pediatr Adolesc Med 1995;149:1113–7.

99. Gebhart D. Tympanostomy tubes in the otitis media prone child. Laryngoscope 981;91:849–66.

100. Gonzalez C, Arnold JE, Woody EA, et al. Prevention of recurrent acute otitis media: chemoprophylaxis versus tympanostomy tubes. Laryngoscope 1986;96:1330–4.

101. Kleinman LC, Kosecoff J, Dubois RW, et al. The medical appropriateness of tympanostomy tubes proposed for children younger than 16 years in the United States. JAMA 1994;271:1250–5.

102. Bluestone CD, Klein JO. The appropriateness of tympanostomy tubes for children. JAMA 1995;273:697–701.

103. Bluestone CD, Klein JO, Gates GA. "Appropriateness of tympanostomy tubes". Setting the record straight. Arch Otolaryngol Head Neck Surg 1994;120:1051–53.

104. Paradise JL, Bluestone CD, Rogers K, et al. Efficacy of adenoidectomy for recurrent otitis media in children previously treated with tympanostomy tube placement: results of parallel randomized and nonrandomized trials. JAMA 1990; 263:2066–73.

105. Mandel EM, Rockette HE, Bluestone CD, et al. Myringotomy with and without tympanostomy tubes for chronic otitis media with effusion. Arch Otolaryngol Head Neck Surg 1989;115:1217–24.

106. Mandel EM, Rockette HE, Bluestone CD, et al. Efficacy of myringotomy with and without tympanostomy tubes for chronic otitis media effusion. Pediatr Infect Dis J 1992;11:270–2.

107. Grundfast KM. A review of the efficacy of systemically administered decongestants in the prevention and treatment of otitis media. Otolaryngol Head Neck Surg 1981;89:432-439.

108. Bahal N, Nahata M. Recent advances in the treatment of otitis media. J Clin Pharm Therap 1992;17:201–15.

109. Cantekin E, Mandel E, Bluestone C. Lack of efficacy of a decongestant-antihistamine combination for otitis media with effusion ("secretory" otitis media) in children. N Engl J Med 1983;308:297–301.

110. Mandel EM, Rockette HE, Bluestone CD, et al. Efficacy of amoxicillin with and without decongestant-antihistamine for otitis media with effusion in children. N Engl J Med 1987;316:432–7.

111. Rosenfeld RM, Mandel EM, Bluestone CD. Systemic steroids for otitis media with effusion in children. Arch Otolaryngol Head Neck Surg 1991;117:984–9.

112. Howie VM, Ploussard JH, Sloyer J. The "Otitis-prone" condition. Am J Dis Child 1975;129:676–8.

113. Marchant CD, Shurin PA, Turczyk VA, et al. Course and outcome of otitis media in early infancy: a prospective study. J Pediatr 1984;104:826–31.

114. Teele DW, Klein JO, Rosner B. Epidemiology of otitis media during the first seven years of life in children in Greater Boston: a prospective cohort study. J Infect Dis 1989;160:83–94.

CHAPTER 7

Asthma

Patricia Parkin, MD, FRCPC
Norma Goggin, MBBCh, MRCP

Asthma and wheezing in childhood are common, burdensome problems. In the United States, Weitzman and colleagues have reported that the prevalence of childhood asthma has increased from 3.1 percent in 1981, to 4.3 percent in 1988.[1] In Canada, the prevalence of asthma has increased from 2.5 percent in 1978 to 1979, to 3.1 percent in 1983 to 1984, to 11.2 percent in 1994 to 1995.[2] Hospital admissions for asthma have also increased. Strachan and colleagues reported a 100 percent increase in the rate of admission for childhood asthma in south London, United Kingdom, since 1978.[3] Since the mid-1960s, asthma hospitalizations among children aged 0 to 14 years increased ten-fold in New Zealand, eight-fold in Australia, six-fold in England and Wales, four-fold in Canada, and three-fold in the United States.[4] Weiss and colleagues reported similar findings, citing rates of hospitalization among children aged 0 to 4 years increasing almost three-fold between 1980 to 1990.[5] In Canada, To and colleagues reported that the observed increasing trend in admissions for asthma among Ontario children in the 1970s and 1980s stabilized in the early 1990s. The declining admission rates were largely caused by the lower admission rates among school-aged children from 5 to 17 years. However, in younger children (0 to 4 years), hospital admissions for asthma continued to increase between 1989 and 1992.[6] Studies from the United States have similarly reported increasing asthma hospitalization rates in this subgroup of very young children.[7,8]

The relationship between wheezing episodes in early childhood and the development of asthma has been studied by Martinez and colleagues.[9] A cohort of 1,246 newborns was followed prospectively. At the age of 6 years, approximately half the children had had wheezing attacks at least once. Of these, approximately one-third had the episode in the first 3 years, but not between 3 and 6 years (transient early wheezing); approximately one-third had no wheezing in the first 3 years, but had wheezing at 6 years (late-onset wheezing); and approximately one-third had wheezing both before 3 years of age and at 6 years of age (persistent wheezing). Factors associated with persistent wheezing (as compared with those who never had wheezing) were found to include eczema, rhinitis apart from colds, maternal asthma, Hispanic ethnic background, male gender, and maternal smoking.

The definition of asthma in childhood remains controversial. In the development of a consensus statement,[10] it has been suggested that the definition has varied depending on the purposes for which it has been sought and has included perspectives from epidemiologists, clinicians, immunologists, physiologists, and pathologists. The definition recommended is as follows: "Recurrent wheezing and/or persistent coughing in a setting where asthma is likely and other rarer conditions have been excluded. With increasing age, particularly beyond 3 years, the diagnosis of asthma becomes progressively more definitive and beyond 6 years of age, the National Heart Lung and Blood Institute (NHLBI) definition can be accepted. This incorporates the concept of asthma as primarily a disease of airway inflammation, in which eosinophils and mast cells are prominent, producing recurrent episodes of cough and wheeze, often associated with increased bronchial hyper-responsiveness and reversible airflow limitation."

Furthermore, as clearly articulated by Taussig,[11] the diagnosis of asthma in infants and young children with persistent or recurrent wheezing remains an art. In that context, he suggests that ". . . the diagnosis of asthma should be entertained for infants and young children who have a history of recurrent wheezing with multiple triggers, prolonged and severe symptoms following viral infections, evidence for underlying atopy, a family history of atopy/asthma, and perhaps, biochemical evidence of atopy . . . Caution needs to be exercised regarding both the under- and over-diagnosis of asthma which makes the entire issue of infantile wheezing a most complicated subject for the clinician caring for infants."

Several groups have worked to develop a consensus regarding guidelines for diagnosis and management of asthma.[10,12–14]

ACUTE ASTHMA MANAGEMENT (SEE TABLE 7–1)

Inhaled Beta$_2$-Agonists

Efficacy and Safety

Short-acting, inhaled beta$_2$-agonists are the first-line therapy in the management of acute asthma attacks. In practice, salbutamol (or albuterol) is the most commonly used inhaled beta$_2$-agonist. The principal action of beta-agonists is to stimulate pulmonary receptors that relax bronchial smooth muscle and decrease airway resistance. Administration of short-acting beta-adrenergic agents by inhalation leads to a very rapid response, generally within a few minutes after inhalation, and the effect lasts for 3 to 4 hours. Inhalation is the route of administration of choice. Only about 10 percent of an inhaled dose actually enters the lungs; much of the remainder is swallowed. Delivery of the drug to the distal airways depends on the size of the particles in the aerosol and respiratory parameters such as inspiratory flow rate, tidal volume, breath-holding time, and airway time. These parameters will change and hence the dose of drug administered, depending on whether the drug is delivered as wet particles by a nebulizer or as preformed aerosols by a metered-dose inhaler (MDI). The main benefit of inhalation therapy, compared with administration by the oral or intravenous route, is that high levels of the drug can be delivered more effectively to the airways, giving the desired therapeutic result with minimal side effects.[15,16]

Inhaled selective beta$_2$-agonist therapy is recommended as first-line treatment for acute asthma in children.[12,14] Beta$_2$-agonists elicit dose-related bronchodilatation.[17,18] Therefore, it is desirable to use the maximum possible dose that does not cause unacceptable side effects. In addition, high doses of inhaled salbutamol are needed in acute asthma because only about 10 percent of the dose actually reaches the lungs.[16,18] It has been suggested that in patients with markedly increased smooth muscle tone, more frequent administration of beta$_2$-agonists may be more effective than less frequently administered doses.[19–21] However, few studies have been performed to determine, first, the efficacy and safety of frequent administration of inhaled salbutamol and, second, the optimal dose in children.

One relevant study suggested that frequent inhalation of nebulized salbutamol was beneficial in children with acute asthma.[22] Thirty-three children, aged 6 to 17 years, attending the emergency department with an acute attack of asthma, were entered into one of two treatment groups. Group 1 patients received salbutamol 0.15 mg/kg, up to a maximum of 5 mg, at 1-hour intervals for a total of three doses. The second group of patients (group 2) were given salbutamol 0.15 mg/kg initially, then 0.05 mg/kg at 20-minute intervals in a total of six doses. The primary outcome measure was forced expiratory volume in 1 second (FEV$_1$), expressed as percent of predicted value (PPV). Baseline severity was similar in both groups, as measured by FEV$_1$ (31 percent in group 1 versus 30 percent in group 2). Both groups had a similar response at 20 minutes to the initial dose of salbutamol (FEV$_1$: 44.5 percent in group 1 versus 46.7 percent in group 2). Thereafter, all the patients in group 2 (frequent doses) continued to improve during the first hour, whereas 30 percent in group 1 (hourly doses) showed deterioration of at least 15 percent in FEV$_1$ prior to the next dose. The overall outcome for both groups, as demonstrated by final FEV$_1$ was not significantly different. The results did

Table 7–1 Management of Acute Childhood Asthma

Condition	Intervention	Quality of Evidence	Recommendation
Acute asthma	High-dose, frequently administered, beta$_2$-agonists are efficacious	I	A
	High-dose, frequently administered, beta$_2$-agonists are safe	I	A
	Delivery of bronchodilator by metered-dose inhaler with spacer as compared with nebulizer are equally efficacious	I	A
	Addition of up to three doses of ipratropium bromide to beta$_2$-agonists in children with severe asthma exacerbation seen in the emergency department are efficacious	I	A
	Addition of ipratropium bromide to beta$_2$-agonists in children admitted to hospital is not efficacious	I	D
	Addition of oral corticosteroids to beta$_2$-agonists in children over 1 year seen in the emergency department is efficacious	I	A
	Addition of oral corticosteroids as compared with addition of intravenous corticosteroids to beta$_2$-agonists in the emergency department is equally efficacious	I	A
	Addition of aminophylline to inhaled beta$_2$-agonists and corticosteroids in children with moderate and severe exacerbation is not efficacious	I	E

generate several important hypotheses, namely, that compared with the more usual hourly regimen, frequent (every 20 minutes) administration of nebulized salbutamol results in an earlier maximal response and prevents deterioration between doses in the initial treatment of acute asthma in children.

Subsequently, a randomized controlled trial (RCT) confirmed that frequently administered, nebulized beta$_2$-agonist therapy was both safe and effective in treating severe, acute asthma in children.[23] This study also contributed important information regarding the optimal dose of the drug. Thirty-two children, aged 5 to 17 years, presenting to the emergency department for treatment of a severe, acute asthma exacerbation were enrolled in the study. All patients received the same first dose of salbutamol (0.15 mg/kg, to a maximum of 5 mg). Patients were then randomly assigned to receive either high-dose (0.15 mg/kg per dose) or low-dose (0.05 mg/kg per dose) nebulized salbutamol for six additional doses at 20-minute intervals. The severity of the attack, as measured by baseline FEV$_1$ was similar between the groups (29.3 percent [high-dose group] versus 32.4 percent [low-dose group]). Compared with the low-dose regimen, the high-dose regimen resulted in significantly greater improvement in FEV_1, between the start and the end of the study. The difference between the groups in the change in mean FEV_1 was statistically significant, beginning 60 minutes after the commencement of the study. The mean percentage increase in FEV_1 from the first treatment to the end of the study was 34.5 percent in the high-dose group versus 9.6 percent in the low-dose group ($p < .05$). The authors concluded that high-dose, frequently administered, nebulized salbutamol is effective in treating severe, acute asthma in children.

In addition to efficacy, the safety of high-dose, frequently administered beta$_2$-agonists was addressed in these studies. This form of treatment produced no additional side effects compared with conventional beta$_2$-agonist therapy. Side effects were mild, infrequent, and of short duration. Tremor was the most common side effect in all groups of patients, and the incidence was greater in the high-dose groups.[23] However, the tremor was mild and subsided quickly after therapy. No apparent increase in the occurrence of nausea, vomiting, or hyperactivity was observed in subjects receiving high-dose, frequently administered salbutamol. In three studies, with a cumulative sample size of 98 children, there were no clinically important adverse effects, specifically tachycardia, palpitations, or arrhythmias.[22–24]

Efficacy of Mode of Delivery

Inhaled beta$_2$-agonists can be delivered either as wet particles by nebulizers or as preformed aerosols by MDIs, with or without holding chambers. Advantages and disadvantages of each involve such factors as efficiency, simplicity, cost, the need for supervision, and coordination issues. Metered-dose inhalers are compact, portable, less expensive, and require less time for use. Various spacer devices, which can be interposed between the MDI and the mouth, can overcome the difficulty in coordinating inspiration with MDI actuation. Furthermore, it has been shown that spacer devices attached to MDIs provide better aerosol deposition in the lungs.[25]

In spite of these advantages, until recently, young children who required inhalation therapy used nebulizers exclusively, as they lacked the coordination required to effectively use MDIs.[26] It has been shown that MDIs attached to spacing devices provide as effective nebulization as in adults with acute asthma.[27,28] In children with stable asthma, the use of spacer devices has been reported to provide equivalent or greater improvement in lung function, in comparison with the use of an MDI alone or a nebulizer.[29,30]

Three well-designed studies have compared the effectiveness of bronchodilator delivery by an MDI with spacer with that by a nebulizer in children with an acute exacerbation of asthma.[31–33] Two of the studies were conducted in the emergency department and the third in the inpatient setting.

Kerem and colleagues enrolled 33 children, aged 6 to 14 years, who presented to the emergency department for treatment of mild to moderately severe asthma exacerbation.[31] Patients were randomized to receive an active drug (albuterol) either by an MDI-spacer or by a nebulizer. Patients were treated with aerosolized albuterol or placebo by an MDI-spacer, followed immediately by albuterol or placebo administered by nebulizer with oxygen. The dose ratio for albuterol delivery by MDI-spacer versus nebulizer was 1:5. Outcome measures included a clinical score, respiratory rate, oxygen saturation, and FEV_1, measured at baseline and at 10, 20, and 40 minutes after treatment. No significant differences were noted for any of these parameters, except for heart rate, between the groups during the 40-minute study period. The heart rate increased in the nebulizer group and decreased in the MDI-spacer group ($p < .05$). The investigators concluded that spacers and nebulizers are equally effective means of delivering beta$_2$-agonists to children with acute asthma.

Chou and colleagues also conducted an RCT in an emergency department and included children aged 2 years and older presenting with an acute asthma exacerbation.[32] One hundred and fifty-two children were randomized to receive standard doses of albuterol by an

MDI-spacer or by a nebulizer. Dosing intervals and other medications were determined by the treating physician. The main outcome measures included changes in asthma severity score (pulmonary index), oxygen saturation, and peak expiratory flow rate (PEFR) in children 5 years or older. These were measured before each treatment and at the time of final disposition. There were no significant differences between the groups in the main outcome measures, leading to the conclusion that MDIs with spacers are an effective alternative to nebulizers for treatment of children with acute asthma exacerbations. There were some interesting findings in the secondary outcomes. In terms of rate of hospital admissions, there were no differences between the groups (5.6 percent in the spacer group versus 6.2 percent in the nebulizer group; $p = 0.89$). However, it was noted that children in the spacer group did spend less time receiving treatment in the emergency department compared with the nebulizer group (66 minutes versus 103 minutes, $p < .001$). It was found that the nebulizer group had a significantly greater mean percent increase in heart rate at disposition compared with the spacer group (15 percent versus 5 percent, $p < .001$).

The lack of evidence in preschool aged (1 to 5 years) children with asthma led Parkin and colleagues to evaluate the effectiveness of MDI-spacers in young children, using an RCT design.[33] Sixty children (mean age 35 months), hospitalized with moderate, acute exacerbation of asthma were enrolled in the study. Patients were randomized to receive bronchodilators by nebulizer or by MDI-spacer. The children randomized to the nebulizer received salbutamol 0.15 mg/kg/dose (maximum 5 mg). The dose ratio for salbutamol by MDI-spacer versus nebulizer was 1:4. The dosing interval of inhaled bronchodilators was determined by the attending physician. All patients received systemic corticosteroids. This was a single-blind study, that is, only the research nurse who measured the outcomes was blinded. The primary outcome measure was a valid, reliable clinical asthma score (measured on a scale of 0 to 10), specifically developed for this population of children less than 5 years of age, hospitalized with an acute exacerbation of asthma.[34] This was measured at baseline and every 12 hours for the first 60 hours of hospitalization. The groups did differ on baseline severity, as measured by the clinical asthma score (MDI-spacer versus nebulizer: 5.7 versus 4.8, $p = .02$). Nine patients allocated to the MDI-spacer group crossed over to the nebulizer group. The intention-to-treat analysis, adjusted on the baseline clinical asthma score difference, showed no significant difference between the groups in the clinical asthma score over time ($p = .54$). The results of this trial suggest that delivery of bronchodilators by an MDI-spacer is as effective as that by a nebulizer in hospitalized young asthmatics.

Anticholinergics

Anticholinergic agents produce bronchodilation by inhibiting cholinergic activation of airway smooth muscle and blocking cholinergic reflex bronchoconstriction. They are not first-line bronchodilators but may provide some additive benefit when combined with inhaled beta$_2$-agonists. Ipratropium bromide, a quaternary ammonium derivative of atropine, is the most commonly used anticholinergic agent in clinical practice. In contrast to atropine, it is a water-soluble compound that is poorly absorbed across biologic membranes. The limited bioavailability of ipratropium accounts for its relative bronchoselectivity when taken by inhalation. The compound is locally effective, with minimal systemic absorption (and hence minimal unwanted systemic anticholinergic effects) from the inhaled or swallowed aerosol droplets. The onset of action of ipratropium is somewhat slower than that of a beta-adrenergic agent, but the duration of its effect is longer. Peak bronchodilation typically occurs 30 to 90 minutes after inhalation, as compared with 5 to 15 minutes with an adrenergic agent. Some bronchodilator response does occur very rapidly after inhalation; 50 percent of the maximal response occurs within 3 minutes and 80 percent within 30 minutes. Significant effects may persist for more than 4 hours.[35–37] The bronchodilation achieved at peak effect is less than that achieved with an adrenergic agent.[38]

Ipratropium bromide is remarkably free of unwanted side effects. In particular, it does not affect respiratory mucociliary clearance, urinary flow, or intraocular tension.[35] There have been isolated reports of ocular complications (ie, prolonged pupillary dilation), when nebulized ipratropium bromide has escaped from the face mask and been absorbed locally into the eye.[39] However, in a study of 20 children with asthma, who had no pre-existing ocular abnormalities, Watson and colleagues concluded that nebulized ipratropium bromide did not significantly increase intraocular pressures or affect pupillary size or pupillary response.[40] Unfavorable interactions between ipratropium and other drugs used for treating asthma have not been reported.

In school-aged children, administration of ipratropium bromide by nebulizer has been reported to produce a dose-dependent bronchodilation that becomes significant at the 75 microgram dose level.[41] A plateau was reached at 75 to 250 micrograms. To avoid subtherapeutic doses, the authors have recommended a dosage regimen of 250 micrograms in children with asthma. This dose has been used safely in wheezy children as young as 5 months of age.[42] Tolerance (tachyphylaxis) to ipratropium, a receptor antagonist, has been sought but not found.[43]

Studies of the effectiveness of a combination of ipratropium bromide and a beta$_2$-adrenergic agonist in adults with an acute exacerbation of asthma have produced conflicting results. While some studies have found inhaled anticholinergics to be effective bronchodilators in acute asthma, others have reported no additional benefits when they are combined with beta-adrenergic agonists. Three studies, set in the emergency department, have reported that combination therapy with sympathomimetic and anticholinergic agents is more efficacious than nebulized sympathomimetic therapy alone.[44–46] In contrast, two large, well-designed, multicenter trials have failed to demonstrate a significant additive benefit of nebulized ipratropium bromide to nebulized beta$_2$-agonists in the emergency department setting.[47,48]

Three studies have looked at the effectiveness of the addition of ipratropium bromide in adults admitted to hospital with an acute asthma exacerbation.[49–51] Valid conclusions cannot be drawn from the inpatient studies. Methodologic problems include low power, short duration of follow-up, and infrequent administration of inhaled bronchodilators.

Numerous RCTs have examined the efficacy of the addition of anticholinergics to beta$_2$-agonists for treating acute asthma in children and adolescents. A meta-analysis of RCTs up to 1992 concluded that there was a 12 percent greater improvement in percentage predicted FEV$_1$ with anticholinergic use but no reduction in hospital admission.[52] Several new trials have been completed since 1992, and the results have been summarized in a systematic review.[53] The majority of studies have been conducted in the emergency department setting.

Ten relevant RCTs were included in the systematic review.[53] Six of these were of high methodological quality.[54] Most trials considered children and adolescents with severe exacerbations, one studied children with mild to moderate asthma,[55] and two failed to describe the baseline severity of their patients' asthma.[56,57] Co-intervention with corticosteroids was infrequent. Most studies only included children aged 5 years and older. This directly reflected the fact that the main outcome variable used was pulmonary function test measurements. Respiratory resistance measured by forced oscillation was used in one trial of children aged 3 to 17 years.[55] Clinical scores were used for the youngest patients in two trials.[56,58]

Five trials with a total number of 453 patients examined the efficacy of adding a single dose of 250 micrograms of ipratropium bromide to beta$_2$-agonists. No reduction in hospitalization was observed when pooling the two trials reporting this outcome (relative risk 0.93, 95 percent confidence interval 0.65 to 1.32).[55,59] Significant group differences in lung function were documented at 60 minutes and at 120 minutes after the dose of anticholinergics, both favoring anticholinergic use.[57,59,60] No group difference was observed in the study examining the intervention in children with mild to moderate exacerbations.[55]

Five trials, with a total of 366 children, examined the effects of multiple doses of combined ipratropium bromide and beta$_2$-agonists in a fixed protocol. The maximum number of doses studied was three. Pooling of the trials contributing data on hospital admission, showed a 30 percent reduction in hospital admission rate in favor of the combination treatment (RR 0.72, 95 percent CI 0.53 to 0.99).[59,61,62] A parallel improvement in lung function was noted 60 minutes after the last combined inhalation. A difference in group means of 9.66 percent (95 percent CI 5.65 to 13.68 percent) was observed when improvement was reported as change in percentage predicted FEV$_1$.[59,62,63] In the one study where anticholinergics were systematically added to every beta$_2$-agonist inhalation, irrespective of asthma severity, no group differences were observed for the few available outcomes.[56]

The conclusions of the systematic review suggest that the addition of multiple doses of inhaled anticholinergics to beta$_2$-agonist therapy seems indicated in the emergency department management of children and adolescents with severe exacerbations of asthma. Two more RCTs have been published since the completion of the systematic review.[64,65] Both were conducted in the emergency department setting, and both included younger children. Patients in both studies were treated with frequent, high-dose, nebulized albuterol and received systemic corticosteroid therapy within 20 minutes of commencing treatment in the emergency department.

Zorc and colleagues[65] randomized 427 children to receive either ipratropium bromide (250 mg/dose) or normal saline with each of the first three nebulized albuterol doses. The overall mean time to discharge was 28 minutes shorter in the ipratropium group compared with controls (185 versus 213, $p = .001$). The ipratropium group received fewer doses of nebulized albuterol compared with controls (median: 4 versus 3, $p < .01$). Admission rates did not differ significantly between the groups (ipratropium versus control: 18 percent versus 22 percent; $p = .33$).

Qureshi and colleagues[64] enrolled 480 children, aged 2 to 18 years, in this randomized, double-blind, placebo-controlled trial. All patients were treated with frequent, high-dose, nebulized albuterol and received oral corticosteroid therapy within 20 minutes of commencing treatment in the emergency department. Children randomized to the treatment group received 500 mg (2.5 mL) of ipratropium bromide with the second and third doses of albuterol; children in the control group received 2.5 mL of normal saline at these times. Overall, the rate of hospitalization (the primary outcome) was lower in the ipratropium group than in the control group (27.4 percent versus 36.5 percent, $p = .05$). There was no significant difference between the groups for patients with moderate asthma (10.1 percent versus 10.7 percent). For patients with severe asthma, the addition of ipratropium significantly reduced the need for hospitalization (37.5 percent versus 52.6 percent, $p = .02$). Although a higher dose of ipratropium was used than in the previous pediatric studies, no adverse effects were reported in any of the participants.

In conclusion, in the initial management of school-aged children and adolescents with severe exacerbations of asthma (< 55 percent of predicted FEV$_1$), the addition of multiple doses (up to three studied) of anticholinergics to beta$_2$-agonist therapy is safe, improves lung function, and reduces the hospital admission rate. In children with mild to moderate asthma exacerbations, there is no apparent benefit from adding a dose of anticholinergics to beta$_2$-agonists.

Three trials have been conducted in the inpatient setting. Storr and Lenney enrolled 138 children hospitalized because of an acute asthma exacerbation.[66] The patients ranged in age from 11 months to 15 years. Patients were randomized to receive nebulized salbutamol (5 mg/dose) or a combination of nebulized salbutamol (5 mg/dose) and ipratropium bromide (250 micrograms/dose). Nebulizers were given within set limits at the discretion of the nursing staff. The main outcome measures were length of hospitalization, number of nebulizer doses required, and PEFR. There were no significant differences between the groups in the mean length of hospital stay in days (salbutamol versus combination; 2.8 versus 3.0). The mean number of nebulized doses received per patient was 8.6 in the salbutamol group and 9.3 in the combination group. These differences were not significant. Only 39 of the 138 study patients were able to reliably carry out spirometry. The authors concluded that the 23 children who had severe airway obstruction (PEFR < 50 percent at baseline) responded better to salbutamol alone, whereas mild airway obstruction (PEFR > 75 percent) responded better to the combination of salbutamol and ipratropium bromide. The results of this study, even if they were valid, are not generalizable to current practice as bronchodilators were used infrequently (approximately every 6 to 8 hours) and corticosteroids were not given to all patients.

In the second inpatient study, Rayner and colleagues studied 37 children with acute asthma.[67] All patients received nebulized salbutamol at 4-hour intervals. Patients then received either nebulized ipratropium or placebo 30 minutes after the salbutamol sequentially at 8–hour intervals. There were no significant differences between the groups in clinical scores, PEFR, or length of hospital stay.

In the third inpatient study, Goggin and colleagues[68] undertook a double-blind, randomized, placebo-controlled trial. Eighty children (1 to 18 years), admitted to hospital with acute exacerbation of asthma were randomized to receive either nebulized ipratropium, 250 microgram/dose or nebulized normal saline. All children received nebulized salbutamol and systemic corticosteroids. The dosing interval of the study drug was matched with the salbutamol dosing interval. Over time, there were no differences between groups in the clinical asthma score (repeated measures ANOVA $p = .07$) in FEV_1 (repeated measures ANOVA $p = .63$). There were no differences between groups in the secondary outcomes: oxygen saturation, mean number of doses of inhaled study drug, mean time (hours) to an inhaled drug dosing interval of 4 hours, and mean length of hospital stay (hours).

In conclusion, there is no strong evidence to support continuing ipratropium bromide in the inpatient management of acute asthma exacerbations.

The reporting of adverse and side effects in the above studies was variable. No apparent increase in the occurrence of nausea, tremor, or vomiting was observed in patients treated in the emergency department with either single or multiple doses of ipratropium bromide. Clinically important adverse effects, such as tachycardia or hypertension, were reported too infrequently to permit any conclusions in the systematic review.

It has been suggested that anticholinergic drugs are useful in the treatment of infants and young children with wheezing and that infants generally respond better to this form of treatment than they do to beta$_2$-agonists. A recent systematic review attempted to determine whether there is evidence to support the use of anticholinergic therapy in the treatment of wheezing in children under the age of 2 years.[69] Six RCTs were identified, which were undertaken in three different settings (emergency department, inpatient, and home). The studies used a variety of delivery systems, doses, and dosing regimes. Outcomes varied in all studies. The results of the review do not support the uncritical use of anticholinergic agents for the treatment of wheezing in infancy. In the emergency department setting, one study was able to identify a reduction in the need for additional therapy 45 minutes after ipratropium plus beta$_2$-agonist versus beta$_2$-agonist alone.[70] No benefits were observed in a second study in the same setting.[71] The authors of the review conclude that a large placebo-controlled study with carefully chosen outcome criteria may be able to identify benefits in terms of a reduction in symptom severity not identified in the studies published to date.

Corticosteroids

The use of corticosteroids in the management of acute asthma exacerbations has been a subject of debate since the publication of the first major article revealing the beneficial effects of intravenous steroids in acute asthma.[72] Recent advances have increased our knowledge about the role of inflammation in the pathophysiology of asthma, making it appear theoretically justifiable to use corticosteroids in the treatment of asthma. The anti-inflammatory actions of corticosteroids include blockade of the late reaction to allergen and reduction of airway hyper-responsiveness. Corticosteroids also suppress the generation of cytokines, recruitment of airway eosinophils, and release of inflammatory mediators.[12]

The overall conclusion from reviewing the adult literature is that corticosteroids are efficacious in the management of acute asthma. All studies reviewed here are RCTs, and all patients received concomitant bronchodilator therapy. A trial conducted in the inpatient setting found a significant improvement in FEV_1 at 24 hours in patients treated with intravenous methylprednisolone compared with placebo. The small sample size (n = 20) limits the conclusions of this study.[73] Two RCTs found that patients treated with corticosteroids in the emergency department and continued on an 8-day course of oral steroids had a reduced relapse rate compared with patients treated with placebo.[74,75] Stein and colleagues found that the early use of steroids in the emergency department did not affect hospital admission rates. However, the overall admission rate in the study was low (18 percent).[76] A similar study did find a significant reduction in hospitalization rate in patients treated with intravenous methylprednisolone compared with placebo (19 percent versus 47 percent, $p < .003$).[77]

The most recent clinical trials in children have shown a beneficial effect of corticosteroids when they are used early in the management of those with an acute exacerbation of asthma. Storr and colleagues randomized 140 patients with acute asthma to receive oral prednisolone or placebo.[78] Thirty percent of the prednisolone group, compared with 3 percent of the placebo group, were discharged at the first review at 5 hours ($p < .0001$).

A randomized, placebo-controlled trial of intramuscular methylprednisolone in 74 young children (aged 7 to 54 months) showed a significant improvement in clinical scores and a significant reduction in hospitalization in the group receiving corticosteroid compared with the group receiving placebo.[79] All patients received concomitant nebulized beta$_2$-agonist therapy. Benefits were seen within 3 hours of administration of corticosteroid, which supports early treatment. The authors also concluded that very young infants benefit from such therapy as well.

The efficacy of corticosteroids was further supported in a trial conducted by Scarfone and colleagues.[80] Seventy-five patients, aged 1 to 17 years, were randomized to receive oral prednisolone or placebo. All patients received frequently administered nebulized albuterol, for up to a maximum of 4 hours. Patients in the oral prednisone group, compared with the placebo group, had greater improvement in pulmonary index, based on clinical evaluation, and a lower admission rate (31 percent versus 49 percent, $p = .10$).

Connett and colleagues conducted a similar randomized trial in 70 children.[81] In addition to randomization to prednisolone or placebo, patients were also randomized to receive either high-dose, frequently administered bronchodilators or less frequently administered salbutamol. It was found that the group receiving prednisolone and more intensive treatment with bronchodilators had significantly higher PEFRs at 4 hours compared with other groups and also had increased likelihood of discharge. The authors conclude that the addition of corticosteroids to optimal bronchodilator treatment produces an independent quantifiable effect on lung function.

The short courses of systemic corticosteroids used in these studies appear to be relatively free of side effects. The main disadvantage of the oral route is the bitter taste of prednisolone. However, very few patients vomited the medication. These studies have included children as young as 1 year and as old as 18 years of age. They have also included a wide range of acute asthma severity in children. The more recent studies also included optimal bronchodilator therapy, which is the recommended first-line treatment for acute asthma. Therefore, these results are applicable to the majority of children who present to pediatricians and emergency departments for treatment of acute asthma.

Corticosteroids, given by the intramuscular or intravenous route, have been shown to be efficacious in the management of acute asthma exacerbations in young children.[79,82] Scarfone and colleagues demonstrated that, compared with placebo, oral prednisolone reduced hospitalization rates.[80] A meta-analysis combining adult and pediatric studies concluded that there is no evidence to suggest that one route improves pulmonary function more than the other.[83]

Barnett and colleagues designed a double-blind RCT to specifically address this question.[84] Forty-nine patients, aged 18 months to 18 years, who presented to the emergency department with moderate to severe asthma exacerbation were enrolled in the trial. They were randomized to receive oral methylprednisolone or intravenous methylprednisolone 30 minutes after the initial treatment with nebulized beta$_2$-agonists. All patients received frequent, high-dose nebulized beta$_2$-agonists. They were also treated with intravenous aminophylline. There were no differences between the groups in any of the outcomes measured at 4 hours after treatment. The principal outcome was hospital admission, and 48 percent of the oral group were admitted, compared with 50 percent of the intravenous group ($p = .88$). The relatively high admission rates in both groups may reflect the severity of the illness in the patients enrolled in the study. The results of this study suggest that the administration of corticosteroids by the oral route is as efficacious as by the intravenous route in children with acute asthma. Oral administration offers several advantages over the IV or IM routes, particularly in the pediatric age group, as it is painless and less frightening for children.

Short courses of oral corticosteroids are recommended in asthma guidelines for adults and children. In children, the recommended dose of prednisolone or an equivalent is 1 to 2 mg per kg once daily (maximum 40 to 60 mg).[12,14] A recent study has been conducted to specifically evaluate three doses of the oral corticosteroid, prednisolone, in children admitted to hospital with acute asthma.[85] Children, aged 1 to 15 years, were randomized to receive one of three prednisolone doses: 0.5 mg, 1.0 mg, or 2.0 mg per kg in a single daily dose, up to a maximum daily dose of 60 mg. All children were treated with nebulized bronchodilators, according to the usual hospital protocol. There were no significant differences between the groups in the measures of asthma severity over time, median duration of hospitalization, and median number of doses of nebulized therapy. No side effects attributable to prednisolone therapy was noted in any of the three treatment groups. During the 2 weeks following discharge, there were no differences in symptom scores, use of bronchodilators, and re-admission rates between the groups. The results suggest that the lower dose of 0.5mg/kg/day of prednisolone is as efficacious as higher doses in treating an acute exacerbation of asthma. It will be important to see if this result is confirmed in future studies of larger sample size.

There have been no studies comparing different timings of administration of corticosteroids. However, in trials designed to evaluate the efficacy of corticosteroid therapy, administration has been early in the management of acute asthma, as early as 30 minutes after presentation. The benefits of corticosteroids have been documented within 4 hours of their administration. Therefore, it is recommended that corticosteroids be used in the early phase of emergency department management. Prednisolone or equivalent 1 to 2 mg/kg in one daily dose for 5 to 10 days is the currently recommended dose, although further research is needed regarding the optimum dose.

Methylxanthines

Theophylline and aminophylline have been popular medications for both acute and chronic asthma for over 50 years. They have proven efficacy as bronchodilators in asthma and formerly were considered first-line therapy. Theophylline has a narrow therapeutic index, and adverse effects such as tremor, nausea, vomiting, tachycardia, headaches, and abdominal pain occur frequently in patients treated for acute asthma exacerbations. More toxic effects, including arrhythmias and seizures, have also been reported. This necessitates frequent blood sampling to monitor serum levels, which increases the level of discomfort for the patient. Significant drug interactions also occur. The introduction of newer pharmacologic agents and concerns about the toxicity of theophylline have recently contributed to its decreased use.[86]

Controlled trials of aminophylline in acute asthma management in adults have had conflicting results. In the emergency department, aminophylline appears to provide no additional benefit over optimal inhaled beta$_2$-agonist therapy and may have increased adverse effects.[87–89] One emergency department study did show a reduction in the rate of admission to hospital.[90] The addition of intravenous theophylline in hospitalized adults remains controversial.[91,92]

Seven RCTs have been undertaken in children. In an early study in 1971, Pierson and colleagues showed that in children hospitalized with acute asthma, intravenous aminophylline provided additional benefit when added to a regimen of hydrocortisone and sympathomimetic drugs.[93] Although this study showed a benefit from aminophylline, sympathomimetic drugs that are currently outmoded were used in the trial. Therefore, its relevance and generalizability to current clinical practice is questionable.

More recently, five well-designed randomized, placebo-controlled, double-blind trials have failed to demonstrate any benefit from adding aminophylline to inhaled beta$_2$-agonists and systemically administered corticosteroids in children hospitalized with mild to moderate acute exacerbation of asthma.[94–98] Three of the studies included children as young as 2 years.[95,97,98] In all five studies, patients were randomized to receive either intravenous infusion of aminophylline or a placebo. All patients received nebulized beta$_2$-agonists and systemic corticosteroids. The primary outcome measure was length of hospital stay in two studies,[94,97] improvement in FEV$_1$ in the study by Carter and colleagues,[96] and clinical scores in the other two studies.[95,98] There were no differences between the groups in outcome measures in the five clinical trials.

In summary, these trials provide evidence that the addition of aminophylline to inhaled beta$_2$-agonists and systemically administered corticosteroids does not enhance improvement of children admitted to hospital with a mild to moderate exacerbation of asthma. The most likely explanation for the lack of added benefit from aminophylline in these studies is the difference between the sympathomimetic drugs currently used and those used in earlier work.[93] Modern beta-agonists are selective for beta$_2$-receptors, act for longer periods, and are probably used in larger equivalent doses than their predecessors, such as isoproterenol and isoprenaline.

The previously described trials excluded severely ill children. Subsequently, a large, well-conducted RCT that included children with severe acute asthma has been reported.[99] The aim of this study was to determine whether children with severe acute asthma treated with large doses of inhaled salbutamol, inhaled ipratropium, and intravenous steroids are conferred any further benefits by the addition of aminophylline given intravenously. A total of 163 children, aged 1 to 19 years, admitted to hospital with severe, acute asthma were enrolled in the study. Patients were randomized to receive intravenous aminophylline infusion or sterile water (placebo) infusion. All patients were given standard care for the institution, which included frequent nebulized salbutamol, nebulized ipratropium bromide every 4 to 6 hours, and systemic corticosteroids. The need for intravenous salbutamol was determined by the medical staff directly looking after the patient. There were no differences between the groups in length of hospital stay. The mean length of stay for the placebo group was 2.87 days and for the aminophylline group 2.69 days. Aminophylline did confer clinically and statistically significant early benefits on airway function (up to 6 hours) and oxygenation (up to 24 hours). At the dose used, it was associated with a significant risk of nausea (43 percent increased frequency) and vomiting (48 percent increased frequency). In conclusion, in children with severe, acute asthma unresponsive to maximum treatment with beta$_2$-agonists and systemic corticosteroids, aminophylline does not confer additional benefits on the ultimate outcome. It has been shown to confer an early additional benefit on airway function and a more sustained benefit on oxygenation, but at the cost of a high frequency of adverse effects. On the basis of these findings, the authors recommend that clinicians should use treatments with a lower risk of adverse effects in such patients. They conclude their discussion by commenting that aminophylline has a role in the emergency treatment of severe acute asthma, when other treatments have been unsuccessful.

LONG-TERM ASTHMA MANAGEMENT (SEE TABLE 7–2)

Corticosteroids

Efficacy of Long-Term Inhaled Steroids

Airway inflammation appears to be a key factor in the development of airway hyper-responsiveness in individuals with asthma. Therefore, anti-inflammatory therapy has become a cornerstone of long-term management of children with moderate to severe asthma. Calpin and colleagues[100] undertook a systematic review of the literature. Twenty-four randomized double-blind, placebo-controlled trials (from 1973 to 1996) of prophylactic inhaled steroid therapy for childhood asthma were identified.[101–124] In total, 1,087 children were studied in the 24 clinical trials, with study sample sizes ranging from 18 to 258 children. Thirteen (57 percent) of the trials involved school-aged children, whereas 10 (42 percent) involved preschool-aged children (age was not specified in one study). Five of the trials (22 percent) involved children with oral steroid–dependent asthma only. Several different inhaled steroids were used as the experimental treatment (betamethasone valerate, beclomethasone dipropionate, flunisolide, budesonide, and fluticasone propionate). There was variation in the daily dose delivered (150 micrograms to 2 mg) and the delivery device used (metered-dose inhaler, nebulizer, nebuhaler, disk inhaler). The median duration of steroid use was 8 weeks (range 4 to 88 weeks). Improvement in the following outcome measures were calculated: total symptom score, cough score, wheeze score, beta-agonist use, oral steroid use, and PEFR. The overall weighted relative improvement in the mean total symptom score (inhaled steroid versus placebo) was 50 percent (95 percent CI: 49 percent, 51 percent); the overall weighted relative decrease in mean concomitant beta-agonist use (inhaled steroid versus placebo) was 37 percent (95 percent CI: 36 percent, 38 percent); the overall weighted relative decrease in mean concomitant oral steroid use (inhaled steroid versus placebo) was 68 percent (95 percent CI: 66 percent, 70 percent); the overall weighted absolute improvement in mean PEFR (inhaled steroid versus placebo) was 38 L/min (95 percent CI: 34.3 L/min, 41.7 L/min). This systematic review demonstrated that prophylactic inhaled steroids are effective, compared with placebo, in improving both clinical and laboratory outcomes in children.

Since the review by Calpin and colleagues,[100] several large, long-term studies have further examined the efficacy of inhaled corticosteroids. Price and colleagues[125] followed up 123 asthmatic children aged 4 to 10 years for 12 months. Children were randomized to receive inhaled fluticasone propionate 100 micrograms daily or sodium cromoglycate 80 micrograms daily, and there was a significant treatment effect in favor of fluticasone (see below for further discussion on sodium cromoglycate). In three studies (total n = 485), each 12 months in duration, beclomethasone 400 micrograms daily has been found to be more effective than salmeterol 100 micrograms daily (see below for further discussion on long-acting beta$_2$-adrenergic-receptor agonists [salmeterol]).[126–128]

Finally, the relative efficacy of different inhaled corticosteroids has been examined in a few clinical trials. For children with mild to moderate asthma requiring medium dose

Table 7–2 Management of Chronic Childhood Asthma

Condition	Intervention	Quality of Evidence	Recommendation
Mild chronic asthma	Inhaled sodium cromoglycate as compared with placebo is efficacious	I	A
Mild to severe chronic asthma	Prophylactic inhaled corticosteroids as compared with placebo are efficacious	I	A
Mild to moderate chronic asthma	Prophylactic inhaled corticosteroids as compared with salmeterol are more efficacious	I	A
Mild to severe chronic asthma	Prophylactic inhaled corticosteroids as compared with sodium cromoglycate are more efficacious	I	A
Moderate to severe chronic asthma	Addition of inhaled salmeterol to inhaled corticosteroids as compared with inhaled corticosteroids alone is equally efficacious	I	D
Moderate to severe chronic asthma	Medium-dose inhaled fluticasone propionate as compared with beclomethasone dipropionate is more efficacious	I	B
Severe chronic asthma	High-dose inhaled fluticasone propionate as compared with budesonide is more efficacious	I	B
Mild to severe chronic asthma	Inhaled beclomethasone dipropionate as compared with placebo is associated with moderate growth impairment. Patients/parents should be informed and growth monitored	I	A
Moderate to severe chronic asthma	Inhaled fluticasone propionate as compared with beclomethasone dipropionate and budesonide is associated with less growth impairment	I	B
Moderate to severe chronic asthma	Oral leukotriene modifiers as compared with placebo are efficacious. However, there is no evidence regarding efficacy as compared with inhaled corticosteroids, and little evidence with respect to safety	I	D

inhaled corticosteroid, fluticasone propionate 200 micrograms daily has been found to be more effective than beclomethasone dipropionate 400 micrograms daily.[129] In children requiring high-dose inhaled corticosteroid, fluticasone propionate 400 micrograms daily has been found to be more effective than budesonide 800 micrograms daily.[130] Barnes and colleagues[131] have undertaken a meta-analysis to determine the relative efficacy and systemic effects of different inhaled corticosteroids. The meta-analysis included seven trials (n = 1,980) comparing fluticasone propionate with budesonide and seven trials (n = 1,584) comparing fluticasone propionate with beclomethasone dipropionate in both adult and pediatric patients. The authors found fluticasone propionate to be more effective than budesonide and as effective as beclomethasone dipropionate in improving PEFR. Cortisol suppression associated with fluticasone propionate and beclomethasone dipropionate was similar; cortisol suppression associated with budesonide was greater than that associated with fluticasone propionate. The authors concluded that fluticasone propionate has a better efficacy to safety ratio as compared with older inhaled corticosteroids.

Growth in Children Receiving Long-Term Inhaled Steroids

There has been considerable concern and controversy regarding the potential role of steroids on the growth of children. Allen and colleagues[132] undertook a meta-analysis of the effect of oral and inhaled corticosteroids on growth. They conducted a literature search for a 37-year period up to January 1993. Studies were included if they reported the number of children with asthma receiving corticosteroids that were at or above their expected height as well as the number of children with asthma receiving corticosteroids who were below their expected height. Only studies that measured attained height over the period of the study were included. Studies using short-term determinations of "growth" (for example, knemometry) and studies using inferential statistics were excluded. Twenty-one studies were identified.[133–153] The specific corticosteroid used in each study was classified as inhaled beclomethasone dipropionate, oral prednisone, or other oral corticosteroids. As several studies included patients with more than one classification of corticosteroids, the 21 studies yielded 29 tests (12 inhaled beclomethasone dipropionate, 7 oral prednisone, and 10 other oral corticosteroids) of the association between corticosteroid use and growth. For the studies that included patients using inhaled beclomethasone dipropionate, the median daily dosage was 400 micrograms/day (range 200 micrograms/day to 875 micrograms/day); only one study used a dosage greater than 800 micrograms/day; the median duration of treatment was between 1.6 and 2.1 years (range 0.2 to 5.8 years); the median age was between 9.1 and 9.4 years (range 7.5 to 12.5 years); half the studies included children with mild to moderate asthma, and half included children with severe asthma. For each study, the number of children below the expected height was compared with the number of children at or above the expected height, using chi-square tests. The chi-square test was then transformed into an effect size, using the product moment correlation (r). A positive correlation ($+r$) indicates that the number of children at or above their expected height was greater than the number of children below their expected height; a negative correlation ($-r$) indicates that the number of children at or above their expected height was smaller than the number of children below their expected height. Oral prednisone therapy showed a significantly moderate tendency to be associated with shorter height than expected ($r = -0.295$). Other oral corticosteroid therapy showed a significantly weak tendency to be associated with shorter than expected ($r = -0.260$). Inhaled beclomethasone dipropionate therapy showed a significantly moderate tendency to be associated with normal stature ($r = +0.423$). For children receiving inhaled beclomethasone dipropionate, there was an inverse relationship between age and growth, whereby children younger than 11.2 years showed no growth impairment, and children older than 11.2 years showed growth impairment; there was no significant association between growth and higher doses (but only one study used doses greater than 800 micrograms/day), longer duration of therapy, more severe asthma. The authors concluded that children and their families should be informed that inhaled moderate-dose (that is, less than 600 micrograms/day) beclomethasone dipropionate therapy is unlikely to have a clinically significant effect on linear growth and should be considered safe; that there remains a risk for idiosyncratic responses leading to significant growth impairment; and that careful monitoring of the linear growth of children with asthma treated with inhaled corticosteroids is warranted.

Several long-term studies of inhaled corticosteroids, in which height velocity has been measured, have been undertaken since the review by Allen and colleagues.[132] Four studies[126,127,154,155] have compared beclomethasone dipropionate with placebo or another asthma therapy (salmeterol or theophylline) over 7 to 12 months. All studies (total n = 597) found that growth in children receiving approximately 400 micrograms daily of beclomethasone dipropionate was restricted (mean growth in the four studies ranged from 3.96 cm/year to 4.7 cm/year) as compared with placebo or another asthma therapy (mean growth in the four studies ranged from 5.04 cm/year to 6.27 cm/year). In a further study of 177 children, Verberne and colleagues[128] found that children receiving 800 micrograms daily of beclomethasone dipropionate had an even greater growth restriction (3.6 cm/year) than two groups of children receiving 400 micrograms daily of beclomethasone dipropionate (4.5 cm/year and 5.1 cm/year).

Growth restriction has not been found in three long term studies of fluticasone proprionate.[125,130,156] Price and colleagues[125] studied 123 children over 12 months randomized to receive fluticasone proprionate 100 micrograms daily as compared with sodium cromoglycate. Growth was 6.0 cm/year versus 6.5 cm/year in the fluticasone proprionate and sodium cromoglycate groups, respectively. Allen and colleagues[156] studied 325 children over 12 months randomized to receive fluticasone proprionate 100 micrograms daily, fluticasone proprionate 200 micrograms daily or placebo. Growth was 5.91 cm/year, 5.67 cm/ year, and 6.1 cm/year in the fluticasone proprionate 100 micrograms daily, fluticasone proprionate 200 micrograms daily and placebo groups, respectively. Ferguson and colleagues[130] studied 333 children who required high-dose inhaled steroids over 20 weeks. The children were randomized to receive fluticasone proprionate 400 micrograms daily or budesonide 800 micrograms daily. In a subgroup of 154 children whose heights had been measured by stadiometry, the adjusted mean growth was 3.31 cm/20 weeks in the group receiving fluticasone proprionate 400 micrograms daily, as compared with 1.99 cm/20 weeks in the group receiving budesonide 800 micrograms daily.

These studies suggest that in school-aged children who require inhaled corticosteroid to control their asthma symptoms, growth restriction is more often associated with beclomethasone dipropionate and budesonide than fluticasone proprionate. This is supported by a meta-analysis by Barnes and colleagues,[131] which included seven trials (n = 1,980) comparing fluticasone propionate with budesonide, and seven trials (n = 1,584) comparing fluticasone propionate with beclomethasone dipropionate in both adult and pediatric patients. The authors found that cortisol suppression associated with fluticasone propionate and beclomethasone dipropionate was similar; cortisol suppression associated with budesonide was greater than that associated with fluticasone propionate.

Suppression of growth hormone is thought to be an important factor associated with growth suppression in children receiving corticosteroid therapy. Since growth hormone is secreted in a circadian rhythm (with several peaks at night), it has been hypothesized that growth suppression may be reduced if inhaled corticosteroids could be administered in the morning, rather than both in the morning and in the evening. In a recent study, Heuck and colleagues[157] compared short-term leg growth (using knemometry) and markers of collagen turnover during treatment with 800 micrograms of inhaled budesonide administered once daily in the morning and 400 micrograms administered twice daily. Twenty-four children aged 5.6 to 12.5 years (mean age 9.2 years) were randomized in a double-blind, two-period, cross-over trial with treatment periods of 4 weeks and a 1-week wash-out period. Mean lower leg length and markers of collagen turnover were suppressed during twice-daily administration as compared with once-daily morning administration. When boys and girls were analyzed separately, it was found that the difference remained significant in boys but not in girls. In an accompanying editorial, Brook[158] recommended the following precautions when interpreting the results of this study: there is controversy about the use of knemometry in studies of growth of children, given that growth in children may be saltatory (jumping) in nature;

the study did not address the issue of the efficacy of once-daily dosing on asthma control; the difference between boys and girls may have been due to the fact that the median age of the boys was likely older than the median age of the girls, and hence the association may have been due to age as much as gender. Finally, Brook[158] notes that "asthma is a killing disease, but nobody died of being short. I urge clinicians first and foremost to aim at optimal disease control; children with uncontrolled asthma grow poorly anyway ... physicians [might] attempt to titrate treatment regimens, trying to give a larger dose of steroid in the morning. As long as they achieve symptom control, they may well have a better growth outcome in the short term."

Sodium Cromoglycate

Sodium cromoglycate inhibits mast cell degranulation, thereby inhibiting the release of mediators of both immediate and late bronchoconstrictive reactions to allergens. The primary advantage of sodium cromoglycate is its minimal side effects. Sodium cromoglycate is recommended for children with frequent episodic symptoms requiring inhaled beta$_2$-adrenergic agonists and those who require stepped-up therapy.[10,12]

Several investigators have examined the efficacy of sodium cromoglycate in school-aged children. The effectiveness of sodium cromoglycate has been established in several placebo-controlled trials including over 350 school-aged children with asthma.[159–166] Effectiveness and safety have been supported in a large, multicenter, randomized, double-blind, placebo-controlled, cross-over study of 276 school-aged children with chronic asthma.[167] Two additional large placebo-controlled studies, which included both school-aged children and adults, have demonstrated the effectiveness of sodium cromoglycate.[168,169] Sodium cromoglycate has been found to be at least as effective as theophylline,[170–174] possibly with fewer side effects. More recently, it has been shown that chronic asthma is better controlled when sodium cromoglycate is used alone or in combination with terbutaline than when the beta-agonist is used alone.[175] Furthermore, the addition of sodium cromoglycate has permitted the reduction of inhaled steroids in children with mild to moderate asthma.[176]

In several small trials, inhaled corticosteroid therapy has been found to be more effective than sodium cromoglycate.[177–183] More recently, Price and Weller studied 225 asthmatic children aged 4 to 12 years. Children were randomized to 50 micrograms of inhaled fluticasone propionate twice daily or 20 mg of inhaled sodium cromoglycate four times daily for 8 weeks. Children receiving inhaled fluticasone propionate demonstrated superior outcomes with significantly better morning and evening percentage predicted PEFRs, and percent of symptom-free days and nights. There were no differences in FEV$_1$ or relief medication used. Subsequently, Price and colleagues[125] followed up 123 asthmatic children aged 4 to 10 years for 12 months. These children were randomized to receive inhaled fluticasone propionate 100 micrograms daily or sodium cromoglycate 80 micrograms daily. Patients were reassessed after 8 weeks of treatment. Those with uncontrolled asthma (defined a priori) were either switched to fluticasone if they were receiving sodium cromoglycate or were withdrawn from the study. After the first 8 weeks of therapy, 22 of 70 (31 percent) children randomized to receive sodium cromoglycate failed to respond to treatment and were switched to fluticasone. Five of 52 (10 percent) patients randomized to receive fluticasone were withdrawn due to poor asthma control. At 1 year, there were no significant differences in height velocity between groups. The mean height velocity was 6.0 cm/year in the fluticasone group, and was 6.5 cm/year in the sodium cromoglycate group. The mean morning percentage of predicted PEFR expressed as change from baseline in percentage points was significantly better in the children that received fluticasone. At 12 months the estimated treatment difference was 7.3 percentage points in favor of fluticasone ($p = .01$).

In summary, in school-aged children, the evidence suggests that sodium cromoglycate is superior to placebo or "as needed" beta$_2$-agonists, and is at least as effective as theophylline in the management of asthma. Therefore, for many children with asthma who require long-term treatment, sodium cromoglycate may provide an effective and safe alternative to corticosteroids and theophylline. However, several studies have shown that inhaled corticosteroids are more effective than sodium cromoglycate, and one study provides evidence that low-dose inhaled fluticasone is more effective than inhaled sodium cromoglycate, with no associated impact on growth. Hence, the current recommendation to step up therapy with the addition of sodium cromoglycate to intermittent inhaled beta$_2$-adrenergic agonists for those children with frequent episodic symptoms and then to replace sodium cromoglycate with low-dose steroid if there is an insufficient response within 6 weeks,[10] appears to be evidence-based.

Additional clinical trials in infants and preschool-aged children with asthma or wheezing have shown mixed results. The two most rigorous studies have found no difference between sodium cromoglycate and placebo over 6 to 10 weeks in children less than 1 year of age,[185] and children 1 to 4 years of age.[186] Several less rigorous studies have suggested that sodium cromoglycate is superior to placebo in preschool-aged children.[187–189] Two other studies have compared sodium cromoglycate with oral theophylline. Glass and colleagues[190] found that neither sodium cromoglycate nor oral theophylline was different from placebo on most measures of symptom control over an 8-week period in children 1 to 4 years of age. Newth and colleagues[191] found that both sodium cromoglycate and oral theophylline are at least equally effective over an 8-week period in children 1 to 4 years of age but did not compare them with placebo. Finally, De Baets and colleagues[192] studied a small group of preschool-aged children (n = 15, age range 43 to 66 months) in a cross-over trial of sodium cromoglycate compared with inhaled beclomethasone over a 2-month period. It was found that children receiving beclomethasone had significantly fewer wheezing exacerbations, but there was no difference in bronchial responsiveness as measured by airway resistance.

In summary, the evidence in preschool-aged children is less clearly supportive of the effectiveness of sodium cromoglycate. However, an approach similar to that recommended for school-aged children (that is, stepping up to addition of sodium cromoglycate and further addition of inhaled corticosteroid if there is no improvement) appears to be supported by the best available evidence.

Long-Acting Beta$_2$-Adrenergic-Receptor Agonists (Salmeterol)

Salmeterol is a long-acting beta$_2$-agonist. The bronchodilator activity of salmeterol lasts for up to 12 hours, as compared with 4 to 5 hours of that of short-acting beta$_2$-agonists. Several studies in children 4 to 16 years,[193–196] and an overview[197] of studies in children and adults comparing salmeterol with placebo or salmeterol with salbutamol have been undertaken. These studies suggest that salmeterol 50 micrograms twice daily provides more effective protection from bronchoconstriction than placebo or "as needed" salbutamol. There has been considerable controversy regarding the potential for the development of tolerance to this protective effect with long-term use and a possible rebound increase in bronchial hyperresponsiveness on stopping treatment. In a 12-month randomized, double-blind trial of salmeterol 50 micrograms twice daily as compared with placebo plus "as needed" salbutamol, von Berg and colleagues[196] have shown that the improvement in lung function is maintained over time without evidence of the development of tolerance. These studies included children receiving concomitant inhaled corticosteroids, and approximately 50 percent continued to receive inhaled corticosteroid therapy throughout the trials. Given that inhaled corticosteroids are the medication of choice for long-term management of asthma, studies comparing inhaled corticosteroids with salmeterol are critical to understanding the role of salmeterol in long-term management. Three studies[126–128] have evaluated salmeterol compared with and in combination with inhaled corticosteroids.

Simons and colleagues[126] performed a randomized, double-blind, parallel-group comparison of beclomethasone 200 micrograms twice daily, salmeterol 50 micrograms twice daily, and placebo twice daily for 1 year in 241 children (age range 6 to 14 years) with mild persistent asthma. Use of corticosteroids within 3 months before enrollment was an exclusion criterion. At baseline, the average age of the study group was 9.3 ± 2.4 years; 25 percent received other asthma medications (cromolyn sodium, nedocromil, theophylline, regular beta$_2$-agonists); the FEV$_1$ (percent of predicted) ranged from 92 ± 13 to 96 ± 16. Airway responsiveness (as assessed using repeated measures analysis of variance of a methacholine challenge) was significantly better in the beclomethasone group as compared with the salmeterol group (p = .003) and the placebo group (p <.001). The effect of salmeterol and placebo on airway hyper-responsiveness did not differ significantly. Spirometric studies improved significantly in both the beclomethasone and salmeterol groups as compared with the placebo group. Control of asthma symptoms was significantly better in the beclomethasone group as compared with placebo. The height increased by 3.96 cm in the beclomethasone group, which was significantly less than the height increases in the placebo group (5.04 cm, p = .018) and the salmeterol group (5.4 cm, p = .004). The results of this study confirm that inhaled beclomethasone is effective for long-term control. However, the authors note that for children with mild persistent asthma, as in this study, one faces a difficult choice between an inhaled beclomethasone, which provides excellent control with the potential impact upon growth, and salmeterol, which provides less effective control (but better than placebo) but no impact on growth.

Verberne and colleagues[127] performed a double-blind study of salmeterol 50 micrograms twice daily and beclomethasone 200 micrograms twice daily in 67 children 6 to 16 years of age with mild to moderate asthma for 1 year. These children had not used inhaled corticosteroids in the previous 6 months. At randomization, the children were approximately 10.5 years, with a mean FEV$_1$ percentage predicted of 82.0 ± 13.9 (salmeterol) and 84.4 ± 16.7 (beclomethasone). After 1 year, the mean difference in FEV$_1$ between treatment groups was 14.2 percent predicted (95 percent CI 8.3, 20.0, p < .0001) in favor of the beclomethasone group. Asthma exacerbations, for which prednisolone was needed, were more frequent in the salmeterol group (17 versus 2). The mean increase in height was 6.1 cm (95 percent CI 5.3, 6.9) in the salmeterol group, compared with 4.7 cm (95 percent CI 4.0, 5.3) in the beclomethasone group (p = .007). The results of this study suggest that treatment with a moderate dose of beclomethasone (400 micrograms/day) is superior to salmeterol in children with mild to moderate asthma. The authors recommend that salmeterol should not be used as monotherapy.

In a subsequent study, Verberne and colleagues[127] performed a randomized double-blind study of beclomethasone 400 micrograms/day plus salmeterol, beclomethasone 400 micrograms/day, and beclomethasone 800 micrograms/day in 177 children 6 to 16 years of age with mild to moderate asthma for 1 year. These children had used inhaled corticosteroids between 200 and 800 micrograms daily for at least 3 months before the start of the study. At randomization, the children were approximately 11 years old, with a mean FEV$_1$ percent predicted ranging from 87.4 ± 12.3 and 89.7 ± 11.8. After 1 year, there were no significant differences between groups in FEV$_1$, PD20 methacholine, symptom scores, and exacerbation rates. The mean increase in height was 5.1 cm (95 percent CI 4.5, 5.7) in the beclomethasone 400 micrograms/day plus salmeterol group, 3.6 cm (95 percent CI 3.0, 4.2) in the beclomethasone 800 micrograms/day group, and 4.5 cm (95 percent CI 3.8, 5.2) in the beclomethasone 400 micrograms/day group. The results of this study suggest that there is no benefit to adding either salmeterol or more beclomethasone to a daily dose of 400 micrograms beclomethasone in children with mild to moderate asthma.

The role of salmeterol in the management of exercise-induced asthma has been studied in adolescents. Green and Price[198] studied 13 children, aged 8 to 15 years, in a randomized, double-bind, cross-over, placebo-controlled trial. The FEV$_1$ measured after a standard exercise test at 1, 5, and 9 hours after treatment was significantly better among children who had received a single 50 microgram dose of salmeterol than those children who had received placebo. In a longer-term study of effectiveness of salmeterol over 28 days, Simons and colleagues[199] showed that on day 1, salmeterol was effective in protecting the subjects from exercise-induced asthma both 1 hour and 9 hours after treatment. However, by day 28, salmeterol was effective 1 hour after treatment but less so at 9 hours after treatment. This suggested to the authors that with daily use, tolerance to the effects of salmeterol may develop.

In summary, the evidence suggests that, although salmeterol 50 micrograms twice daily provides significant improvement in lung function as compared with placebo or "as needed" salbutamol, beclomethasone 400 micrograms/day is more effective than salmeterol. However, beclomethasone therapy is associated with a potential impact on growth. The evidence that salmeterol, in addition to beclomethasone 400 micrograms/day, provides even greater asthma control is mixed. Hence, clinicians may wish to consider the addition of salmeterol for children receiving optimal inhaled corticosteroid therapy but continue to experience symptoms requiring frequent bronchodilator therapy. Salmeterol may also play a role in the management of exercise-induced asthma; intermittent use of salmeterol appears useful in protecting against exercise-induced asthma, but daily doses may result in the development of tolerance. Salmeterol should not be used as a rescue medication, and its role in long-term monotherapy is controversial.

Leukotriene Modifiers

Leukotrienes are fatty acids that are formed from arachidonic acid that is released from the cell-membrane phospholipids.[200,201] Leukotrienes promote vascular permeability, tissue edema, and mucus secretion and are potent bronchoconstrictors. Antileukotriene drugs are either receptor antagonists, or enzyme inhibitors. Several large randomized, double-blind, placebo-controlled trials in adults demonstrate that this new class of antiasthma drugs provide significantly greater asthma control, as compared with placebo.[202–206]

Three studies have been undertaken in children. Knorr and colleagues[207] and Kemp and colleagues[208] have studied montelukast. Pearlman and colleagues[209] have studied zafirlukast. Both these new drugs are leukotriene D4 receptor antagonists.

Knorr and colleagues[207] undertook a randomized, double-blind, placebo-controlled trial of oral montelukast 5 mg chewable tablet once daily at bedtime in 336 children 6- to 14-years of age. During the 8-week trial, children were able to use "as needed" short-acting $beta_2$-agonists and were allowed to continue to use concomitant inhaled corticosteroids if they were already receiving this therapy. At baseline, the median age was 11 years, 37 percent were receiving concomitant inhaled corticosteroid, and the mean FEV_1 was 72 percent predicted. Children in the montelukast group experienced a 8.23 percent increase in FEV_1 from baseline (95 percent CI 6.33 to 10.13 percent) as compared with 3.58 percent increase in FEV_1 from baseline in the placebo group (95 percent CI 1.29 to 5.87 percent). Secondary outcome measures were also significantly improved in the montelukast group, including use of "as needed" $beta_2$-agonist, asthma exacerbations, and quality of life. The effects of montelukast were consistent across genders, history of allergic rhinitis, concomitant inhaled corticosteroid use, and age group (6 to 11 years as compared with 12 to 14 years). Montelukast had a rapid onset of action within 1 day of dosing. Common adverse events were headache, upper respiratory tract infection, pharyngitis, and abdominal pain. However, these did not differ significantly from those of the placebo group.

In a second study Kemp and colleagues[208] studied 27 children, 6 to 14 years of age, with evidence of exercise-induced asthma. In a randomized, double-blind, placebo-controlled, cross-over study, children received montelukast 5 mg chewable tablet or placebo once daily in the evening for 2 days. The children underwent an exercise challenge 20 to 24 hours after the second dose. Montelukast was superior to placebo on two measures of protection against exercise-induced asthma: the change in FEV_1 from before exercise through the 60 minutes after exercise and the postexercise maximum FEV_1 percent fall from the pre-exercise baseline. The maximum percent fall in FEV_1 was 18 percent ± 13 percent in the montelukast group, compared with 26 percent ± 14 percent in the placebo group.

Pearlman and colleagues[209] studied 39 children, 6 to 14 years of age, with evidence of exercise-induced asthma. In two parallel randomized, double-blind, placebo-controlled, three-way cross-over studies, children received zafirlukast at four dosage levels (5 mg, 10 mg, 20 mg, and 40 mg). Each dosage was administered 4 hours prior to the exercise challenge. The maximum percent fall in FEV_1 was 8.7 to 11.1 percent in the zafirlukast groups, compared with 16.3 to 17.1 percent in the placebo group. All dosages conferred protection from exercise-induced asthma, but an optimal dose was not identified.

These early studies of leukotriene receptor antagonists (LTRA) in children, along with studies in adults, suggest that these new antiasthma drugs will play a role in the management of children with asthma. How effective these drugs will be in longer-term trials, and in comparison with other established therapies, such as inhaled corticosteroids, sodium cromoglycate, and short- and long-acting beta-agonists, remains to be seen. Although there are currently no large comparative trials, it appears that their efficacy is similar to that of the well-established drugs. Furthermore, the safety profile of LTRAs is not well established, and whether compliance is improved with oral therapy, as compared with inhaled therapy, is not known. Further evidence is required on which clinicians may base their decisions regarding the appropriate role of LTRAs. Until then, it is suggested that the LTRAs be employed in managing the child with difficult-to-control asthma, where the addition of a steroid-sparing medication to low-dose inhaled steroids might be considered before use of higher-dose steroids. Or, they may be used in the child who cannot or will not take inhaled steroids.[210] In an accompanying editorial, Kercsmar notes that there are still miles to go before these new drugs find their appropriate places in the management of childhood asthma.[210]

REFERENCES

1. Weitzman M, Gortmaker S, Sobol A, Perrin J. Recent trends in the prevalence and severity of childhood asthma. JAMA 1992;268(19):2673–7.

2. Millar WJ, Hill BG. Childhood asthma. Health Reports 1998;10(3):9–21.

3. Strachan DP, Anderson HR. Trends in hospital admission rates for asthma in children. Br Med J 1992;304(6830):819–20.

4. Mitchell EA, Borman B. Demographic characteristics of asthma admissions to hospitals. N Z Med J 1986;99:576–9.

5. Weiss KB, Gergen PJ, Wagener DK. The changing epidemiology of asthma morbidity and mortality. Ann Rev Publ Health 1993;14:491–513.

6. To T, Dick P, Feldman W, Hernandez R. A cohort study on childhood asthma admissions and readmissions. Pediatrics 1996;98(2):191–5.

7. Gergen PJ, Weiss KB. Changing patterns of asthma hospitalization among children: 1979 to 1987. JAMA 1990;264(13):1688–92.

8. Goodman DC, Stukel TA, Chang C. Trends in pediatric asthma hospitalization rates: regional and socioeconomic differences. Pediatrics 1998;101:208–13.

9. Martinez FD, Wright AL, Taussig LM, et al. Asthma and wheezing in the first six years of life. N Eng J Med 1995;332(3):133–8.

10. Warner JO, Naspitz CK. Third international pediatric consensus statement on the management of childhood asthma. Pediatr Pulmonol 1998;25(1):1–17.

11. Taussig LM. Wheezing in infancy: When is it asthma? Pediatr Pulmonol 1997;(Suppl 16):90–1.

12. National Heart Lung and Blood Institute. Expert panel report 2: guidelines for the diagnosis and management of asthma. Bethesda, MD: National Institutes of Health; 1997.NIH publication no. 97–4051.

13. Ernst P, FitzGerald JM, Spier S. Canadian Asthma Consensus Conference summary of recommendations. Can Respir J 1996;3(2):89–100.

14. British Thoracic Society, The National Asthma Campaign, The Royal College of Physicians of London in association with the General Practitioner in Asthma Group, The British Association of Accident and Emergency Medicine, The British Paediatric Respiratory Society, The Royal College of Paediatrics and Child Health. The British guidelines on asthma management 1995, review and position statement. Thorax 1997;52(Suppl 1):S1–21.

15. Pavia D, Thomson ML, Clarke SW, et al. Effect of lung function and mode of inhalation on penetration of aerosol into the human lung. Thorax 1977;32:194–7.

16. Newhouse M, Dolovich M. Control of asthma by aerosols. N Engl J Med 1986;315:870–4.

17. Popa VT, Werner P. Dose-related dilation of airways after inhalation of metaproterenol sulfate. Chest 1976;70:205–11.

18. Nelson HS, Specter SL, Whitsett TL, et al. The bronchodilator response to inhalation of increasing doses of aerosolized albuterol. J Allergy Clin Immunol 1983;72:371–5.

19. Stenfield GM, Hodson ME, Clark SW, et al. Patterns of response to isoprenaline in asthma patients. Br J Dis Chest 1975;69:273.

20. Rebuck AS, Read J. Assessment and management of severe asthma. Am J Med 1971;51:788–98.

21. Chaieb JA, Kamburoff PL, Prime FJ. Effect of a repeated dose of terbutaline by inhalation. Curr Med Resp Opin 1974;5:275–80.

22. Robertson C, Smith F, Beck R, Levison H. Response to frequent low doses of nebulized salbutamol in acute asthma. J Pediatr 1985;106:672–4.

23. Schuh S, Parkin P, Rajan A, et al. High- versus low-dose, frequently administered, nebulized albuterol in children with severe, acute asthma. Pediatr 1989;83:513–8.

24. Schuh S, Reider M, Canny G, et al. Nebulized albuterol in acute childhood asthma: comparison of two doses. Pediatrics 1990;86:509–13.

25. Newman S, Millar A, Lennard-Jones T, et al. Improvement of pressurized aerosol deposition with nebuhaler spacer device. Thorax 1984;39:935–41.

26. Canny G, Levison H. Childhood asthma: a rational approach to treatment. Ann Allergy 1990;64:406–15.

27. Morgan MD, Singh BV, Frame MH, Williams SJ. Terbutaline aerosol given through pear spacer in acute severe asthma. Br Med J Clinical Research Edition 1982;285:849–50.

28. Idris A, McDermott M, Raucci J, et al. Emergency department treatment of severe asthma: metered dose inhaler plus holding chamber is equivalent in effectiveness to nebulizer. Chest 1993;103:665–72.

29. Gurwitz D, Levison H, Mindorff C, et al. Assessment of a new device (Aerochamber) for use with aerosol drugs in asthmatic children. Ann Allergy 1983;50:166–70.

30. Rivlin J, Mindorff C, Reilly P, Levison H. Pulmonary response to a bronchodilator delivered from three inhalation devices. J Pediatr 1984;104:470–3.

31. Kerem E, Levison H, Schuh S, et al. Efficacy of albuterol administered by nebulizer versus spacer device in children with acute asthma. J Pediatr 1993;123:313–7.

32. Chou K, Cunningham S, Crain E. Metered-dose inhalers with spacers vs nebulizers for pediatric asthma. Arch Pediatr Adolesc Med 1995;149:201–5.

33. Parkin P, Saunders N, Diamond S, et al. Randomised trial spacer vs nebulizer for acute asthma. Arch Dis Child 1995;72:239–40.

34. Parkin P, MacArthur C, Saunders N, et al. Development of a clinical asthma score for use in hospitalized children between 1 and 5 years of age. J Clin Epidemiol 1996;49:821–5.

35. Gross N. Ipratropium bromide. N Engl J Med 1988;319:486–94.

36. Bryant D, Rogers P. Effect of ipratropium bromide nebulizer solution with and without preservatives in the treatment of acute and stable asthma. Chest 1992;102:742–7.

37. Firstater E, Mizrachi E, Topilsky M. The effect of vagolytic drugs on airway obstruction in patients with bronchial asthma. Ann Allergy 1981;46:332–5.

38. Ruffin R, FitzGerald J, Rebuck A. A comparison of the bronchodilator activity of Sch 1000 and salbutamol. J Allergy Clin Immunol 1977;59:139–41.

39. Jannun D, Mickel S. Anisocoria and aerosolized anticholinergics. Chest 1986;90:148–9.

40. Watson W, Shuckett P, Becker A, Simons F. Effect of nebulized ipratropium bromide on intraocular pressures in children. Chest 1994;105:1439–41.

41. Davis A, Vickerson F, Worsley, et al. Determination of dose-response relationship for nebulized ipratropium in asthmatic children. J Pediatr 1984;105:1002–5.

42. Hodges I, Groggins R, Milner A, Stokes G. Bronchodilator effect of inhaled ipratropium bromide in wheezy toddlers. Arch Dis Child 1981;56:729–32.

43. Gross N. Anticholinergic agents. In: Weiss EB, Stein M, editors. Bronchial asthma: mechanism and therapeutics, 3rd ed. Boston: Little Brown; 1993.p.876–83.

44. O'Driscoll B, Taylor R, Horsley M, et al. Nebulized salbutamol with and without ipratropium bromide in acute airflow obstruction. Lancet 1989;1:1418–20.

45. Rebuck A, Chapman K, Abboud R, et al. Nebulized anticholinergic and sympathomimetic treatment of asthma and chronic obstructive airways disease in the emergency room. Am J Med 1987;82:59–64.

46. Garrett J, Town G, Rodwell P, Kelly A. Nebulized salbutamol with and without ipratropium bromide in the treatment of acute asthma. J Allergy Clin Immunol 1997;100:165–70.

47. Karpel J, Schacter N, Fanta C, et al. A comparison of ipratropium and albuterol vs albuterol alone for the treatment of acute asthma. Chest 1996;110:611–6.

48. FitzGerald J, Grunfeld A, Pare P, et al. The clinical efficacy of combination nebulized anticholinergic and adrenergic bronchodilators vs nebulized adrenergic bronchodilator alone in acute asthma. Chest 1997;111:311–5.

49. Ward M, Fentem P, Roderick Smith W, Davies D. Ipratropium bromide in acute asthma. Br Med J 1981;282:598–600.

50. Bryant D. Nebulized ipratropium bromide in the treatment of acute asthma. Chest 1985;88:24–9.

51. Higgins R, Stradling J, Lane D. Should ipratropium bromide be added to beta-agonists in treatment of acute severe asthma? Chest 1988;94:718–22.

52. Osmond M, Klassen T. Efficacy of ipratropium bromide in acute childhood asthma: a meta-analysis. Acad Emerg Med 1995;2:651–6.

53. Plotnick L, Ducharme F. Should inhaled anticholinergics be added to beta 2-agonists for treating acute childhood and adolescent asthma? A systematic review. Br Med J 1998;317:971–7.

54. Jadad A, Moore R, Carroll D, et al. Assessing the quality of reports of randomized controlled trials: is blinding necessary? Control Clin Trials 1995;134:1–12.

55. Ducharme F, Davis G. Randomized controlled trial of ipratropium bromide and frequent low doses of salbutamol in the management of mild and moderate acute pediatric asthma. J Pediatr 1998;133:479–85.

56. Guill M, Maloney M, DuRant R. Comparison of inhaled metaproterenol, inhaled atropine sulfate, and their combination in treatment of children with acute asthma. Ann Allergy 1987;59:367–71.

57. Phanichyakam P, Kraisarin C, Sasisakulporn C. Comparison of inhaled terbutaline and inhaled terbutaline plus ipratropium bromide in acute asthmatic children. Asian Pac J Allergy Immunol 1990;8:45–8.

58. Cook J, Fergusson D, Dawson K. Ipratropium and fenoterol in the treatment of acute asthma. Pharmatherapeutica 1985;4:383–6.

59. Schuh S, Johnson D, Callahan S, et al. Efficacy of frequent nebulized ipratropium bromide added to frequent high-dose albuterol therapy in severe childhood asthma. J Pediatr 1995;126:639–45.

60. Beck R, Robertson C, Galdes-Sebaldt M, Levison H. Combined salbutamol and ipratropium bromide by inhalation in the treatment of severe acute asthma. J Pediatr 1985;107:605–8.

61. Reisman J, Galdes-Sebalt M, Kazim F, et al. Frequent administration by inhalation of salbutamol and ipratropium bromide in the initial management of severe acute asthma in children. J Allergy Clin Immunol 1988;81:16–20.

62. Qureshi F, Zaritsky A, Lakkis H. Efficacy of nebulized ipratropium in severe asthmatic children. Ann Emerg Med 1997;29:205–11.

63. Watson W, Becker A, Simons F. Comparison of ipratropium solution, fenoterol solution, and their combination administered by nebulizer and face mask to children with acute asthma. J Allergy Clin Immunol 1988;82:1012–8.

64. Qureshi F, Pestian J, Davis P, Zaritsky A. Effect of nebulized ipratropium on the hospitalization rates of children with asthma. N Engl J Med 1998;339:1030–5.

65. Zorc JJ, Pusic MV, Ogborn CJ, et al. Ipratropium bromide added to asthma treatment in the pediatric emergency department. Pediatrics 1999;103:748–52.

66. Storr J, Lenney W. Nebulized ipratropium and salbutamol in asthma. Arch Dis Child 1986;61:602–3.

67. Rayner R, Cartlidge P, Upton C. Salbutamol and ipratropium in acute asthma. Arch Dis Child 1987;62:840–1.

68. Goggin N, Parkin PC, Macarthur C. The efficacy of the addition of ipratropium bromide to salbutamol and corticosteroid therapy in children hospitalized with an acute exacerbation of asthma [abstract]. Proceedings of the APS/SPR/APA 1998 Annual Meeting.

69. Everard M, Kurian M. Anti-cholinergic drugs for wheeze in children under the age of two years. In: Ducharme FM, Jones P, editors. Airways module of The Cochrane Database of systematic

reviews. Available in The Cochrane Library. The Cochrane Collaboration. Issue 4 (Updated Quarterly). Oxford: Update Software, 1999.

70. Naspitz C, Sole D. Treatment of acute wheezing and dyspnea attacks in children under 2 years old: inhalation of fenoterol plus ipratropium bromide versus fenoterol. J Asthma 1992;29:253–8.

71. Schuh S, Johnson D, Canny G, et al. Efficacy of adding nebulized ipratropium bromide to nebulized albuterol therapy in acute bronchiolitis. Pediatrics 1992;90:920–3.

72. Medical Research Council. Controlled trial of effects of cortisone acetate in status asthmaticus. Lancet 1956;2:803–6.

73. Fanta C, Rossing T, McFadden EJ. Glucorticoids in acute asthma: a critical controlled trial. Am J Med 1983;74:845–51.

74. Fiel S, Swartz M, Glanz K, Francis M. Efficacy of short-term corticosteroid therapy in outpatient treatment of acute bronchial asthma. Am J Med 1983;75:259–62.

75. Chapman K, Verbeek P, White J, Rebuck A. Effect of a short course of prednisone in the prevention of early relapse after the emergency room treatment of acute asthma. N Engl J Med 1991;324:788–94.

76. Stein L, Cole R. Early administration of corticosteroids in emergency room treatment of acute asthma. Ann Intern Med 1990;112:822–7.

77. Littenberg B, Gluck E. A controlled trial of methylprednisolone in the emergency treatment of acute asthma. N Engl J Med 1986;314:150–2.

78. Storr J, Barreell E, Barry W, et al. Effect of a single oral dose of prednisolone in acute childhood asthma. Lancet 1987;I:879–82.

79. Tal A, Levy N, Bearman J. Methylprednisolone therapy for acute asthma in infants and toddlers; a controlled clinical trial. Pediatrics 1990;86:350–6.

80. Scarfone R, Fuchs S, Nager A, Shane S. Controlled trial of oral prednisone in the emergency department treatment of children with acute asthma. Pediatrics 1993;92:513–8.

81. Connett G, Warde C, Wooler E, Lenney W. Prednisolone and salbutamol in the hospital treatment of acute asthma. Arch Dis Child 1994;70:170–3.

82. Younger R, Gerber P, Herrod H, et al. Intravenous methylprednisolone efficacy in status asthmaticus of childhood. Pediatrics 1987;80:225–30.

83. Rowe B, Keller J, Oxman A. Effectiveness of steroid therapy in acute exacerbations of asthma: a meta-analysis. Am J Emerg Med 1992;10:301–10.

84. Barnett P, Caputo G, Baskin M, Kuppermann N. Intravenous versus oral corticosteroids in the management of acute asthma in children. Ann Emerg Med 1997;29:212–7.

85. Langton Hewer S, Hobbs J, Reid F, Lenney W. Prednisolone in acute childhood asthma: clinical responses to three dosages. Respir Med 1998;92:541–6.

86. Weinberger M, Hendeles L. Theophylline in asthma. N Engl J Med 1996;334:1380–8.

87. Fanta C, Rossing T, McFadden EJ. Treatment of acute asthma: is combination therapy with sympathomimetics and methylxanthines indicated? Am J Med 1986;80:5–10.

88. Rossing T, Fanta C, Goldstein D, et al. Emergency therapy of asthma: comparison of the acute effects of parenteral and inhaled sympathomimetics and infused aminophylline. Am Rev Respir Dis 1980;122:365–71.

89. Murphy D, McDermott M, Rydman R, et al. Aminophylline in the treatment of acute asthma when beta$_2$-adrenergics and steroids are provided. Arch Intern Med 1993;153:1784–8.

90. Wrenn K, Slovis C, Murphy F, Greenberg R. Aminophylline therapy for acute bronchospastic disease in the emergency room. Ann Intern Med 1991;115:241–7.

91. Self T, Abou-Shala N, Burns R, et al. Inhaled albuterol and oral prednisone therapy in hospitalised adult asthmatics. Does aminophylline add any benefit? Chest 1990;98:1317–21.

92. Huang D, O' Brien R, Harman E, et al. Does aminophylline benefit adults admitted to the hospital for an acute exacerbation of asthma? Ann Intern Med 1993;119:1155–60.

93. Pierson W, Bierman C, Stamm S, VanArsdel P. Double-blind trial of aminophylline in status asthmaticus. Pediatrics 1971;48:642–6.

94. Strauss R, Wertheim D, Bonagura V, Valacer D. Aminophylline therapy does not improve outcome and increases adverse effects in children hospitalized with acute asthmatic exacerbations. Pediatrics 1994;93:205–10.

95. DiGiulio G, Kercsmar C, Krug S, et al. Hospital treatment of asthma: Lack of benefit from theophylline given in addition to nebulized albuterol and intravenously administered corticosteroid. J Pediatr 1993;122:464–9.

96. Carter E, Cruz M, Chesrown S, et al. Efficacy of intravenously administered theophylline in children hospitalized with severe asthma. J Pediatr 1993;122:470–6.

97. Needleman J, Kaifer M, Nold J, et al. Theophylline does not shorten hospital stay for children admitted for asthma. Arch Pediatr Adolesc Med 1995;149:206–9.

98. Bien J, Bloom M, Evans R, Specker B, et al. Intravenous theophylline in pediatric status asthmaticus. Clin Peds 1995;34:475–81.

99. Yung M, South M. Randomised controlled trial of aminophylline for severe acute asthma. Arch Dis Child 1998;79:405–10.

100. Calpin C, MacArthur C, Stephens D, et al. Effectiveness of prophylactic inhaled steroids in childhood asthma: a systematic review of the literature. J Allergy Clin Immunol 1997;100:452–7.

101. Frears JF, Wilson LC, Friedman M. Betamethasone 17-valerate by aerosol in childhood asthma. Arch Dis Child. 1973;48(11):856–63.

102. Howard K, Jacoby N. Betamethasone valerate treatment of steroid dependent children. Postgrad Med J 1974;50(Suppl 4):41–4.

103. Taylor B, Norman A. Betamethasone valerate treatment of steroid dependent children. Postgrad Med J 1974;50(Suppl 4):44-49.

104. Lovera J, Collins-Williams C, Bailey J. Beclomethasone dipropionate by aerosol in the treatment of asthmatic children. Postgrad Med J 1975;51(Suppl 4):94-98.

105. Klein R, Waldman D, Kershner H. Treatment of chronic childhood asthma with beclomethasone dipropionate aerosol. I. A double-blind crossover trial in nonsteroid-dependent patients. Pediatrics 1977;60:7-13.

106. Richards W, Platzker A, Church J, et al. Steroid-dependent asthma treated with inhaled beclomethasone dipropionate in children. Ann Allergy 1978;41:274–7.

107. Hiller E, Groggin R, Lenney W, et al. Beclomethasone dipropionate powder inhalation treatment in chronic childhood asthma. Prog Respir Res 1981;17:285–9.

108. Shapiro G, Izu A, Furukawa C, et al. Short-term double-blind evaluation of flunisolide aerosol for steroid-dependent asthmatic children and adolescents. Chest 1981;80:671–5.

109. Meltzer E, Kemp J, Orgel A, Izu A. Flunisolide aerosol in the treatment of steroid dependent asthma in children. Pediatrics 1982;69:340–5.

110. Orgel H, Meltzer E, Kemp J. Flunisolide aerosol in the treatment of steroid-dependent asthma in children. Ann Allergy 1983;51:21–5.

111. Webb M, Milner A, Hiller E, Henry R. Nebulized beclomethasone dipropionate suspension. Arch Dis Child 1986;61:1108–10.

112. Storr J, Lenney C, Lenney W. Nebulized beclomethasone dipropionate in pre-school asthma. Arch Dis Child 1986;61:270–3.

113. Katz R, Rachelefsky G, Siegel S, et al. Twice-daily beclomethasone dipropionate in the treatment of childhood asthma. J Asthma 1986;23:1–7.

114. Gleeson J, Price J. Controlled trial of budesonide given by the nebuhaler in pre-school children with asthma. Br Med J 1988;298:163–6.

115. Carlsen K, Leegaard J, Larsen S, Orstavik J. Nebulized beclomethasone dipropionate in recurrent obstructive episodes after acute bronchiolitis. Arch Dis Child 1988;63:1428–33.

116. van Bever H, Schuddinck L, Wojciechowski M, Stevens W. Aerosolized budesonide in asthmatic infants: a double blind study. Pediatr Pulmonol 1990;9:177–80.

117. Bisgaard H, Nunck S, Nielsen J, et al. Inhaled budesonide for treatment of recurrent wheezing in early childhood. Lancet 1990;336:649–51.

118. Piacentini G, Sette L, Peroni D, et al. Double-blind evaluation of effectiveness and safety of flunisolide aerosol for treatment of bronchial asthma in children. Allergy 1990;45:612–6.

119. van Essen-Zandvliet E, Hughes MD, Waalkens HJ, et al. Effects of 22 months of treatment with inhaled corticosteroids and/or beta$_2$-agonists on lung function, airway responsiveness, and symptoms in children with asthma. Am Rev Respir Dis 1992;146:547–54.

120. Noble V, Ruggins N, Everard M, Milner A. Inhaled budesonide for chronic wheezing under 19 months of age. Arch Dis Child 1992;67:285–8.

121. Ilangovan P, Pedersen S, Godfrey J, et al. Treatment of severe steroid dependent pre-school asthma with nebulized budesonide suspension. Arch Dis Child 1993;68:356–9.

122. Mackenzie C, Weinberg E, Tabachnik E, et al. A placebo controlled trial of fluticasone propionate in asthmatic children. 1993;152:856–60.

123. Connett GJ, Warde C, Wooler E, Lenney W. Use of budesonide in severe asthmatics aged 1-3 years. Arch Dis Child 1993;69:351–5.

124. de Blic J, Delacourt C, Le Dourgeois M, et al. Efficacy of nebulized budsonide in treatment of severe infantile asthma: a double-blind study. J Allergy Clin Immunol 1996;98:14–20.

125. Price JF, Russell G, Hindmarsh PC, et al. Growth during one year of treatment with fluticasone propionate or sodium cromoglycate in children with asthma. Pediat Pulmonol 1997;24:178–86.

126. Simons EF. A comparison of beclomethasone, salmeterol, and placebo in children with asthma. N Engl J Med 1997;337:1659–65.

127. Verberne AA, Frost C, Roorda RJ, et al. One year treatment with salmeterol compared with beclomethasone in children with asthma. Am J Respir Crit Care Med 1997;156:688–95.

128. Verberne AA, Frost C, Duiverman EJ, et al. Addition of salmeterol versus doubling the dose of beclomethasone in children with asthma. Am J Respir Crit Care Med 1998;158:213–9.

129. Gustafsson P, Tsanakas J, Gold M, et al. Comparison of the efficacy and safety of inhaled fluticasone propionate 200 micrograms/day with inhaled beclomethasone dipropionate 400 micrograms/day in mild and moderate asthma. Arch Dis Child1993;69(2):206–11.

130. Ferguson AC, Spier S, Manjra A, et al. Efficacy and safety of high-dose inhaled steroids in children with asthma: a comparison of fluticasone propionate with budesonide. J Pediatr 1999;134:422–7.

131. Barnes NC, Hollett C, Harris TA. Clinical experience with fluticasone propionate in asthma: a meta-analysis of efficacy and systemic activity compared with budesonide and beclomethasone dipropionate at half the micrograms dose or less. Respir Med 1998;92:95–104.

132. Allen DB, Mullen M, Mullen B. A meta-analysis of the effect of oral and inhaled corticosteroids on growth. J Allergy Clin Immunol 1994;93:967–76.

133. Kerribijin KF. Beclomethasone dipropionate in long-term treatment of asthma in children. Pediatr 1976;89:821–6.

134. Kuzemko J. Growth velocity in children on oral corticosteroids and betamethasone valerate aerosol. Postgrad Med J 1974;50(Suppl 4):38–40.

135. Balfour-Lynn L. Growth and childhood asthma. Arch Dis Child 1986;61:1049–55.

136. Godfrey S, Konig P. Treatment of childhood asthma for 13 months and longer with corticosteroid aerosol. Arch Dis Child 1974;49:591–6.

137. Godfrey S, Balfour-Lynn L, Tooley M. A three to five year follow-up of the use of aerosol steroid beclomethasone dipropionate in childhood asthma. J Allergy Clin Immunol 1978;62:335–9.

138. Bager B, Engstrom I, Kraepelien S. Long-term treatment with corticosteroids in children. Scandanavian J Resp Dis 1977(Suppl 101):189–96.

139. Bahn GL, Gwynn CM, Smith JM. Growth and adrenal function of children on prolonged beclomethasone dipropionate treatment. Lancet 1980;1:96–7.

140. Brown HM, Bhowmik M, Jackson FA, Thantrey N. Beclomethasone dipropionate aerosols in the treatment of asthma in childhood. Practitioner 1980;224:847–51.

141. Chang KC, Miklich DR, Barwise G, et al. Linear growth of chronic asthmatic children: the effects of disease and various forms of steroid therapy. Clin Allergy 1982;12:369–78.

142. Delacourt C, Chomienne F, de Blic J, et al. Preservation of growth velocity in asthmatic children treated with high doses of inhaled beclomethasone dipropionate [abstract]. Eur Respir J 1991;4:593s.

143. Dutau G, Rochiccioli P. Corticotropic testing during long-term beclomethasone dipropionate treatment in asthmatic children. Poumon et Le Coeur 1978;34:247–53.

144. Falliers C, Tan L, Szentivanti J, et al. Childhood asthma and steroid therapy as influences on growth. Am J Dis Child 1963;105:127–37.

145. Francis R. Long-term belcomethasone dipropionate aerosol therapy in juvenile asthma. Thorax 1976;31:309–14.

146. Graff-Lonnevig V, Kraepelien S. Long-term treatment with beclomethasone dipropionate aerosol in asthmatic children, with special reference to growth. Allergy 1979;34:57–61.

147. Morris H. Growth and skeletal maturation in asthmatic children: effect of corticosteroid treatment. Pediatr Res 1975;9:579–83.

148. Reimer L, Morris H, Ellis E. Growth of asthmatic children during treatment with alternate day steroids. J Allergy Clin Immunol 1975;55:224–31.

149. Smith J. Long-term steroid treatment in asthmatic children. Ann Allergy 1965;23:492–6.

150. Tarada J. Experience in long-term use of Aldecin (BDP inhaler). Jpn Pharmacol Ther 1981;9:1607–19.

151. VanMetre T, Neirmann W, Rosen LJ. A comparison of the growth suppressive effect of cortisone, prednisone, and other adrenal cortical hormones. J Allergy 1960;31:531–42.

152. Varsano I, Volovitz B, Malik H, Amir Y. Safety of one year of treatment with budesonide in young children with asthma. J Allergy Clin Immunol 1990;85:914–20.

153. Westphal O. Growth hormone levels in children during long-term treatment with corticosteroids. Acta Paediatr Scand 1968;182:56–62.

154. Tinkelman DG, Reed CE, Nelson HS, Offord KP. Aerosol beclomethasone dipropionate compared with theophylline as primary treatment of chronic, mild to moderately severe asthma in children. Pediatrics 1993;92:64–77.

155. Doull IJ, Freezer NJ, Holgate ST. Growth of prepubertal children with mild asthma treated with inhaled beclomethasone dipropionate. Am J Respir Crit Care Med 1995;151:1715–9.

156. Allen DB, Bronsky EA, LaForce CF, et al. Growth in asthmatic children treated with fluticasone propionate. J Pediatr 1998;132:472–7.

157. Heuck C, Wolters OD, Kollerup G, et al. Adverse effects of inhaled budesonide (800 μg) on growth and collagen turnover in children with asthma: a double-blind comparison of once-daily versus twice-daily administration. J Pediatr 1998;133:608–12.

158. Brook CG. Short stature never killed anybody. J Pediatr 1998;133:591–2.

159. Morrison Smith J, Devey GF. Clinical trial of disodium cromoglycate in treatment of asthma in children. Br Med J 1968;2:340–4.

160. Hyde JS, Buranakul B, Vithayasai V. Effect of cromolyn sodium on childhood asthma. Ann Allergy 1970;28(10):449–58.

161. Collins-Williams C, Chiu AW, Lamenza C, et al. Treatment of bronchial asthma with disodium cromoglycate (Intal) in children. Ann Allergy 1971;29(12):613–20.

162. Silverman M, Connolly NM, Balfour-Lynn L, Godfrey S. Long-term trial of disodium cromoglycate and isoprenaline in children with asthma. Br Med J 1972;3:378–81.

163. Fox ZR, Brickman HF, Beaudry PH, et al. Response to disodium cromoglycate in children with chronic asthma. Can Med Assoc J 1972;106:975–9.

164. Friday GA, Facktor MA, Bernstein RA, Fireman P. Cromolyn therapy for severe asthma in children. Pediatrics 1973;83(2):299–304.

165. Crisp J, Ostrander C, Giannini A, et al. Cromolyn sodium therapy for chronic perennial asthma. A double-blind study of 40 children. JAMA 1974;229(7):787-789.

166. Marks MB. Therapeutic efficacy of cromolyn in childhood asthma. Am J Dis Child 1974;128:301–4.

167. Berman BA, Fenton MM, Girsh LS, et al. Cromolyn sodium in the treatment of children with severe, perennial asthma. Pediatrics 1975;55(5):621–9.

168. Eigen H, Reid JJ, Dahl R, et al. Evaluation of the addition of cromolyn sodium to bronchodilator maintenance therapy in the long-term management of asthma. J Allergy Clin Immunol 1987;80:612–21.

169. Blumenthal MN, Selcow J, Spector S, et al. A multicenter evaluation of the clinical benefits of cromolyn sodium aerosol by metered-dose inhaler in the treatment of asthma. J Allergy Clin Immunol 1988;81:681–7.

170. Hambleton G, Weinberger M, Taylor J, et al. Comparison of cromoglycate (cromolyn) and theophylline in controlling symptoms of chronic asthma. A collaborative study. Lancet 1977;1(8008):381–5.

171. Edmunds AT, Carswell F, Robinson P, Hughes AO. Controlled trial of cromoglycate and slow-release aminophylline in perennial childhood asthma. Br Med J 1980;281:842.

172. Selcow JE, Mendelson L, Rosen JP. A comparison of cromolyn and bronchodilators in patients with mild to moderately severe asthma in an office practice. Ann Allergy 1983;50:13–8.

173. Springer C, Goldenberg B, Dov B, Godfrey S. Clinical, physiologic, and psychologic comparison of treatment by cromolyn or theophylline in childhood asthma. J Allergy Clin Immunol 1985;76:64–9.

174. Furukawa CT, Shapiro GG, Bierman W, et al. A double-blind study comparing the effectiveness of cromolyn sodium and sustained-release theophylline in childhood asthma. Pediatrics 1984;74(4):453–59.

175. Shapiro GG, Furukawa CT, Pierson WE, et al. Double-blind evaluation of nebulized cromolyn, terbutaline, and the combination for childhood asthma. J Allergy Clin Immunol 1988;81:449–54.

176. Petersen W, Karup-Pedersen F, Friis B, et al. Sodium cromoglycate as a replacement for inhaled corticosteroids in mild-to-moderate childhood asthma. Allergy 1996;51:870–5.

177. Kuzemko JA, Bedford S, Wilson L, Walker S. A comparison of betamethasone valerate aerosol and sodium cromoglycate in children with reversible airways obstruction. Postgrad Med J 1974;50:53–8.

178. Hiller EJ, Milner AD. Betamethasone 17 valerate aerosol and disodium chromoglycate severe childhood asthma. Br J Dis Chest 1975;69(2):103–6.

179. Mitchell I, Paterson IC, Cameron SJ, Grant IWB. Treatment of childhood asthma with sodium cromoglycate and beclomethasone dipropionate aerosol singly and in combination. Br Med J 1976;2:457–8.

180. Ng SH, Dash CH, Savage SJ. Betamethasone valerate compared with sodium cromoglycate in asthmatic children. Postgrad Med J 1977;53:315–20.

181. Sarsfield JK, Sugden E. A comparative study of betamethasone valerate aerosol and sodium cromoglycate in children with severe asthma. Practitioner 1977;218(1303):128–32.

182. Francis RS, McEnery G. Disodium cromoglycate compared with beclomethasone dipropionate in juvenile asthma. Clin Allergy 1984;14:537–40.

183. Kraemer R, Sennhauser F, Reinhardt M. Effects of regular inhalation of beclomethasone dipropionate and sodium cromoglycate on bronchial hyper-reactivity in asthmatic children. Acta Paediatr Scand 1987;76:119–23.

184. Price JF, Weller PH. Comparison of fluticasone propionate and sodium cromoglycate for the treatment of childhood asthma (an open parallel group study). Respir Med 1995;89(5):363–8.

185. Furfaro S, Spier S, Drblik SP, et al. Efficacy of cromoglycate in persistently wheezing infants. Arch Dis Child 1994;71(4):331–4.

186. Bertelsen A, Andersen JB, Busch P, et al. Nebulized sodium cromoglycate in the treatment of wheezy bronchitis. Allergy 1986;41:266–70.

187. Hiller JE, Milner AD, Lenney W. Nebulized sodium cromoglycate in young asthmatic children. Arch Dis Child 1977;52:875–6.

188. Henry RL, Hiller EJ, Milner AD, et al. Nebulized ipratropium bromide and sodium cromoglycate in the first two years of life. Arch Dis Child 1984;59:54–7.

189. Cogswell JJ, Simpkiss MJ. Nebulized sodium cromoglycate in recurrently wheezy preschool children. Arch Dis Child 1985;60(8):736–8.

190. Glass J, Archer LN, Adams W, Simpson H. Nebulized cromoglycate, theophylline, and placebo in preschool asthmatic children. Arch Dis Child 1981;56(8):648–51.

191. Newth CJ, Newth CV, Turner JA. Comparison of nebulized sodium cromoglycate and oral theophylline in controlling symptoms of chronic asthma in pre-school children: a double blind study. Austral N Z J Med 1982;12(3):232–8.

192. De Baets F, Van Daele S, Franckx H, Vinaimont F. Inhaled steroids compared with disodium cromoglycate in preschool children with episodic viral wheeze. Pediatr Pulmonol 1998;25:361–6.

193. Russell G, Williams DAJ, Weller P, Price JF. Salmeterol xinafoate in children on high dose inhaled steroids. Ann Allergy Asthma Immunol 1995;75:423–8.

194. Verberne AA, Hop WC, Creyghton FB, et al. Airway responsiveness after a single dose of salmeterol and during four months of treatment in children with asthma. J Allergy Clin Immunol 1996;97:938–46.

195. Weinstein SF, Pearlman DS, Bronsky EA, et al. Efficacy of salmeterol xinafoate powder in children with chronic persistent asthma. Ann Allergy Asthma Immunol 1998;81:51–8.

196. von Berg A, De Blic J, La Rosa M, et al. A comparison of regular salmeterol vs "as required" salbutamol therapy in asthmatic children. Respir Med 1998;92:292–9.

197. Verberne A, Fuller R. An overview of nine clinical trials of salmeterol in an asthmatic population. Respir Med 1998;92:777–82.

198. Green CP, Price JF. Prevention of exercise induced asthma by inhaled salmeterol xinafoate. Arch Dis Child 1992;67(8):1014–7.

199. Simons EF, Gerstner TV, Cheang MS, Math M. Tolerance to the bronchoprotective effect of salmeterol in adolescents with exercise-induced asthma using concurrent inhaled glucocorticoid treatment. Pediatrics 1997;99:655–9.

200. Rachelefsky G. Childhood asthma and allergic rhinitis: the role of leukotrienes. J Pediatr 1997;131:348–55.

201. Horwitz RJ, Microgramsill KA, Busse WW. The role of leukotriene modifiers in the treatment of asthma. Am J Respir Crit Care Med 1998;157:1363–71.

202. Spector SL, Smith LJ, Glass M. Effects of 6 weeks of therapy with oral doses of ICI 204,219, a leukotriene D4 receptor antagonist, in subjects with bronchial asthma. ACCOLATE Asthma Trialists Group. Am J Respir Crit Care 1994;150(3):618–23.

203. Israel E, Rubin P, Kemp JP, et al. The effect of inhibition of 5-lipoxygenase by zileuton in mild-to-moderate asthma. Ann Intern Med 1993;119(11):1059–66.

204. Israel E, Cohn J, Dube L, Drazen JM. Effect of treatment with zileuton, a 5-lipoxygenase inhibitor, in patients with asthma. A randomized controlled trial. Zileuton Clinical Trial Group. JAMA 1996;275(12):931–6.

205. Reiss TF, Chervinsky P, Dockhorn RJ, et al. Montelukast, a once-daily leukotriene receptor antagonist, in the treatment of chronic asthma. Arch Intern Med 1998;158:1213–20.

206. Leff JA, Busse WW, Pearlman D, et al. A leukotriene-receptor antagonist, for the treatment of mild asthma and exercise-induced bronchoconstriction. N Engl J Med 1998;339:147–52.

207. Knorr B, Matz J, Bernstein JA, et al. Montelukast for chronic asthma in 6-14-year-old children. JAMA 1998;279:1181–6.

208. Kemp JP, Dockhorn RJ, Shapiro GG, et al. Montelukast once daily inhibits exercise-induced bronchoconstriction in 6-14-year old children with asthma. J Pediatr 1998;133:424–8.

209. Pearlman DS, Ostrom NK, Bronsky EA, et al. The leukotriene D4-receptor antagonist zafirlukast attenuates exercise-induced bronchoconstriction in children. J Pediatr 1999;134:273–9.

210. Kercsmar CM. Leukotriene receptor antagonist treatment of asthma: are we there yet? J Pediatr 1999;134:256–9.

CHAPTER 8

Pneumonia and Bronchiolitis

Kevin B. Laupland, MD
H. Dele Davies, MD, MSc, FRCPC

Acute lower respiratory infection (LRI), which is mainly manifested as bronchiolitis and pneumonia, is the most common cause of hospitalization in young children. Bronchiolitis is an inflammation of the bronchioles and clinically presents as acute onset of wheezing in a young child (usually under 2 years of age) with rhinorrhea, dyspnea, indrawing, or cough. Bronchiolitis typically occurs as a result of a viral infection and resolves with supportive measures alone. Pneumonia affects children of all ages and involves lung parenchymal infection, usually with consolidation of the airspace. It is diagnosed when a child has an acute illness with fever, cough, tachypnea, and hypoxia with an infiltrate identified on chest radiography. Pneumonia has a broad range of causes and may demonstrate a complicated course. This chapter focuses on the epidemiology, etiology, diagnosis, and treatment of bronchiolitis and acute uncomplicated pneumonia in previously healthy children.

EPIDEMIOLOGY

In North America, lower respiratory tract infections, the majority of which are pneumonia and bronchiolitis, are most common in the first year of life, with an annual incidence of 240 episodes per 1,000 infants compared with an average 134 episodes per 1,000 children under 15 years of age.[1–3] Bronchiolitis is usually a mild illness that occurs in young children less than 6 months old.[2] In a prospective cohort study of 253 healthy full-term infants, 7 percent of children followed up for the first 2 years of life were diagnosed with bronchiolitis, and 1 percent required hospitalization.[4] On the basis of observations that children with bronchiolitis often have subsequent episodes of wheezing after their acute illness, many investigators have suggested that bronchiolitis may lead to increased rates of lung disease later in life.[4–7] However, it is also possible that an attack of bronchiolitis may be more commonly manifested in those children already predisposed to develop asthma. There have been no prospective studies adequately designed to address this question.

Pneumonia occurs with an incidence of 30 to 45 per 1,000 children under 5 years of age; it is less common in 5 to 9 year olds (16 to 22 per 1,000) and in older children (7 to 16 per 1,000).[2,3,8,9] Hospitalization rates for pneumonia are much higher than for bronchiolitis. In some pneumonia series, up to 50 percent of children are admitted to hospital, with the rates being highest in young children.[2,8,10,11] The mortality rates for pneumonia and bronchiolitis among healthy children in the developed countries are low, but the rates are higher in the developing countries, where case fatality rates in rural areas may be greater than 10 percent.[7,8,12–15] It is estimated that every year, five million children in the developing countries die from pneumonia.

ETIOLOGY

The etiology of bronchiolitis is usually viral, but there is a broad range of infectious agents reported to cause pneumonia, and defining a cause has been difficult for several reasons. First, many studies do not strictly define the criteria for pneumonia and therefore the agent responsible is unclear[2,3,16–18] Second, while organisms are identified in up to 80 percent of bronchiolitis cases, an agent is demonstrated in only about 50 percent of pneumonia cases.[2,3,7,9–11,16–26] Third, few population-based, prospective studies have been reported, with the majority of the published literature being either hospital or clinic based, which may not represent true rates in the general population.[8,16,22,24,27] Finally, there is no "gold standard" for the determination of etiology for lower respiratory tract infections. Cultures of bronchoalveolar lavage fluid and percutaneous lung aspirate fluid are highly specific for bacterial etiology, but they are not very sensitive (30 to 80 percent); because of the invasiveness of the procedure, they are not routinely available.[28–31] As a result, indirect measures are usually used to determine etiology, which may lead to false-positive conclusions. Therefore, the relative importance of each etiologic agent in lower respiratory tract infections should be regarded as estimates.

Age appears to be the best predictor of etiology. Lower respiratory infections occurring in the first week of life are usually perinatally acquired, being vertically transmitted from the maternal genital tract. These are pneumonias caused most commonly by group B Streptococcus, *Escherichia coli* and other gram-negative enteric organisms, and *Listeria monocytogenes*. Other perinatally acquired pathogens include *Chlamydia trachomatis, Ureaplasma urealyticum*, and cytomegalovirus. These organisms cause bronchiolitis or a "pneumonitis syndrome" in 2-week to 3-month old infants, characterized by the onset of cough and tachypnea without fever but with interstitial infiltrates identified on chest radiography.[7,19–21]

Pneumonia and bronchiolitis in infancy after the first few weeks of life are usually the result of viral infection. Respiratory syncytial virus (RSV) is by far the most common, causing up to 80 percent of all cases, but parainfluenza types 1, 2, and 3, adenovirus, and influenza are occasionally responsible.[2,11,17,21,32]. Respiratory syncytial virus often causes outbreaks in winter to early spring, and parainfluenza virus tends to occur in late summer and fall.[3] Bacteria do not cause bronchiolitis. Although pneumonia in this age group is typically viral, *Streptococcus pneumoniae* is an occasional etiologic agent, particularly in the setting of severe disease.

Pneumonia in older infants and children up to 5 years of age is most commonly caused by respiratory viruses and *Streptococcus pneumoniae* and much less likely by *Mycoplasma pneumoniae* and the *Chlamydiae* sp.[2,3,10,11,16,22] Pneumonia in school-age children is most likely due to *M. pneumoniae, S. pneumoniae*, and *C. pneumoniae*, and much less likely a result of respiratory viruses.[3,8,9,11,16]

Streptococcus pneumoniae is a cause of pneumonia in all age groups, and this etiology should be considered in any severe pneumonia. Other bacterial causes may include group A streptococci, *Staphylococcus aureus*, and *Hemophilus influenzae* (including type b in nonvaccinated or asplenic children). Aspiration pneumonia should be considered in a patient with a history of gastrointestinal reflux, altered level of consciousness, seizure disorder, nasogastric tube feeds, or periodontal disease, as this increases the risk for mixed infections with oral anaerobes, gram-negative organisms, and *S. aureus* in severe cases.[33,34] It is not uncommon in pneumonia to identify more than one agent.[8,10,11,17,22–24,35]

There are numerous other infectious and noninfectious etiologies that need to be considered in the differential diagnosis of pneumonia.[36] Tuberculosis may be a cause of LRI, and risk factors include being immunocompromised, aboriginal, immigrants from endemic areas, and poor socioeconomic status. Patients with cystic fibrosis are typically infected with *S. aureus, Pseudomonas aeruginosa* or *Burkholderia cepacia*. Patients infected with human immunodeficiency virus (HIV) are at risk for the usual pathogens but also for tuberculosis, *Pneumocystis carinii*, cytomegalovirus, and fungal infections. Coccidioidomycosis may occur in patients living in or traveling to the southwestern United States and histoplasmosis in the eastern United States and Canada, respectively. Exposure to birds may suggest *Chlamydia psittaci*, and exposure to goats and sheep may suggest *Coxiella burnetti*. Noninfectious illnesses that may present similar to infectious pneumonia include hypersensitivity pneumonitis, bronchiolitis obliterans, vasculitis, connective tissue disease, pulmonary fibrosis, and drug reactions.

DIAGNOSIS

The diagnosis of LRI involves clinical assessment and often laboratory testing and chest radiography. The goal is to correctly identify whether lower respiratory tract disease exists, to differentiate bronchiolitis from pneumonia, and to gain insight into a potential etiology. Bronchiolitis is suggested when a child under 2 years of age has an acute illness characterized by airway obstruction with wheezing. The presence of consolidation on chest radiography, if performed, defines coexisting pneumonia.[21] The clinical presentation of pneumonia varies with age. "Typical pneumonias" may occur at any age, are classically attributed to a bacterial etiology, and are characterized by rapid onset of high fever, productive sputum, leukocytosis or leukopenia in severe cases, and lobar consolidation on chest radiography. "Atypical pneumonias," including the infant "pneumonitis syndrome", tend to present more insidiously with little or no fever, dry cough, a normal white blood cell count or mild lymphopenia, and diffuse interstitial infiltrates on chest radiogram.[19,20] This pattern is suspicious for viral, chlamydial, or mycoplasmal etiology. Conjunctivitis is present in about 50 percent of children with pneumonia due to *Chlamydia trachomatis*.[20] Despite these classic patterns, at least three studies have demonstrated the poor ability of clinical criteria, chest radiography, and laboratory criteria such as ESR and cross-reactive protein to reliably distinguish between viral and bacterial pneumonias (level II D).[10,37,38]

Clinical Examination

History taking and physical examination are an inexpensive first step in the evaluation of patients with bronchiolitis and pneumonia. This clinical examination, however, is limited by variability among clinicians and by the generally low sensitivity and specificity of clinical signs for lower respiratory tract infection.[9,39–50] The diagnosis of bronchiolitis is a clinical one based on a typical presentation of an infant with wheezing, intercostal indrawing, and tachypnea. Because this diagnosis is clinical, the sensitivity and specificity of certain clinical findings are difficult to define. However, the interobserver reliability of the cardinal sign of wheezing in the diagnosis of bronchiolitis is somewhat low, with a mean kappa value of 0.31 noted in one study.[47] In contrast, the diagnosis of pneumonia is made by positive findings on chest radiography. The sensitivity and specificity of clinical findings in the radiologic diagnosis of pneumonia have been well studied and are shown in Table 8–1 (Level II).[9,39–50]

To rule out pneumonia, clinical findings appear to be most useful in combination. The World Health Organization has suggested that when the patients present with cough and tachypnea, a respiratory rate of more than 50 breaths per minute in infants 2 to 11 months of age and more than 40 breaths per minute in children aged 12 months or more can be used for diagnosing pneumonia.[51] This algorithm has a sensitivity of approximately 70 to 86 percent and a specificity of 50 to 80 percent in diagnosing pneumonia.[40,48,51,52] If there is no respiratory distress, tachypnea, crackles, or decreased breath sounds, pneumonia is accurately excluded clinically (level II).[9,39–41,45,49]

Clinical signs to detect hypoxia are specific but are not sensitive and therefore not helpful in ruling out hypoxia. Cyanosis is a specific sign of severe hypoxia and has good interobserver reliability (>90 percent), but is insensitive (<20 percent) for detection of mild hypoxia (level II).[42,43,48,53] In infants less than 1 year of age, the combined findings of normal attentiveness, consolability, respiratory effort, color, and movement accurately rules out hypoxia (level II).[54] Compared with oximetry, clinical findings are insensitive for predicting severity of disease.[13,47,53,55,56] However, there is considerable interobserver variation in the assessment of oximetry measurements (kappas of 0.31 to 0.7).[42]

Table 8–1. Diagnostic Utility of Clinical Signs in Children with Pneumonia

Study (Reference)	No. of Patients Total	Age Range	No. patients with Pneumonia	Appearance		Tachypnea		Retraction		Crackles	
				sns*	spc†	sns*	spc†	sns*	spc†	sns*	spc†
Berman et al[43]	90	<4 mo	63			62	63				
Leventhal[45]	133	3 mo–15 y	26	92	15	81	60	35	82	44	80
Zukin et al[39]	125	<17 y	18			50	68	17	84	57	75
Grossman et al[41]	155	<19 y	51	67	40	64	54			43	77
Taylor et al[40]	576	<2 y	42			75	70				
Dai[48]	541	<5 y	341			50	71	9	93	62	48
Korppi[50]	201	<16 y	127			62		44		36	78
Singhi[49]	226	<2 mo	91			78	97	46	100		

Adapted from Jadavji T, Law B, Lebel MH, et al. A practical guide for the diagnosis and treatment of pediatric pneumonia. Can Med Assoc J 1997;156(Suppl):S703–11.

*sns = sensitivity in percent

†spc = specificity in percent

Laboratory Tests

Laboratory testing may be helpful in confirming the presence of infection and in identifying the causative agent. However, different investigators have different definitions for laboratory cut-offs for abnormality, which limits comparison between studies. Furthermore, the causes of lower respiratory tract infection are poorly defined, and tests for etiology in general are of low yield and have only limited use clinically.

Complete blood counts are commonly ordered in an attempt to differentiate viral infection from bacterial infection but have limited usefulness in this regard. In general, bacterial infections are associated with high white blood cell counts with a left shift and normal counts, or mild lymphopenia suggests a nonbacterial cause. However, severe bacterial pneumonias may be associated with leukopenia or a normal count.[10,22,23,38] Levels of the erythrocyte sedimentation rate and cross-reactive protein tend to be higher in bacterial pneumonias, although they have low diagnostic utility (low sensitivity and specificity).[10,37,38,41,44,57] Indications for use of these tests are based on clinical impression alone (level III C).

Specific tests for etiology include cultures, antigen testing, serology, and isolation of genetic material. There are no studies demonstrating that testing for the specific etiology of pneumonia or bronchiolitis in the outpatient setting leads to better outcome than empiric therapy alone. We recommend that specific tests be reserved only for situations in which it is important to identify the causative agent, such as in hospitalized patients with moderate to severe disease or with deterioration, in immunocompromised hosts or children on immunosuppressive agents, and in outbreak management in homes or institutions (level III B).

Blood cultures are considered diagnostic (100 percent specific) for etiology when positive in the setting of an acute pneumonia but are highly insensitive, identifying a pathogen in approximately 10 percent of cases only.[11,28,31] Percutaneous lung puncture aspirates are diagnostic when positive, but this procedure is rarely performed in the developed countries because of its invasiveness.[28,30,31] Bronchoalveolar lavage cultures are considered strong evidence for causation but are rarely performed in uncomplicated cases of pneumonia.[29] Sputum gram stain and culture have low specificity because of the potential for colonizing organisms from the upper respiratory tract to be cultured, which may result in a false-positive diagnosis, and the difficulty in obtaining specimens from children.[28] The specificity of this test may be increased by the identification of fewer than 10 squamous cells and more than 25 white blood cells per high-powered microscopic field on sputum microscopy. *Mycoplasma pneumoniae* can be isolated from the throat or nasopharyngeal cultures of children with pneumonia and is rarely present in asymptomatic individuals. However, the culture test is not widely available.

Bacterial antigen testing has been investigated as a diagnostic tool and appears to be more sensitive than blood culture. However, this increased sensitivity is offset by decreased specificity, as these antigen tests are often positive in the setting of noninvasive infections such as otitis media.[35,37,58–60] Serology may correctly identify an infectious etiology but is not practical for clinical decision making when paired samples are required. In the serologic diagnosis of pneumococcal infections, immune complex detection appears to be more sensitive than antigen and antibody assays.[61] Mycoplasma serology is accurate for diagnosis in the acute phase, and techniques include detection of cold agglutinins and specific antibody tests using enzyme-linked immunosorbent assays (ELISA) and complement fixation (CF) assays. The cold agglutinin test detects an IgM autoantibody that agglutinates human red blood cells at 4°C. The sensitivity of the test for *M. pneumoniae* pneumonia is between 30 to 75 percent for cold agglutinin titers > 1:32.[62] They usually appear towards the end of the first week and persist up to 3 months. The ELISA test is more sensitive and specific than the CF test. It detects the P1 protein surface antigen from purified *M. pneumoniae* organisms and can detect IgG and IgM antibodies. Complement fixation titers persist for a long time, and a four-fold rise in titers is necessary to confirm acute infection. Up to 60 percent of children less than 4 years of age may not have any CF antibodies against *M. pneumoniae*.[62]

Chlamydia trachomatis is best diagnosed by isolating the organism in tissue culture from a specimen obtained by nasopharyngeal aspiration or use of a cotton- or Dacron-tipped aluminium swab.[63,64] If conjunctivitis is present, scrapings of the conjunctiva should also be obtained. Many antigen detection methods exist for diagnosing *C. trachomatis* infections, including direct fluorescent antibody (DFA), ELISA, polymerase chain reaction (PCR), and nucleic acid probes. The most widely used tests are DFA and ELISA. Direct fluorescent antibody has sensitivities of 33 to 85 percent and specificity of 75 to 93 percent, while ELISA has an 87 percent sensitivity and 92 percent specificity for nasopharyngeal specimens compared with culture.[65–67] A four-fold rise in IgG antibodies or positive IgM antibody test using microimmunofluorescence (MIF) can also be used for confirmation of infection.

Detection of RSV is best accomplished by nasopharyngeal wash with culture. However, antigen testing using ELISA or DFA testing is very sensitive and specific compared with culture (sensitivity 80 to 90 percent, specificity 95 percent) and has the benefit of being rapid.[68,69] Other respiratory viruses may be cultured, but this has little therapeutic implication as no specific treatment is available.[70]

Radiography

Chest radiography (CXR) is considered the "gold standard" investigation for detecting the presence or absence of pneumonia. However, it is poor at identifying a specific cause. Classically, lobar alveolar infiltrates occur with bacterial pneumonia and viral illnesses, and "atypicals" cause diffuse infiltrates and peribronchial thickening, but these patterns are not reliable to differentiate between these etiologies (level II).[10,37,44,71–75] The identification of cavities or large pleural effusions do not occur with viral etiologies alone. Hilar adenopathy suggests infection with *M. pneumoniae*, *Mycobacterium tuberculosis*, or fungi, although noninfectious etiologies such as neoplasms and sarcoidosis may demonstrate this finding. Patients with bronchiolitis may have a normal CXR but commonly have hyperinflation, bronchial thickening, perihilar linear opacities, and atelectasis.[76–80]

Although the CXR is considered the gold standard for diagnosing lower respiratory tract disease, there are significant problems with interpretation of the films. There is considerable interobserver variability in CXR interpretation of various features of lower respiratory disease, with kappa values of 0.3 to 0.8 reported for interobserver variation, with the best agreement in assessment of hyperinflation (level II).[74,80,81] The finding of consolidation and the assessment of disease of the airspace appear to be reliable with kappa values for interobserver variability of 0.79 and 0.91, respectively, reported in one study.[81] Radiologists' interpretations of CXR findings may be influenced by the clinical information provided to them that may lead to overcall and overtreatment as suggested in one study.[82]

Despite the widespread use of chest radiography, there is only limited literature examining its clinical value. One study has demonstrated that routine chest radiography does not affect the outcome of mild lower respiratory tract infections in children (level I E).[83] In this trial, 522 children aged 2 to 59 months with cough and tachypnea, but without severe disease that manifested as chest indrawing, cyanosis, stridor, and altered level of consciousness, were randomized to management with or without a CXR. Although there was a slightly higher (61 percent versus 52 percent) rate of antibiotic use in the CXR group, there were no differences in time to recovery or subsequent use of health care facilities.[83] Thus, there appears to be limited clinical utility in performing routine chest radiography in children with bronchiolitis or in suspected pneumonias in children treated as outpatients.[82,83] For inpatients admitted with a clinical diagnosis of bronchiolitis, chest radiography is not helpful in assessing severity (level II E).[84] It has been suggested that CXR be obtained in bronchiolitis only when the need for the intensive care unit is being considered, when there has been an unexpected deterioration in the child's condition, or the child has an underlying cardiac or pulmonary disorder.[84] When radiography is performed in previously healthy children with acute respiratory illness, the lateral radiographic view appears to add only minimal sensitivity to the posteroanterior CXR and does not need to be ordered routinely in this setting (level II D).[85]

TREATMENT

There are considerable differences in the approach to the treatment of bronchiolitis and pneumonia. Bronchiolitis is caused by viruses, and supportive care alone usually suffices; however, pneumonia is often more severe and may be caused by a broad range of organisms, for which there is efficacious antimicrobial therapy. The majority of lower respiratory tract infections in children older than 3 months of age do not require inpatient management. Unlike the adult population, where expert evidence-based guidelines have been developed to aid in the decision whether to admit or not, the decision in children is based on individual physician clinical judgment alone.[86] Factors that may be considered in this decision include severity of disease, age (the risk being higher in very young children), hypoxia, dehydration, coexistent medical conditions, distance from medical care, requirement for intravenous medication, and perceived competence of the parents to manage the condition at home.[9,87] The specific treatments for bronchiolitis and pneumonia are discussed in the following sections.

Bronchiolitis

There is no consensus on the optimal treatment of bronchiolitis, and there is marked regional variation in practice.[88–90] Treatment usually involves supportive care with oxygen and hydration. The use of bronchodilators, corticosteroids, ribavirin, and immunoglobulin is reviewed below.

Bronchodilators

As a result of the variable results of numerous randomized trials, there has been considerable debate over the value of bronchodilators in the management of bronchiolitis.[91,92] Most of these trials have had small numbers of patients enrolled, and meta-analyses have been reported independently by two groups in an attempt to summarize the results of these studies.[91,92] Kellner and colleagues identified eight randomized controlled trials of bronchodilator agents (β_2-agonists [albuterol, salbutamol] and/or ipratropium in two studies) in children with first-time wheezing and found a modest benefit in the clinical score but no effect on the rate of hospitalization.[91] Flores and Horwitz performed meta-analysis on five trials of β_2-agonists in the outpatient treatment of bronchiolitis and found no differences in the rates of hospitalization but a small (1.2 percent) but statistically significant increase in oxygen saturation in the treatment group.[92] Thus, β_2-agonists offer some clinical benefit in the treatment of bronchiolitis, but this effect is small (level I B). Trials published subsequent to these meta-analyses do not appear to change these conclusions.[93–96] We recommend offering this therapy to infants with bronchiolitis in the outpatient setting. Patients who fail to respond to β_2-agonist treatment and subsequently require hospitalization, in effect, demonstrate a lack of efficacy of these agents. For this reason and because of potential adverse reactions, β_2-agonist treatment is not recommended in hospitalized children.

Bronchodilating agents other than β_2-agonists have been investigated in the treatment of bronchiolitis with variable results. Ipratropium does not offer significantly increased bronchodilation in combination with β_2-agonists (level I D).[97,98] No evidence exists to support the use of theophylline (level III C).[99] Epinephrine is superior to both placebo and β_2-agonists in the acute treatment of bronchiolitis.[100–104] In one double-blind randomized trial that compared nebulized epinephrine and albuterol in the treatment of infants with bronchiolitis treated in the emergency room, those treated with epinephrine were much less likely to require hospital admission (33 percent versus 81 percent).[101] There is good evidence to support the use of nebulized epinephrine as the initial bronchodilator agent for children with bronchiolitis (level I A).

Corticosteroids

Since the pathogenesis of bronchiolitis involves small airway inflammation, corticosteroids have been investigated as treatment agents. Most of the initial trials in the 1960s showed no benefit with oral or parenteral steroids.[105–109] Some of these studies also had a co-intervention in that they treated the patients with antibiotics during the time of receipt of steroids or placebo.[105,108] One trial involving 32 hospitalized infants aged 1 to 12 months found later that the combination of salbutamol and intramuscular dexamethasone was much better than either drug alone or placebo with more than twice the rate of improvement, but this study included 13 patients with an admission diagnosis of "asthma," and 7 with a diagnosis of "wheezing associated respiratory illness."[110] Since then, there have been several well-designed, placebo-controlled, randomized trials of steroid therapy in previously healthy infants with an initial episode of wheezing and admitted with bronchiolitis, but these studies have shown no benefit (level I E).[111–114] One trial that enrolled very ill patients (26 percent ventilated) found that among 14 ventilated patients, those who received steroids had a significantly shorter hospital stay.[115] This issue needs further evaluation in a larger trial, but critically ill patients with bronchiolitis may derive some benefit from systemic corticosteroid therapy (level I B). Data on whether inhaled steroids given after an episode of bronchiolitis reduce subsequent wheezing episodes are conflicting, as all the studies were either not powerful enough to show a difference due to small sample size, or included infants with recurrent wheezing or those in whom RSV was not identified (level I C)[116–119].

Ribavirin

The large majority of cases of bronchiolitis are caused by infection with RSV; as such, ribavirin, a guanosine analogue that has activity against this virus, has been investigated in the treatment of bronchiolitis and pneumonia. Most studies of ribavirin effectiveness do not clearly define between these two lower respiratory tract infections, and therefore this section also includes studies of pneumonia caused by RSV.

The use of ribavirin has been controversial.[120–122] Early randomized trials showed improved clinical severity scores and oxygenation in patients randomized to ribavirin therapy, although there were no differences in hospitalization stays.[123–127] Later, Smith and colleagues demonstrated that ventilated patients treated with ribavirin had decreased ventilation duration, requirements for oxygen, and hospital stays as compared with placebo.[128] However, in this trial as well as many others, water was used as the placebo, which may have worsened the bronchospasm and made ribavirin appear more effective.[123–128] Meert and colleagues performed a randomized trial in 41 mechanically ventilated patients with ribavirin and saline placebo and found no differences in outcome.[129] Similarly, other reports have suggested no benefit for ribavirin in the treatment of RSV bronchiolitis and pneumonia.[130–133]

In an attempt to summarize the results of randomized controlled trials of ribavirin treatment, Randolph and Wang performed a systematic overview of the literature.[134] When they applied meta-analysis to three trials, ribavirin was not shown to significantly decrease either mortality or respiratory deterioration, although there were trends towards these effects.[124,128,129,134] There is no evidence to support the routine use of ribavirin in RSV lower respiratory tract infections, and its high cost and possible occupational exposure risks should be considered (level I C). Although there is no experimental evidence, there is expert opinion that certain groups of at-risk or severely ill patients should be considered for ribavirin use.[120] In the setting of RSV as the proven etiological agent, prophylactic use of antibiotics is not indicated because of the low risk for bacterial super-infection of approximately 1 percent (level II E).[135]

Immune globulin

On the basis of the observation that high-titer circulating antibody to RSV appears to confer protection from RSV lower respiratory infection, passive immunization with immunoglobulin (IG) has been investigated in the treatment of bronchiolitis and pneumonia. However, randomized trials have not shown a benefit for pooled intravenous IG (IVIG) or for preparations with high-titer RSV antibodies (RSV-IVIG) in the treatment of acute RSV infections in either high-risk or previously healthy children (level I E).[136–138]

The role of immunoglobulin treatment is more important in the prevention than in the treatment of RSV infections in high-risk children.[139,140] Conditions that predispose to severe RSV lower respiratory tract disease include prematurity, bronchopulmonary dysplasia (BPD), compromised immune status, and congenital heart disease.[141–143] Low-titer pooled IVIG is not effective in reducing the number and severity of lower respiratory tract infections (level I E).[144] However, large randomized controlled trials of prevention in young children (<2 years) with bronchopulmonary dysplasia or prematurity (<36 weeks) have demonstrated significant benefit with RSV-IVIG, given monthly at a dose of 750 mg/kg intravenously during the RSV season (level I A).[145–147] When used in children with congenital heart disease, RSV-IVIG showed a trend toward reducing the rate of hospitalization in acyanotic disease but higher hospitalization rates and statistically significant increase of surgically related severe events in infants with cyanotic heart disease.[148] Thus, this product is currently contra-indicated in infants with cyanotic heart disease (level I D).[139,140] Furthermore, there is a need to defer immunization with measles-mumps-rubella (MMR) and varicella vaccines for 9 months after the last dose of RSV-IVIG because of interference.

The humanized monoclonal antibody to RSV, palivizumab, has been investigated in a worldwide, randomized, placebo controlled trial involving 1,502 infants.[149] It was shown to be of benefit in premature infants (<36 weeks) and those with BPD, reducing hospitalization rates overall by 55 percent and reducing the number of days of hospitalization due to RSV infections compared with placebo (level I A).[149] It is given at 30-day intervals, starting at the beginning of the RSV season, as five intramuscular doses (15 mg/kg). This drug has the advantage of not being a blood product and does not interfere with MMR and varicella vaccinations, but the disadvantage is that it does not offer any protection against other viruses.[139] Furthermore, because it is given intramuscularly, it obviates the need for long clinic visits and potential fluid overload associated with intravenous infusions with RSV-IVIG. Palivizumab has not been compared with RSV-IVIG in a randomized trial. Despite the effectiveness of these agents, their use may be limited by their high cost.[150]

Pneumonia

The treatment of pneumonia consists of supportive care and the use of antimicrobial agents, when appropriate. When the infecting pathogen is known, specific narrow-spectrum treatment with an antimicrobial agent with activity against that organism is indicated. Most commonly the pathogen is unknown, and empirical treatment may be employed when a bacterial etiology is suggested or if the child is severely ill. Empirical treatment is usually directed at the most likely cause of the pneumonia on the basis of age and clinical presentation, although these are not necessarily reliable indicators. Whether or not treated with antimicrobials, it is important to re-evaluate therapy on the basis of the clinical response and the results of tests of etiology and sensitivity to antibiotics. Patients admitted to hospital with presumed bacterial pneumonia are at least initially treated with intravenous antibiotics to ensure adequate systemic drug levels. The step-down to oral antibiotics is a clinical decision, but usually patients with uncomplicated pneumonia who are afebrile, have no diarrhea, and can tolerate oral medication can be stepped down from intravenous therapy after 2 to 4 days.[9,151,152]

There are few randomized trials comparing different antibiotics in the treatment of pneumonia in children; as a result, treatment recommendations rely primarily on expert opinion.[9,36,87] Suggested initial antimicrobial agents for the empirical treatment of acute uncomplicated pneumonia in children are shown in Table 8–2. These suggestions reflect opinions from several published expert guidelines and those of the authors of this chapter.[9,36,87]

Some conclusions may be drawn from the few randomized controlled trials that have been published. Erythromycin and the newer macrolides, clarithromycin and azithromycin, appear to have similar efficacy in the treatment of uncomplicated, community-acquired pneumonia in children older than 2 years (level I).[153–156] The newer macrolides have fewer

Table 8–2. Suggested Initial Empirical Antibiotic Treatment of Children with Acute Uncomplicated Pneumonia

Age	Treatment Outpatient/Not Severe	Treatment Inpatient/Severe	Duration
Neonate (<1 month)	NR*	Ampicillin[†] and gentamicin[‡]	10-14 days
1 to 3 months- "afebrile pneumonia/pneumonitis syndrome"	NR	Erythromycin[§]	10-14 days
1 to 3 months; other pneumonia	NR	Cefuroxime[//] Add cloxacillin[#] if in ICU	10-14 days
3 months to 5 years	Amoxicillin** if bacterial suspected, erythromycin[§] if atypicals suspected[††]	Cefuroxime[//] and erythromycin[§]	7-10 days
5 to 18 years	Erythromycin[§]	Erythromycin[§] and cefuroxime[//] if very sick (requiring intensive unit care)	7 days

* NR outpatient treatment not recommended, hospitalization advised

[†]150 mg/kg/day divided in 4 doses

[‡]2.5 mg/kg/dose given every 8 hours

[§] 40 mg/kg/day divided in 4 doses. Other macrolides (clarithromycin 15mg /kg/day orally in 2 doses for 7 to 10 days or azithromycin 10mg/kg/day orally once a day for 3 days) may be used in cases of known poor gastrointestinal tolerance to erythromycin. Allergic reaction to erythromycin is a contraindication to using any macrolide

[//]150 mg/kg/day divided in 3 doses

[#]150 mg/kg/day divided in 4 doses

**40 mg/kg/day divided in 3 doses

[††]Based on clinical findings. Suspect atypicals in the setting of other family members or close contacts with cough, particularly if index patient or family member/close contact has had cough persisting for >2 weeks.

Table 8–3. Summary of Recommendations for the Diagnosis and Management of Bronchiolitis and Pneumonia.

Condition	Intervention	Level of Evidence	Recom- mendation
Pneumonia/Bronchiolitis	CBC, ESR, C-reactive protein	III	C
Pneumonia/Bronchiolitis (severe)	Specific etiologic tests	III	B
Mild pneumonia	Routine CXR	I	E
Bronchiolitis	Routine CXR	II	E
Acute LRI[*]	Routine lateral CXR	II	D
Bronchiolitis	β_2-agonists	I	B
Bronchiolitis	Ipratropium	I	D
Bronchiolitis	Theophylline	III	C
Bronchiolitis	Epinephrine	I	A
Bronchiolitis (not severe)	Corticosteroids (systemic)	I	E
Bronchiolitis (critically ill)	Corticosteroids (systemic)	I	B
Bronchiolitis	Corticosteroids (inhaled)	I	C
Bronchiolitis	Ribavirin	I	C
Bronchiolitis	Prophylactic antibiotics	II	E
Acute RSV[†] LRI[*]	Pooled IVIG[§]/RSV-IVIG[§]	I	E
RSV[†] LRI[*]	Prophylactic pooled IVIG[§]	I	E
RSV[†] LRI[*] (BPD[‡], prematurity)	Prophylactic RSV- IVIG[§]/ Palivizumab	I	A
RSV[†] LRI[*] (CHD[//])	Prophylactic RSV- IVIG[§]/ Palivizumab	I	D
Pneumonia (>2 years old)	Azithromycin, clarithromycin, or erythromycin	I	A (equivalent)
Aspiration pneumonia	Clindamycin or penicillin	I	A (equivalent)
PRSP[§] pneumonia (not severe)	β-lactam antibiotic	II	B
PRSP[§] pneumonia (severe)	β-lactam antibiotic plus vancomycin	III	A
Measles pneumonia (malnourished)	Vitamin A	I	A

[*]Lower respiratory infection
[†]Respiratory syncytial virus
[‡]Bronchopulmonary dysplasia
[§]Intravenous immunoglobulin
[//]Cyanotic heart disease
[#]Penicillin resistant *Streptococcus pneumoniae*

gastrointestinal-related adverse events, but the cost of erythromycin is considerably less. The adverse events of a 3-day course of azithromycin and a 10-day course of erythromycin were similar in a prospective open randomized study, and both drugs had equal efficacy.[154] However, the power of the study to show differences, if present, was not stated, and the lack of blinding may have led to bias of the clinical evaluation.

There are few data to suggest a difference in efficacy between classes of cephalosporins, or between these agents and ampicillin or amoxicillin. In one open-labeled randomized study involving 62 children with community-acquired lobar/segmental pneumonia, the activities of cefixime (an oral third-generation cephalosporin) and amoxicillin-clavulanate were comparable in the treatment or step-down from parenteral ceftriaxone in suspected bacterial pneumonia.[151] However, the study may not have had sufficient power to show a clinically significant difference, as there was not a priori sample size calculation. There was a trend toward better results in the cefixime recipients at the end of treatment (97 percent cure, 3 percent improvement, and 0 percent failure) versus the amoxicillin-clavulanate group (88 percent cure, 6 percent improvement, and 6 percent failure).

One randomized trial comparing penicillin and clindamycin in the treatment of children aged 6 months to 18 years hospitalized for aspiration pneumonia showed similar effectiveness; it had an 80 percent power to have shown a clinically and statistically significant difference in hospital admission days of 48 hours or more (level I).[157] The addition of an agent with broad-spectrum, gram-negative coverage including that for *Pseudomonas aeruginosa* is suggested in those with severe nosocomially acquired pneumonia or in patients with recent multiple antibiotic exposures (level III B).

There have been recent increases in the rates of pneumonia caused by strains of penicillin-resistant *S. pneumoniae* (PRSP).[158] However, retrospective studies have shown no differences in the outcome of these pneumonias treated with β-lactams, suggesting that β-lactam therapy alone is sufficient for pneumonias caused by PRSP (level II B).[159–162] In patients with severe pneumonia or in those not improving with *S. pneumoniae* resistant (MIC >1 g/mL) to penicillin, addition of vancomycin is prudent (level III A).

There is good evidence to support the use of supplemental vitamin A to decrease mortality in pneumonia following measles in the developing countries, but this condition is rare in the developed countries (level I A).[163,164]

REFERENCES

1. Glezen WP, Denny FW. Epidemiology of acute lower respiratory disease in children. N Engl J Med 1973;288:498–505.

2. Foy HM, Cooney MK, Maletzky AJ, Grayston JT. Incidence and etiology of pneumonia, croup, and bronchiolitis in preschool children belonging to a prepaid medical care group over a four year period. Am J Epidemiol 1973;97:80–92.

3. Murphy TF, Henderson FW, Clyde WA, et al. Pneumonia: an eleven year study in a pediatric practice. Am J Epidemiol 1981;113:12–21.

4. Young S, O'Keefe PT, Arnott J, Landau LI. Lung function, airways responsiveness, and respiratory symptoms before and after bronchiolitis. Arch Dis Child 1995;72:16–24.

5. Pullan CR, Hey EN. Wheezing, asthma, and pulmonary dysfunction 10 years after infection with respiratory syncytial virus in infancy. Br Med J 1982;284:1665–9.

6. Murray M, Webb MSC, O'Callaghan C, et al. Respiratory status and allergy after bronchiolitis. Arch Dis Child 1992;67:482–7.

7. Brasfield DM, Stagno S, Whitley RJ, et al. Infant pneumonitis associated with cytomegalovirus, chlamydia, pneumocystis, and ureaplasma: follow-up. Pediatrics 1987;79:76–83.

8. Heiskanen-Kosma T, Korppi M, Jokinen C, et al. Etiology of childhood pneumonia: serologic results of a prospective, population-based study. Pediatr Infect Dis J 1998;17:986–91.

9. Jadavji T, Law B, Lebel MH, et al. A practical guide for the diagnosis and treatment of pediatric pneumonia. Can Med Assoc J 1997;156(Suppl):S703–11.

10. Turner RB, Lande AE, Chase P, et al. Pneumonia in pediatric outpatients: cause and clinical manifestations. J Pediatr 1987;111:194–200.

11. Claesson BA, Trollfors B, Brolin I, et al. Etiology of community-acquired pneumonia based on antibody responses to bacterial and viral antigens. Pediatr Infect Dis J 1989;8:856–62.

12. Tyeryar FJ, Richardson LS, Belshe RB. Report of a workshop on respiratory syncytial virus and parainfluenza viruses. J Infect Dis 1978;137:835–46.

13. Wang EEL, Law BJ, Stephens D, other members of PICNIC. Pediatric Investigators Collaborative Network on Infections in Canada (PICNIC) prospective study of risk factors and outcomes in patients hospitalized with respiratory syncytial viral lower respiratory tract infection. J Pediatr 1995;126:212–9.

14. World Health Organization. A programme for controlling acute respiratory infections in children: memorandum from a WHO meeting. Bull WHO 1984;62:47–58.

15. Kristensen K, Dahm T, Frederiksen PS, et al. Epidemiology of respiratory syncytial virus infection requiring hospitalization in East Denmark. Pediatr Infect Dis J 1998;17:996-1000.

16. Nohynek H, Eskola J, Laine E, et al. The causes of hospital-treated acute lower respiratory tract infection in children. Am J Dis Child 1991;145:618–22.

17. Wright AL, Taussig LM, Ray CG, et al. The Tucson Children's Respiratory Study. II. Lower respiratory tract illness in the first year of life. Am J Epidemiol 1989;129:1232–46.

18. Loda FA, Clyde WA, Glezen WP, et al. Studies on the role of viruses, bacteria and *M. pneumoniae* as causes of lower respiratory tract infections in children. J Pediatr 1968;72:161–76.

19. Stagno S, Brasfield DM, Brown MB, et al. Infant pneumonitis associated with cytomegalovirus, chlamydia, pneumocystis, and ureaplasma: a prospective study. Pediatrics 1981;68:322–9.

20. Tipple MA, Beem MO, Saxon EM. Clinical characteristics of the afebrile pneumonia associated with *Chlamydia trachomatis* infection in infants less than 6 months of age. Pediatrics 1979;63:192–7.

21. Davies HD, Matlow A, Petric M, et al. Prospective comparative study of viral, bacterial and atypical organisms identified in pneumonia and bronchiolitis in hospitalized Canadian infants. Pediatr Infect Dis J 1996;15:371–4.

22. Korppi M, Heiskanen-Kosma T, Jalonen E, et al. Aetiology of community-acquired pneumonia in children treated in hospital. Eur J Pediatr 1993;152:24–30.

23. Hietala J, Uhari M, Tuokko H, Leinonen M. Mixed bacterial and viral infections are common in children. Pediatr Infect Dis J 1989;8:683–6.

24. Ruuskanen O, Nohynek H, Ziegler T, et al. Pneumonia in childhood: etiology and response to antimicrobial therapy. Eur J Clin Microbiol Infect Dis 1992;11:217–23.

25. Forgie IM, O'Neill KP, LLoyd-Evans N, et al. Etiology of acute lower respiratory tract infections in Gambian children: I. Acute lower respiratory tract infections in infants presenting at the hospital. Pediatr Infect Dis J 1991;10:33–41.

26. Forgie IM, O'Neill KP, LLoyd-Evans N, et al. Etiology of acute lower respiratory tract infections in Gambian children: II. Acute lower respiratory tract infection in children ages one to nine years presenting at the hospital. Pediatr Infect Dis J 1991;10:42–7.

27. Ausina V, Coll P, Sambeat M, et al. Prospective study on the etiology of community-acquired pneumonia in children and adults in Spain. Eur J Clin Microbiol Infect Dis 1988;7:348–54.

28. Silverman M, Stratton D, Diallo A, Egler LJ. Diagnosis of acute bacterial pneumonia in Nigerian children: value of needle aspiration of lung and countercurrent immunophoresis. Arch Dis Child 1977;52:925–31.

29. Grigg J, van denBorre C, Malfroot A, et al. Bilateral fiberoptic bronchoalveolar lavage in acute unilateral lobar pneumonia. J Pediatr 1993;122:606–8.

30. Mimica I, Donoso E, Howard JE, Lederman GW. Lung puncture in the etiological diagnosis of pneumonia. A study of 543 infants and children. Am J Dis Child 1971;122:278–82.

31. Garcia de Olarte D, Trujillo H, Uribe A, Agudelo N. Lung puncture-aspiration as a bacteriologic diagnostic procedure in acute pneumonias of infants and children. Clin Pediatr 1971;10:346–50.

32. Henderson FW, Clyde WA, Collier AM, et al. The etiologic and epidemiologic spectrum of bronchiolitis in pediatric practice. J Pediatr 1979;95:183–90.

33. Finegold SM. Aspiration pneumonia. Rev Infect Dis 1991;13;S737–42.

34. Brook I, Finegold SM. Bacteriology of aspiration pneumonia in children. Pediatrics 1980;65:1115–20.

35. Paisley JW, Lauer BA, McIntosh K, et al. Pathogens associated with acute lower respiratory tract infection in young children. Pediatr Infect Dis J 1984;3:14–9.

36. Wang EEL, Long SS. Acute uncomplicated pneumonia. In: Long SS, Pickering LK, Prober CG, editors. Principles and practice of pediatric infectious diseases. New York: Churchill Livingstone; 1997 p.250–7.

37. Isaacs D. Problems in determining the etiology of community-acquired childhood pneumonia. Pediatr Infect Dis J 1989;8:143–8.

38. Nohynek H, Valkeila E, Leinonen M, Eskola J. Erythrocyte sedimentation rate, white blood cell count, and serum C-reactive protein in assessing etiologic diagnosis of acute lower respiratory infections in children. Pediatr Infect Dis J 1995;14:484–90.

39. Zukin DD, Hoffman JR, Cleveland RH, et al. Correlation of pulmonary signs and symptoms with chest radiographs in the pediatric age group. Ann Emerg Med 1986;15:792–6.

40. Taylor JA, DelBeccaro M, Done S, Winters W. Establishing clinically relevant standards for tachypnea in febrile children younger than 2 years. Arch Pediatr Adolesc Med 1995;149:283–7.

41. Grossman LK, Caplan SE. Clinical, laboratory and radiological information in the diagnosis of pneumonia in children. Ann Emerg Med 1988;17:43–6.

42. Wang EEL, Law BJ, Stephens D, et al. Study of interobserver reliability in clinical assessment of RSV lower respiratory illness: a Pediatric Investigators Collaborative Network on Infections in Canada (PICNIC) study. Pediatr Pulmonol 1996;22:23–7.

43. Berman S, Simoes EAF, Lanata C. Respiratory rate and pneumonia in infancy. Arch Dis Child 1991;66:81–4.

44. Korppi M, Kiekara O, Heiskanen-Kosma T, Soimakallio S. Comparison of radiological findings and microbial aetiology of childhood pneumonia. Acta Paediatr 1993;82:360–3.

45. Leventhal JM. Clinical predictors of pneumonia as a guide to ordering chest roentgenograms. Clin Pediatr 1982;21:730–4

46. Godfrey S, Edwards RHT, Campbell EGM, et al. Repeatability of physical signs in airway obstruction. Thorax 1969;24:4–9.

47. Wang EEL, Milner RA, Navas L, Maj H. Observer agreement for respiratory signs and oximetry in infants hospitalized with lower respiratory infections. Am Rev Respir Dis 1992;145:106–9.

48. Dai Y, Foy HM, Zhu Z, et al. Respiratory rate and signs in roentgenographically confirmed pneumonia among children in China. Pediatr Infect Dis J 1996;14:48–50.

49. Singhi S, Dhawan A, Kataria S, Walia BNS. Clinical signs of pneumonia in infants under 2 months. Arch Dis Child 1994;70:413–7.

50. Korppi M. Physical signs in childhood pneumonia. Pediatr Infect Dis J 1995;14:405–6.

51. Programme for the control of acute respiratory infections. Case management of acute respiratory infections in children in developing countries. Report of a working group meeting. Geneva: World Health Organization; 1984. WHO/RSD/85.15.

52. Cherian T, John TJ, Simoes EAF, et al. Evaluation of simple clinical signs for the diagnosis of acute lower respiratory tract infection. Lancet 1988;2:125–8.

53. Simpson H, Flenley DC. Arterial blood-gas tensions and pH in acute lower respiratory-tract infections in infancy and childhood. Lancet 1967;1:7–12.

54. Margolis PA, Ferkol TW, Marsocci D, et al. Accuracy of the clinical examination in detecting hypoxemia in infants with respiratory illness. J Pediatr 1994;124:552–60.

55. Hall CB, Hall WJ, Speers DM. Clinical and physiological manifestations of bronchiolitis and pneumonia. Outcomes of respiratory syncytial virus. Am J Dis Child 1979;133:798–802.

56. Shann F, Barker J, Poore P. Clinical signs that predict death in children with severe pneumonia. Pediatr Infect Dis J 1989;8:852–5.

57. Korppi M, Heiskanen-Kosma T, Leinonen M. White blood cells, C-reactive protein and erythrocyte sedimentation rate in pneumococcal pneumonia in children. Eur Respir J 1997;10:1125–9.

58. Rusconi F, Rancilio L, Assael BM, et al. Counterimmunoelectrophoresis and latex particle agglutination in the etiologic diagnosis of presumed bacterial pneumonia in pediatric patients. Pediatr Infect Dis J 1988;7:781–5.

59. Ramsey BW, Marcuse EK, Foy HM, et al. Use of bacterial antigen detection in the diagnosis of pediatric lower respiratory tract infections. Pediatrics 1986;78:1–9.

60. Michaels RH, Poziviak CS. Countercurrent immunoelectrophoresis for the diagnosis of pneumococcal pneumonia in children. J Pediatr 1976;88:72–4.

61. Korppi M, Leinonen M. Pneumococcal immune complexes in the diagnosis of lower respiratory infections in children. Pediatr Infect Dis J 1998;17:992–5.

62. Broughton RA. Infections due to *Mycoplasma pneumoniae* in childhood. Pediatr Infect Dis J 1986;71–85.

63. Ripa K, Mardh P. Cultivation of *Chlamydia trachomatis* in cyclohexamide treated McCoy cells. J Clin Microbiol 1977;6:328–31.

64. Smith T, Weed L. Evaluation of calcium alginate-tipped aluminum swabs transported in Culturettes® containing ampoules of 2-sucrose phosphate medium for recovery of *Chlamydia trachomatis*. Am J Clin Pathol 1983;80:213–5.

65. Bell TA, Kuo C, Stamm WE, et al. Direct fluorescent monoclonal antibody stain for rapid detection of infant *Chlamydia trachomatis* infections. Pediatrics 1984;74:224–8.

66. Roblin PM, Hammerschlag MR, Cummings C, et al. Comparison of two rapid microscopic methods and culture for detection of *Chlamydia trachomatis* in ocular and nasopharyngeal specimens from infants. J Clin Microbiol 1989;27:968–70.

67. Hammerschlag MR, Roblin PM, Cummings C, et al. Comparison of enzyme immunoassay and culture for diagnosis of chlamydial conjunctivitis and respiratory infections in infants. J Clin Microbiol 1987;25:2306–8.

68. Michaels MG, Serdy C, Barbadora K, et al. Respiratory syncytial virus: a comparison of diagnostic modalities. Pediatr Infect Dis J 1992;11:613–6.

69. Reina J, Ros MJ, DelValle JM, et al. Evaluation of direct immunofluorescence, dot-blot enzyme immunoassay, and shell-vial culture for detection of respiratory syncytial virus in patients with bronchiolitis. Eur J Clin Microbiol Infect Dis 1995;14:1018–20.

70. Rabalais GP, Stout GG, Ladd KL, Cost KM. Rapid diagnosis of respiratory syncytial viral infections by using a shell viral assay and monoclonal antibody pool. J Clin Microbiol 1992;30:1505–8.

71. Condon VR. Pneumonia in children. J Thorac Imaging 1991:6:31–44.

72. Tew J, Calenoff L, Berlin B. Bacterial or nonbacterial pneumonia: accuracy of radiographic diagnosis. Radiology 1977;124:607–12.

73. Courtoy I, Lande AE, Turner RB. Accuracy of radiographic differentiation of bacterial from nonbacterial pneumonia. Clin Pediatr 1989;28:261–4.

74. McCarthy PL, Speisel SZ, Stashwick CA, et al. Radiographic findings and etiologic diagnosis in ambulatory childhood pneumonias. Clin Pediatr 1981;20:686–91.

75. Bettenay FAL, de Campo JF, McCrossin DB. Differentiating bacterial from viral pneumonias in children. Pediatr Radiol 1988;18:453–4.

76. Wohl M, Chernick V. Bronchiolitis. Am Rev Respir Dis 1978;118:759–81.

77. Osbourne D. Radiologic appearance of viral disease of the lower respiratory tract in infants and children. Am J Roentgenol 1978;130:29–33.

78. Erikson J, Nordshus T, Carlsen KH, et al. Radiological findings in children with respiratory syncytial virus infection: relationship to clinical and bacteriological findings. Pediatr Radiol 1986;16:120–2.

79. Wildin SR, Chonmaitree T, Swischuk LE. Roentgenographic features of common pediatric viral respiratory tract infections. Am J Dis Childhood 1988;142:43–6.

80. Coblentz CL, Babcook CJ, Alton D, et al. Observer variation in detecting the radiologic features associated with bronchiolitis. Invest Radiol 1991;26:115–8.

81. Davies HD, Wang EEL, Manson D, et al. Reliability of the chest radiograph in the diagnosis of lower respiratory infections in young children. Pediatr Infect Dis J 1996;15:600–4.

82. Kramer MS, Roberts-Brauer R, Williams RL. Bias and 'overcall' in interpreting chest radiographs in young febrile children. Pediatrics 1992;90:11–3.

83. Swingler GH, Hussey GD, Zwarenstein M. Randomised controlled trial of clinical outcome after chest radiograph in ambulatory acute lower-respiratory infection in children. Lancet 1998;351:404–8.

84. Dawson KP, Long A, Kennedy J, Mogridge N. The chest radiograph in acute bronchiolitis. J Paediatr Child Health 1990;26:209–11.

85. Lamme T, Nijhout M, Cadman D, et al. Value of the lateral radiologic view of the chest in children with acute pulmonary illness. Can Med Assoc J 1986;134:353–6.

86. Fine MJ, Auble TE, Yealy DM, et al. A prediction rule to identify low-risk patients with community-acquired pneumonia. N Engl J Med 1997;336:243–50.

87. Schutze GE, Jacobs RF. Management of community-acquired bacterial pneumonia in hospitalized children. Pediatr Infect Dis J. 1992;11:160-4.

88. Kimpen JLL, Schaad UB. Treatment of respiratory syncytial virus bronchiolitis: 1995 poll of members of the European Society for Pediatric Infectious Diseases. Pediatr Infect Dis J 1997;16:479–81.

89. Wang EEL, Law BJ, Boucher FD, et al. Pediatric Investigators Collaborative Network on Infections in Canada (PICNIC) study of admission and management variation in patients hospitalized with respiratory syncytial viral lower respiratory tract infection. J Pediatr 1996;129:390–5.

90. Law BJ, De Carvalho V, Pediatric Investigators Collaborative Network on Infections in Canada. Respiratory syncytial virus in infections in hospitalized Canadian children: regional differences in patient populations and management practices. Pediatr Infect Dis J 1993;12:659–63.

91. Kellner JD, Ohlsson A, Gadomski AM, Wang EEL. Efficacy of bronchodilator therapy in bronchiolitis: a meta-analysis. Arch Pediatr Adolesc Med 1996;150:1166–72.

92. Flores G, Horwitz RI. Efficacy of β_2-agonists in bronchiolitis: a reappraisal and meta-analysis. Pediatrics 1997;100:233–9.

93. Dobson JV, Stephens-Groff SM, McMahon SR, et al. The use of albuterol in hospitalized infants with bronchiolitis. Pediatrics 1998;101:361–8.

94. Cengizlier R, Saraclar Y, Adalioglu G, Tuncer A. Effect of oral and inhaled salbutamol in infants with bronchiolitis. Acta Paediatrica Japonica 1997;39:61–3.

95. Chowdhury D, Al Howasi M, Khalil M, et al. The role of bronchodilators in the management of bronchiolitis: a clinical trial. Ann Tropic Paediatr 1995;15:77–84.

96. Can D, Inan G, Yendur G, et al. Salbutamol or mist in acute bronchiolitis. Acta Paediatrica Japonica 1998;40:252–5.

97. Schuh S, Johnson D, Canny G, et al. Efficacy of adding nebulized ipratropium bromide to nebulized albuterol therapy in acute bronchiolitis. Pediatrics 1992;90:920–3.

98. Wang EEL, Milner R, Allen U, Maj H. Bronchodilators for treatment of mild bronchiolitis: a factorial randomised trial. Arch Dis Child 1992;67:289–93.

99. Brooks LJ, Cropp GJA. Theophylline therapy in bronchiolitis. Am J Dis Child 1981;135:934–6.

100. Sanchez I, DeKoster J, Powell RE, et al. Effect of racemic epinephrine and salbutamol on clinical score and pulmonary mechanics in infants with bronchiolitis. J Pediatr 1993;122:145–51.

101. Menon K, Sutcliffe T, Klassen TP. A randomized trial comparing the efficacy of epinephrine to salbutamol in acute bronchiolitis. J Pediatr 1995;126:1004–7.

102. Reijonen T, Korppi M, Pitkakangas S, et al. The clinical efficacy of nebulized racemic epinephrine and albuterol in acute bronchiolitis. Arch Pediatr Adolesc Med. 1995;149:686–92

103. Lowell DI, Lister G, Von Koss H, McCarthy P. Wheezing in infants: the response to epinephrine. Pediatrics 1987;79:939–45.

104. Kristjansson S, Lodrup Carlsen KC, Wennergren G, et al. Nebulized racemic adrenaline in the treatment of acute bronchiolitis in infants and toddlers. Arch Dis Child 1993;69:650–4.

105. Connolly JH, Field CMB, Glasgow JFT, et al. A double blind trial of prednisolone in epidemic bronchiolitis due to respiratory syncytial virus. Acta Pediatr Scand 1969;58:116–20.

106. Dabbous IA, Tkachyk JS, Stamm SJ. A double blind study of the effects of corticosteroids in the treatment of bronchiolitis. Pediatrics 1966;37:477–84.

107. Leer JA, Green JL, Heimlich EM, et al. Corticosteroid treatment in bronchiolitis: a controlled collaborative study in 297 infants and children. Am J Dis Child 1969;117:495–503.

108. Sussman S, Grossman M, Magoffin R, Schieble J. Dexamethasone (16 alpha-methyl, 9 alpha-fluoroprednisolone) in obstructive respiratory tract infection in children, a controlled study. Pediatrics 1964;34:851–5.

109. Oski FA, Salitsky S, Barness LA. Steroid therapy in bronchiolitis: a double blind study. [abstract] Am J Dis Child. 1961;102:759.

110. Tal A, Bavilski C, Yohai D, et al. Dexamethasone and salbutamol in the treatment of acute wheezing in infants. Pediatrics. 1983;71:13–8.

111. De Boeck K, Van der Aa N, Van Lierde S, et al. Respiratory syncytial virus bronchiolitis. A double blind dexamethasone efficacy study [Abstract]. Am J Respir Crit Care Med 1994;149:345.

112. Roosevelt G, Sheehan K, Grupp-Phelan J, et al. Dexamethasone in bronchiolitis: a randomised controlled trial. Lancet. 1996;348:292-5.

113. Klassen TP, Sutcliffe T, Watters LK, et al. Dexamethasone in salbutamol treated inpatients with acute bronchiolitis: a randomized, controlled trial. J Pediatr 1997;130:191–6.

114. Springer C, Bar-Yishay E, Uwayyed K, et al. Corticosteroids do not affect the clinical or physiological status of infants with bronchiolitis. Pediatr Pulmonol 1990;9:181–5.

115. van Woensel JBM, Wolfs TFW, van Aalderen WMC, et al. Randomised double blind placebo controlled trial of prednisolone in children admitted to hospital with respiratory syncytial virus bronchiolitis. Thorax 1997;52:634-7.

116. Reijonen T, Korppi M, Kuikka L, Remes K. Anti-inflammatory therapy reduces wheezing after bronchiolitis. Arch Pediatr Adolesc Med 1996;150:512–7.

117. Carlsen KH, Leegaard J, Larsen S, Orstavik I. Nebulized beclomethasone dipropionate in recurrent obstructive episodes after acute bronchiolitis. Arch Dis Child 1988;63:1428–33.

118. Goodwin A. An uncontrolled assessment of nebulized budesonide in the treatment of acute infantile bronchiolitis. Br J Clin Res 1995;6:113–9.

119. Richter H, Seddon P. Early nebulized budesonide in the treatment of bronchiolitis and the prevention of post bronchiolitic wheezing. J Pediatr 1988;132:849–53.

120. Committee on Infectious Diseases, American Academy of Pediatrics. Reassessment of the indications for ribavirin therapy in respiratory syncytial virus infections. Pediatrics 1996;97:137–40.

121. Mitchell I, Joffe A, Newth CJL. Ribavirin. Red Book Committee recommendations questioned. Pediatrics 1995;95:319.

122. Wald ER, Dashefsky B. Ribavirin. Red Book Committee recommendations questioned. Pediatrics 1994;94:672–3.

123. Taber LH, Knight V, Gilbert BE, et al. Ribavirin aerosol treatment of bronchiolitis associated with respiratory syncytial virus infections in infants. Pediatrics 1983;72:613–8.

124. Rodriguez WJ, Kim HW, Brandt CD, et al. Aerosolized ribavirin in the treatment of patients with respiratory syncytial virus disease. Pediatr Infect Dis J 1987;6:159–63.

125. Hall CB, McBride JT, Walsh EE, et al. Aerosolized ribavirin treatment of infants with respiratory syncytial viral infection. A randomized double-blind study. N Engl J Med 1983;308:1443–7.

126. Hall CB, McBride JT, Gala CL, et al. Ribavirin treatment of respiratory syncytial viral infection in infants with underlying cardiopulmonary disease. JAMA 1985;254:3047–51.

127. Groothius JR, Woodkin KA, Katz R, et al. Early ribavirin treatment of respiratory syncytial viral infection in high risk children. J Pediatr 1990;117:792–8.

128. Smith DW, Frankel LR, Mathers LH, et al. A controlled trial of aerosolized ribavirin in infants receiving mechanical ventilation for severe respiratory syncytial virus infection. N Engl J Med 1991;325:24–9.

129. Meert KL, Sarniak AP, Gelmini MJ, Lieh-Lai MW. Aerosolized ribavirin in mechanically ventilated children with respiratory syncytial virus lower respiratory tract disease: a prospective, double blind, randomized trial. Crit Care Med 1994;22:566–72.

130. Law BJ, Wang EL, MacDonald N, et al. Does ribavirin impact on the hospital course of children with respiratory syncytial virus (RSV) infection. An analysis using the pediatric investigators collaborative network on infections in Canada (PICNIC) RSV database. Pediatrics 1997;99:E7

131. Moler FW, Steinhart CM, Ohmit SE, Stidham GL. Effectiveness of ribavirin in otherwise well infants with respiratory syncytial virus-associated respiratory failure. J Pediatr 1996;128:422–8.

132. Long CE, Voter KZ, Barker WH, Hall CB. Long term follow-up of children hospitalized with respiratory syncytial virus lower respiratory tract infection and randomly treated with ribavirin or placebo. Pediatr Infect Dis J 1997;16:1023–8.

133. Janai HK, Harris HR, Zaleska M, et al. Ribavirin effect on pulmonary function in young infants with respiratory syncytial virus bronchiolitis. Pediatr Infect Dis J 1993;12:214–8.

134. Randolph AG, Wang EEL. Ribavirin for respiratory syncytial virus lower respiratory tract infection: a systematic overview. Arch Pediatr Adolesc Med 1996;150:942–7.

135. Hall CB, Powell KR, Schnabel KC, et al. Risk of secondary bacterial infection in infants hospitalized with respiratory syncytial viral infection. J Pediatr 1988;113:266–71.

136. Rodriguez WJ, Gruber WC, Welliver RC, et al. Respiratory syncytial virus (RSV) immune globulin intravenous therapy for RSV lower respiratory tract infection in infants and young children at high risk for severe RSV infection. Pediatrics 1997;99:454–61.

137. Rodriguez WJ, Gruber WC, Groothius JR, et al. Respiratory syncytial virus immune globulin treatment of RSV lower respiratory tract infection in previously healthy children. Pediatrics 1997;100:937–42.

138. Hemming VG, Rodriguez W, Kim HW, et al. Intravenous immunoglobulin treatment of respiratory syncytial virus infections in infants and young children. Antimicrob Agents Chemother 1987;31:1882–6.

139. Committee on Infectious Diseases and Committee on Fetus and Newborn, American Academy of Pediatrics. Prevention of respiratory syncytial virus infections: indications for the use of palivizumab and update on the use of RSV-IGIV. Pediatrics 1998;102:1211–6.

140. Committee on Infectious Diseases and Committee on Fetus and Newborn, American Academy of Pediatrics. Respiratory syncytial virus immune globulin intravenous: indications for use. Pediatrics 1997;99:645–50.

141. Groothius JR, Gutierrez KM, Lauer BA. Respiratory syncytial virus infection in children with bronchopulmonary dysplasia. Pediatrics 1988;82:199–203.

142. MacDonald NE, Hall CB, Suffin SC, et al. Respiratory syncytial viral infections in infants with congenital heart disease. N Engl J Med 1982;307:397–400.

143. Hall CB, Powell KR, MacDonald NE, et al. Respiratory syncytial virus infections in children with immunocompromised immune function. N Engl J Med 1986;315:77–81.

144. Meissner HC, Fulton DR, Groothius JR, et al. Controlled trial to evaluate protection of high-risk infants against respiratory syncytial virus disease by using standard intravenous immune globulin. Antimicrob Agents Chemother 1993;37:1655–8.

145. The PREVENT Study Group. Reduction of respiratory syncytial virus hospitalization among premature infants and infants with bronchopulmonary dysplasia using respiratory syncytial virus immune globulin prophylaxis. Pediatrics 1997;99:93–9.

146. Groothius JR, Simoes EAF, Levin MJ, et al. Prophylactic administration of respiratory syncytial virus immune globulin to high-risk infants and young children. New Engl J Med 1993;329:1524–30.

147. Groothius JR, Simoes EAF, Hemming VG. Respiratory Syncytial Virus Immune Globulin Study Group. Respiratory syncytial virus (RSV) infection in preterm infants and the protective effects of RSV immune globulin (RSVIG). Pediatrics 1995;95:463–7.

148. Simoes EAF, Sondheimer HM, Top FH, et al. Respiratory syncytial virus immune globulin for prophylaxis against respiratory syncytial virus disease in infants and children with congenital heart disease. J Pediatr 1998;133:492–9.

149. The IMPACT-RSV Study Group. Palivizumab, a humanized respiratory syncytial virus monoclonal antibody, reduces hospitalization from respiratory syncytial virus infection in high-risk infants. Pediatrics 1998;102:531–7.

150. Robbins JM, Tilford JM, Jacobs RF, et al. A number-needed-to-treat analysis of the use of respiratory syncytial virus immune globulin to prevent hospitalization. Arch Pediatr Adolesc Med 1998;152:358–66.

151. Amir J, Harel L, Eidlitz-Markus T, Varsano I. Comparative evaluation of cefixime versus amoxicillin-clavulanate following ceftriaxone therapy of pneumonia. Clin Pediatr 1996;629–33.

152. Dagan R, Syrogiannopoulos G, Ashkenazi S, et al. Parental-oral switch in the management of paediatric pneumonia. Drugs 1994;47:43–51.

153. Block S, Hedrick J, Hammerschlag MR, et al. *Mycoplasma pneumoniae* and *Chlamydia pneumoniae* in pediatric community-acquired pneumonia: comparative efficacy and safety of clarithromycin vs. erythromycin ethylsuccinate. Pediatr Infect Dis J 1995;14:471–7.

154. Roord JJ, Wolf BHM, Goossens MMHT, Kimpen JLL. Prospective open randomized study comparing efficacies and safeties of a 3-day course of azithromycin and a 10-day course of erythromycin in children with community-acquired acute lower respiratory tract infections. Antimicrob Agents Chemother 1996;40:2765–8.

155. Chien SM, Pichotta P, Siepman N, Chan CK. Treatment of community acquired pneumonia. A multicenter, double-blind, randomized study comparing clarithromycin with erythromycin. Canada-Sweden Clarithromycin Pneumonia Study Group. Chest 1993;103:697–701.

156. Tarlow MJ, Block SL, Harris J, Kolokathis A. Future indications for macrolides. Pediatr Infect Dis J 1997;16:457–62.

157. Jacobson SJ, Griffiths K, Diamond S, et al. A randomized controlled trial of penicillin vs clindamycin for the treatment of aspiration pneumonia in children. Arch Pediatr Adolesc Med 1997;151:701–4.

158. Bradley JS, Kaplan SL, Klugman KP, Leggiadro RJ. Consensus: management of infections in children caused by *Streptococcus pneumoniae* with decreased susceptibility to penicillin. Pediatr Infect Dis J 1995;14:1037–41.

159. Freidland IR. Comparison of the response to antimicrobial therapy of penicillin-resistant and penicillin-susceptible pneumococcal disease. Pediatr Infect Dis J 1995;14:885–90.

160. Pallares R, Linares J, Vadillo M, et al. Resistance to penicillin and cephalosporin and mortality from severe pneumococcal pneumonia in Barcelona, Spain. N Engl J Med 1995;333:474–80.

161. Tan TQ, Mason EO, Barson WJ, et al. Clinical characteristics and outcome of children with pneumonia attributable to penicillin-susceptible and penicillin-nonsusceptible *Streptococcus pneumoniae*. Pediatrics 1998;102:1369–75.

162. Silverstein M, Bachur R, Harper MB. Clinical implications of penicillin resistance among children with pneumococcal bacteremia. Pediatr Infect Dis J 1999;18:35–41.

163. Hussey GD, Klein M. A randomized controlled trial of vitamin A in children with severe measles. N Engl J Med 1990;323:160–4.

164. Kjolhede CL, Chew FJ, Gadomski AM, Marroquin DP. Clinical trial of vitamin A as adjuvant treatment for lower respiratory tract infections. J Pediatr 1995;126:807–12.

CHAPTER 9

Croup

Mark Elliott Feldman, MD, FRCPC

Croup (acute laryngotracheobronchitis) is a common childhood illness caused by viral infection resulting in inflammation of the upper airway. The syndrome is characterized by a hoarse "barking" cough and varying degrees of stridor with dyspnea. The majority of children with croup are mildly and transiently symptomatic and managed as outpatients. On occasion, croup may be severe and result in upper airway obstruction, with respiratory failure requiring endotracheal intubation.[1,2]

BURDEN OF SUFFERING

Children with croup frequently present to doctors' offices and to the emergency department (ER). Among children less than 6 years of age, the annual incidence of croup is approximately 3 per 100.[3] Admission rates vary from 1.5 to 21 percent of children identified with croup, depending on whether the studied patients present to primary or tertiary care facilities.[1,2] The mean length of hospital stay for children with croup in the province of Ontario has been about 2 days with a corresponding cost of approximately Canadian $1,200 per admitted child.[4] As many as 5 percent of children hospitalized with croup have required endotracheal intubation.[1,2] This latter statistic, however, was reported prior to currently recommended treatment strategies described below.

MAKING THE DIAGNOSIS: SIGNS, SYMPTOMS, AND SETTING

Most children with croup presenting to hospitals do so between 6 months and 4 years of age and most often in the fall and winter months. Croup commonly starts suddenly at night or may develop insidiously over days (80 percent of children who present to hospital do so after office hours).[2]

Children with croup may or may not have coryza; among emergency room patients with croup, only 19 percent do. They may or may not have fever; only 14 percent of children with croup who present to hospital have a high fever.[2]

Respiratory distress is a common feature in croup. Just over half the children who present to the hospital with croup have stridor. Chest wall retractions are seen in about a third of children with croup who present to the hospital.[2]

The hoarse quality of the cough of croup is similar to the barking of a seal. The cough is so characteristic that a provisional diagnosis can often be made even while the patient is in the waiting room. A diagnosis of croup may be made when this cough is the only sign of illness. However, all that barks is not croup.

BEWARE

Most cases of croup can be effectively managed by family physicians, pediatricians, and casualty officers. Young children with acute upper airway problems that mimic croup often have conditions that require the specialized care of anesthetists and ear, nose and throat (ENT) surgeons in conjunction with a pediatrician. Red flags indicating that the cough and stridor may not be due to croup include the following.

High Fever

Although as many as 1 in 7 children with viral croup may have a high fever (discussed earlier), one should also consider rare bacterial airway infections such as epiglottitis or bacterial tracheitis, both of which are life-threatening conditions. However, most children who present with high fever and otherwise typical croup do, in fact, have croup and do not have epiglottitis or bacterial tracheitis. Epiglottitis has become particularly rare among children immunized against *Haemophilus* influenza type B.[5] Other signs to consider are discussed below.

Drooling

Dysphagia is not a feature of croup. Children with epiglottitis typically have such severe dysphagia that they cannot even swallow their saliva.

Sudden Deterioration after a Typical Course of Croup

Bacterial tracheitis is a rare complication of croup. It is caused by bacterial superinfection (most commonly *Staphylococcus aureus*) of the airways of children with croup.[6] Such children develop a greater degree of airway obstruction and become systemically ill.

Choking Episode

Foreign body aspiration into the upper airway may be the cause of a hoarse cough and stridor, with (or without) a clear history of a choking episode. The foreign body may be radiolucent, making diagnosis even more difficult. A high index of suspicion is necessary, and early referral for endoscopy to an ENT surgeon is warranted when there is a history to suggest foreign body aspiration or when the symptoms of croup are resistant to therapy.

Young Age or Recurrent Symptoms

If younger than 6 months of age, consider congenital airway abnormalities complicated by intercurrent illness. Congenital subglottic hemangiomata, for example, may present for the first time with stridor during an upper respiratory tract infection in infants as old as 4 months of age.[7] Other entities to consider with early and recurrent symptoms include laryngomalacia, tracheal webs and clefts, vascular rings with airway compression, and gastroesophageal reflux disease with recurrent aspiration.

INVESTIGATIONS

When there is a strong clinical suspicion of croup, laboratory tests and radiography do not aid in diagnosis. The white blood count may be high (in 16 percent of cases) or normal.[2] Radiography will yield a positive diagnosis of croup in only one-third of true cases and will yield an incorrect diagnosis of epiglottitis in about one-quarter of cases of croup. Conversely, in children who truly have epiglottitis, chest radiography yields a positive diagnosis in also only about one-third of true cases of epiglottitis and yields an incorrect diagnosis of croup in about one-quarter of cases of epiglottitis.[8] Chest radiography does not appear to alter management decisions in children with a clinical diagnosis of croup.[9]

Investigations may be helpful only if the presentation is atypical and an alternative diagnosis is being considered. Bacterial airway infections are rare but, if present, are immediately life threatening. Such patients should not be sent for radiography without a secured airway; thus, immediate consultation with a pediatrician, anesthetist, and ENT surgeon is prudent, if epiglottitis or bacterial tracheitis are being considered.

TREATMENT

After 30 years of controversy surrounding the effectiveness of corticosteroids in the treatment of croup,[10–21] the clear benefits of intramuscular dexamethasone for children hospitalized with croup was finally established by the end of the 1980s.[22-24] Other croup treatments such as mist therapy and inhaled epinephrine had received less attention. During the past several years, inhaled and oral corticosteroids have also been advocated for use in children with croup and have been recommended for outpatients with mild-to-moderate croup as well as for more severe croup affecting hospitalized children. The purpose of this review is to evaluate the evidence of the benefits and risks of various modalities of therapy for children with croup and to develop recommendations for physicians who provide care for such children.

DATA IDENTIFICATION

MEDLINE was searched for relevant articles published between 1966 and 1998. MeSH terms used were "croup," "random allocation," and "double-blind method;" text words were "clinical," "trial," "prospective-," "random," "croup," "laryngotracheitis," "laryngotracheobronchitis," "tracheolaryngobronchitis," and "pseudocroup," followed by a manual search of bibliographies. An independent search was conducted by an experienced medical librarian. A third MEDLINE search was conducted (because of a paucity of controlled trials concerning mist therapy), using text words "mist" and "humid-" and eliminating MeSH headings and text words concerned with study design.

DATA SELECTION

In 1980, because of controversy concerning corticosteroid use in croup, Tunnessen and Feinstein[21] made specific recommendations about the methodologic rigor necessary for croup therapy studies to be meaningful. Previous studies were criticized because of (1) inadequate diagnostic criteria, (2) nonrandom allocation of treatment, (3) inadequate criteria for pretreatment severity, (4) inadequate drug dosage (5) unequal supplemental treatments, (6) inappropriate outcomes measured, (7) inadequate post-therapeutic examination, and (8) unblinded ascertainment of outcome.

Articles assessing the value of corticosteroids or epinephrine were rejected, if allocation to treatment or control groups was not truly randomized or if outcomes were measured by unblinded observers. A high value was assigned to treatments that obviate hospitalization, shorten hospital stay, reduce the need for artificial airway support, or reduce the need for supplemental medical treatments. A lesser value was assigned to treatments that reduce the perceived work of breathing as measured by clinical severity rating scales or "croup scores" because croup scores are surrogate measures of morbidity.

Studies were evaluated using the levels of evidence described by the Canadian Task Force on the Periodic Health Examination.[25] Graded recommendations about therapy were based on the burden of illness as well as on the level of evidence regarding a therapy's effectiveness and its adverse effects.

CROUP SCORES

The Westley croup score (Table 9–1)[26] or modified variants are frequently used in studies concerning therapy for croup. A modified Westley summative croup score has been shown to be reliable (inter-rater agreement achieving a weighted kappa of 0.95).[27] This croup score has also been shown to be valid and sensitive to change when correlated with global assessments of croup severity and a similar scale correlated well with tracheal lumen caliber.[28]

MANOEUVRES

Humidification in "croup tents" has long been standard therapy for children presenting to the ER with croup. If there is little improvement or if there is respiratory distress, inhaled racemic epinephrine may be used. Corticosteroids such as intramuscular dexamethasone are

Table 9–1 Westley Croup Score

Level of consciousness		
	Normal (including sleep)	0
	Disoriented	5
Cyanosis		
	None	0
	Cyanosis with agitation	4
	Cyanosis at rest	5
Stridor		
	None	0
	When agitated	1
	At rest	2
Air entry		
	Normal	0
	Decreased	1
	Markedly decreased	2
Retractions		
	None	0
	Mild	1
	Moderate	2
	Severe	3

widely used, and more recently, oral dexamethasone or inhaled budesonide have become treatment options.

Humidification

The presumed beneficial effects of mist therapy are mediated through the reduction of inflammation caused by mucosal drying and the reduction of the viscosity of airway secretions.[29] "Steam kettle" and "steam bath" treatments have long been recommended for outpatients with croup. However, reports of children presenting with scalds[30] have led most advocates of humidity treatment to recommend cool mist therapy. "Mist tents" may be upsetting to infants, make it difficult for the health-care providers to see the child, require separation of mother and child, and incur some equipment expenditure. High humidity can be delivered by "mist sticks" (simple tubing held to the child's face), which may be less distressing. Sasaki and colleagues reported improved airflow in kittens with partial airway obstruction when they breathed increased humidity.[31] In children, however, only one study[32] has compared high humidity with room air in a controlled trial. Unfortunately, the sample size was inadequate (n = 9), the method of randomization unclear, and the outcome measured by unblinded observers. This study did not demonstrate any benefit to mist therapy.

Clearly, at present, there is poor evidence to include or exclude the use of mist therapy in the treatment of croup, and decisions to use this treatment should be based on other grounds.

Inhaled Epinephrine

Only one RCT has failed to demonstrate improved croup scores among children with croup who are treated with inhaled epinephrine. This study showed a trend toward improvement but lacked a sufficient sample size to draw meaningful conclusions.[33] For children with croup who have at least mild respiratory distress (stridor, retractions, or diminished air entry), inhaled epinephrine has been shown to lead to improved croup scores within 10 to 30 minutes. This beneficial effect of racemic epinephrine may be transient and a "rebound" or "relapse phenomenon" is often seen within 2 hours.[26,34,35,36]

Improved croup scores have been demonstrated, whether the epinephrine is administered by intermittent positive pressure (IPP) breathing devices[23,26,34] or by simple nebulization.[35] A small cohort study[37] and a small RCT[36] did not demonstrate an advantage of the IPP device over nebulization for the administration of epinephrine. Racemic (R) epinephrine is the traditional form of epinephrine used for croup but L-epinephrine is more available, less expensive, and has been shown to have similar efficacy to racemic epinephrine, in one RCT with a reasonable large sample size.[38] Kuusela and colleagues demonstrated that for hospitalized children with croup, repeated doses of inhaled epinephrine administered by a positive pressure breathing device may decrease hospital stay by approximately 1 day. This advantage, however, was found to be less pronounced in patients who had received dexamethasone, for whom hospital stay is already much shorter.[23] This study of R-epinephrine is the only one that has reported an important beneficial outcome other than improved croup scores. Other croup studies have not examined the effect of repeated doses of inhaled epinephrine on hospital stays.

Studies of inhaled epinephrine may suffer from an unblinding effect because racemic epinephrine formulations have a distinct odor. Furthermore, inhaled epinephrine, upon inhalation, can cause noticeable blanching of the skin of a child's face. Most studies address the former concern by formulating the placebo to have a similar odor. The latter issue, however, is more difficult to approach.

Adverse Effects

Although no croup study demonstrated excess morbidity in R-epinephrine treated children, rare events may have been missed.

Recommendations

For life-threatening croup, a strong recommendation (A) can be made because even transient clinical improvement may be life saving. Because of concerns about the transient efficacy of inhaled epinephrine and concerns surrounding the use of surrogate outcome measures and potential unblinding in trials of R-epinephrine, there is at best only fair evidence to recommend the routine use of R-epinephrine in mild or moderate croup (recommendation B). The summary of studies of inhaled epinephrine is provided in Table 9–2.

Corticosteroids

Intramuscular Dexamethasone

To help settle the longstanding "croup-steroid" controversy, Kairys and colleagues, in 1989, published a meta-analysis of studies (1966 to 1983) of corticosteroid treatment for children with croup.[22] They concluded that the odds ratio of having a significant clinical improvement after treatment (as measured by various scoring systems) at 12 hours is 2.25 and by 24 hours is 3.19 (ie, treated patients were two to three times more likely to improve than were children given placebo). The odds ratio for requirement of endotracheal intubation, if treated with corticosteroids, was found to be 0.21 (95 percent CI 0.05, 0.84), that is, treated children were only one-fifth as likely to need intubation. Six of the nine corticosteroid trials, evaluated in the meta-analysis, studied IM dexamethasone; one studied oral dexamethasone, one prednisolone, and one IV methylprednisolone.

Since 1989, when this meta-analysis was published, more evidence demonstrating the effectiveness of intramuscular dexamethasone has been published. Kuusela and colleagues

Table 9–2 Summary of Studies of Inhaled Epinephrine for the Treatment of Croup

Study	Level of Evidence	Study Sample (n)	Dose & Delivery	Outcome (p<.05)	Pretreatment Criteria & Comments
Gardner et al, 1973	RCT (Level I)	20	0.5 mL of 2.25% RE in NS nebulized	Improved croup score "following treatment"	Did not achieve statistical significance (but study lacked sufficient power to exclude a significant benefit)
Taussig et al, 1975	RCT (Level I)	13	0.25 mL of 2.25% RE in NS by IPPB	Significantly improved croup score at 10 min	
Westley et al, 1978	RCT (Level I)	20	0.5 mL of 2.25% RE in NS by IPPB	Significantly improved croup scores at 10 and 30 min	Criterion for treatment: "stridor at rest" (croup score 3 to 6)*
Kuusela et al, 1988	RCT (Level I)	37	0.25 mL/5 kg of 2.25% RE in NS by IPPB	Significantly improved croup scores and shortened hospital stay by ~1 day (repeated doses)	Criterion for treatment: "strong stridor" 4 study arms (IM dexamethasone, epinephrine, both and placebo); multiple doses needed; `less advantage in those treated with dexamethasone
Kristjansson, 1994	RCT (Level I)	54	0.5 mg/kg RE in NS by nebulizer	Significantly improved croup score at 30 min	Criterion for treatment: "stridor at rest" (croup score ≥2)

RE = R-epinephrine; NS = ; IPPB = intermittent positive pressure breathing

showed an important reduction in croup scores at 6 and 12 hours as well as a reduction in hospital stay by approximately 2 days.[23] The study by Super and colleagues showed a significantly decreased need for racemic epinephrine (OR = 0.14) and reduced croup scores.[24] Johnson and colleagues showed a reduction in hospitalization rate and croup scores.[39]

Oral Dexamethasone

Of the studies examining dexamethasone in the meta-analysis by Kairys and colleagues, only one evaluated the use of oral dexamethasone. It showed that in children with an initial croup score of >4, an important improvement (croup score of ≤1 by 6 hours) occurred in 70 percent of the treatment group but in only 40 percent of the placebo group.[18] More recently, in 1995, Geelhoed and colleagues demonstrated in a double-blind RCT that children with croup who presented with stridor and retractions and who were treated with 0.6 mg/kg of oral dexamethasone were twice as likely as the controls to be discharged.[40] In addition, in the treated group, as compared with the controls, a croup score of ≤1 was achieved 6 hours earlier and they were discharged home 8 hours earlier. Furthermore, they were much less likely to require supplemental racemic epinephrine treatments than were controls.

In their next study of croup, the authors showed that 0.15 mg/kg of dexamethasone was as effective as 0.6 mg/kg, with a power of 80 percent to detect a 20 percent difference in the use of supplemental racemic epinephrine or a 100 percent difference in length of hospital stay.[41] One might argue that a type II error, given these parameters, is not sufficiently unlikely (ie, a larger sample size may have given a different result). In fact, the meta-analysis by Kairys and colleagues demonstrated that studies using a minimum of 0.3 mg/kg of dexamethasone were more likely to show a beneficial effect.

For outpatients who present to the ER with milder croup, oral dexamethasone in a dose of 0.15 mg/kg[42] (as well as higher dose IM dexamethasone)[43] has been shown to decrease the need for return to hospital.

Other Systemic Corticosteroids

Two of the nine studies included in the meta-analysis by Kairys and colleagues evaluated steroids other than dexamethasone, but one of these (using oral prednisolone) had not been randomized.[10] The other used a probably inadequate dose of methylprednisolone and was not able to demonstrate a beneficial effect.[12]

Massicotte and Tetreault, however, in 1973, published a double-blind RCT of intravenous methylprednisolone for the treatment of croup, but this study was not included in the meta-analysis of Kairys and colleagues because it was not published in English.[44] The authors compared methylprednisolone with placebo using 4 mg/kg/dose and found the treatment group to have significantly better croup scores by 4 hours.

Inhaled Budesonide

Husby and colleagues demonstrated in a double-blind RCT that for children with moderate to severe croup (modified Westley croup score of >5), inhaled budesonide given in a single dose of 2 mg, compared with placebo, reduced croup scores and overall clinical impressions of croup severity. Improvements were seen as early as 2 hours after treatment.[45]

Klassen and colleagues demonstrated that for less severe croup (modified Westley croup score ≥ 2) budesonide, compared with placebo, decreased croup scores by 4 hours, enabled earlier discharge from the emergency department, and decreased the number of hospital admissions.[27] To prevent 1 such hospitalization in this study, 5 children would be the number needed to treat.

In their next study, Klassen and colleagues demonstrated that among children who had received oral dexamethasone, inhaled budesonide conferred additional reductions in croup scores, compared with croup scores among children who had received dexamethasone alone.[46] The number of dexamethasone-treated children with croup who needed to be treated with budesonide to achieve an important added improvement in croup score was 4 children.

Klassen and colleagues subsequently compared inhaled budesonide, oral dexamethasone, and the combination of the two and found similar clinical improvements. They concluded that oral dexamethasone was the preferred treatment because of its greater availability, ease of administration, and lower cost.[47]

Geelhoed and colleagues, in 1995, had also compared nebulized budesonide with oral dexamethasone. Both led to important reductions in croup scores, R-epinephrine use, and duration of hospitalization, when compared with placebo. No significant difference was demonstrated in outcomes between the oral dexamethasone group and the inhaled budesonide group.[40]

Johnson and colleagues showed that intramuscular dexamethasone conferred a greater reduction in croup scores than did inhaled budesonide.[39]

Table 9–3 Summary of Studies of Corticosteroids for the Treatment of Croup

Study	Level of Evidence	Study Sample	Dose & Delivery	Outcome*
Kairys et al, 1966–1983	Meta-analysis of RCTs (level I)	1,286 children from RCTs	Minimum dose of 0.3 mg/kg of dex or equivalent	Clinical improvement (as measured by various scoring systems) by 12 h (OR=2.25), by 24 h (OR=3.19) Reduction in endotracheal intubation (OR=0.21)
Massicotte & Tetreault, 1973	RCT (level I)	42 children	4 mg/kg/dose (0, 4 & 8 h) of IV methylprednisolone	Lower croup scores at 4 & 8 h, but not at 14 or 20 h
Kuusela & Vesikari, 1988	RCT (level I)	72 children with a "dyspnoea score" of 3 (in 4 arms; dex, epi, dex & epi, placebo)	0.6 mg/kg IM dex	Lower croup scores at 6 & 12 h. Decreased average length of stay by 42 h (from ~3.8 to 2 days)
Super et al, 1989	RCT (level I)	29 children with a modified Westley croup score of > or = 3	0.6 mg/kg IM dex	Lower croup scores at 12 h Reduction in use of racemic epinephrine (OR=0.14)
Husby et al, 1993	RCT (level I)	36 children with a modified Westley croup score of > 5	2 mg of nebulized budesonide	Lower croup scores (delta 4) at 2 h and improved global impression of severity
Klassen et al, 1994	RCT (level I)	54 children with a modified Westley croup score of > or = 2	2 mg of nebulized budesonide	Lower croup scores at 4 h and improved global impression of severity Shorter ER stay and fewer children requiring hospitalization (no. needed to treat = 5)
Geelhoed et al, 1995	RCT (level I)	87 children (30 placebo, 23 dex, 27 budesonide) with a minimum croup score of 3	1st arm: 0.6 mg/kg oral dex 2nd arm: 2 mg nebulized budesonide	Decreased average length of stay by 6-8 h. Reduction in use of racemic epi [0/23 as compared to 6/30 controls] {similar results found with oral dex & inhaled budesonide}

Cruz et al, 1995	RCT (level I)	38 outpatient children with a modified Westley croup score of > or = 2	0.6 mg/kg IM dex	Clinical improvement at 24 h telephone interview [OR=3.8]
Geelhoed et al, 1996	RCT (level I)	96 outpatient children with very mild croup (score = 0.9)	0.15 mg/kg oral dex	Reduction of return visits with croup (0/48 vs. 8/48 controls) OR for returning for any reason = 0.5
Klassen et al, 1996	RCT (level I)	50 children who had received 0.6 mg/kg of oral dexamethasone for croup	2 mg of nebulized budesonide	Lower croup scores at 4 h (number needed to treat for a two-point croup score improvement = 4)
Klassen et al, 1998	RCT (level I)	198 children with a modified Westley croup score of > or = 2	1st arm: 2 mg of nebulized budesonide 2nd arm: 0.6 mg oral dex 3rd arm: both	No difference between oral dex or inhaled budesonide or combination therapy
Johnson et al, 1998	RCT (level I)	144 children with moderately severe croup (score > or = 3)	1st arm: 4 mg of nebulized budesonide 2nd arm: 0.6 mg IM dex	Both superior to placebo in decreasing the hospitalization rate IM dex achieved lower croup scores than did inhaled budesonide

dex = dexamethasone; epi = epinephrine;
*All values statistically significant to p value less than 0.05.

Table 9–4 Summary of Maneuvers, Effectiveness, Levels of Evidence and Recommendations for the Treatment of Children Presenting to the ER with Croup

Manoeuver	Effectiveness	Level of Evidence	Recommendation
Humidified air (mist therapy)	No good data of effectiveness available • one RCT with inadequate sample size[23] • animal studies[25]		Poor evidence for the use of mist for croup, and recommendations may be made on other grounds (C)
Inhaled epinephrine [0.05 mL/kg of 2.25% R-epi in 4 cc saline or 0.5 mg/kg of L-epinephrine in single or repeated doses for respiratory distress	• Transiently improved croup scores (delta>2) in moderate to severe croup (score>2) • Repeated doses shorten hospital stay in moderate to severe croup by ~1 day	Improved croup score • Randomized controlled trials (RCT)[2,18,28,29] (level 1) Shorter hospitalization • RCT[2] (level 1)	There is good evidence to support the recommendation (A) that the manoeuver be considered for children with severe croup Fair evidence to support recommendation (B) for manoeuver in mild to moderate croup
(and) Budesonide (single dose of nebulized budesonide, 2 mg)	• Improved croup score within 2 to 4 h (number needed to treat=3) • Reduction in hospital admissions (number needed to treat, to prevent one hospitalization=5) • Improved overall global assessment • Decreased need for racemic epinephrine (number needed to treat=4) • Shorter hospital stay by ~7 h	RCTs[19,33,38] (level 1)	There is good evidence to support the recommendation (A) that the manoeuver be considered for children with mild, moderate, and severe croup
(or) Oral dexamethasone (range of 0.15 mg/kg to 0.6 mg/kg dose, given in a single dose)	• Improved croup score and shorter hospital stay (similar to budesonide) • Decreased need for racemic epinephrine (number needed to treat=4) • Decreased need for return to hospital	RCTs[33,35] (level I)	There is good evidence to support the recommendation (A) that the manoeuver be considered for children with mild and moderate croup
(or) Intramuscular dexamethasone 0.6 mg/kg/dose, given in a single dose)	• Improved croup score at 6, 12 and 24 h (OR~2 to 3) • Fewer intubations (OR=0.21) • Less use of racemic epinephrine (OR=0.14) • Shorter hospital stay by ~2 days	Meta-analysis[1] RCTs[2,3,26] (level I)	There is good evidence to support the recommendation (A) that the manoeuver be considered for children with mild, moderate and severe croup

Adverse Effects of a Single Dose of Corticosteroid

Although no croup study has demonstrated excess morbidity in corticosteroid-treated children, rare events may be missed. Some children may find it very upsetting to be forced to swallow oral medications and may, in fact, not tolerate oral dexamethasone for this reason. Others may find having to sit with a mask of nebulized budesonide more upsetting, while still others would find the pain of an intramuscular dexamethasone administration to be more distressing. Which route of administration is the least unpleasant to children has not yet been established.

Recommendations

Intramuscular dexamethasone, oral dexamethasone, and inhaled budesonide, each has been shown to confer important clinical benefits when administered to children with mild, moderate, or severe croup. Strong recommendations can be made for the routine use of any one of these corticosteroids for the treatment of children with croup presenting to the emergency room with even mild respiratory distress (corresponding to croup scores ≥1 by various scoring systems). The dosage of inhaled budesonide should be 2 mg. The dosage of dexamethasone that appears to be effective ranges from 0.15 to 0.6 mg/kg. The choice of corticosteroid and route to be administered should be individualized for the patient and treatment setting. The summary of the studies of corticosteroids for the treatment of croup is provided in Table 9–3.

SUMMARY OF RECOMMENDATIONS

There is poor evidence to recommend the use of mist therapy for children with croup, and decisions to treat may be made on other grounds (recommendation C). For children with croup who present to the emergency room with mild, moderate, or severe respiratory distress (Westley croup score of ≥1), there is good evidence to recommend treatment with inhaled budesonide (2 mg), oral dexamethasone, or IM dexamethasone (0.15 to 0.6 mg/kg) (recommendation A). For children with moderately severe croup, there is good evidence to choose IM dexamethasone (0.6 mg/kg) (recommendation A).

In addition to corticosteroid treatment, inhaled epinephrine may be used (0.05 mL/kg of 2.25 percent R-epinephrine or 0.5 mg/kg of L-epinephrine in 4 cc saline). There is fair evidence to recommend inhaled epinephrine for mild to moderate croup in single or repeated doses (recommendation B) and good evidence to recommend inhaled epinephrine for the treatment of severe, life-threatening croup (recommendation A). A summary of recommendations for the treatment of children with croup presenting to the ER is provided in Table 9–4.

RESEARCH QUESTIONS

Is mist therapy useful? The longstanding tradition of using mist therapy for the treatment of croup may well be warranted, but this remains to be established. Are repeated administrations of inhaled epinephrine truly beneficial for children with less severe croup (analogous to repeated salbutamol administrations for children with asthma)? For mild-to-moderate croup, is inhaled budesonide or oral dexamethasone better tolerated?

REFERENCES

1. Skolnik NS. Treatment of croup. Am J Dis Child 1989;143:1045–9.

2. Sendi KS, Crysdale WS, Yoo J. Tracheitis: outcome of 1,700 cases presenting to the emergency department during two years. J Otolaryngol 1992;21(1):20–4.

3. Denny GW MT, Clyde WA Jr, Collier AM, Henderson FW. Croup: an 11-year study in a pediatric practice. Pediatrics 1983;71:871–6.

4. To T YW. Hospitalizations for croup in Ontario. Clin Invest Med 1994;17:A25.

5. Gonzalez Valdepena H, Wald ER, Rose E, et al. Epiglottitis and *Haemophilus influenzae* immunization: the Pittsburgh experience—a five-year review. Pediatrics 1995;96(3 Pt 1):424–7.

6. Brook I. Aerobic and anaerobic microbiology of bacterial tracheitis in children. Pediatr Emerg Care 1997;13(1):16–8.

7. Kiff KM, Mok Q, Dunne J, Tasker RC. Steroids for intubated croup masking airway haemangioma. Arch Dis Child 1996;74:66–7.

8. Stankiewicz JA, Bowes AK. Croup and epiglottitis: a radiologic study. Laryngoscope 1985;95(10):1159–60.

9. Dawson KP, Steinberg A, Capaldi N. The lateral radiograph of neck in laryngo-tracheo-bronchitis (croup). J Qual Clin Pract 1994;14(1):39–43.

10. Martensson B, Nilson G, Torbjar JE. The effect of corticosteroids in the treatment of pseudo-croup. Acta Otolaryngol 1960;158(Suppl):62–9.

11. Novik A. Corticosteroid treatment of non-diptheritic croup. Acta Otolaryngol 1960;158(Suppl):20–3.

12. Eden AN, Larkin VDP. Corticosteroid treatment of croup. Pediatrics 1964;33:768–9.

13. Sussman S, Grossman M, Magoffin R, Schieble J. Dexamethasone (16 alpha-methyl, 9 alpha-fluoroprednisolone) in obstructive respiratory tract infections in children. Pediatrics 1964;34:851–5.

14. Skowron PN, Turner JAP, McNaughton GA. The use of corticosteroid (dexamethasone) in the treatment of acute laryngotracheitis. Can Med Assoc J 1966;94:528–31.

15. Eden AN, Kaufman A, Yu R. Corticosteroid and croup. JAMA 1967;200:133–4.

16. James JA. Dexamethasone in croup. Am J Dis Child 1969;117:511.

17. Lepzig B, Oski FA. A prospective randomized study to determine the efficacy of steroids in the treatment of croup. J Pediatr 1979;94:194–6.

18. Muhlendahl KE, Kahn D, Spohr HL, Dressler F. Steroid treatment of pseudo-croup. Helv Paediatr Acta 1982;37:431–6.

19. Koren G, Frand M, Barzilay Z, Macleod SM. Corticosteroid treatment of laryngotracheitis versus spasmodic croup in children. Am J Dis Child 1983;137:941–4.

20. Hawkins DB. Corticosteroids in the management of laryngotracheobronchitis. Otolaryngol Head Neck Surg 1980;88:207–10.

21. Tunnessen WW, Feinstein AR. The steroid-croup controversy: an analytic review of methodologic problems. J Pediatr 1980;96:751–6.

22. Kairys SW, Olmstead EM, O'Connor GT. Steroid treatment of laryngotracheitis. A meta-analysis of the evidence from randomized trials. Pediatr 1989;83:683–93.

23. Kuusela A, Vesikari T. A randomized double-blind, placebo-controlled trial of dexamethasone and racemic epinephrine in the treatment of croup. Acta Paediatr Scand 1988;77:99–104.

24. Super DM, Cartelli NA, Brooks LJ, et al. A prospective randomized double-blind study to evaluate the effect of dexamethasone in acute laryngotracheitis. J Pediatr 1989;115:323–9.

25. Goldbloom RB. The periodic health examination: 1. Introduction. Can Med Assoc J 1986;134:721–3.

26. Westley CR, Cotton EK, Brooks JG. Nebulized racemic epinephrine by IPPB for the treatment of croup: a double-blind study. Am J Dis Child 1978;132:484–7.

27. Klassen TP, Feldman ME, Watters LK, et al. Nebulized budesonide for children with mild-to-moderate croup. N Engl J Med 1994;331:285–9.

28. Corkey CWB, Barker GA, Edmonds JF, et al. Radiographic tracheal diameter measurements in acute infectious croup: an objective scoring system. Crit Care Med 1981;9:587–90.

29. Henry R. Moist air in the treatment of laryngotracheitis. Arch Dis Child 1983;58:577.

30. Greally P, Cheng K, Tanner MS, Gield DJ. Children with croup presenting with scalds. Br Med J 1990;301:113.

31. Sasaki CT, Suzuki M. The respiratory mechanism of aerosol inhalation in the partially obstructed airway. Pediatrics 1977;59:689-94.

32. Bourchier D, Dawson KP, Fergusson DM. Humidification in viral croup: a controlled trial. Austral Paediatr J 1984;20:289–91.

33. Gardner HG, Powell KR, Roden VJ, Cherry JD. The evaluation of racemic epinephrine in the treatment of infectious croup. Pediatr 1973;52:52–5.

34. Taussig LM, Castro O, Beaudry PH, et al. Treatment of laryngotracheobronchitis (croup). Am J Dis Child 1975;129:790–3.

35. Kristjansson S, Berg-Kelly K, Winso E. Inhalation of racemic adrenaline in the treatment of mild and moderately severe croup. Clinical symptom score and oxygen saturation measurements for evaluation of treatment effects. Acta Paediatrica 1994;83:1156–60.

36. Fogel JM, Berg IJ, Gerber MA, Sherter CB. Racemic epinephrine in the treatment of croup: nebulization alone versus nebulization with intermittent positive pressure breathing. J Pediatr 1982;101:1028–31.

37. Zach M. Pseudokrupptherapie durch einfach Epinephrinvernebelung. Erste Erfahrungen. Monatsschrift Kinderheilkunde 1984;129:168–70.

38. Waisman Y, Klein BL, Boenning DA, et al. Prospective randomized double-blind study comparing L-epinephrine and racemic epinephrine aerosols in the treatment of laryngotracheitis (croup). Pediatrics 1992;89:302–6.

39. Johnson DW, Jacobson S, Edney P, et al. A comparison of nebulized budesonide, intramuscular dexamethasone and placebo for moderately severe croup. N Engl J Med 1998;339(8):498–503.

40. Geelhoed GC, MacDonald WBG. Oral and inhaled steroids in croup: a randomized placebo-controlled trial. Pediatr Pulmonol 1995;20:355–61.

41. Geelhoed GC, MacDonald WBG. Oral dexamethasone in the treatment of croup: 0.15 mg/kg versus 0.3 mg/kg versus 0.6 mg/kg. Pediatr Pulmonol 1995;20:362–8.

42. Geelhoed GC, Turner J, MacDonald WBG. Efficacy of a small single dose of oral dexamethasone for outpatient croup: a double blind, placebo controlled clinical trial. Br Med J 1996;313:140–2.

43. Cruz MN, Stewart G, Rosenberg N. Use of dexamethasone in the outpatient management of acute laryngotracheitis. Pediatrics 1995;96:220–3.

44. Massicotte P, Tetreault L. Evaluation de la methylprednisolone dans le traitement des laryngites aigues de l'enfant. Union Med Can 1973;102:2064.

45. Husby S, Agertoft L, Mortensen S, Pedersen S. Treatment of croup with nebulised steroid (budesonide): a double-blind, placebo controlled study. Arch Dis Child 1993;68:352–5.

46. Klassen TP, Watters LK, Feldman ME, et al. The efficacy of nebulized budesonide in dexamethasone-treated outpatients with croup. Pediatrics 1996;97:463–6.

47. Klassen TP, Craig WR, Moher D, et al. Nebulized budesonide and oral dexamethasone for treatment of croup. JAMA 1998;279(20):1629–32.

CHAPTER 10

Common Cardiovascular Problems

Brian W. McCrindle, MD, MPH, FRCPC

Cardiovascular disease remains a leading cause of mortality and morbidity in the developed countries, and widespread experience with this often sudden and silent killer fuels a great deal of anxiety in the general population. Since cardiovascular signs or symptoms are common during childhood but true pathology is relatively rare, one of the primary tasks of the physician is to effectively and efficiently differentiate those children with cardiovascular disease from those with benign or functional complaints. Concomitant with this, if no significant pathology is suspected or confirmed, the physician must provide sufficient reassurances and education to address misperceptions and prevent cardiac "nondisease"—unnecessary restrictions imposed in the absence of pertinent pathology.

This chapter will address common symptoms and signs encountered by the primary care physician, and will focus on evidence to guide evaluation and management of heart murmurs, chest pain, and syncope in children.

HEART MURMURS

Fundamentals of Heart Murmur Evaluation

History and physical examination remain the foundation of the initial evaluation of heart murmurs. Specific areas regarding history include symptoms of cardiac disease, such as failure to thrive and poor feeding with diaphoresis, tachypnea, and dyspnea; decreased exercise tolerance and easy fatigueability; chest pain and palpitations; and dizziness and syncope. However, symptoms generally are of limited usefulness in differentiating heart murmurs and are more likely to be associated with noncardiac conditions or to be benign or functional in nature.[1] A family history of cardiovascular disease or sudden death should be sought, although such a history is also of limited usefulness. Having a parent with congenital heart disease only increases the risk of heart disease in the child minimally, and innocent murmurs continue to predominate. Associated physical signs such as cyanosis and clubbing, a precordial bulge or increased precordial activity, and altered peripheral pulses suggest pathology but are almost certainly associated with heart murmurs that are easily recognized as pathologic. McCrindle and colleagues showed that findings on auscultation predominated in the differentiation of heart murmurs in ambulatory children.[1]

Since the major key to differentiating pathologic heart murmurs from innocent ones primarily is careful auscultation, complete characterization of the heart sounds and murmur is essential. Conditions for auscultation must be optimized, including minimizing extraneous noises. A well-maintained stethoscope, with intact tubing and no cracks in the diaphragm or bell, and clean, snug-fitting ear pieces will ensure that sound is optimally conducted from the patient to the listener. Patient cooperation is essential, and auscultation may be performed early in the examination with the patient sitting in the parent's lap, if necessary. Auscultation should be performed widely across the chest, back, and neck and may include the head and abdomen. Selective and focused listening is necessary to differentiate important subtleties of the heart sounds, particularly the intensity and splitting of the components of the second heart sound. Extra sounds such as clicks and opening snaps should be noted.

The murmur must be completely described. The intensity or loudness of the murmur is graded from I to VI and the presence of a palpable thrill noted. The quality of the murmur can be an important clue, with the vibratory or pure frequency murmurs more likely to be innocent and the harsh or mixed frequency murmurs more likely related to turbulent bloodflow and cardiac pathology. The timing of the murmur in the cardiac cycle is important. Diastolic murmurs occur during ventricular relaxation and likely represent flow in venous structures, antegrade flow across the atrioventricular valves or regurgitant flow across the semilunar valves and may not be heard throughout diastole. Systolic murmurs may begin in the isovolumic contraction phase of systole (thereby usually pansystolic) and represent unguarded flow from the ventricle into the lower pressure chambers, such as with a ventricular septal defect or atrioventricular valve regurgitation. Systolic murmurs that do not begin until the ejection phase of systole and thereby occur only when blood is being ejected from the ventricle are most commonly related to flow across the ventricular outflow tracts and beyond. The farther the site of murmur production from the heart, the more likely it is to take on a continuous quality, with ongoing flow heard into diastole. Notable exceptions include murmurs that may not begin until midsystole, such as with mitral valve prolapse or dynamic forms of subaortic obstruction. The point of maximal intensity or loudness of the murmur must be localized, together with other areas to which the sound appears to radiate. Provocative and postural manouvers can be particularly useful to differentiate pathologic murmurs from innocent ones, since innocent murmurs are more likely to be sensitive to variations in pressure and flow patterns. A murmur is not completely characterized until all the blanks in the following statement are completed: "This is a (loudness grade) out of 6, (quality) (timing) murmur heard best at (point of maximal intensity) and radiates to (radiation) and changes with (provocative or postural maneuvers)."

McCrindle and colleagues tested clinical assessment characteristics and documented six cardinal clinical signs that could be used to accurately differentiate pathologic murmurs from innocent ones. These include four murmur characteristics—grade III or greater intensity, harsh quality, pansystolic and heard best at the second left intercostal space—and the presence of a click or an abnormality of the second heart sound. The presence of any one of these characteristics predicted the presence of cardiac pathology with a sensitivity of 95 percent and a specificity of 61 percent. However, the study was performed in an ambulatory pediatric cardiology referral clinic, and the performance of these cardinal signs in other settings is unknown.

Innocent Heart Murmurs

The majority of murmurs heard in clinical practice will be innocent murmurs, and their differentiation from pathologic murmurs can often be made on the presence of positive findings. While the mechanism of sound production in almost all pathologic murmurs is that of turbulent bloodflow with the simultaneous production of multiple frequency noises, the etiology of most innocent murmurs has been less completely characterized. The prevailing theories would suggest that these noises are produced by laminar flow at increased velocities, which sets up purer frequency vibrations in vascular structures. There is some evidence to support that the common Still's murmur is produced by this mechanism in the presence of high normal left ventricular outflow velocities across a low normal diameter outflow tract.[2–6]

Innocent murmurs can be broadly classified into four main types, each with its own specific characteristics .[7–9] Carotid or brachiocephalic arterial bruits are felt to arise from abrupt directional changes of bloodflow from the aortic arch into the head and neck arteries. It is most commonly heard in children between the ages of 2 and 10 years and can be best described as a grade I or II, harsh-ejection systolic murmur, heard best over the supraclavicular region in the neck (often more prominent on the right) with radiation below the clavicles. The murmur is accentuated with exercise or fever and is diminished with hyperextension of the shoulders backwards with the chin held upright. It may be confused with murmurs related to left-sided obstructive lesions or wrongly assumed to represent carotid vessel disease.

The venous hum is felt to be due to flow within the jugular venous system. It is most commonly heard in children between the ages of 3 to 8 years and can be best described as a grade I or II (although variable), soft or blowing murmur, most commonly continuous with diastolic accentuation, heard best in the supra- and subclavicular regions with radiation to the neck and base. This murmur is very responsive to postural maneuvers and may be diminished in the supine position or with gentle pressure over the jugular veins in the supraclavicular fossae. It is most commonly confused with murmurs related to patent ductus arteriosus or arteriovenous malformations.

The pulmonic outflow murmur is felt to be due to vibrations produced in the right ventricular outflow tract and pulmonary artery trunk. It is most commonly heard in children between the ages of 8 to 16 years and can be best described as a grade I or II, vibratory or soft-ejection systolic murmur, heard best at the left base with very little radiation; it is accentuated by exercise, supine position, Valsalva's maneuver, or in patients with very thin and narrow chests. It is most commonly confused with atrial septal defect, anomalous pulmonary venous drainage or right-sided obstructive lesions. A very common variant occurs in the neonate when closure of the ductus arteriosus requires that the entire right-sided output must make an acute turn from the pulmonary trunk into relatively small left and right pulmonary arteries. This is usually referred to as physiologic peripheral pulmonary stenosis and is characterized by the radiation of the murmur into the axilla. It is often confused with patent ductus arteriosus, ventricular septal defect, and both right- and left-sided obstructive lesions.

Perhaps the most prevalent type of innocent murmur is the left ventricular outflow murmur or Still's murmur, produced by high-normal velocity flow across a low-normal diameter left ventricular outflow tract. It is most commonly heard between the ages of 2 and 7 years and is best described as a grade I or II, vibratory ejection systolic murmur heard best between the apex and the lower left sternal border with little radiation; it is increased by exercise, fever, and supine position and diminished with sitting or standing. It is most commonly confused with a ventricular septal defect, mitral valve regurgitation, or left-sided obstructive lesions. This murmur causes more anxiety among pediatric cardiologists, since it may sound exactly like the murmur of some forms of subaortic stenosis, which are exceedingly rare, and Still's murmur, which is extremely common.

Utility of Clinical Assessment

There have been several prospective cohort studies performed in pediatric cardiology outpatient practice settings that have confirmed the high degree of accuracy of clinical assessment by pediatric cardiologists in the differentiation of heart murmurs in children (Table 10–1). All studies used echocardiography as the criterion against which clinical assessment was evaluated. The study by McCrindle and colleagues[1] used multiple logistic regression analysis to identify six cardinal clinical signs that were independently associated with the presence of pathology. The presence of any one of these signs detected by a pediatric cardiologist predicted the presence of pathology with a sensitivity of 95 percent and specificity of 61 percent.

There is less evidence regarding the accuracy of clinical assessment by providers other than pediatric cardiologists. A standardized assessment of cardiac auscultatory skills of internal medicine and family practice trainees showed an accuracy of only 20 percent.[16] Smythe and colleagues[10] reported that when the referring physician felt that pathology was present, this was confirmed in 75 percent of cases at assessment by a pediatric cardiologist. McCrindle and colleagues[17] showed a strong correlation between referring physicians' esti-

Table 10–1 The Accuracy of Physicians in Differentiating Innocent and Pathologic Heart Murmurs

Reference	Design	Setting	Observers	Criterion	Proportion with Cardiac Lesions	Sens* %	Spec* %
Newburger[13] 1983	Prospective cohort	Consultation Clinic	Academic pediatric cardiologists	M mode echocardiograhy and follow-up	103/280 (37%)	96	97
Geva[14] 1988	Prospective cohort	Consultation clinic	Academic pediatric cardiologists	2D echocardiography	46/100 (46%)	87	96
Smythe[10] 1990	Prospective cohort	Consultation clinic	Academic pediatric cardiologists	2D echocardiography with color Doppler	45/161 (28%)	91	96
Hanson[15] 1995	Prospective cohort	Not specified	General pediatricians	2D echocardiography with color Doppler	23/100 (23%)	65	90
McCrindle[1] 1996	Prospective cohort	Consultation clinic	Academic pediatric cardiologists	2D echocardiography with color Doppler	74/222 (33%)	92	94
Du[12] 1997	Prospective cohort	Neonatology unit	Senior pediatricians	2D echocardiography with color Doppler	(Neonates) 97/116 (84%)	99	26
Haney[11] 1998	Diagnostic maneuver assessment	Continuing medical education session	General pediatricians	Cardiology consultation and echocardiography	16/37 (43%)	82	72

Sens = sensitivity; Spec = specificity

*Patients categorized as having possible heart disease were combined with the no–heart disease categories.

mates of the likelihood that the child with a murmur had pathology and subsequent confirmation at the time of pediatric cardiology assessment. Rushford and colleagues[18] found that, of patients referred for cardiology assessment, more of the patients were found to have pathology if they had been referred by pediatricians than by general practitioners. However, the suspected diagnosis offered by the referring physician was correct for 84 percent of patients referred by general practitioners versus only 41 percent of patients referred by pediatricians. In a recent study of general pediatricians who were assessed in a setting similar to a pediatric cardiology ambulatory clinic, where about 35 to 50 percent of patients assessed will have cardiac pathology, the mean sensitivity of clinical assessment was 82 percent with a mean specificity of 72 percent.[11] The performance of general practitioners and pediatricians in their own office practices, where the likelihood of cardiac pathology is very low, needs to be assessed.

Strategies for Evaluation and Referral

The implications of diagnostic characteristics associated with clinical assessment are twofold. An inadequate sensitivity implies that there will be a greater number of false negatives or missed disease. This has the potential to cause undue morbidity in terms of the potential for ventricular failure, arrhythmias, pulmonary vascular obstructive disease, and risk of endocarditis. Fortunately, the sensitivity of clinical assessment by pediatric cardiologists in referral settings (where the prevalence of pathology is relatively high) consistently ranges above 95 percent, and the types of lesions missed are clinically insignificant and usually resolve spontaneously, although some may represent a low risk of endocarditis.[1] However, the sensitivity of other types of providers practicing in acute and primary care settings, where the prevalence of pathology might be expected to be substantially lower, may be less optimal. This may be important in that these types of providers are the ones who make the decision to refer for further consultation or evaluation, and thus there may be a greater potential for significant missed disease or delayed diagnosis.

An inadequate specificity of clinical assessment results in a high rate of false positives, with undue patient and parental anxiety and a greater reliance on further consultation and diagnostic testing, with important cost implications. The combination of a high level of concern and misperceptions about heart disease in the general public, together with a false-positive diagnosis of heart disease, however trivial, can lead to a state of "cardiac nondisease," in which unwarranted anxiety and physical restrictions are imposed on the child in the absence of pathology.[19] Misperceptions are common. Scanlon[20] showed in a well-child-care clinic that 78 percent of parents were unable to define a heart murmur and viewed it as an actual cardiac lesion. McCrindle and colleagues[21] showed in a pediatric cardiology ambulatory clinic that only 16 percent of parents could correctly define a heart murmur as a sound made by the heart and that there were ongoing concerns and misperceptions despite pediatric cardiology consultation with echocardiography documenting the absence of pathology.

A high rate of false positives also increases health-care costs, since these patients will require further consultation and diagnostic testing to correctly exclude the presence of pathology. When pathology is suspected on clinical assessment, either correctly or incorrectly, several strategies may be employed—the physician may elect to continue to follow up the patient, refer directly for diagnostic testing, or refer for consultation. Continued follow-up is warranted if the physician judges the likelihood of pathology to be very low, as a murmur is often first heard during an acute illness episode when the patient is febrile or anemic and therefore in a hyperdynamic state that may accentuate an innocent murmur. McCrindle and colleagues,[17] in a study of factors prompting referral for pediatric cardiology assessment of a heart murmur, showed that the situation most often cited at the time of referral was that the murmur had not been previously heard and that this scenario was more common when the patient was not familiar to the referring physician. Also, many referrals were made for reasons related to parental anxiety and request and medicolegal concerns. Clearly, there is a need for all levels of physicians to more effectively educate and address parental and patient concerns related to heart murmurs to prevent cardiac nondisease and unwarranted requests for referral and testing. Strategies to achieve this have not been well studied. McCrindle and colleagues[21] showed that pediatric cardiology consultation with echocardiography was effective in reducing misperceptions and anxiety in the majority of parents. Scanlon[20] showed that the use of an instructional fact sheet was effective in reducing parental anxiety and increasing knowledge.

While echocardiography remains the criterion for detecting functional and structural cardiac abnormalities, the usefulness of electrocardiography and chest radiography has been less well studied. Temmerman and colleagues[22] showed that the routine use of chest radiography did not contribute much useful information to clinical assessment. In contrast, Swenson and colleagues,[23] in a prospective study of referrals for pediatric cardiology assessment of heart murmur or chest pain, concluded that the use of both electrocardiography and chest radiography appeared to increase the accuracy of clinical assessment alone, although not all patients underwent echocardiography. Birkabaek and colleagues[24] found that the differentiation of heart disease in children with heart murmurs by chest radiography showed a sensitivity of 30 percent with a specificity of 86 percent, with low reproducibility and accuracy between radiologists' interpretations.

The role of echocardiography in the evaluation of children with heart murmurs remains controversial. There have now been several studies that have shown that clinical assessment alone by a pediatric cardiologist is adequate to exclude the presence of cardiac pathology. Echocardiography is, however, very useful in specifying the exact anatomic diagnosis and its severity in those patients suspected of having cardiac pathology.[1,10,12,25] A recent study by Danford and colleagues[25] of pediatric cardiologists showed that the clinical specification of minor ventricular septal defects was very accurate, but that of intermediate or major defects was inaccurate. A further study showed diagnostic inaccuracies in the specification of pulmonary stenosis.[26] Given the higher relative cost of echocardiography versus pediatric cardiology consultation, the more cost-effective strategy for diagnostic evaluation is consultation, provided the consultant does not routinely use echocardiography and relies primarily on clinical assessment.[27]

Many physicians, however, may wish to refer directly for echocardiography. This strategy is suboptimal for several reasons. While echocardiography in the hands of a pediatric cardiologist is a highly effective diagnostic tool in assessing cardiac structure and function in children, its accuracy as performed by radiologists and cardiologists for adults is less well known. Hurwitz and colleagues[28] showed that only 52 percent of echocardiography performed in pediatric patients by laboratories for adults were technically adequate and interpreted correctly. Many repeat studies were necessary, and many children would have not required echocardiography if referred directly to the pediatric cardiologist. The referring physician is often left to interpret the echocardiographic report. Echocardiography is a highly sensitive tool, and subtle normal findings may be interpreted as indicating significant pathology by those untrained in pediatric cardiology. This includes physiologic amounts of valvar regurgitation, normal anatomic variants such as persistent left superior vena cava to coronary sinus, the presence of a closing ductus arteriosus and a tiny patent foramen ovale in a newborn, and many trivial lesions that might be expected to resolve spontaneously. Improper interpretation and communication may lead to undue physician and parental anxiety and cardiac nondisease. Clearly, if physicians opt for an "echo first" strategy, they must be aware of the quality of the echocardiographic study and be able to appropriately interpret and respond to its findings.

Cardiology consultation remains the most cost-effective strategy for the confirmatory assessment of patients felt to have pathology. However, the qualifications of the consultant physician must be carefully considered. Assessment of children by a cardiologist for adults, or another physician type, may not be as optimal as that by a pediatric cardiologist. The cost-effectiveness of this strategy applies only if the consultant does not perform routine echocardiography on all patients.

The Primary Care Physician's Role in the Management of Cardiac Pathology

A few patients with heart murmurs will be found to have cardiac pathology. Management of these patients requires the concerted effort of a team, of which the primary care physician is an integral member and where he plays an important role (Table 10–2).

Recommendations

Evidence-based recommendations for heart murmur assessment are given below:

Condition	Intervention	Quality of Evidence	Recommendation
1. Presumed innocent murmur	Watchful waiting	II-2	B
2. Clinical assessment features present that suggest a pathologic murmur	Referral to a pediatric cardiologist for clinical assessment; echocardiography at the cardiologist's discretion	II-2	A

Summary

1. Clinical assessment by a pediatric cardiologist can accurately differentiate innocent murmurs from pathologic ones with a high degree of sensitivity and specificity.
2. The accuracy of clinical assessment by other types of providers (eg, general practitioners and general pediatricians) in the differentiation of heart murmurs in children remains controversial.
3. For murmurs for which there is sufficient suspicion of pathology, pediatric cardiology consultation represents the most cost-effective strategy.

CHEST PAIN

The prevalence of chest pain in the general pediatric population is unknown, although it has been reported to account for 0.14 to 0.6 percent[30,31] of visits by children to the emergency department. The significance of the symptom of chest pain to the patient or the parent depends on many factors that may influence the mode of presentation. Clearly, many children and adolescents with chest pain do not see physicians, others present electively to primary care physicians, and some to emergency departments, and some are referred to a pediatric cardiologist or other subspecialist. Pediatric cardiologists are often involved because of underlying cardiac anxiety, although a cardiac cause is unusual.

Pathophysiology

An understanding of the pathophysiology of chest pain provides an important insight to guide differential diagnoses, investigation, and management. Chest pain can be defined as either cutaneous or visceral. As the skin is richly innervated with pain receptors, cutaneous or chest wall pain is often described as sharp, stabbing, well localized and reproducible, and of brief duration, with no relation to activity. In contrast, as the viscera are poorly innervated, visceral pain is often described in terms of a pressure sensation (gripping, crushing, burning, aching, dull) and is poorly localized or may be referred to other areas.

Table 10–2 The Role of the Primary Care Physician in the Management of the Patient with Significant Cardiac Disease

1. Monitor growth and development and help to ensure adequate nutrition.

2. Monitor for signs and symptoms of worsening congestive heart failure or cyanosis.

3. Monitor the medical management of the patient:
   • Serum digoxin levels for those patients receiving digoxin
   • Serum electrolytes for those patients receiving diuretics
   • Serum creatinine and urea for those patients receiving angiotensin converting enzyme inhibitors
   • Appropriate dosage adjustments with significant changes in patient weight

4. Ensure that endocarditis prophylaxis guidelines are being followed.

5. Provide for ancillary vaccinations (eg, pneumococcus, influenza) as appropriate.

6. Monitor and reinforce compliance with clinic visits, medications, and restrictions

7. Provide ancillary education to parents and patients to address misperceptions and inappropriate anxiety.

Etiology

While chest pain in children is usually benign, the physician is faced with the problem of pinpointing the cause from a rather long and diverse list of differential diagnoses, of which idiopathic is the most common (Table 10–3). Although chest pain of cardiac origin is very infrequent in children, it gains importance in that some of the underlying conditions can be life threatening. Cardiac chest pain results from either metabolic imbalance (ischemia) or from irritation of serosal surfaces (ie, the pericardium). The mechanism of chest pain in myocarditis and cardiomyopathy, arrhythmias, and mitral valve prolapse is less well understood. Even children with documented underlying structural heart disease are more likely to have chest pain of noncardiac, rather than cardiac, origin. Woolf and colleagues[32] noted that 14 of 17 adolescents with chest pain and mitral valve prolapse had abnormal findings on gastroesophageal evaluation, with resolution of symptoms upon treating the underlying gastroesophageal cause. Tunaoglu and colleagues[33] noted that 4 of 10 children with cardiac disease evaluated for chest pain had cardiac lesions of mild severity and not expected to be associated with chest pain. Fyfe and colleagues[34] noted a cardiac cause in only 4 of 24 children with congenital heart lesions and chest pain.

Chest pain in pulmonary conditions may be caused by pleural irritation or inflammation or by musculoskeletal strain in association with dyspnea or coughing. The majority of pulmonary causes will be evident on clinical assessment, with the exception of exercise-induced asthma. Nudel and colleagues[35] performed exercise testing in 147 children with complaints of exercise-associated chest pain, and cardiac disease was excluded with testing. Exercise-induced asthma was subsequently diagnosed as the cause of the chest pain in 14 patients (10 percent). Izumi and colleagues[36] performed a case-control study of methacholine challenge, and noted significant bronchial reactivity in 20 of 32 patients (63 percent) with idiopathic chest pain versus 3 of 27 normal controls (11 percent), with reproduction of the chest pain in 8 cases.

Gastroesophageal conditions can be an underdiagnosed cause of chest pain and most commonly relate to esophageal inflammation or spasm. Berezin and colleagues[37] reported that of 27 children previously diagnosed with idiopathic chest pain, 21 (78 percent) had a gastrointestinal cause on specific evaluation, with all symptoms resolving with appropriately directed treatment. In a further study, Berezin and colleagues[38] reported that of 60 children with atypical chest pain (none of whom had symptoms of heartburn or esophagitis), 45 were

Table 10–3 Causes of Chest Pain

Idiopathic
    Pleurodynia
    Texidor's twinge/precordial catch
Psychogenic
    Anxiety/hyperventilation
    Depression
    Conversion disorder/somatization
Musculoskeletal
    Chest wall or muscular trauma or strain
    Costochondritis
    Slipping rib syndrome/xiphoid pain
    Tietze's syndrome
Pulmonary
    Asthma
    Pneumonia
    Pleuritis
    Bronchitis/severe cough
    Pneumothorax/pneumomediastinum
    Pulmonary embolism
Cardiac
    Pericarditis/myocarditis
    Arrhythmias
    Mitral valve prolapse
    Cardiomyopathy
    Congenital coronary anomaly
        Anomalous origin of the left coronary artery/coronary ostial stenosis
        Coronary artery fistula
        Coronary artery compression
    Acquired coronary abnormality
        Kawasaki disease
        Homozygous familial hypercholesterolemia
        Metabolic disorders
    Severe ventricular outflow obstruction
    Aortic aneurysm or dissection
Gastrointestinal
    Gastroesophageal reflux/esophagitis
    Esophageal spasm
    Esophageal foreign body
    Gastritis
    Biliary colic
    Pancreatitis
Other Organic
    Sickle cell disease/vaso-occlusive crisis
    Bone tumors
    Herpes zoster
    Breast pain

diagnosed with esophagitis, with reproduction of chest pain symptoms in 18 patients after intraesophageal acid infusion (Bernstein test). Berezin and colleagues[39] further reported that upon gastroesophageal evaluation of 16 children with asthma and chronic chest pain, 11 were found to have esophagitis, attributed to gastroesophageal reflux in all 7 patients who were tested, with a positive Bernstein test in 4 patients. Glassman and colleagues[40] reviewed the results of esophageal manometry and esophagogastroscopy in 83 children referred with chest pain and noted abnormalities in 43 percent, including esophagitis only in 15, esophageal dysmotility only in 13, and both in 8 patients. Treatment of esophagitis was more successful than treatment of esophageal spasm.

Musculoskeletal chest pain usually relates to trauma, strain, or irritation of chest wall structures and is relatively easy to differentiate on clinical assessment alone. Costochondritis is a specific cause of musculoskeletal pain characterized by palpable tenderness over the costochondral or chondrosternal junctions of the anterior upper chest without swelling or deformity. It is often preceded, sometimes after a prolonged interval, by an upper respiratory infection or by exercise and is self-limited.

Psychogenic chest pain most commonly relates to anxiety or stress and less frequently to psychiatric illness such as depression or conversion disorder. Psychogenic pain may represent an increased awareness and altered perception of minor chest sensations, precipitated or exacerbated by stressful events, recent cardiac experiences in others, or a predisposition to somatization in the family. Asnes and colleagues[41] evaluated 36 children (24 females) with presumed psychogenic chest pain, referred from a total of 123 children presenting with chest pain, to a pediatric clinic. A family history of chest pain was noted in 47 percent, other recurrent somatic complaints in 56 percent, and sleep disturbances in 30 percent of patients. A specific stressful situation could be identified in the majority. Tunaoglu and colleagues[33] reported that when 74 of 100 children referred to a cardiology clinic for evaluation of chest pain were interviewed by a child psychiatrist, abnormal psychiatric findings were noted in 55 (74 percent) patients. Anxiety was noted in 15 patients, conversion disorder in 14, depression in 11, somatization disorder in 6, avoidance disorder in 5, and behavioral disorders in 4 patients.

Hyperventilation syndrome is believed to be a common form of psychogenic chest pain in adolescents. Herman and colleagues[42] described a series of 34 patients, 13 with associated anxiety, 5 with severe psychopathology, 5 with reactive-situational hyperventilation, 5 with postexertional hyperventilation, and 6 patients with no associated factors. At follow-up, 12 of 30 patients (40 percent) continued to have hyperventilation episodes into adulthood, with many patients having other ongoing chronic symptoms. Joorabchi[43] reported some success in treating these types of patients with propranolol to relieve the somatic sensations of anxiety.

The likelihood of each cause of the chest pain depends on the setting to which the child has presented or been referred (Table 10–4).[29–31,33,44–47] Patients with chest pain who are referred to a pediatric cardiologist are more likely to have pain that is chronic in nature;[33] although still uncommon, a cardiac cause is more prevalent in this than in other settings, and more interestingly, the chest pain reported is often not related to the cardiac disease noted. Idiopathic causes appear to predominate. In general pediatric settings, particularly in the emergency department, trauma and other musculoskeletal causes are prevalent, with respiratory causes less so, and idiopathic causes continuing to predominate. Knowledge of the spectrum of causes in particular settings may help to focus information gathering.

However, from the above discussion, it is clear that the diagnosis of idiopathic chest pain is being challenged as many patients, upon specific investigation, are found to have asthma, esophageal disease, or psychogenic etiologies. It is also evident that the designation of idiopathic causes may have been applied either due to a lack of careful history or physical examination, or due to a lack of suggestive specific findings on clinical assessment. It is not known what proportion of children previously felt to have idiopathic chest pain may have a treatable underlying etiology. Driscoll and colleagues[44] noted that 9 of 13 patients (69 percent) with idiopathic chest pain continued to have chest pain at 4 to 8 weeks after assessment. Fyfe and colleagues[34] noted persistence of chest pain at follow-up in 29 percent of children with idiopathic chest pain. Selbst[45] noted that on follow-up of 60 of 267 children evaluated in a pediatric emergency room for chest pain, 35 (58 percent) still had the symptom. Rowland and colleagues,[48] in a follow-up study of 31 of 44 children evaluated in a pediatric cardiology clinic

Table 10-4 Frequency of Causes of Chest Pain in Published Series

Reference	Design	Setting	Study Population	Cardiac (%)	Musculo-Skeletal (%)	Pulmonary (%)	Idiopathic (%)	Psychogenic (%)	Gastro-Intestinal (%)	Other (%)
							Causes of Chest Pain			
Driscoll[44] 1976	Prospective cohort	All outpatient clinics	n=43 all ages	–	33	12	45	–	–	10
Pantell[47] 1983	Prospective cohort	Adolescent outpatient clinic	n=100 adolescents	1	31	2	39	20	2	5
Selbst[45] 1985	Retrospective chart review	Pediatric emergency department	n=267 all ages	3	29	12	28	17	7	4
Selbst[30] 1988	Prospective cohort	Pediatric emergency department	n=407 all ages	4	29	21	21	9	4	11
Rowe[31] 1990	Prospective cohort	Pediatric emergency department	n=325 all ages	2	43	28	12	5	8	2
Kaden[46] 1991	Retrospective cohort	Pediatric cardiology consultation	n=25 adolescents	22	8	4	52	8	–	6
Zavaras[29] 1992	Retrospective chart review	Pediatric emergency department	n=134 all ages	19	16	10	20	6	7	15
Tunaoglu[33] 1995	Prospective cohort	Pediatric cardiology consultation	n=100 all ages	10	–	–	33	55	1	1

and diagnosed with idiopathic chest pain, reported that 45 percent had persistent symptoms. Selbst and colleagues[49] followed 149 of 407 children evaluated in a prospective study and noted resolution of chest pain in 57 percent. There were some diagnostic changes during follow-up, such as change from an organic to non-organic cause (psychogenic or idiopathic) in 39 patients and a new organic cause diagnosed in 12 patients. The high rates of persistence of idiopathic chest pain suggest that these patients need ongoing follow-up and may benefit from more specific investigations to ensure that a treatable cause has not been missed.

One specific type of chest pain legitimately remains idiopathic—the precordial catch syndrome. This condition can be identified by the specific description of the pain, which is of acute onset and very brief duration, sharp, and well localized along the left sternal border or beneath the left breast, any grade of intensity, unrelated to any provoking factors, often worsened with inspiration, and not related to hyperventilation. Pickering[50] described 17 patients with this syndrome, many of whom had underlying cardiac disease that was not felt to be the cause of the pain or an innocent heart murmur. Anxiety was felt to be a significant factor.

Clinical Assessment

A detailed history and physical examination are paramount in making a diagnosis and directing further investigation in the majority of patients. Specific features of the chest pain to be elicited on history include a detailed description of the duration, quality, and location of the pain and exacerbating and relieving factors. Description of the relation or response of the pain to activity, time of day, eating or drinking, movement or position, breathing, and cold or stress should also be obtained. Associated symptoms such as dyspnea, anxiety, abdominal pain, cough, vomiting, fever, dysphagia, syncope, dizziness, and palpitations, as well as any recent episodes of injury or overexertion, should be noted. Associated or previous medical conditions and medication use (both prescribed and illicit) should be sought. A family history of early, sudden, or unexplained death and cardiovascular conditions should be obtained. Psychosocial factors can play an important part in maximizing or minimizing the patient's or parent's pain perception and influence the interpretation and significance of the chest pain episodes. Specific areas to address include the patient's and parent's reactions to episodes, associated symptoms or signs of anxiety, previous or current stressful events, cardiac events or disease in family members, associated psychosomatic symptoms such as headaches and chronic abdominal pain, and symptoms or signs indicative of depression. It is important to understand the underlying concerns that are causing the patient to seek medical attention. Kaden and colleagues[46] showed in a case-control study of adolescents that there were no differences between cases and controls regarding patient knowledge of possible etiologies of chest pain; nonetheless, 68 percent of patients attributed their chest pain to heart disease and were more concerned about their heart than were the controls. Interestingly, 48 percent of the patients had heart murmurs.

A careful physical examination is likely to be helpful in differentiating some causes of chest pain. General observation for the degree of distress or hyperventilation or signs of chronic disease, with evaluation of vital signs and temperature, should be done. Features suggestive of a specific syndrome should be sought (eg, Marfan syndrome). Examination should not be limited to the thorax; rashes or bruises should be noted, and careful examination of the abdomen should be done. Observation for chest wall deformities and careful palpation of the chest wall, as well as having the patient demonstrate any movements that elicit or exacerbate the pain, are very useful for differentiating musculoskeletal causes. Percussion of the chest and auscultation of the lungs for wheezes, crackles, rubs, or diminished breath sounds may suggest a pulmonary cause. Cardiac auscultation may reveal murmurs, rubs, diminished heart sounds, or rhythm irregularities, although the presence of a murmur in association with chest pain still implies, on rare occasions, the presence of cardiac pathology. In published series, physical examination is most likely to be normal regardless of the setting to which the patient presents, with murmurs more likely in patients referred to pediatric cardiologists[33] and chest wall tenderness more likely in patients seen in an emergency department.[29–31,47]

Evaluation

Several studies have reported on the limited usefulness of ancillary testing in the evaluation of chest pain in children.[29–31,45] Laboratory evaluation is best reserved only for investigation of a specific cause suspected from history and physical examination. Regardless of physical findings, patients with a history of syncope, chest pain on exertion, palpitations, known structural or functional heart disease, or a positive family history of cardiomyopathy or sudden death require further cardiologic evaluation and, regardless of historical features, patients with unexplained tachycardia, fever, or physical abnormalities suggestive of pulmonary or cardiac disease require further evaluation. The routine or confirmatory use of electrocardiography, chest radiography, and laboratory tests is not warranted. Selbst[45] noted that of 267 children evaluated in an emergency department 28 percent had chest radiography (7 percent abnormal) and 37 percent had electrocardiography (9 percent abnormal). Selbst and colleagues[30] noted in a further prospective study of 407 children that 34 percent had chest radiography (27 percent abnormal), 47 percent had electrocardiography (16 percent abnormal), and 34 percent had echocardiography (12 percent abnormal). Abnormalities were either minor or expected, with the exception of 12 newly diagnosed cases of mitral valve prolapse (4 without any physical signs); the authors, however, conclude that the incidence of mitral valve prolapse in children with chest pain does not differ from that in asymptomatic children. Rowe and colleagues[31] evaluated 325 children in a pediatric emergency department with chest radiography in 50 percent (11 percent abnormal) and electrocardiography in 18 percent (10 percent abnormal). Horton and colleagues[51] reported the use of electrocardiography in a pediatric emergency department and noted abnormalities in 8 of 38 patients (21 percent) with chest pain. Electrocardiograms were obtained in 15 patients in whom the pain was reproducible on palpation (all normal). The interpretations of the electrocardiograms by emergency department staff were altered in 40 percent upon review by a pediatric cardiologist.

Recommendations

Evidence-based recommendations for chest pain assessment are given below:

Condition	Intervention	Quality of Evidence	Recommendation
1. Presumed functional or idiopathic chest pain of an acute nature	Ongoing follow-up and specific investigation as directed by changes in clinical assessment	II-2	B
2. Chest pain associated with palpitations, syncope, or underlying cardiac disease	Referral to a pediatric cardiologist for clinical assessment; echocardiography and further investigation at the cardiologist's discretion	II-2	A
3. Chest pain with a specific underlying cause suggested by clinical assessment	Investigation and referral as suggested by the clinical assessment	II-2	A
4. Chronic functional or idiopathic chest pain	Consider investigation for psychiatric cause, asthma, or gastroesophageal pathology	II-2	B

Summary

1. Chest pain in children represents a benign disorder, with the incidence of life-threatening underlying cardiac disease being extremely rare.
2. The majority of causes of chest pain can be differentiated on clinical assessment alone, with only limited and directed use of ancillary testing.
3. Patients without a clear underlying cause (idiopathic) require ongoing follow-up and may merit more specific investigation to exclude occult asthma, esophageal disease, or psychogenic causes.

SYNCOPE

Syncope is a sudden, transient loss of consciousness and, although common and usually benign, elicits a great deal of anxiety in patients, families, and physicians. Syncope may result in injury or is infrequently associated with a significant risk of sudden death. In the only population-based study, Driscoll and colleagues[52] defined an annual incidence of syncope coming to medical attention of 125.8/100,000 persons aged 22 years or less, with a peak between ages 15 to 19 years. However, many pediatric patients with isolated syncopal episodes do not present to medical attention, and the true incidence is probably much greater, with estimates as high as 50 percent of adolescents experiencing at least one episode.[53] The algorithms for the evaluation and management of childhood syncope are changing rapidly and remain controversial.

Pathophysiology and Etiology

While the underlying cause of syncope is sudden, transient, and diffuse cerebral malfunction due to a sudden impairment and deficiency in the delivery of vital substrates to the brain, the mechanisms by which this state can be produced fall into three broad categories (Table 10–5). The most common causes relate to abnormalities of autonomic control, which affect circulatory function, vascular volume, and vascular tone through various reflex mechanisms. This is generally known as vasovagal syncope and results from a sudden loss of vasomotor tone with peripheral pooling, decreased central vascular volume, and subsequent systemic hypotension (known as the vasodepressor response). It often leads to a sudden decrease in ventricular volume, which through a catecholamine response and its withdrawal elicits a ventricular mechanoreceptor reflex with vagally mediated paradoxic bradycardia (known as the cardioinhibitory response). In these situations, bloodflow to the brain is acutely decreased, with near-syncope or syncope. The relative contribution of these two responses to syncope in children is variable and often disputed. These responses can also be exacerbated by chronic excessive vagal tone (as seen in some healthy adolescents and conditioned athletes), acute excessive vagal tone (as seen in situational syncope, such as with cough and stretching), orthostatic changes that diminish baseline vascular volume (such as blood loss and dehydration), and impairments of oxygen delivery (such as in anemia). Since these patients have little to find on physical examination (occasionally sinus bradycardia, postural hypotension), the diagnosis is usually suggested by the history. Breath-holding spells or pallid syncope in infants and toddlers may relate to autonomic mechanisms, and patients with a history of these episodes may be more prone to develop typical vasovagal syncope at an older age.

Cardiac causes of syncope are uncommon but are of particular concern because the syncopal episode may be a marker for sudden death. Syncope is seen in relation to cardiac lesions that severely limit systemic ventricular filling (cardiac tamponade, pulmonic stenosis, pulmonary hypertension, pulmonary vein stenosis, atrial myxoma, mitral stenosis) or outflow (hypertrophic cardiomyopathy, aortic outflow obstruction). In these circumstances, syncope may be due to restricted cardiac output itself or a result of restricted output impairing myocardial oxygen delivery and leading to ventricular dysfunction or arrhythmias. These

Table 10–5 Causes of Syncope in Children

Autonomic Causes
    Vasovagal syncope
    Excessive vagal tone
    Reflex or situational syncope
    Breath-holding or pallid syncope
    Hypovolemia
        Acute: blood loss, dehydration
        Chronic: idiopathic, diuretic use
    Orthostatic hypotension
        Idiopathic
        Post-exertion
Cardiac Abnormalities
    Restricted systemic ventricular filling
        Cardiac tamponade: hemopericardium, pericardial effusion
        Pulmonary outflow obstruction
        Pulmonary hypertension
        Pulmonary venous obstruction
        Atrial myxoma
        Mitral stenosis
    Systemic ventricular outflow obstruction
        Hypertrophic cardiomyopathy
        Aortic outflow obstruction
    Coronary artery abnormalities
        Congenital: anomalous left coronary artery from the pulmonary trunk
        Acquired: Kawasaki disease
    Myocardial abnormalities
        Myocarditis
        Cardiomyopathy
    Arrhythmias
        Tachyarrhythmias
            Supraventricular tachycardias
            Long QT syndrome
            Ventricular tachycardias
        Bradyarrhythmias
            Atrioventricular block
            Sinus node dysfunction
Noncardiac Abnormalities
    Convulsive syncope
    Syncopal migraine
    Hypoglycemia
    Psychologic disorders: hysteric faints, malingering, hyperventilation syndrome
    Drugs: antihypertensive drugs, cocaine, alcohol

cardiac causes are almost uniformly evident on physical examination. Rarely, coronary artery abnormalities in children may cause myocardial ischemia with syncope.

Both bradyarrhythmias (by diminished cardiac output) and tachyarrhythmias (by diminished ventricular filling or ineffective ventricular ejection) can lead to syncope and occur both in the setting of structural or repaired heart disease and normal hearts. Structural heart disease is evident on clinical assessment, and the presence of arrhythmias may exacerbate the hemodynamic effects of restrictive or obstructive defects. Arrhythmias in structurally normal hearts may relate to supraventricular tachycardias (sometimes associated with pre-excitation), cardiomyopathy and myocarditis, medications, or illicit drug use. Complete or high-grade heart block may be congenital or a complication of Lyme carditis. Long QT syndrome can lead to sudden ventricular tachyarrhythmias with syncope, convulsive syncope, or sudden death. Prolongation of the QTc (QT interval corrected for heart rate) can be congenital (sporadic or inherited) or acquired (electrolyte disturbance, central nervous system abnormalities, medications).

Noncardiac causes of syncope represent a heterogenous group of etiologies. Seizure disorder is often in the differential diagnosis of syncope in children, and common syncopal episodes, such as vasovagal syncope, may sometimes be associated with tonic-clonic movements, which may be termed convulsive syncope. Hypoglycemia, hyperventilation, and hysteria are also rare causes of syncope.

There have been few studies characterizing the different causes of syncope in different settings (Table 10–6).[52,54,55]

Clinical Assessment

Careful history taking often suggests the etiology or an appropriate line of investigation. The number, timing, and duration of episodes should be sought. The circumstances at the time of the episode give important clues, such as the environment, patient's position (standing most common), exertion, illness, or stressors. Associated prodromal symptoms such as lightheadedness, nausea, or warmth may suggest a vasovagal cause. An associated history of chest pain or palpitation must be taken seriously. Witnesses of the episode can give important information, particularly regarding tonic-clonic movements or other findings. Information concerning medication use should be sought. A careful family history of syncope, seizures, or sudden death should be elicited, and the presence of other family members with a diagnosis of cardiomyopathy or long QT syndrome should be noted.

On physical examination, heart rate and blood pressure should be assessed, with the patient in the sitting and supine positions. Signs of structural heart disease should be sought on palpation of the pulses and precordium, percussion, and auscultation. Postural maneuvers with auscultation may unmask signs of hypertrophic cardiomyopathy or mitral valve prolapse. Neurologic examination may point to abnormalities associated with seizures or epilepsy.

Evaluation

Routine laboratory tests are not generally indicated. Electrocardiography is generally recommended as part of the evaluation of patients with all types of syncope. Abnormal atrial or ventricular forces may suggest underlying structural heart disease, and abnormalities of ST segments and T waves may suggest a myocardial abnormality (cardiomyopathy or myocarditis) or ischemia (coronary artery abnormality). Evidence of pre-excitation (Wolff-Parkinson-White) includes the presence of a short PR interval with a delta wave. Abnormalities of conduction should be noted, although episodic arrhythmias are usually not noted on routine electrocardiography. The QTc interval should be measured as a marker for long QT syndrome, although its sensitivity and specificity and the technique of proper measurement continue to be debated. Echocardiography and exercise testing should be reserved for patients with evidence suggesting a cardiac cause of syncope. Table 10–7 lists characteristics of patients with syncope who merit more detailed and intensive evaluation.

There has been an increasing interest and role for tilt-table testing in the evaluation of syncope in children, particularly for those with atypical or recurrent episodes. While there are many variations on test protocol, in general, the patient is placed in the supine position for a period of time on a table with a footboard; then, while being monitored, the patient is brought into a 60 to 90° head-up position for a defined period or until syncope or presyncope is induced. The purpose of the study is to identify patients with a tendency to vasovagal syncope or an exaggeration of the normal autonomic responses previously described. Pongiglione and colleagues[56] evaluated 20 normal children with syncope, with production

Table 10-6 Causes of Syncope in Published Series

Reference	Design	Setting	Study Population	Causes of Chest Pain								
				Vaso-vagal (%)	Cardio-inhibitory (%)	Mixed Response (%)	Orthostatic Hypotension (%)	Reflex (%)	Neuro-logic (%)	Psycho-logic (%)	Other (%)	Unknown (%)
Pratt[54] 1989	Prospective cohort	Pediatric emergency department	n=40 Children	50	—	—	20 (anemia 5%)	—	13	—	5	—
Lerman-Sagie[55]1976	Prospective cohort	Pediatric emergency department	n=58 Children	54	22	7	—	5	—	3	—	9
Driscoll[52] 1997	Population-based study	All sources of medical care	n=151 Children and adolescents (1987 to 1991)	69	—	—	1	4	2	3	19	8

Table 10–7 Patients with Syncope that Merit Referral for Further Evaluation

---

Patients with:
- Recurrent syncope
- Exercise or exertional syncope
- Syncope associated with chest pain
- Syncope associated with palpitations
- Pathologic cardiovascular findings on clinical assessment
- Abnormalities on electrocardiography
- Neurologic abnormalities or findings
- Family history of sudden death
- Family history of seizures
- Family history of cardiomyopathy
- Atypical syncopal episodes

---

of symptoms in 14 (70 percent). The exaggerated response elicited by tilt-testing was felt to be cardioinhibitory in 3 patients, vasodepressor in 2, and mixed in 11 patients. Thilenius and colleagues[57] evaluated 35 normal adolescents with syncope, with positive responses in 24 (69 percent) and borderline results in 3 patients. Beta blockade resulted in normal tilt-table response in 5 of 6 patients who were retested. Lerman-Sagle and colleagues[58] performed a case-control study and noted positive tests in 6 (40 percent) of 15 adolescents with syncope and none of the 10 normal controls. Ross and colleagues[59] performed orthostatic testing (tilt testing without the table) in 104 children with syncope with a positive result (syncope) in 47 (45 percent), and normal results in 12 normal controls. Oslizlok and colleagues[60] likewise performed orthostatic testing in 209 children with positive results in 122 (58 percent), 5 of whom were felt to have isolated exaggerated cardioinhibitory responses. Balaji and colleagues[61] performed orthostatic testing in 162 children with a positive result in 100 (62 percent), with isolated cardioinhibitory syncope in 11 patients. Fludrocortisone and salt were used in 84 patients in the orthostatic positive group, with resolution of symptoms in 55 (65 percent) and improvement in 14 (17 percent). As there have been concerns about the reproducibility of tilt testing in adults, Fish and colleagues[62] performed repeat testing after a 25- to 30-minute recovery period in 21 children, with a positive result initially, and symptoms again produced in 18 patients. In addition, the pattern of response was different between the two tests in 7 patients.

The evaluation of patients with suspected arrhythmia as a cause of their syncope is somewhat problematic. Clearly, the goal is to correlate the patient's heart rhythm with the occurrence of the syncopal episode. Ambulatory Holter monitoring can be useful in identifying more frequent occult episodes of arrhythmia but can only be used for a limited period. Event recorders are a more long-term means of capturing heart rhythm at the time of syncopal episodes but are dependent on patient compliance. There has been some recent interest in an implantable loop recorder, which is implanted surgically in a subcutaneous pocket and activated by the patient or family member at the time of an event to store preceding and concurrent electrocardiographic recordings, although there are no reports of its use in children.

Treatment

All patients with worrisome syncope require ongoing follow-up. Patients with vasovagal syncope should be counseled regarding avoidance of precipitating circumstances and how to recognize and respond to prodromal symptoms to prevent episodes or injury. In many patients, recurrent vasovagal syncope resolves spontaneously during follow-up; therefore, assessments of therapeutic strategies must incorporate placebo or comparative groups. Treatment with salt supplementation and fludrocortisone is an accepted first-line therapy.

Although there are case series of treatment with beta-blockers, alpha-agonists, disopyramide, and scopolamine, there are no reports in children with control groups. Scott and colleagues[63] compared atenolol with fludrocortisone in a randomized study of pediatric vasovagal syncope and showed no difference in episode scores at 6 months. Treatment of other forms of syncope is directed at the underlying cause.

Recommendations

Evidence-based recommendations for evaluation of syncope are given below.

Condition	Intervention	Quality of Evidence	Recommendation
1. Typical isolated autonomic syncopal episode	Clinical assessment only, electrocardiography and reassurance	III	B
2. Syncope associated with exercise, palpitations, chest pain, or underlying cardiac disease	Referral to a pediatric cardiologist for clinical assessment; echocardiography and further investigation at the cardiologist's discretion	II-2	A
3. Syncope associated with a family history of sudden death, seizures, or cardiomyopathy	Referral to a pediatric cardiologist for clinical assessment; echocardiography and electrophysiologic testing at the cardiologist's discretion	II-2	A
4. Recurrent autonomic syncopal episodes	Referral to a pediatric cardiologist for clinical assessment; orthostatic tilt testing; treatment with avoidance maneuvers, ±salt, ±fludrocortisone	II-2	B
5. Atypical syncopal episodes	Referral to a pediatric cardiologist for clinical assessment; consider orthostatic tilt testing, psychiatric evaluation; ongoing follow-up	III	B

Summary

1. The cause of syncope in the majority of children can be differentiated on the basis of clinical assessment and surface electrocardiography, with treatment directed at the underlying cause.
2. Orthostatic and tilt-table testing have a role in the evaluation of atypical or recurrent syncope.

REFERENCES

1. McCrindle BW, Shaffer KM, Kan JS, et al. Cardinal clinical signs in the differentiation of heart murmurs in children. Arch Pediatr Adolesc Med 1996;150:169–74.

2. Schwartz ML, Goldberg SJ, Wilson N, et al. Relations of Still's murmur, small aortic diameter and high aortic velocity. Am J Cardiol 1986;57:1344–8.

3. Sholler GF, Celermajer DS, Whight CM. Doppler echocardiographic assessment of cardiac output in normal children with and without innocent precordial murmurs. Am J Cardiol 1987;59:487–8.

4. Klewer SE, Connerstein RL, Goldberg SJ. Still's-like innocent murmur can be produced by increasing aortic velocity to a threshold value. Am J Cardiol 1991;68:810–2.

5. Donnerstein RL, Thomsen VS. Hemodynamic and anatomic factors affecting the frequency content of Still's murmur. Am J Cardiol 1994;74:508–10.

6. Van Oort A, Hopman J, De Boo T, et al. The vibratory innocent heart murmur in school-children: a case-control Doppler echocardiographic study. Pediatr Cardiol 1994;15:275–81.

7. McNamara DG. The pediatrician and the innocent heart murmur. Am J Dis Child 1987;141:1161.

8. Rosenthal A. How to distinguish between innocent and pathologic murmurs in childhood. Pediatr Clin NA 1984;31:1229–40.

9. Sapin SO. Recognizing normal heart murmurs: a logic-based mnemonic. Pediatrics 1997;99:616–9.

10. Smythe JF, Teixeira OHP, Vlad P, et al. Initial evaluation of heart murmurs: are laboratory tests necessary? Pediatric 1990;86:497–500.

11. Haney I, Feldman W, Ipp M, McCrindle BW. Accuracy of clinical assessment by general pediatricians in differentiating heart murmurs in children [abstract]. Pediatr Res 1998; 43(Pt 2):111A.

12. Du Z-D, Roguin N, Barak M. Clinical and echocardiographic evaluation of neonates with heart murmurs. Acta Paediatrica 1997; 86:752–6.

13. Newburger JW, Rosenthal A, Williams RG, et al. Noninvasive tests in the initial evaluation of heart murmurs in children. N Engl J Med1983;308:61–4.

14. Geva T, Hegesh J, Frand M. Reappraisal of the approach to the child with heart murmurs: is echocardiography mandatory? Internat J Cardiol 1988;19:1070150–13.

15. Hansen LK, Birkebaek NH, Oxhoj H. Initial evaluation of children with heart murmurs by the non-specialized paediatrician. Eur J Pediatr 1995;154:15–7.

16. Mangione S, Nierman LZ. Cardiac auscultatory skills of internal medicine and family practice trainees. A comparison of diagnostic proficiency. JAMA 1997;278:717–22.

17. McCrindle BW, Shaffer KM, Kan JS, et al. Factors prompting referral for cardiology evaluation of heart murmurs in children. Arch Pediatr Adol Med 1995;149:1277–9.

18. Rushford JA, Wilson N. Should general pediatricians have access to pediatric cardiologists? Br Med J 1992;305:1264–5.

19. Bergman AB, Stamm SJ. The morbidity of cardiac nondisease in schoolchildren. N Engl J Med 1967; 276:1008–13.

20. Scanlon JW. Do parents need to know more about innocent murmurs? Experience with an instructional fact sheet. Clin Pediatr 1971;10:23–6.

21. McCrindle BW, Shaffer KM, Kan JS, et al. An evaluation of parental concerns and misperceptions about heart murmurs. Clin Pediatr 1995;34:25–31.

22. Temmerman AM, Mooyaart EL, Taverne PP. The value of the routine chest roentgenogram in the cardiologic evaluation of infants and children. A prospective study. Eur J Pediatr 1991;150:623–6.

23. Swenson JM, Fischer DR, Miller SA, et al. Are chest radiographs and electrocardiograms still valuable in evaluating new pediatric patients with heart murmurs or chest pain? Pediatrics 1997;99:1–3.

24. Birkabaek NH, Hansen LK, Elle B, et al. Chest roentgenogram in the evaluation of heart defect in asymptomatic infants and children with a cardiac murmur: reproducibility and accuracy. Pediatrics 1999;103:e15.

25. Danford DA, Martin AB, Fletcher SE, et al. Children with heart murmurs: can ventricular septal defect be reliably diagnosed without an echocardiogram? J Am Coll Cardiol 1997; 30:243–6.

26. Danford DA, Salaymeh KJ, Marcin AB, et al. Pulmonary stenosis: defect-specific diagnostic accuracy of heart murmurs in children. J Pediatr 1999;134:76–81.

27. Danford DA, Nasir A, Gumbiner C. Cost assessment of the evaluation of heart murmurs in children. Pediatrics 1993;91:365–8.

28. Hurwitz RA, Caldwell RL. Should pediatric echocardiography be performed in adult laboratories? Pediatrics 1998;102:e15.

29. Zavaras-Angelidou KA, Weinhouse E, Nelson DB. Review of 180 episodes of chest pain in 134 children. Pediatr Emerg Care 1992;8:189–93.

30. Selbst SM, Ruddy RM, Clark BJ, et al. Pediatric chest pain: a prospective study. Pediatrics 1988;82:319–23.

31. Rowe BH, Dulberg CS, Peterson RG, et al. Characteristics of children presenting with chest pain to a pediatric emergency department. Can Med Assoc J 1990;143:388–94.

32. Woolf PK, Gewitz MH, Berezin S, et al. Noncardiac chest pain in adolescents and children with mitral valve prolapse. J Adolesc Health 1991;12:247–50.

33. Tunaoglu FS, Olgunturk R, Akcabay S, et al. Chest pain in children referred to a cardiology clinic. Pediatr Cardiol 1995;16:69–72.

34. Fyfe DA, Moodie DS. Chest pain in pediatric patients presenting to a cardiac clinic. Clin Pediatr 1984;23:321–4.

35. Nudel DB, Diamant S, Brady T, et al. Chest pain, dyspnea on exertion, and exercise induced asthma in children and adolescents. Clin Pediatr 1987;26:388–92.

36. Izumi N, Haneda N, Mori C. Methacholine inhalation challenge in children with idiopathic chest pain. Acta Paediatrica Japonica 1992;34:441–6.

37. Berezin S, Medow MS, Glassman MS, Newman LJ. Chest pain of gastrointestinal origin. Arch Dis Child 1988;63:1457–60.

38. Berezin S, Medow MS, Glassman MS, Newman LJ. Use of the intraesophageal acid perfusion test in provoking nonspecific chest pain in children. J Pediatr 1989;115:709–12.

39. Berezin S, Medow MS, Glassman MS, Newman LJ. Esophageal chest pain in children with asthma. J Pediatr Gastroent Nutr 1991;12:52–5.

40. Glassman MS, Medow MS, Berezin S, Newman LJ. Spectrum of esophageal disorders in children with chest pain. Digest Dis Sci 1992;37:663–6.

41. Asnes RS, Santulli R, Bemporad JR. Psychogenic chest pain in children. Clin Pediatr 1981;20:788–91.

42. Herman SP, Stickler GB, Lucas AR. Hyperventilation syndrome in children and adolescents: long-term follow-up. Pediatrics 1981;67:183–7.

43. Joorabchi B. Expressions of the hyperventilation syndrome in childhood. Studies in management, including an evaluation of the effectiveness of propranolol. Clin Pediatr 1977;16:1110–5.

44. Driscoll DJ, Glicklich LB, Gallen WJ. Chest pain in children: a prospective study. Pediatrics 1976;57:648–51.

45. Selbst SM. Chest pain in children. Pediatrics 1985;75:1068–70.

46. Kaden GG, Shenker IR, Gootman N. Chest pain in adolescents. J Adolesc Health 1991;12:251–5.

47. Pantell RH, Goodman BW. Adolescent chest pain: a prospective study. Pediatrics 1983;71:881–7.

48. Rowland TW, Richards MM. The natural history of idiopathic chest pain in children. A follow-up study. Clin Pediatr 1986;25:612–4.

49. Selbst SM, Ruddy R, Clark BJ. Chest pain in children. Follow-up of patients previously reported. Clin Pediatr 1990;29:374–7.

50. Pickering D. Precordial catch syndrome. Arch Dis Child 1981;56:401–3.

51. Horton LA, Mosee S, Brenner J. Use of the electrocardiogram in a pediatric emergency department. Arch Pediatr Adolesc Med 1994;148:184–8.

52. Driscoll DJ, Jacobsen SJ, Porter CJ, Wollan PC. Syncope in children and adolescents. J Am Coll Cardiol 1997;29:1039–45.

53. Hannon DW, Knilans TK. Syncope in children and adolescents. Curr Prob Pediatr 1993;23:358–84.

54. Pratt JL, Fleisher GR. Syncope in children and adolescents. Pediatr Emerg Care 1989;5:80–2.

55. Lerman-Sagie T, Lerman P, Mukamel M, et al. A prospective evaluation of pediatric patients with syncope. Clin Pediatr 1994;33:67–70.

56. Pongiglione G, Fish FA, Strasburger JF, Benson DWJ. Heart rate and blood pressure response to upright tilt in young patients with unexplained syncope. J Am Coll Cardiol 1990;16:165–70.

57. Thilenius OG, Quinones JA, Husayni TS, Novak J. Tilt test for diagnosis of unexplained syncope in pediatric patients. Pediatrics 1991;87:334–8.

58. Lerman-Sagie T, Rechavia E, Strasberg B, et al. Head-up tilt for the evaluation of syncope of unknown origin in children. J Pediatr 1991;118:676–9.

59. Ross BA, Hughes S, Anderson E, Gillette PC. Abnormal responses to orthostatic testing in children and adolescents with recurrent unexplained syncope. Am Heart J 1991;122:748–54.

60. Oslizlok P, Allen M, Griffin M, Gillette P. Clinical features and management of young patients with cardioinhibitory response during orthostatic testing. Am J Cardiol 1992;69:1363–5.

61. Balaji S, Oslizlok PC, Allen MC, et al. Neurocardiogenic syncope in children with a normal heart. J Am Coll Cardiol 1994;23:779–85.

62. Fish FA, Strasburger JF, Benson DWJ. Reproducibility of a symptomatic response to upright tilt in young patients with unexplained syncope. Am J Cardiol 1992;70:605–9.

63. Scott WA, Pongiglione G, Bromberg BI, et al. Randomized comparison of atenolol and fludrocortisone acetate in the treatment of pediatric neurally mediated syncope. Am J Cardiol 1995;76:400–2.

CHAPTER 11

Abdominal Pain in Children

Hema Patel, MD, FRCPC, MSc

Abdominal pain, acute or chronic, is a common pediatric complaint. Although the patho-physiology of pain production and perception is becoming better understood,[1,2] abdominal discomfort remains a complex, often nonspecific symptom. Nonetheless, in a minority of children, abdominal pain represents an important indicator of disease. In this chapter, the most common causes of abdominal pain in children are discussed, and the clinical features ("red flags") that differentiate benign, self-limited conditions from those requiring prompt diagnosis and/or intervention are highlighted. Wherever possible, the level of supporting evidence is indicated, along with appropriate references. The aim is to provide a practical, evidence-based approach to the treatment of the child with abdominal pain.

ACUTE ABDOMINAL PAIN

Acute abdominal pain has been aptly defined as pain severe enough to require an urgent medical assessment; this may be a pain of new onset or of increased intensity on a background of chronic discomfort.[1] Two recent cross-sectional surveys have shown that acute abdominal pain accounts for 4 to 5 percent of pediatric outpatient encounters.[3,4] Most of the acute abdominal pains in children have a non-specific etiology. The heterogeneic nature of acute abdominal pain has been highlighted by the study by Scholer and colleagues of 1,141 American children aged 2 to 12 years with acute, nontraumatic abdominal pain. In this survey, the most frequent final diagnoses included upper respiratory tract infection/pharyngitis/viral syndrome/febrile illness (59 percent), abdominal pain of unknown etiology (15.6 percent), gastroenteritis (10.9 percent), bronchitis/asthma (2.6 percent), pneumonia (2.3 percent), constipation (2.0 percent) and urinary tract infection (1.6 percent). Acute appendicitis was diagnosed in 10 children (0.9 percent); 3 of whom were diagnosed on a repeat visit to the pediatric emergency department.[4]

Although the vast majority of children with acute abdominal pain have an underlying medical diagnosis such as those listed above, surgically correctable causes of pain do require prompt recognition and intervention. The three most common surgical emergencies in children with abdominal pain are (1) incarcerated inguinal hernia, (2) intussusception, and (3) appendicitis. The first two conditions primarily occur in infants and young children, while appendicitis is the most common surgical emergency in school-aged children.

Inguinal hernias most often are diagnosed in the first few months of life. Boys are affected six to nine times more often than are girls; similarly, preterm infants are at a higher risk compared with term infants (level III).[5,6] Unlike umbilical hernias, inguinal hernias rarely, if ever, resolve spontaneously.[5–7] The caregiver usually reports seeing an intermittent, smooth, firm mass in the groin, scrotal, or labial area. The mass is pronounced when the infant cries, coughs, or strains. Often, the hernia is first observed while the infant is being bathed.[7,8] Survey studies (level III) indicate that the overall incidence of inguinal hernias in children varies between 0.8 to 4.4 percent.[5–9] Of these children, approximately 10 to 30 percent have hernias that become incarcerated and/or strangulated.[8–10] Because of this risk, coupled with the lack of spontaneous resolution, surgical repair is recommended in any infant with an inguinal hernia.[5–7]

Incarcerated hernias are seen most frequently in infants, with a peak incidence at 2 to 3 months of age; these difficult-to-reduce hernias represent a surgically urgent situation.[10] Affected infants develop crampy abdominal pain, irritability, and vomiting. Early vomiting is usually nonbilious; bilious vomiting may occur as the bowel obstruction persists.[2] Physical signs include the presence of a firm inguinal mass; abdominal distention is a later finding.[7-10] As an incarcerated hernia becomes strangulated (ischemic), the overlying groin skin may appear erythematous or purplish in color. At this point, infants may appear systemically ill, with dehydration and tachycardia.[2] An urgent surgical consultation is warranted for any child with an incarcerated hernia, with or without evidence of strangulation. In most children, the incarcerated hernia can be reduced with Trendelenburg positioning and gentle pressure on the hernial sac. Concomitant traction of the external inguinal ring is recommended. Definitive operative repair can then take place on a semielective basis over the next 12 to 24 hours.[7] Of course, operative repair is required immediately if reduction of the hernia sac is unsuccessful.

Laboratory investigations play a minor role in the diagnosis and therapy of inguinal hernias. Clinical history and physical examination are the diagnostic gold standards. Herniography, with radiopaque contrast media injected into the peritoneal cavity, is rarely performed. Abdominal radiography is of ancillary benefit in the detection and confirmation of bowel obstruction in those with incarcerated hernias. Specific findings of interest include air fluid levels in bowel loops and free air secondary to bowel perforation. Because the earliest clinical symptoms in infants with incarceration of an inguinal hernia are nonspecific (irritability and pain) and may mimic many other medical conditions, a careful physical examination, with the infant fully undressed, is crucial.

Intussusception, or telescoping of the bowel, is the second most common cause of bowel obstruction in children aged 2 months to 5 years.[11] The peak incidence has been reported to be between 4 and 10 months of age (level III).[12] In 95 percent of affected children, the intussusception occurs at the ileocecal junction.[11,12] The etiology of intussusception remains unknown in approximately 95 percent of children,[13] though it has long been hypothesized that hypertrophied lymphoid tissue in the gastrointestinal Peyer's patches act as a lead point to the bowel invagination. In the minority of children with a defined lead point, the most common cause of intussusception is a Meckel's diverticulum (level III).[13] Children with Henoch-Schönlein purpura (HSP) and cystic fibrosis are known to be at a higher risk for intussusception.[14] Older children with intussusception are more likely than preschool-aged children to have a pathologic leading edge, such as a lymphoma, polyp, or other mass lesions.[11,12]

The classic clinical triad of colicky intermittent abdominal pain, vomiting, and currant jelly (bloody) stool appears in only 10 to 20 percent of all children with intussusception.[15] Characteristically, the infant has intermittent severe crying spells. Often, during these episodes, the legs are drawn up with the hips in flexion. In between these periods, the infant may appear quite normal. An infant may also present with nonspecific findings such as lethargy, pallor, and shock.[11] A preliminary study of 88 infants with intussusception quantified the positive predictive value (PPV) of the following clinical symptoms and signs: right upper quadrant abdominal mass (PPV=94 percent), grossly bloody stool (PPV=80 percent), blood on rectal examination (PPV=78 percent) and the classic triad described above (PPV=100 percent).[15] The PPV is a clinically useful measure that indicates the proportion of patients with a positive test who truly have the condition being evaluated. The negative predictive value (NPV) indicates the proportion of patients with a negative test who truly do not have the condition.[16]

The air-contrast enema has been accepted as the diagnostic and therapeutic gold standard for intussusception. This procedure is as effective and has a lower complication rate compared with the previously used barium contrast enema method (level I,[17] level II,[18] and level III).[19] In the past, plain radiography had been advocated as a first-line investigation in infants suspected as having a bowel intussusception (level III).[20,21] Unfortunately, plain radiography identifies a characteristic lucent right upper quadrant mass in only 49 percent of infants with true intussusception.[20] As well, a small proportion (2.3 percent) of normal infants have a similar finding (false-positive diagnosis).[20]

Ultrasound imaging, when conducted by an experienced operator, in infants with equivocal findings is helpful in the diagnosis of intussusception.[15] In one prospective study of 245 infants with suspected intussusception, ultrasonographic findings (target/doughnut sign/pseudokidney sign) had a PPV of 92.6 percent with an NPV of 97.4 percent.[15] Because classic clinical findings show similarly high PPVs, ultrasonography appears to be most useful in infants with suspected intussusception but without specific diagnostic features. Ultrasonographic evaluation would likely create an unnecessary delay in intervention in infants with an obvious clinical diagnosis; these infants should proceed directly to air-contrast enema treatment.

Acute appendicitis is the most common surgical emergency of childhood, with a peak incidence between 10 and 12 years of age.[2] Clinical examination by an experienced physician remains the gold standard of diagnosis. The classic presentation of appendicitis includes (1) a prodrome of constant, vague epigastric or periumbilical pain, frequently followed by nonbilious vomiting, (2) progressive pain migration to the right lower quadrant of the abdomen, and (3) low-grade fever.[22] Anorexia, nausea, and diarrhea may also occur. In children, subtle evidence of accompanying peritoneal irritation includes (1) limping while walking, (2) hesitancy/refusal to change position or to be examined, and (3) a history of discomfort during the ride to hospital. Gentle percussion over the right lower quadrant has been advocated as a sensitive indicator of appendicitis.[2,23]

In children with a classic clinical presentation of acute appendicitis, no further tests are indicated.[22–24] Unfortunately, few children have unequivocal clinical findings; furthermore, in infants and preschool-aged children, presenting symptoms and signs are subtle and often nonspecific. Not surprisingly, in the under–3-year-olds, the proportion of those with a perforated appendix at the time of diagnosis is approximately 60 percent.[24] As well, up to 50 percent of children in this age group may have a false-positive diagnosis, that is, a normal appendix found at the time of surgery (level III).[24]

Because of the inherent difficulty in clinical diagnosis in both children and adults, clinicians have searched for predictive factors. Here, we will review the predictive values for (1) specific clinical signs and symptoms, (2) the white blood cell count (WBC), (3) the neutrophil count (PMN), (4) C-reactive protein (CRP), (5) plain radiography of the abdomen, and (6) ultrasonographic evaluation.

Wagner and colleagues conducted a systematic review of the significance of clinical findings in patients with acute appendicitis.[22] Ten cohort and cross-sectional surveys were selected as providing the best available information (level II-2, III).[22] These studies, which included adults as well as children, involved a total of 5,275 patients. Data from children alone were not provided. A summary of the pooled results is provided in Table 11–1. The "sensitivity" of each characteristic is a measure of the true positive rate,[16] that is, if the value is high (close to 1.00), the presence of the feature makes acute appendicitis likely. In other words, high sensitivity means that the false-negative rate is low. The "specificity" of each characteristic is a measure of the true negative rate,[16] that is, if the value is high (close to 1.00) and the feature is absent, the patient is more likely not to truly have acute appendicitis.

These results (see Table 11–1)[22] indicate that the presence of abdominal wall rigidity, classic pain migration to the right lower quadrant, and a positive psoas sign are helpful features in ruling in acute appendicitis. In contrast, the absence of right lower quadrant pain, the presence of pain *after* vomiting, and a previous history of similar pain are all helpful in ruling out the diagnosis of acute appendicitis. The presence or absence of anorexia, nausea, vomiting, or rectal tenderness, in isolation, are not particularly helpful in diagnosis.

Table 11–1 Summary of Clinical Examination Operating Characteristics for Appendicitis

Clinical Characteristic	Sensitivity	Specificity
Right lower quandrant pain	0.81	0.53
Abdominal wall rigidity	0.27	0.83
Classic pain migration	0.64	0.82
Pain before vomiting	1.00	0.64
Positive psoas sign	0.16	0.95
Fever	0.67	0.79
Rebound tenderness test	0.63	0.69
Guarding	0.74	0.57
No similar pain previously	0.81	0.41
Rectal tenderness	0.41	0.77
Anorexia	0.68	0.36
Nausea	0.58	0.37
Vomiting	0.51	0.45

While Wagner and colleagues reviewed studies of both children and adults, smaller retrospective case-series have focused on children alone.[23,24] The difficulty in the diagnosis of acute appendicitis in children was highlighted by the overall observed incidence (18 to 30 percent) of appendiceal perforation at the time of surgery.[23,24] Neither study was able to clearly identify useful risk factors. Reynolds and colleagues found that 7 percent of children with true appendicitis were evaluated on more than one occasion before the diagnosis was made.[23] Clearly, clinical observation and re-evaluation are key diagnostic aids.

The white blood cell count (WBC), the neutrophil count (PMN), and C-reactive protein (CRP) have been evaluated, alone and in combination, for their predictive value in making the diagnosis of acute appendicitis. In a retrospective case series of 90 preschool-aged children, operated on for suspected appendicitis, the WBC and PMN counts were of no help in distinguishing appendicitis with perforation, appendicitis without perforation, and no appendicitis (level III).[24] Not surprisingly, the CRP was found to be statistically higher in those children with perforation.[24] Of note, this study did not evaluate the WBC, PMN, or CRP levels in children with suspected appendicitis who were observed but not operated upon.

In a prospective descriptive study of 204 adults and children with suspected appendicitis (100 had appendectomy, 104 were observed), an elevated WBC showed a sensitivity of 83 percent with an NPV of 88 percent (level III).[25] In combination, an elevated WBC or PMN count or CRP value had a PPV of only 37 percent. In contrast, the NPV was 100 percent in the small group of patients having normal values for all three measures (WBC, PMN, and CRP). Thus, those patients with equivocal clinical findings and completely normal values for the WBC, PMN and CRP may deserve a period of observation and re-evaluation versus immediate surgery. It is important to re-emphasize that individuals with clear clinical findings should proceed directly to operative repair; laboratory testing is not diagnostically helpful in these instances.

Plain radiography of the abdomen is of limited use in the detection of most surgical diseases in children, including acute appendicitis. In a prospective descriptive study of 354 children 15 years of age and younger who had abdominal films taken in the emergency department, only 29 (8 percent) had findings suggestive of major disease (for example, appendicitis, intussusception, mechanical bowel obstruction) (level III).[26] Specifically, the low utility of plain abdominal radiography in patients with appendicitis is well documented. One pediatric study found that the abdominal radiography in 90 percent of children with true appendicitis was normal or had noncontributory incidental findings (level III).[27]

Lastly, ultrasound evaluation has been used as a diagnostic aid for acute appendicitis. As in infants with intussusception, the value of ultrasonography is primarily in children with equivocal clinical findings. Likewise, the validity of the study is directly dependent upon the skill and experience of the ultrasonographer. Positive ultrasonographic findings include the presence of an enlarged (>6 to 8 mm in diameter), immobile, noncompressible, blind-ending tubular structure with a hypoechoic lumen.[28] Paired with serial clinical re-examination, it appears that ultrasound imaging can significantly reduce the current rate of unnecessary appendectomies; in children, this rate ranges between 30 and 46 percent.[29] Prospective, descriptive studies have shown that ultrasonography has a PPV of 86 to 93.6 percent (sensitivity of 89.7 to 94 percent) and an NPV of 97 to 98 percent (specificity 89 to 98.2 percent) (level III).[30–32] In children with poorly visualized appendices or those with perforation, ultrasonography has shown less diagnostic value.

Clearly, the serial clinical examination remains the diagnostic gold standard for acute appendicitis in children. Ultrasonography and laboratory evaluations are indicated as diagnostic aids in children with equivocal findings. Importantly, clinical findings should dictate management, even in the face of negative ultrasonographic or laboratory findings. Similarly, in the child with a clinical diagnosis of acute appendicitis, neither ultrasonographic studies nor laboratory results are likely to alter or improve the care provided.[33]

In summary, acute abdominal pain is a common pediatric problem. Most children have spontaneously resolving, self-limited pain. Although truly serious underlying conditions are rare, diagnosis can be particularly difficult in the preverbal or noncooperative child. Clinical experience has shown that the "red flags" shown in Table 11–2 are worth careful consideration (level III).[1,2,23,34] Observation, re-evaluation, and targeted investigations are key to the management of the child with acute abdominal pain of uncertain etiology.

CHRONIC OR RECURRENT ABDOMINAL PAIN

Chronic abdominal pain is more correctly defined as recurrent abdominal pain, as most children experience pain-free episodes between times of abdominal pain. As with acute abdominal pain, recurrent pain is exceedingly common. Various population-based surveys have reported that 10 to 15 percent of school-aged children experience recurrent abdominal pain; in 9 to 11-year-olds, estimates have been as high as 30 percent.[35–38] The syndrome of recurrent abdominal pain (RAP) of childhood, first described in the late 1950s by Apley and Naish, continues to account for the vast majority of school-aged children with chronic abdominal pain.[39] Approximately 90 percent of children with chronic abdominal pain referred to a pediatric tertiary care center have a diagnosis of RAP (level III).[37] Taking into account the effect of referral bias, almost all children with recurrent abdominal pain seen in the primary care setting will have this relatively benign diagnosis.[40] Chronic constipation affects approximately 5 percent of children with recurrent pain seen in the primary care setting and up to 25 percent of those evaluated in a tertiary care environment.[41–43]

Of the more serious but less common disorders, inflammatory bowel disease (IBD) is an important condition that requires prompt recognition and intervention.[44] In children, IBD comprises Crohn's disease and ulcerative colitis. There is an overall incidence of 4 to 6 cases per 1,000 with a peak age-at-onset between 10 and 30 years. Approximately 20 percent

Table 11–2 Clinical Red Flags in the Assessment of Acute Abdominal Pain in Children

Red Flag	Interpretation
Severe abdominal pain without other symptoms	Less likely that the etiology is related to a viral illness or associated diagnosis, for example, otitis media
Pain awakening the child from sleep	Indicates severity of pain; has been noted to occur in children with appendicitis, intussusception
Absence of high fever	Although many children with appendicitis may have a low grade fever (38 to 38.5°C), high fever (>38.5°C) is unusual and is more consistent with an acute infectious process
Vomiting after abdominal pain	Children with gastroenteritis often have vomiting preceding or concurrently with abdominal pain; those with appendicitis are more likely to have abdominal pain as an initial feature
Vomiting for >24 hours, without diarrhea	The common diagnosis of viral gastroenteritis becomes less likely without the presence of diarrhea
Bilious or feculent vomiting	Abnormal, until proven otherwise; indicative of bowel obstruction, usually a late finding
Asymmetric or localized pain	Focality may indicate a specific diagnosis, for example, hepatitis with right upper quandrant pain, appendicitis with right lower quandrant pain
Previous history of abdominal surgery	Increases the risk of bowel obstruction secondary to adhesions
Specific peritoneal signs (rebound tenderness, abnormal gait, difficulty with movement)	Indicate peritoneal irritation secondary to an inflammatory or traumatic abdominal event, for example, acute appendicitis
Any history or evidence of trauma (motor vehicle accident, abdominal bruising)	Requires careful evaluation, signs and symptoms of specific injuries may be delayed in appearance; non-abdominal injuries and nonaccidental causes need to be considered
More than two visits to a health care facility for the same episode of abdominal pain	A significant proportion of children with appendicitis or intussusception are diagnosed on second and subsequent emergency department visits; a complete clinical re-assessment is required each time
Inability to do an adequate examination (noncooperative child)	A resistant child may be experiencing severe abdominal discomfort and/or peritoneal irritation; clinical assessment is vital to the evaluation
Systemic features of shock (poor perfusion, pallor, cool extremities, tachycardia, lethargy)	Young infants with incarcerated hernias or intussusception may present in this manner; once resuscitation has been initiated, the underlying cause requires identification

of all individuals with IBD are younger than 20 years of age.[44,45] There are many other serious, but rarer, causes of recurrent abdominal pain; the red flags indicating such serious conditions are listed in Table 11–3.[36–38] Children with one or more red flag features deserve diagnostic investigations beyond the careful clinical examination. Here, the diagnosis and management of the two most common causes of chronic abdominal pain, RAP and chronic constipation, are discussed in more detail.

Recurrent abdominal pain has been defined as paroxysmal, periumbilical abdominal discomfort, occurring at least three times, over a period of 3 months, in a child between the ages of 4 and 16 years. The pain is characteristically severe enough to interfere with daily activities.[39] Children with RAP are otherwise healthy and demonstrate normal growth and development. Because an underlying pathology is not evident in most children with RAP, this pain has been described as being "functional" in nature.[38] The pain is often vague in description; a minority of children may provide a highly detailed account of the discomfort.[36] Autonomic symptoms such as pallor, nausea, vomiting, tachycardia, and perspiration occur in many children.[36,38,39] Apley and Naish reported the following frequencies of associated symptoms: pallor (38 percent), vomiting (22 percent), headache (23 percent), and subsequent sleepiness or lethargy (26 percent).[39] There are no specific inciting or relieving factors for the pain of RAP. Typically, pain episodes last 1 to 3 hours and do not wake the child from sleep.[36–39] Continuous pain has been described in less than 10 percent of patients.[38] By definition, the pain is periumbilical and does not radiate in location. Between exacerbations, the child is completely well.

In the past, clinicians believed that in children with RAP, underlying psychological dysfunction was the primary etiology of the condition. Although a clear stress factor can be identified in many children , the pain is considered a real entity and not simply a tool for primary or secondary gain. Currently, it is felt that children with RAP are a heterogeneic group with disordered gastrointestinal motility and/or abdominal visceral hypersensitivity.[38]

Stress factors for children may be subtle and unrecognized by the parents. Commonly, these include school tensions (learning difficulties, school bullies, peer problems, student-teacher conflicts), changes in the environment (new sibling, new school, new neighbourhood), and family problems (parental marital difficulties, health problems in another family member, parental unemployment, changes in family structure). A detailed social history is an important component in the evaluation of the child with RAP.

Importantly, the child with RAP has no associated red flag features (see Table 11–3). Specifically, there is no history of weight loss, diarrhea, fever, or growth arrest.[36–39] The child's physical examination, including a rectal examination and test for occult blood, is also normal. Given the high prevalence of RAP in school-aged children, the yield of laboratory tests or imaging studies in children with no red flag features is extremely low. Specifically, several case-series studies have shown that abdominal ultrasonography is of no diagnostic value.[46,47] Thus, the diagnosis of RAP is made on the basis of consistent historical findings and a normal physical examination.

Although children with RAP are physically healthy, the condition carries significant psychosocial morbidity. Survey studies (level III) have shown that 90 percent of children are absent from school regularly, with 28 percent of children missing more than 10 percent of school days.[38] Beyond these educational problems, children with RAP often have dysfunctional relationships with peers and family. In the 30 to 50 percent of children who have pain continuing into adolescence and adulthood, associated anxiety and depression or other psychiatric illness have been found (level III)[35] (level II).[48]

Therapy for children with RAP has centered on affirmation of good health and minimization of the sick role. This type of cognitive-behavioral family intervention has been tested against routine pediatric care in one controlled trial involving 44 children.[49] In this study, both groups improved significantly over time; children who received behavioral ther-

Table 11–3 Clinical Red Flags in Children with Recurrent Abdominal Pain

Red Flag*	Interpretation
Any abnormality of growth: weight loss, poor weight gain, height deceleration, short stature	Suggests an underlying organic pathology including, for example: inflammatory bowel disease (IBD), malabsorption
Evidence of anemia: pallor	Children with IBD commonly present with a microcytic, hypochromic anemia and elevated erythrocyte sedimentation rate
Occult or frankly bloody stools	50 to 60 percent of children with IBD present with this feature; consider infectious causes also
Extraintestinal symptoms: conjunctivitis, uveitis, fever, rash, arthralgias or arthritis, recurrent apthous ulcers (mouth sores)	Any one of these features consistent with IBD in children, may also indicate other systemic disease (connective tissue diseases, malignancy, chronic infections)
Perianal disease: anal fissure, perianal fistula, perirectal ulceration	Consistent with Crohn's disease, may also be found in ulcerative colitis and children with immunocompromising conditions
Organomegaly	Does not occur in children with RAP
Onset of pain before age 5 years	RAP is unusual in preschool-aged children, likewise a new onset of pain after 12 years is suspicious of an underlying disorder
Anorexia	Uncommon in children with RAP
Abdominal pain localized away from the umbilicus	Suggests a focal cause of pain and requires further investigation
Nocturnal pain that awakens the child from sleep	May indicate hyperacidity or ulcerative disease, also occurs in children with IBD
Frequent vomiting	Although nausea and occasional vomiting are common in children with RAP, regular or protracted vomiting may indicate obstructive disease
Changes in bowel function: diarrhea, incontinence	Suggestive of underlying organic pathology
Associated features of dysuria, urgency, urinary incontinence, past medical history of urinary tract infections	An underlying renal abnormality may be present
Significant family history of chronic illness	Familial tendency for IBD, and in many rare causes of chronic abdominal pain, for example: pancreatitis, sickle cell disease, lactose intolerance, porphyria

*The presence of any one red flag indicates that further evaluation and follow-up are required. If inflammatory bowel disease is suspected, initial investigations might include complete blood count (CBC) with ESR, serum protein and albumin, fresh stool samples for blood, leukocytes, and culture for bacteria and parasites. Endoscopy and mucosal biopsy are the diagnostic gold standards for both Crohn's disease and ulcerative colitis. Referral to a gastroenterologist is advised.

apy had less interference of their daily activities by pain. Not suprisingly, the researchers found that those children who developed active self-coping skills to manage the pain were most likely to do well in the long term.[49]

In the only other controlled trial for therapy of RAP, Feldman and colleagues found that children treated for 6 weeks with 10 g of fiber in specially made cookies had significantly fewer episodes of abdominal pain than the children who were randomized to receive placebo cookies.[50] This study was double blinded. As in adults with irritable bowel syndrome (IBS), supplementary fiber appears to help a proportion of children with RAP, including those without a clear history of constipation. The mechanism of this benefit remains unclear.

In summary, RAP is the most common cause of chronic abdominal pain in school-aged children. The diagnosis is based on a normal physical examination and a consistent history. These children have normal growth and development and none of the red flag features listed in Table 11–3. Investigations are unnecessary in this selected group but are indicated if any red flags are present. Therapy includes (1) identification and intervention for obvious stress factors, (2) reassurance of health, (3) pain management techniques (including prompt return to school), (4) a 6 to 8-week dietary trial of high fiber and (5) follow-up with the health-care provider.

Constipation, defined as infrequent or difficult evacuation of feces, is another common cause of recurrent abdominal pain in children.[51] Information from population prevalence data suggests that 95 percent of healthy children have at least one bowel movement every 1 to 2 days; these stools are normally soft and easy to pass.[52–55] More than 95 percent of constipated children have "idiopathic" or "primary" constipation, where no underlying pathology for the problem (ie, anatomic, neurologic, endocrine, metabolic, or pharmacologic) is found.[56] Inadequate dietary fiber, excessive colonic fluid absorption, and delayed gastrointestinal motility have all been proposed as contributors to the condition.[41] In many children, there is a strong family history of similar bowel problems.

The diagnosis of constipation is primarily based on clinical evaluation and includes historical features such as infrequent bowel movements associated with abdominal pain, painful defecation due to large or hard bowel movements, and overflow fecal soiling.[41,42,56] Children with idiopathic constipation are otherwise healthy and show no limitations in growth. Evidence of excessively retained stool may be determined by palpable abdominal stool or the finding of hard stool in the rectum on digital examination. A dilated rectum reflects the chronicity of the constipation. A rectal examination positive for these features is both highly sensitive and specific to the condition of constipation (level III).[57] Occasionally, an anal fissure may be present. The anal tone, deep tendon reflexes, and gait are all normal in children with idiopathic constipation.

Investigations play a minor role in the diagnosis of constipation in most children. Children with clear clinical features require no further testing. Although abdominal radiography has been advocated to measure constipation severity,[58–60] the correlation between radiographic findings and clinical features is poor.[57,61,62] Additionally, the presence of stool seen on the abdominal radiograph may be normal; thus a diagnosis of constipation made solely on radiologic findings is potentially misleading.[61]

Rarely, in children with atypical or difficult-to-treat constipation, further diagnostic testing may be warranted. Gut transit time measurements may be made with radiopaque markers and serial abdominal radiography.[41] Anal manometry studies may indicate dysfunctional rectal and anal muscular function.[41]

Therapy for idiopathic constipation includes dietary and behavioral modification and pharmacologic interventions. Dietary recommendations involve an increase in fluids and fiber. As with any dietary intervention, specific examples of suitable foods and quantities should be provided to children and their families. Behavioral modification strategies include regular toilet sitting times during the day and positive feedback techniques. Pharmacologic therapies can be broadly classified into oral and rectal agents. Oral treatments include lubricants (mineral oil), osmotic agents (lactulose), promotility agents (cisapride), laxatives, and cathartics (senna preparations). Rectal therapies include suppositories and enemas.

Although all therapies appear effective to some extent, no single therapy appears to be the best. As well, there are only a limited number of comparative studies available (levels I to II-1).[63–68] Oral medications have not been directly compared with rectally administered treatments in controlled trials. Enemas are used frequently,[42,56,69] even though they have long been considered by parents and gastroenterologists as excessively invasive therapy.[70–73] Enema use may produce electrolyte abnormalities; rarely, these result in death.[74]

Dietary interventions are usually the first line of therapy, and in many children, this treatment is sufficient for resolution of abdominal pain and constipation. High-fiber foods such as bran, whole grains, beans, lentils, fruits, and vegetables are recommended. Prune juice is high in fiber and becomes more palatable to children when mixed with fruit juice or made into popsicles. The effect of fiber supplementation has been examined in several case-series studies of children with severe constipation (level III)[42,56,75,76] and in one randomized controlled trial (level I).[68] Because fiber was an adjunctive treatment in almost all studies, it is difficult to clearly estimate the effectiveness of this form of therapy. Nonetheless, it remains a nutritional and safe form of therapy. As well, the benefits of fiber supplementation in constipated adults have been well established.[76,77] In healthy, nonconstipated children, the American Academy of Pediatrics recommends a daily fiber intake of 0.5 g/kg;[78] values for children with constipation have not been clearly established, though the margin of safety appears wide.

Behavioral modification strategies in children with chronic constipation include regular toilet sitting (10 minutes after each meal) and positive reinforcement of compliant behavior (use of star charts, parental praise, and rewards).[63,64,67] Educational programs for parents and children have routinely been incorporated into such programs. Three controlled trials have shown limited benefit in children treated with such behavioral therapy plus laxative therapy versus those treated with either therapy alone (levels I to II-1).[63,64,67] It is important to note that all studies examining behavioral modification therapy have focused on the group of children with severe constipation and encopresis. Encopresis is defined as the passage of fecal material in a socially unacceptable manner; in most children, this involves soiling of the underwear. The majority of children with encopresis have a longstanding history of chronic constipation.

There is no definitive pharmacologic therapy for constipation in children. In addition to the wide variety of medications available, the dosage of each medication also varies significantly; most clinicians titrate the dosage according to the clinical response of the child. Six controlled trials of various medications have been conducted in children with severe constipation, many of whom were also encopretic (levels I to II-1).[63–68] No single therapy appeared uniquely effective, but it is clear that further research in this area is indicated.

Mineral oil, a heavy, colorless oil, is an intestinal lubricant which historically has been the most commonly used medication for constipation in children. The oil is given in a dose of 1 to 5 mL/kg/day by mouth and is available in flavored or unflavored form. Because of a potential risk of pulmonary aspiration and chemical pneumonitis, this medication is generally not recommended in children with swallowing dysfunction or in those less than 1 year of age. It is otherwise an inert substance. Concern regarding the malabsorption of fat-soluble vitamins associated with this therapy has diminished as measured serum levels of these vitamins appear normal in American children treated with the oil for up to 4 months with up to 5.4 mL/kg/day.[79]

In summary, idiopathic constipation in a common cause for recurrent abdominal pain in children. The diagnosis is confirmed clinically; a dilated or impacted rectal ampulla is highly specific to the diagnosis. Children with idiopathic constipation are otherwise physically healthy and appropriately developed. Specific dietary interventions are a reasonable first-line therapy in the primary care setting. Behavioral modification strategies and pharmacologic interventions are indicated as the severity of the condition increases. Although no single medication appears superior to others, the pediatric experience with mineral oil is most extensive. As with all chronic conditions, education, reassurance, and follow-up are important components of the care provided to the child with constipation.

Table 11–4 Summary of Interventions for Specific Conditions Causing Abdominal Pain

Condition	Intervention	Quality of Evidence	Recommendation
Reducible inguinal hernia	Therapeutic: referral to surgeon, promptly but not urgently	III	A-B
Incarcerated inguinal hernia	Therapeutic: emergency referral to surgeon	III	A*
Intussusception, with clinical suspicion	Diagnostic and therapeutic: air-contrast enema	I, II, III	A
Intussusception, with clinical uncertainty	Diagnostic: ultrasound examination by a trained and experienced operator	III	B
Appendicitis, with clinical suspicion	Diagnostic and therapeutic: appendectomy	III	A*
Appendicitis, with clinical uncertainty	Diagnostic: serial clinical examination	II-2, III	A
	Diagnostic: plain abdominal radiography	III	D
	Diagnostic: laboratory investigations (see text for specific tests)	III	C
	Diagnostic: ultrasound examination by a trained and experienced operator	III	B
Recurrent abdominal pain	Diagnostic: ultrasound examination in children with no "red flag" features	III	D
	Therapeutic: cognitive-behavioral family intervention	II-1	A
	Therapeutic: high-fiber diet	I	A
Idiopathic constipation	Diagnostic: plain abdominal radiography	III	D
	Therapeutic: high-fiber diet	I, III	A

*Given the potential risks and benefits to the child, the intervention is strongly recommended, even in the absence of higher-grade evidence.

Summary

Abdominal pain is a common pediatric problem, whether the discomfort is acute or chronic. In the vast majority of children, these pains are self-limited and require little in the way of investigation beyond a careful clinical assessment. Specific attention to red flag features will help to identify those children who require more extensive diagnostic evaluations. Evidence-based interventions for specific conditions are summarized in Table 11–4. For all children with abdominal pain, re-evaluation and follow-up are key components in the overall management of the condition.

References

1. Boyle JT. Abdominal pain. In: Walker WA, Durie PR, Hamilton JR, editors. Pediatric gastrointestinal disease, Vol 1, 2nd ed. St. Louis: Mosby; 1996. p. 205–26.

2. Irish MS, Pearl RH, Caty MG, Glick PL. The approach to common abdominal diagnoses in infants and children. Pediatr Clin N Am 1998;45(4):729–72.

3. Britt H, Bridges-Webb C, Sayer GP, et al. The diagnostic difficulties of abdominal pain. Austral Fam Phys 1994;23:375–7.

4. Scholer SJ, Pituch K, Orr DP, Dittus RS. Clinical outcomes of children with acute abdominal pain. Pediatrics 1996;98(4):680–5.

5. Grosfeld JL. Hernias in children. In: Spitz L, Coran AG, editors. Rob and Smith's Pediatric surgery. 5th ed. London: Chapman and Hall Medical; 1995. p. 222–38.

6. Lloyd DA, Rintala RJ. Inguinal hernia and hydrocele. In: O'Neill JA, Rowe MI, Grosfeld JL, editors. Pediatric surgery, Vol 2, 5th ed. St. Louis: Mosby; 1998. p. 1071–86.

7. Kapur P, Caty MG, Glick PL. Pediatric hernias and hydroceles. Pediatr Clin N Am 1998;45(4):773–89.

8. Scherer LR, Grosfeld JL. Inguinal hernia and umbilical anomalies. Pediatr Clin N Am 1993;40(6):1121–6.

9. Rescorla FJ, Grosfeld JL. Inguinal hernia repair in the perinatal period and early infancy: clinical considerations. J Pediatr Surg 1984;19:832–7.

10. Rowe MI, Clatworthy HW. Incarcerated and strangulated hernias in children. Arch Surg 1970;101:136–9.

11. Stevenson RJ, Ziegler MM. Abdominal pain unrelated to trauma. Pediatr Rev 1993;14(8):302–11.

12. Mason JD. The evaluation of acute abdominal pain in children. Emerg Med Clin N Am 1996;14(3):629–43.

13. Ong NT, Beasley DW. The leadpoint in intussusception. J Pediatr Surg 1990;25:640–3.

14. Choong DK, Beasley SW. Intra-abdominal manifestations of Henoch-Schönlein purpura. J Paediatr Child Health 1998;34(5):405–9.

15. Harrington L, Connolly B, Hu X, et al. Ultrasonographic and clinical predictors of intussusception. J Pediatr 1998;132(5):836–9.

16. Streiner DL, Norman GR. PDQ Epidemiology. 2nd ed. St. Louis: Mosby-Year Book Inc.; 1996.

17. Meyer JS, Dangman BC, Buonomo C, Berlin JA. Air and liquid contrast agents in the management of intussusception: a controlled, randomized trial. Radiology 1993;188(2):507–11.

18. Palder SB, Ein SH, Stringer DA, Alton D. Intussusception: barium or air? J Pediatr Surg 1991;26(3):271–5.

19. Ein SH, Palder SB, Alton DJ, Daneman A. Intussusception: toward less surgery? J Pediatr Surg 1994;29(3):433–5.

20. Lee JM, Kim H, Byun JY, et al. Intussusception: characteristic radiolucencies on the abdominal radiograph. Pediatric Radiology 1994;24(4):293–5.

21. Smith DS, Bonandio WA, Losek JD, et al. The role of abdominal x-rays in the diagnosis and management of intussusception. Pediatr Emerg Care 1992;8(6):325–7.

22. Wagner JM, McKinney WP, Carpenter JL. Does this patient have appendicitis? JAMA 1996;276(19):1589–94.

23. Reynolds SL. Missed appendicitis in a pediatric emergency department. Pediatr Emerg Care 1993;9(1):1–3.

24. Paajanen H, Somppi E. Early childhood appendicitis is still a difficult diagnosis. Acta Paediatr 1996;85:459–62.

25. Dueholm S, Bagi P, Bud M. Laboratory aid in the diagnosis of acute appendicitis. A blinded, prospective trial concerning diagnostic value of leukocyte count, neutrophil differential count and C-reactive protein. Dis Colon Rectum 1989;32(10):855–9.

26. Rothrock SG, Green SM, Hummel CB. Plain abdominal radiography in the detection of major disease in children: a prospective analysis. Ann Emerg Med 1992;21(12):1423–9.

27. Campbell JPM, Gunn AA. Plain abdominal radiographs and acute abdominal pain. Br J Surg 1988;75:554–6.

28. Sivit CJ. Diagnosis of acute appendicitis in children: spectrum of sonographic findings. AJR Am J Radiol 1993;161:147–52.

29. Hoffmann J, Rasmussen OO. Aids in the diagnosis of acute appendicitis. Br J Surg 1989;76:774–9.

30. Schwerk WB, Wichtrup B, Ruschoff J, et al. Acute and perforated appendicitis: current experience with ultrasound-aided diagnosis. World J Surg 1990;14:271–6.

31. Vignault F, Filiatrault D, Brandt ML, et al. Acute appendicitis in children: evaluation with US. Radiology 1990;176(2):501–4.

32. Rioux M. Sonographic detection of the normal and abnormal appendix. AJR Am J Radiol 1992;158:773–8.

33. Wilcox RT, Traverso LW. Have the evaluation and treatment of acute appendicitis changed with new technology? Surg Clin N Am 1997;77(6):1355–68.

34. Davenport M. Acute abdominal pain in children. Br Med J 1996;312:498–501.

35. Hyams JS, Burke G, Davis PM, et al. Abdominal pain and irritable bowel syndrome in adolescents: a community-based study. J Pediatr 1996;129(2):220–6.

36. Oberlander TF, Rappaport LA. Recurrent abdominal pain during childhood. Pediatr Rev 1993;14(8):313–9.

37. Pearl RH, Irish MS, Caty MG, Glick PL. The approach to common abdominal diagnoses in infants and children. Pediatr Clin N Am 1998;45(6):1287–326.

38. Boyle JT. Recurrent abdominal pain: an update. Pediatr Rev 1997;18(9):310–21.

39. Apley J, Naish N. Recurrent abdominal pains: a field study of 1,000 school children. Arch Dis Child 1958;33:165–70.

40. Feldman W, Rosser W, McGrath P. Recurrent abdominal pain in children. Can Fam Physician 1988;34:629–30.

41. Rosenberg AJ. Constipation and encopresis. In: Wyllie R, Hyams JS, editors. Pediatric gastrointestinal disease: pathophysiology, diagnosis, management. Philadelphia: W.B. Saunders Company; 1993. p. 198–208.

42. Loening-Baucke V. Constipation in early childhood: patient characteristics, treatment and long-term follow-up. Gut 1993;34:1400–4.

43. Abrahamian FP, Lloyd-Still JD. Chronic constipation in childhood: a longitudinal study of 186 patients. J Pediatr Gastroenterol Nutr 1984;3(3):460–7.

44. Israel EJ. Inflammatory bowel disease. In: Dershewitz RA, editor. Ambulatory pediatric care, Vol 1, 2nd ed. Philadelphia: J.B. Lippincott Company; 1993. p. 415–8.

45. Winesett M. Inflammatory bowel disease in children and adolescents. Pediatr Ann 1997;26(4):227–34.

46. Shanon A, Martin DJ, Feldman W. Ultrasonographic studies in the management of recurrent abdominal pain. Pediatrics 1990;86(1):35–8.

47. Wewer V, Strandberg C, Paerregaard A, Krasilnikoff PA. Abdominal ultrasonography in the diagnostic work-up in children with recurrent abdominal pain. Eur J Pediatr 1997;156:787–8.

48. Hotopf M, Carr S, Mayou R, et al. Why do children have chronic abdominal pain, and what happens to them when they grow up? Population based cohort study. Br Med J 1998;316:1196–200.

49. Sanders MR, Shepherd RW, Cleghorn G, Woodford H. The treatment of recurrent abdominal pain in children: a controlled comparison of cognitive-behavioral family intervention and standard pediatric care. J Consulting Clin Psychol 1994;62(2):306–14.

50. Feldman W, McGrath P, Hodgson C, et al. The use of dietary fiber in the management of simple, childhood, idiopathic, recurrent, abdominal pain. Am J Dis Childhood 1985;139:1216–8.

51. Anderson DM. Dorland's illustrated medical dictionary. 28th ed. Philadelphia: W.B. Saunders Company; 1994.

52. Lemoh JN, Brooke OG. Frequency and weight of normal stools in infancy. Arch Dis Child 1979;54:719–20.

53. Weaver LT, Streiner H. The bowel habits of young children. Arch Dis Child 1984;59:649–52.

54. Colon AR, Jacob LJ. Defecation patterns in American infants and children. Clin Pediatr 1977;16(10):999–1000.

55. Fontana M, Bianchi C, Cataldo F, et al. Bowel frequency in healthy children. Acta Pediatr Scand 1989;78:682–4.

56. Loening-Baucke V. Chronic constipation in children. Gastroenterology 1993;105(5):1557–64.

57. Rockney RM, McQuade WH, Days AL. The plain abdominal roentgenogram in the management of encopresis. Arch Pediatr Adolesc Med 1995;149:623–7.

58. Blethyn AJ, Jones KV, Newcombe R, et al. Radiological assessment of constipation. Arch Dis Child 1995;73:532–3.

59. Barr RG, Levine MD, Wilkinson RH, Mulvihill D. Chronic and occult stool retention. Clin Pediatr 1979;18(11):675–86.

60. Starrveld JS, Pols MA, Van Wijk HJ, et al. The plain abdominal radiograph in the assessment of constipation. Z Gastroenterology 1990;28:335–8.

61. Bewley A, Clancy MJ, Hall JRW. The erroneous use by an accident and emergency department of plain abdominal radiographs in the diagnosis of constipation. Arch Emerg Med 1989;6:257–8.

62. Benninga MA, Buller HA, Staalman CR, et al. Defecation disorders in children, colonic transit time versus the Barr-score. Eur J Pediatr 1995;154:277–84.

63. Berg I, Forsythe I, Holt P, Watts J. A controlled trial of `senekot' in fecal soiling treated by behavioural methods. J Child Psychiatry Psychol 1983;24(4):543–9.

64. Halpern WI. The treatment of encopretic children. Am Acad Child Psychol 1977;16:478–99.

65. Perkin JM. Constipation in childhood: a controlled comparison between lactulose and standardized senna. Curr Med Res Opin 1977;4(8):540–3.

66. Staiano A, Cucchiara S, Andreotti MR, et al. Effect of cisapride on chronic idiopathic constipation in children. Digest Dis Sci 1991;36(6):733–6.

67. Nolan F, Debrelle G, Oberklaid F, Coffey C. Randomised trial of laxatives in treatment of childhood encopresis. Lancet 1991;338:523–7.

68. Sondheimer JM, Gervaise EP. Lubricant versus laxative in the treatment of chronic functional constipation in children: a comparative study. J Pediatr Gastroenterol Nutrition 1982;1(2):223–6.

69. Davidson M, Kugler MM, Bauer CH. Diagnosis and management of children with severe and protracted constipation and obstipation. J Pediatr 1963;62(2):261–75.

70. Gleghorn EE, Heyman MB, Rudolph CD. No-enema therapy for idiopathic constipation and encopresis. Clin Pediatr 1991;30(12):669–72.

71. Sprague-McRae JM, Lamb W, Homer D. Encopresis: a study of treatment alternatives and historical and behavioural characteristics. Nurse Practitioner 1993;18:52–3, 56–63.

72. Beach RC. Management of childhood constipation. Lancet 1996;348:766–7.

73. Fleischer DR. Encopresis, enemas and gold stars. Pediatrics 1978;61:155–6.

74. Martin RR, Lisehora GR, Braxton M. Fatal poisoning from sodium phosphate enema. JAMA 1987;257:2190–2.

75. Clayden GS, Lawson JON. Investigation and management of long-standing chronic constipation in childhood. Arch Dis Child 1976;51:918–23.

76. Snape WJ. The effect of methylcellulose on symptoms of constipation. Clin Thera 1989;11(5):572–9.

77. Muller-Lissner SA. Effect of wheat bran on weight of stool and gastrointestinal transit time: a meta-analysis. Br Med J 1988;296:615–7.

78. Dwyer JT. Dietary fibre for children: how much? Pediatrics 1995;96(Suppl 5):1019–22.

79. Clark JH, Russell GJ, Fitzgerald JF, Nagamori KE. Serum beta-carotene, retinol and alpha-tocopherol levels during mineral oil therapy for constipation. Am J Dis Child 1987;141:1210–2.

CHAPTER 12

Seizure Disorders

Peter Camfield, MD, FRCPC
Carol Camfield, MD, FRCPC

Seizures in children are common and have many causes. This chapter concentrates on spontaneous, unprovoked seizures that tend to recur, as well as febrile seizures. Seizures can be provoked by nearly any acute disturbance to the cerebral neocortex. Provoked seizures, irrespective of the cause, have a very low rate of recurrence, provided that the provoking factor can be treated or avoided. For example, only about 10 percent of people who have seizures provoked by a major head injury will later develop epilepsy.[1]

The decision that a child has had a seizure is almost always based on the history since most seizures are brief and have stopped by the time the child is seen by a physician. Only the history can exclude such disorders as syncope, breath-holding, or vertigo. Even experts interpreting the same history may have difficulty, on occasion, in agreeing on the nature of a child's "event"[2] (level II-2). In our opinion, if the history is unclear, it is less harmful to await a recurrent event than to falsely label a child as having an epileptic disorder.

There are different kinds of seizures, and if seizures are recurrent, there are different types of epilepsy. Seizures can be categorized into partial (or focal) and generalized types. Partial seizures begin in one part of the brain. They are subdivided into simple partial, if consciousness is retained, or complex partial, if consciousness is altered or lost. Generalized seizures arise diffusely all over the brain at once; they can be thought of as a "system failure" or "system overload." The main types of generalized seizures are generalized tonic-clonic, absence, and myoclonic seizures. If a seizure begins in one part of the brain and spreads to involve the entire brain, a partial seizure with secondary generalization is said to have occurred. The patient may have an "aura" followed by a generalized tonic-clonic seizure. The aura is really a simple partial seizure. Therefore, a child with a "grand mal" or generalized tonic-clonic seizure may have had a primarily generalized seizure or a partial seizure with secondary generalization.

When all of the details of a child's seizure disorder are combined with the electroencephalography (EEG), an epilepsy syndrome can usually be defined. The diagnosis of an epilepsy type may assist in understanding the cause and in defining the prognosis. Table 12–1 outlines the main epilepsy syndromes and serves to emphasize the variety of types of epilepsy.[3] The clinician is urged to consider seizures as the result of many different brain processes.

FEBRILE SEIZURES

About 3 to 4 percent of children will have one or more febrile convulsions, making this the most common convulsive event in humans.[4] The usual age range is 6 months to 5 years with a peak age at 18 to 22 months. To make the diagnosis, there must be documented fever and a clear history of a convulsion. It is important to note that syncope in small children may be precipitated by fever[5] (level III).

When a child presents with an ongoing febrile seizure, the first task is to stop the seizure. Intravenous diazepam or lorazepam appear to be roughly equivalent[6] (level I, recommendation A). Although rectal diazepam has not been subjected to a randomized controlled trial

Table 12–1 International classification of epilepsies and epileptic syndromes and related seizure disorders

I.   Localization-related (local, focal, partial) epilepsies and syndromes
    1.1   Idiopathic (with age-related onset)
        Benign childhood epilepsy with centro-temporal spikes
        Childhood epilepsy with occipital paroxysms
        Primary reading epilepsy
    1.2   Symptomatic
        Chronic progressive epilepsia partialis continua
        Syndromes characterized by seizures with specific modes of precipitation
        Temporal lobe epilepsies
        Frontal lobe epilepsies
        Parietal lobe epilepsies
        Occipital lobe epilepsies
    1.3   Cryptogenic

II. Generalized epilepsies and syndromes
    2.1   Idiopathic (with age-related onset)
        Benign neonatal familial convulsions
        Benign neonatal convulsions
        Benign myoclonic epilepsy in infancy
        Childhood absence epilepsy
        Juvenile myoclonic epilepsy
        Epilepsy with grand mal seizures (GTCS) on awakening
        Other generalized idiopathic epilepsies
        Epilepsies with seizures precipitated by specific modes of activation
    2.2   Cryptogenic or symptomatic
        West syndrome
        Lennox-Gastaut syndrome
        Epilepsy with myoclonic-astatic seizures
        Epilepsy with myoclonic seizures
    2.3   Symptomatic
        2.3.1   Non-specific etiology
            Early myoclonic encephalopathy
            Early infantile epileptic encephalopathy with suppression burst
            Other symptomatic generalized epilepsies
        2.3.2   Specific syndromes
            Epileptic seizures complicating other disease states

III. Epilepsies and syndromes undetermined whether focal or generalized
    3.1   With both generalized and focal seizures
        Neonatal seizures
        Severe myoclonic epilepsy of infancy
        Epilepsy with continuous spike waves during slow wave sleep
        Acquired epileptic epilepsies
        Other undetermined epilepsies
    3.2   Without unequivocal generalized or focal features

IV. Special syndromes
    4.1   Situation-related seizures
        Febrile convulsions
        Isolated seizures or isolated status-epilepticus
        Seizures occurring only with acute metabolic or toxic events

(RCT), the nature of status epilepticus and the prompt response to rectal diazepam convince us that it is effective to stop seizures at a dose of 0.5 mg/kg[7] (level III, recommendation B). Rectal lorazepam has been less studied but is apparently effective at 0.1 mg/kg[8] (level III). Once the seizure has stopped, it is very unlikely that it will start again (level III); therefore, we do not usually give further acute medications (recommendation D).

After the seizure has stopped, the physician must take the necessary steps to exclude meningitis. Almost all children with seizures and meningitis have important clinical features that allow them to be distinguished.[9,10] A child with a febrile seizure and who quickly returns to neurologic well-being does not have meningitis and need not be subjected to a lumbar puncture (LP) (recommendation D). Children less than 1 year of age or with suspicious neurologic or physical findings should have an LP done (recommendation A), although the yield is still only about 15 percent[11] (level II-2).

There is good evidence that complete blood count (CBC), electrolytes, and serum glucose provide insufficient yield to be worth measuring (level II-2[11–13] and level III,[14] recommendation D). There is some evidence that children with a first febrile seizure are more likely to have a recurrence within that illness if the serum sodium is lowered[15] (level II-2). This makes a case for checking electrolytes in children with a first febrile seizure, not to help with the acute management but rather to help with prediction of recurrence within that illness (recommendation B).

Neuroimaging studies (CT and MRI) and skull radiography have no value in children with febrile seizures, even complex febrile seizures[14] (level III, recommendation E). The EEG is also of no predictive value in this setting and is not recommended (level III,[14] level II-2,[16] recommendation E).

Families of patients get very upset by febrile seizures, and most parents indicate that they thought that their child was dying during the event[17,18] (level III). Since the child will recover unscathed, much of the acute management must be devoted to parental reassurance. There is no data to indicate the value of admitting the child to the hospital; however, if admission is contemplated, the rationale would be reassurance of parents or further investigation/treatment of the fever. The febrile seizure is no longer an issue. The value of an admission for parental reassurance has not been studied, but the expense of admission and lack of benefit to the child strongly suggest that admission is usually not of value (recommendation D).

Following the febrile seizure, there are two possible sequellae—recurrence of febrile seizures in 30 to 40 percent[19] and epilepsy in 2 to 4 percent.[20] Recurrent febrile seizures can be reasonably predicted by the following risk factors: age of seizure <14 months, low fever at the time of the seizure, a short duration of illness prior to the seizure, and family history of febrile seizures. A child with all four factors has about an 80 percent chance of recurrence, while a child with no risk factors has only about 10 to 15 percent of recurrence.[19,21]

Rigorous antipyretic use does not prevent recurrent febrile seizures. This might sound ridiculous, since fever is a necessary ingredient; however, the literature is very consistent[22–25] (level I, recommendation E).

The most rigorous studies of daily phenobarbital or valproic acid suggest that these medications can reduce recurrences[22,26,27] (level I); however, there is rarely a convincing reason to prescribe daily medication for febrile seizures (recommendation E). A meta-analysis of randomized trials of phenobarbital or valproate disputes their efficacy,[28] although the trials with the most rigorous methodology and compliance are at odds with this conclusion. Compliance is a major confounder. Daily phenobarbital has a high rate of severe behavioral reactions, and there is some evidence that the child's learning abilities may be affected.[26,27] Valproic acid has been associated with fatal hepatitis in small children, possibly at a rate of 1:500.[29] The importance of these side effects and the uncertainty of the efficacy of these medications mean that there is rarely a convincing reason to prescribe daily medication (recommendation D).

Diazepam can be used intermittently in children with febrile seizures. One approach is to use liquid injectable diazepam in a dose of 0.5 mg/kg up to 20 mg given rectally during an actual seizure[30,31] (levels II-2 and II-3). The medication can be drawn up in a small syringe, the needle removed, and the syringe inserted into the rectum, thus obviating the need for a rectal tube. The medication is quickly absorbed, and the seizure stops promptly. Parents using this approach need careful instruction, as an overdose can cause apnea. This approach will prevent prolonged febrile seizures but requires a well-organized family for the child. It may be of some use for those living in very remote areas (recommendation B).

The other approach is to use diazepam at the time of a fever to prevent recurrent febrile seizures. Since a febrile seizure is frequently the initial manifestation of the illness, clearly this approach will never be completely successful. Rectal liquid diazepam 0.5 mg/dose given every 12 hours during the illness is as effective as daily phenobarbital[30] (level I). Oral diazepam at a dose of 0.3 mg/kg every 8 hours during the illness is associated with a modest reduction in febrile seizure recurrence[31] (level I). However, it is necessary to treat 14 children to prevent 1 febrile seizure recurrence.[32] Twenty-five percent of children have side effects from 0.3 mg/kg oral diazepam. In Uhari's study, a lower dose of 0.2mg/kg was shown to be ineffective[23] (level I). We do not recommend this approach to treatment because the rate of seizure reduction is very low and the incidence of side effects very high (recommendation E).

It is fortunate that only 2 to 4 percent of children with a febrile seizure later develop epilepsy.[20] There is no evidence that the febrile seizures actually cause the subsequent epilepsy and likewise no evidence that prevention of febrile seizures prevents subsequent epilepsy.[33] Risk factors noted at the time of a first febrile seizure are associated with an increased risk of subsequent epilepsy. These factors include focal seizure, prolonged febrile seizure, ≥ 2 seizures within an illness, developmental abnormalities at the time of the febrile seizure, and family history of epilepsy. Each of these factors increases the risk of subsequent epilepsy to about 4 to 6 percent. Combinations of the factors increase the risk to about 10 to 15 percent. Thus even in the "high-risk" group, 85 percent of children will not develop epilepsy[20,21] (level II-2). This reassuring information should be kept in mind because as many as 40 percent of children with a first febrile seizure will have a risk factor for subsequent epilepsy[19,20] (level II-2).

AFEBRILE SEIZURES

This section is divided into two parts. The first deals with types of epilepsy that can present with a single seizure. When a child is seen after a first seizure, there are special issues concerning evaluation and treatment. The second part of this section deals with epilepsies that virtually always present with multiple seizures. The issues for evaluation of these are somewhat different, but treatment decisions are usually more straightforward.

Evaluation of a Child with a Single Seizure

Most children presenting with a single seizure have had a generalized tonic-clonic, partial with secondary generalization, or a dramatic complex partial seizure. Simple partial seizures and many complex partial seizures are initially not recognized by parents to be very significant.

Once the child has been stabilized, the clinician must decide if a seizure has occurred and if the seizure was provoked by factors such as CNS infection, head injury, electrolyte disturbance, and hypoglycemia. Usually, the history and physical examination will determine provoking factors, and treatment will flow directly from the diagnosis. A conundrum occurs when there are no clear provoking factors: how much acute investigation is needed?

Lumbar Puncture and Blood Tests

In the absence of fever, there is no clear value for a lumbar puncture[34] (level III). Aside from the detection of meningitis/encephalitis, the LP cannot provide any useful diagnostic information in this setting. If the child is completely well, the chance of CNS infection must be very remote, and therefore there is no need for an LP (recommendation D). Blood work, including electrolytes, calcium, glucose, and urea, rarely gives useful results; however, the literature on children studied with these routine tests is not very extensive[35–37]) (level III). In a well child, there does not seem to be much justification for routine blood work (recommendation D).

Neuroimaging Studies

Brain tumors in children virtually never present with a first unprovoked seizure. After a first unprovoked seizure, brain imaging studies, especially MRI, are abnormal in about 15 percent[38] (level III). Fortunately, most of these abnormalities do not require direct treatment. Their value is a fuller understanding of the cause of the seizure, but their significance in predicting recurrent seizures is unstudied. Conditions that might require immediate neurosurgical intervention, such as intracerebral hemorrhage from an arteriovenous malformation or acute hydrocephalus, are expected to manifest significant clinical findings. It is safe to conclude that a child with a first seizure who has recovered completely rarely benefits from an emergency imaging study (recommendation E). If an imaging study is to be carried out, it can be done electively. In addition, when the EEG (see below) shows evidence of an idiopathic epilepsy, there is no need for an imaging study. If the EEG is normal or shows a focal abnormality, an elective MRI is the best imaging study, although CT will detect most major abnormalities[39] (level II-2). If the child has not recovered from the seizure or there are new neurologic abnormalities on examination, clearly an urgent imaging study is required to exclude such disorders as intracranial hemorrhage, hydrocephalus, or other acute processes. A CT scan is adequate in this acute assessment.

Electroencephalography

Following a first unprovoked seizure, an EEG is always recommended (recommendation A). A single study in adults suggested that the sooner the EEG is performed, the higher the yield will be, with the greatest yield within 24 hours of the seizure[40] (level III). Nonetheless, an EEG should be regarded as an elective investigation. Its role is to help classify the seizure disorder and assist in the prediction of recurrence. The possible increased yield from very early EEG must be balanced with the fact that early EEG recordings may be contaminated by transient postictal slow-wave abnormalities. Such findings may require another later EEG to determine the significance of the slow waves. In most clinical settings, especially outside of normal working hours, emergency EEG is not available. Until there is more evidence for the optimal timing of the EEG, our preference is to delay it until the postictal changes are likely gone, perhaps in 48 hours (recommendation B).

The EEG can give clear evidence of an idiopathic epilepsy, that is, the etiology is genetic and no further work-up is needed. The two most important disorders to consider are benign focal epilepsy of childhood with centro-temporal spikes (benign rolandic epilepsy) and juvenile myoclonic epilepsy.

The presence of spike discharge on EEG after a first seizure increases the risk of recurrence from about 20 percent to about 70 percent[41] (level II-2).

Treatment after a first seizure

After a first unprovoked seizure, about 50 percent of children will never have another seizure[37] (level II-2). The diagnosis of epilepsy is reserved for those with two seizures because the recurrence risk after two seizures is about 80 percent[42,43] (level II-2). Factors that help predict further seizures are neurologic abnormality (or remote symptomatic etiology) and focal seizure and epileptic (spike) discharge on EEG. Remote symptomatic etiology means that the child has a longstanding brain abnormality that has now caused a seizure (for example, a brain malformation or previous severe head injury). With all of these factors, the recurrence risk is about 75 percent; with none, it is about 15 percent.[41,42]

There is little reason to offer antiepileptic medication after a first seizure in childhood (recommendation E). In population-based studies, the rate of recurrence is not altered by the prescription of medication, presumably because of compliance issues[42,44] (level II-2). In randomized trials, the rate of recurrence is decreased but not enough to be medically significant[45,46] (level I). For example, in the largest trial, the recurrence risk for those treated was still 25 percent, compared with 51 percent for the untreated over a 2-year period.[46] This means that treated patients continue to have a high rate of recurrence and must make the same adjustments to lifestyle as those not treated. Those not treated after a first seizure have the same rate of long-term remission as those treated after repeated seizures[47] (level I). Parents need to know that most recurrences happen within a few months of the first seizure and recurrence after 6 months is very uncommon.[42] No studies have addressed the value of restrictions in the child's daily activities; after a first seizure, we do not usually recommend any change[48] (level III, recommendation D).

Approach after Two or More Seizures

When a child presents with a possible first seizure, there is often a history of other more minor but convincing events. Partial seizures may be dismissed by the family as unimportant, until there is a secondarily generalized seizure. A history of less severe events means that the child has epilepsy. Alternatively, a true first seizure may be followed by a second. Once the diagnosis of epilepsy has been made, there are several important considerations that concern investigation and management. The first and most critical decision must be the definition of the child's epilepsy syndrome. The approach to a benign focal epilepsy may be much more relaxed than that to a symptomatic partial epilepsy. To come to a syndrome diagnosis, the history must be evaluated by an expert (recommendation B). The success of an expert in assigning a correct diagnosis of a syndrome has not been compared with the skills of other physicians; however, given that the current classification of epilepsy includes >100 syndromes, it would seem likely that an expert would be more accurate. The EEG and imaging studies must be interpreted in the context of the history.

The evaluation of a child who has had two or more seizures is essentially the same as after the first seizure. If the clinical history and examination, supplemented by the EEG, yield a diagnosis of idiopathic epilepsy, there is no need for brain imaging studies. This means that children with disorders such as benign Rolandic epilepsy or juvenile myoclonic epilepsy do not derive any additional benefit from a CT scan or MRI.

Once there have been two or more seizures, prescription of an antiepileptic drug (AED) may be considered. These medications do not "cure" epilepsy but do suppress seizures. The rate of long-term remission of the epilepsy is the same if treatment is delayed for up to at least 10 seizures[49] (level II-2). Many experts suggest starting medication after two seizures. It is acceptable to wait longer, provided there is no clear "down side" to the child, in terms of excessive supervision or exclusion from normal activities[49] (level II-2, recommendation B).

Initial Medication for Epilepsies that may present with a Single Seizure (once further seizures have occurred)

There is good evidence that carbamazepine and valproic acid are equally effective on the basis of the British "Epiteg" study, an open-label but randomized, multi-centered trial of newly treated children[50] (level I). Phenytoin, valproate, and carbamazepine were equivalent in another randomized trial; however, phenobarbital was inferior because of a much higher rate of unacceptable side effects[51] (level I). The only large, double-blind, comparative trial of antiepileptic drugs (AEDs) in childhood epilepsy is the Canadian Clobazam Trial[52] (level I). This study randomized children in double-blind fashion to clobazam, phenytoin, and carbamazepine. Each drug was equally efficacious as measured by the time retained on medication, although the data for carbamazepine and clobazam were most secure.

Studies in adults suggest that lamotrigine is roughly equivalent to carbamazepine[53] (level I) and vigabatrin is equivalent to carbamazepine[54] (level I).

The bottom line is that many medications are interchangeable at the beginning of treatment. On the basis of relative lack of side effects and ease of use, our personal preference is to use carbamazepine or clobazam first for children with partial epilepsies (partial seizures or partial with secondary generalization) (recommendation B). Although there are no randomized trials, there is a very wide consensus that valproate is best for juvenile myoclonic epilepsy and carbamazepine may exacerbate this disorder (level III, recommendation B).

Evaluation of Epilepsies that Always Present with Multiple Seizures

A variety of epilepsies always present with multiple seizures. The seizure types in these epilepsies include infantile spasms, generalized absence, akinetic (drop) seizures, and myoclonus. The most common epilepsy types are West's syndrome, typical childhood absence, and Lennox-Gastaut syndrome.

If the child is intellectually normal and has absence seizures from the history confirmed by EEG, then there is no need for further evaluation (level III, recommendation A). Absence epilepsy is dealt with separately below.

If the epilepsy with many seizures at presentation is of any other type, a careful search for etiology is needed. Nearly all of these epilepsies have an underlying etiology; they are considered "remote symptomatic," meaning that there is a pre-existing brain problem. Etiologies include diffuse brain injury from neonatal or postnatal hypoxia, developmental brain abnormalities such as neuronal migration problems, or neurocutaneous syndromes such as tuberous sclerosis. Evaluation must include a very careful history and physical examination. A brain imaging study and consultation with an expert are always indicated because the causes may be subtle, the treatment difficult, and there is a high rate of either long-term intractable epilepsy and/or mental handicap (level III, recommendation B).

Treatment depends on the epilepsy type. Perhaps the most complex is infantile spasm. This devastating disorder has its onset in the first year of life. The spasms usually appear in clusters, but the child becomes dull, withdrawn and less interested in life between the seizures. The EEG shows a special pattern called hypsarrhthymia with a chaotic continuous electrical disaster—the spasms are the tip of the iceberg for a very serious condition, and rapid treatment is indicated, even though the long-term mental outcome is nearly always unfavorable. There is evidence from a large open case series[55] (level III), a small randomized placebo-controlled trial[56] (level I), and a comparative trial that vigabatrin is often effective within 1 to 2 days[57] (level I). It is not as powerful as adrenal corticotrophic hormone (ACTH) treatment, where the response rate is >80 percent.[57] Because of the side effects of ACTH, most experts suggest initial treatment with vigabatrin. If it fails to stop the spasms after 48 to 72 hours, then ACTH can be started (recommendation B). The dose of ACTH and length of treatment varies; a low dose of 4 to 5 units/kg/day for a month seems to be as effective as higher doses for most patients.[58] Oral prednisone may also be effective[59] (level III); however, there have not been definitive randomized trials comparing prednisone with ACTH.[58]

For other epilepsies always presenting with repeated seizures, valproic acid is usually the first drug, even though there are no comparative drug trials. Open-label case series have consistently shown reasonable efficacy (level III, recommendation B). Ethosuximide is very effective for absence seizures but has no action against generalized tonic-clonic seizures (level III). A benzodiazepine such as clobazam or nitrazepam, is often started first.

GENERALIZED ABSENCE EPILEPSY

About 10 percent of children with epilepsy have absence seizures ("petit mal"). There are several different types of absence epilepsy but the most common is typical childhood absence epilepsy with onset between ages 3 to 10 years. The children have many seizures a day, and virtually all will have an actual seizure during EEG, which confirms the diagnosis. The ictal EEG pattern is typically generalized 3 Hz spike and wave. The cause of typical childhood absence epilepsy appears to be genetic, although the specific inheritance pattern remains unknown. Once EEG indicates this diagnosis, there is no value in further work-up. Specific medications may be effective for this disorder. Ethosuximide is equivalent to valproic acid for absence epilepsy, although valproate has additional efficacy against generalized tonic-clonic seizures[60] (level I). Also effective are clobazam[61] (level II-1) and lamotrigine[62] (level I, recommendation A). In our opinion, any of these medications may be used.

Routines in Clinical Practice for Antiepileptic Drug Therapy

When a medication is started, there is hope that the seizures will be completely suppressed without side effects. In clinical practice, these two issues need to be balanced. For nearly all AEDs, one can usually expect increased seizure control with an increased dose. Determination of serum levels of AEDs has been used to try to optimize treatment. There are no carefully designed trials to determine the optimal serum level of any AED. In Canada, and likely in all countries, it is possible to have the same level interpreted in one center as subtherapeutic and potentially toxic in another[63] (level III). For patients with controlled seizures, there is evidence that further assessment of serum levels interferes with management. The only randomized trial of this issue indicated that the use of serum levels actually increased side effects without improving seizure control[64] (level I). The "therapeutic range" for all AEDs should be used only as a rough guide for dosing. In general, the dose is correct if there are no seizures and no side effects (recommendation E).

Our current practice is to order very few serum levels. If there is an issue of compliance, it seems that direct questioning of the child and family more often gets useful information than checking blood levels[65] (level III). Since there is a lot of individual sensitivity to the behavioral and cognitive side effects of AEDs, asking about these side effects is likely of greater value than measuring serum levels (recommendation B).

Clinicians are appropriately concerned about severe catastrophic reactions to AEDs. These include liver failure, aplastic anemia, nephritis, and Stevens-Johnson reaction. These reactions are idiosyncratic and are not related to dose, although they tend to occur early in treatment (first few months). None of these reactions can be predicted in asymptomatic patients from screening blood and urine tests[67] (level II-2). There is an important consensus in Canada that screening tests are of no value and may interfere with treatment[68] (level III). We recommend that patients be warned of these reactions and asked to call the physician immediately if such a reaction is suspected. At that time the child can be investigated, as the clinical situation appears to warrant (recommendation E).

Duration of Treatment

Epilepsy in children is often outgrown. For only about 40 percent is it a life-long disorder[68,69] (level II-2). Once a child has had 1 to 2 seizure-free years, it is reasonable to consider stopping medication. Overall, such children have a 60 to 70 percent chance of remaining seizure-free. This percentage is about the same if the seizure-free interval has been 1, 2, 4, or 5 years[70] (level II-2). Therefore, in general, consideration of stopping medication is appropriate once a child has been seizure-free for 1 year[71] (level II-2, recommendation A).

The group of children with the best chance of remaining seizure-free off medication are those with normal intelligence, normal neurologic examination, generalized epilepsy, and age at onset <12 years. This group has a 80 to 90 percent chance of remaining free of further seizures, once off medication. Those with teenage onset of partial seizures in association with neurologic deficits have only a 10 to 15 percent chance of successfully stopping medication[69,70] These children may be candidates for longer treatment.

Recommendations for the treatment of seizure disorders are listed in Table 12–2.

Table 12–2 Recommendations

Condition	Intervention	Level of Evidence	Recommendation
Febrile Seizures			
On-going febrile seizure	Intravenous diazepam or lorazepam	1	A
On-going febrile seizure	Rectal diazepam or lorazepam	III	B
Febrile seizure stopped	Further medication	III	D
Febrile seizure at >1 year and child appears well	Lumbar puncture	III	D
Febrile seizure at <1 year or child of any age appears ill	Lumbar puncture	II-2	A
Febrile seizure work-up	Glucose, CBC, electrolytes	II-2, III	D
Febrile seizure work-up	Serum sodium	II-2	B
Febrile seizure work-up	Skull radiography, CT, or MRI	III	E
Febrile seizure work-up	EEG	III	E
Febrile seizure	Hospital admission	none	D
1. Febrile seizure drug treatment	Antipyretic treatment	I	E
2. Febrile seizure drug treatment	Reduction of recurrences with daily prophylactic AEDs	I	E
3. Febrile seizure drug treatment	Intermittent rectal diazepam during seizure	II-2, II-3	B
4. Febrile seizure drug treatment	Intermittent oral diazepam during febrile illness	I	E
First Afebrile Seizure			
First afebrile work-up	Lumbar puncture	III	D
First afebrile work-up	Glucose, calcium, electrolytes, urea	III	D
First afebrile work-up	Neuro imaging studies	III	E
First afebrile work-up	EEG elective	III	A
First afebrile work-up	EEG in 48 hours	Not studied	D
First afebrile work-up	Treatment	I	E
First afebrile work-up	Restrictions	Not studied	D
Recurrent Afebrile Seizures			
2 or more afebrile seizures	Referral to expert	Not studied	B
2 or more afebrile seizures	Wait to treat	II-2	B

(continued)

Table 12–2 Recommendations *(continued)*

Condition	Intervention	Level of Evidence	Recommendation
Partial epilepsies	Clobazam or carbamazepine	I	B
Juvenile myoclonic epilepsy	Valproate	III	B
Absence seizures, intellectually normal, typical EEG	Further evaluation (neuroimaging studies)	III	E
Multiple generalized afebrile seizures (West's or Lennox-Gastaut syndrome, myoclonic, etc)	Further evaluation needed: history, physical examination, neuroimaging	III	B
Infantile spasms	Vigabatrin 1st, ACTH 2nd	I, I	B
Multiple generalized afebrile seizures	Valproate	III	B
Absence seizures	Ethosuximide, valproate, clobazam, lamotrigine	I, II-1	A
Treated epilepsy	Routine screening AED levels	I	E
Treated epilepsy	Documentation of compliance by history	III	B
Treated epilepsy	Routine screening of blood/urine for severe side effects	II-2, III	E
Afebrile seizures, seizure-free >12 months	Discontinuation of AEDs	II-2	A

AED=antiepileptic drug; CBC=complete blood count; EEG=electroencephalography; CT=computed tomography; MRI=magnetic resonance imaging

REFERENCES

1. Young B, Rapp RP, Norton JA, et al. Failure of prophylactically administered phenytoin to prevent late post-traumatic seizures. J Neurosurg 1983;58:236–41.

2. Van Donselaar CA, Geerts AT, Meulstee J, et al. Reliability of the diagnosis of a first seizure. Neurology 1989;29:267–71.

3. Commission on classification and terminology of the International League Against Epilepsy. Proposal for revised classification of epilepsies and epileptic syndromes. Epilepsia 1989;30:389–99.

4. Nelson KB, Ellenberg JH. Predictors of epilepsy in children who have experienced febrile seizures. N Engl J Med 1976;295:1029–33.

5. Stevenson JBP. Fits and faints. Oxford: MacKeith Press; 1990.

6. Treiman DM, Myers PD, Walton NY, et al. A comparison of four treatments for generalized convulsive status. N Engl J Med 1998;339:792–8.

7. Knudsen FU. Rectal administration of diazepam in solution in the acute treatment of convulsions in infants and children. Arch Dis Child 1979;54:855–7.

8. Appelton R, Sweeney A, Choonara I, et al. Lorazepam vs diazepam in the acute treatment of epileptic seizures and status epilepticus. Dev Med Child Neurol 1995;37:682–8.

9. Offringa M. Seizures associated with fever: management controversies. Sem Pediatr Neurol 1993;1:90–101.

10. Joffe A, McCormich M, DeAngelis C. Which children with febrile seizure need lumbar puncture? Am J Dis Child 1983;137:1153–6.

11. Gerber MA, Berliner BC. The child with a "simple" febrile seizure. Appropriate diagnostic evaluation. Am J Dis Child 1981;135:431–3.

12. Heijbel J, Blom S, Bergfors PG. Simple febrile convulsions: a prospective incidence study and an evaluation of investigations initially needed. Neuropaediatrie 1980;11:45–56.

13. Rutter N, Smales ORC. Role of routine investigations in children presenting with their first febrile convulsion. Arch Dis Child 1977;52:188–91.

14. Provisional Committee on Quality Improvement, Subcommittee on Febrile Seizures. Practice parameter: the neurodiagnostic evaluation of the child with a first simple febrile seizure. Pediatr 1996;97:769–75.

15. Kiviranta T, Airaksinen EM. Low serum sodium levels are associated with subsequent febrile seizures. Acta Ped 1995;84:1372–4.

16. Frantzen E, Lennox-Buchthal M, Nygaard A, Stene J. Longitudinal EEG and clinical study of children with febrile convulsions. Electroencephalogr Clin Neurophysiol 1968;24:197–212.

17. Rutter N, Metcalfe DH. Febrile convulsions: what do parents do? Br Med J 1978;2:1345–6.

18. Balslev T. Parental reactions to a child's first febrile convulsion. Acta Paediatr Scand 1991;80:466–9.

19. Berg AT, Shinnar S, Hauser WA, et al. Predictors of recurrent febrile seizures: a prospective study of the circumstances surrounding the initial febrile seizure. N Engl J Med 1992;327:1122–7.

20. Nelson K, Ellenberg J. Prognosis in children with febrile seizures. Pediatrics 1978;61:720–7.

21. Annegers JF, Hauser WA, Shirts SB, Kurland LT. Factors prognostic of unprovoked seizures after febrile convulsions. N Engl J Med 1987;316:493–8.

22. Camfield PR, Camfield CS, Shapiro S, Cummings C. The first febrile seizure—antipyretic instruction plus either phenobarbital or placebo to prevent a recurrence. J Pediatr 1980;97:16–21.

23. Uhari M, Rantala H, Vainionpaa L, Kurttila R. Effect of acetaminophen and of low dose intermittent diazepam on prevention of recurrences of febrile seizures. J Pediatr 1995;126:991–5.

24. Van Stuijvenberg M, Derksen-Lubsen G, Steyerberg EW, et al. Randomized controlled trial of ibuprofen syrup administered during febrile illnesses to prevent febrile seizure recurrences. Pediatrics 1998;102:51e.

25. Schnaiderman D, Lahat E, Sheffer T, Aladjem M. Antipyretic effectiveness of acetaminophen in febrile seizures: ongoing prophylaxis versus sporadic usage. Eur J Pediatr 1993;152:747–9.

26. Farwell J, Lee YJ, Hirtz DG, et al. Phenobarbital for febrile seizures—effects on intelligence and on seizure recurrence. N Engl J Med 1990;322:364–9.

27. Mamelle N, Pleasse JC, Revol M, Gilly R. Prevention of recurrent febrile convulsions—a randomized therapeutic assay: sodium valproate, phenobarbital and placebo. Neuropediatrics 1984;15:37–42.

28. Newton RW. Randomized controlled trials of phenobarbitone and valproate in febrile convulsions. Arch Dis Child 1988;63:1189–92.

29. Dreifus FE, Santilli N, Langer DH, et al. Valproic acid hepatic fatalities: a retrospective review. Neurology 1987;37:379–85.

30. Knudsen FU, Vestermark S. Prophylactic diazepam or phenobarbitone in febrile convulsions: a prospective, controlled study. Arch Dis Child 1978;53:660–3.

31. Camfield CS, Camfield PR, Smith E, Dooley JM. Home use of rectal diazepam to prevent status epilepticus in children with convulsive disorders. J Child Neurol 1989;4:125–6.

32. Rosman NP, Colton T, Labazzo J, et al. A controlled trial of diazepam administered during febrile illnesses to prevent recurrence of febrile seizures. N Engl J Med 1993;329:79–84.

33. Camfield PR, Camfield CS, Gordon K, Dooley JM. Prevention of Recurrent febrile seizures [editorial]. J Pediatr 1995:129;991–2.

34. Report of the Quality Standards Subcommittee of the American Acadamy of Neurology. Practice parameters: lumbar puncture. Neurology 1993;43:625–7.

35. Eisner RF, Turnbull TL, Howes DS, Gold IW. Efficacy of a "standard" seizure workup in the emergency department. Ann Emerg Med 1986;15:69–75.

36. Turnbull TL, Vanden Hoek TL, Howes DS, Eisner RF. Utility of laboratory studies in the emergency department patient with a new-onset seizure. Ann Emerg Med 1990;19:373–7.

37. Smith RA, Martland T, Lowry MF. Children with seizures presenting to accident and emergency. J Accid Emerg Med 1996;13:54–8.

38. O'Dell C, Shinnar S, Mitnick R, et al. Neuroimaging abnormalities in children with a first afebrile seizure. Epilepsia 1998;38(Suppl 8):184.

39. Kuzneicky RI. Neuroimaging in pediatric epilepsy. Epilepsia 1996;37(Suppl 1):S10–21.

40. King MA, Newton MR, Jackson GD, et al. Epileptology of the first-seizure presentation: a clinical, electroencephalographic and magnetic resonance imaging study of 300 consecutive patients. Lancet 1998;352:1007–11.

41. Berg AT, Shinnar S. The risk of seizure recurrence following a first unprovoked seizure: a meta-analysis. Neurology 1991;41;965–72.

42. Camfield PR, Camfield CS, Dooley JM, et al. Epilepsy after a first unprovoked seizure in childhood. Neurology 1985;35:1657–60.

43. Hauser WA, Rich SS, Lee JR, et al. Risk of recurrent seizures after two unprovoked seizures. N Engl J Med 1998;338:429–34.

44. Hauser WA, Anderson VE, Loewneson RB, McRoberts SM. Seizure recurrence after a first unprovoked seizure. N Engl J Med 1982;307:522–8.

45. Camfield PR, Camfield CS, Dooley J, et al. A randomized study of carbamazepine versus no medication after a first unprovoked seizure childhood. Neurology 1989;39:851–2.

46. First Seizure Trial Group. Randomised clinical trial on the efficacy of antiepileptic drugs in reducing the risk of relapse after a first unprovoked tonic-clonic seizure. Neurology 1993;43:478–82.

47. Musicco M, Beghi E, Solari A, Viani F. Treatment of first tonic-clonic seizure does not improve the prognosis of epilepsy. First Seizure Trial Group. Neurology 1997;49:991–8.

48. Camfield CS, for the Commission of Pediatrics of the International League against Epilepsy. Restrictions for children with epilepsy. Epilepsia 1997;38:1054–7.

49. Camfield CS, Camfield PR, Gordon K, Dooley J. Does the number of seizures before treatment influence ease of control or remission of childhood epilepsy? Not if the number is 10 or less. Neurology 1996;46:41–4.

50. Verity CM, Hosking G, Easter DJ, on behalf of The Pediatric EPITEG Collaborative Group. A multicenter comparative trial of sodium valproate and carbamazepine in pediatric epilepsy. Dev Med Child Neurol 1995;37:97–108.

51. De Silva M, MacArdle B, McGowan M, et al. Randomized comparative monotherapy trial of phenobarbitone, phenytoin, carbamazepine, or sodium valproate for newly diagnosed childhood epilepsy. Lancet 1996;347:709–13.

52. Canadian Clobazam Co-operative Study Group. Clobazam in treatment of Refractory Epilepsy: the Canadian Experience. A retrospective study. Epilepsia 1991;32:407–16.

53. Brodie MJ, Richens A, Yuen AW. Double-blind comparison of lamotrigine and carbamazepine in newly diagnosed epilepsy. UK Lamotrigine/Carbamazepine Monotherapy Trial Group. Lancet 1995;345:476–9.

54. Kalviainen R, Aikia M, Saukkonen AM, et al. Vigabatrin vs carbamazepine in patients with newly diagnosed epilepsy. Arch Neurol 1995;52:989–96.

55. Aicardi J, Mumford JP, Duma C, Wood S. Vigabatrin as initial therapy for infantile spasms: a European retrospective study. Epilepsia 1996;37:638–42.

56. Appleton R. A double-blind study of vigabatrin for infantile spasms 1999 [In press]

57. Vigevano F, Cilio MR. Vigabatrin vs ACTH as first line treatment for infantile spasms: a randomized prospective study. Epilepsia 1997;38:1270–4.

58. Baram TZ, Mitchell WG, Tournay A, et al. High-dose corticotrophin (ACTH) versus prednisone for infantile spasms: a prospective, randomized, blinded study. Pediatrics 1996;97:375–9.

59. Schlumberger E, Dulac O. A simple, effective and well-tolerated treatment regime for West syndrome. Dev Med Child Neurol 1994;36:863–72.

60. Sato S, White BG, Penry JK, et al. Valproic acid vs ethosuximide in the treatment of absence seizures. Neurology 1982;32:157–63.

61. Canadian Clobazam Cooperative Study Group. Clobazam in treatment of refractory epilepsy: the Canadian experience. A retrospective study. Epilepsia 1991;32:407–16.

62. Frank LM, Enlow T, Holmes GL, et al. Lamictal monotherapy for typical absence seizures in children. Epilepsia 1999;40:973–9.

63. Dooley JM, Camfield PR, Camfield CS, et al. The use of antiepileptic drug (AED) levels in children: a survey of Canadian pediatric neurologists. Can J Neurol Sci 1993;20:217–21.

64. Woo E, Chan YM, Yu YL, et al. If a well-stabilized epileptic patient has a subtherapeutic drug level, should the dose be increased? A randomized prospective study. Epilepsia 1988;29:129–39.

65. Schoeman JF, Elyas AA, Brett EM, Lascelles PT. Correlation between plasma carbamazepine 10,11 epoxide concentrations and drug side effects in children with epilepsy. Dev Med Child Neurol 1984;26:756–64.

66. Camfield CS, Camfield PR, Smith E, Tibbles JAR. Asymptomatic children with epilepsy: little benefit from screening for anticonvulsant-induced liver, blood or renal damage. Neurology 1986;36:838–41.

67. Camfield PR, Camfield CS, Dooley J, et al. Routine screening of blood and urine for severe reactions to anticonvulsant drugs in asymptomatic patients is of doubtful value. Can Med Assoc J 1989;140:281–5.

68. Sillanpaa M. Remission of seizures and predictors of intractability in long-term follow-up. Epilepsia 1993;34:930–6.

69. Camfield CS, Camfield PR, Gordon K, et al. Outcome of childhood epilepsy: a population-based study with a simple predictive scoring system for those treated with medication. J Pediatr 1993;122:861–8.

70. Berg AT, Shinnar S. Relapse following discontinuation of anti-epileptic drugs: a meta-analysis. Neurology 1994;44:601–8.

71. Dooley JM, Gordon K, Camfield PR, et al. Discontinuation of anticonvulsant therapy in children free of seizures for 1 year. Neurology 1996;46:969–74.

CHAPTER 13

Headaches in Childhood

J.M. Dooley, MBBCh, FRCPC
K.E. Gordon, MD, MS, FRCPC

Headaches impose a significant burden upon society. They occur in almost 75 percent of children[1,2] and are associated with a total annual cost in the United States in excess of $17 billion.[3] Despite this prevalence, there have been insufficient randomized controlled trials to allow an evidence-based approach to many aspects of childhood headache management. Where such data are not available, the best available evidence is presented.

EPIDEMIOLOGY

Epidemiologic studies of childhood headache are frequently compromised by the selection bias inherent in clinic-based studies and by the tendency of questionnaires to depend on the memories of parents or patients for details.

In 1962, Bille published his landmark paper on headache.[1] This study, consisting of almost 9,000 Scandinavian children, showed that by 7 years of age, approximately 40 percent had experienced headaches and 75 percent by 15 years of age.[1]

Similar prevalence rates have been found in other studies. By 3 years of age, 3 to 8 percent of children will have experienced headache.[5] Headaches occur in 19.5 percent of children at 5 years of age and 37 to 51.5 percent of children at 7 years.[6] In a British prospective study, mothers reported headache during the previous month in 4 percent of their 3-year-old children.[5] The presence of headaches was closely associated with depression as well as marital problems and poor health in the mothers.[5]

The value of historical reports is limited. More recent data suggest an increase in the prevalence of headache in schoolchildren from 14.4 percent in 1974 to 51.5 percent in 1992.[2] The reason for this increase in prevalence is unclear.

When specific headache types are studied, similar trends are seen.

Acute Headache

Acute headaches are usually associated with acute illnesses, such as infection.[7] Few data are available on the incidence or prevalence of illness-related headache. Such headaches may persist for 3 to 4 weeks after the illness and are more common in those with a family history of migraine.[8]

Acute Recurrent Headache

Acute recurrent headaches comprise both migraine and tension-type headaches.

Migraine is slightly more common in boys aged 3 to 7 years, but thereafter, the trend is reversed.[1,9] Migraine prevalence may be increasing. Using the same nine-item questionnaire, migraine prevalence in 7-year-old school children increased from 1.9 percent in 1974[10] to 5.7 percent in 1992.[2] Similar increases were found in both boys and girls. Migraine, therefore, has a prevalence of 1.2 to 3.2 percent at 7 years of age and 4 to 11 percent between 7 and 15 years of age.[1,9,10] A recent meta-analysis has shown that gender accounts for 14 percent of the variance among studies and for approximately 30 percent of the variation when combined with age.[11] When three factors were combined (differences in case definition, age, and sex of the study populations), 70 percent of the variance among studies was explained.[11]

Tension-type headache is reported to be uncommon before 7 years of age.[12,13] This has been disputed by a Finnish population-based study of 6-year-old children, which found a 14.6 percent prevalence of headache that disturbed activity within the preceding 6 months.[14] Among these children, 25 percent were classified as having episodic tension-type headache and 15 percent as having tension-type headache not fulfilling all International Headache Society (IHS) criteria.[14] As in migraine, the prevalence of tension-type headache increases with age. Tension-type headaches, within the previous month, occurred in 27.3 percent of 8 to 9-year-old Finnish children.[15] Clinic-based case studies add more evidence for an increase in tension-type headaches during adolescence, particularly in females.[4,13,16,17].

Cluster headache is extremely rare in childhood, but the exact incidence is unknown. Among adults with cluster headache, childhood onset is reported by 2 percent and adolescent onset by 10 percent.[18]

Chronic Progressive Headache

Chronic progressive headache may be secondary to raised intracranial pressure. Causes of chronic progressive headache have not been well studied. Headache secondary to idiopathic intracranial hypertension (pseudotumor cerebri) is rare. We reported an incidence of this type of headache in childhood of 8.4 per 1,000,000.[19]

Chronic Nonprogressive Headaches

There is increasing evidence that some children experience chronic daily headache.[20] The incidence and prevalence of these headaches are unclear, using current diagnostic criteria.

Impact of Headache

There are inconclusive data regarding the use of health-care resources by children with headache. One study reported physician consultation by only 11.3 percent of 3- to 11-year-olds with migraine.[23] The reasons for not seeking a medical opinion were ignorance of diagnosis, assumption that little could be done to help, and a parental attempt to prevent the learning of illness behavior.[23] In contrast, another study found that 51.8 percent of children aged 11 to 13 years had consulted a doctor because of headache.[24] The children who had consulted a doctor were more likely to report associated nausea and were more likely to come from a densely populated area.[24] They were also more likely to have missed more days from school.[24] Those who visited a doctor wanted (1) the cause to be found, (2) to receive pain relief, and (3) to receive reassurance that they did not have a brain tumor.[25] In one population-based study, tension-type headache was thought to be as worrisome as migraine from the parent's perspective.[14] The impact of headache on school attendance varies among studies. In one study, headache accounted for only 1 percent of school days missed and for school absenteeism in only 3.7 percent of children.[26] In another study, 10 percent of children with migraine missed 1 day of school over a 2-week period, and nearly 1 percent missed 4 days.[27] The recently recognized entity of chronic daily headache has been associated with higher levels of impairment than migraine.[28]

Pathogenesis

As the cerebral cortex itself is insensitive, headache results from stimulation of nerve fibers surrounding the large cerebral vessels, pial vessels, venous sinuses and dura mater.[29] These chiefly unmyelinated nerve fibers arise from the ophthalmic division of the trigeminal ganglion and contain substance P and calcitonin gene-related peptide (CGRP), which are released following trigeminal ganglion stimulation.[30] In the posterior fossa, the nerve fibers arise from the upper cervical dorsal roots.[29]

Acute Headache

Headache is a frequent accompaniment of febrile illness in childhood. The pathogenesis of illness-related headache is believed to be through bacterial and viral toxins, which stimulate the release of endogenous pyrogens such as interleukin-1 and interferon. These pyrogens give rise to headache through the release of prostaglandins and vasoactive peptides.[31]

Acute Recurrent Headache

Migraine was previously considered a solely vascular disorder, involving dilatation of intracranial vessels. Although dilatation of these blood vessels results in pain,[32] the vascular theory did not explain all migraine phenomena, such as the spread of symptoms across vascular territories. The current "neurovascular" theory proposes that migraine is primarily neurogenic, with secondary vascular changes. This hypothesis originated with recognition that migraine can be produced in nonmigraine sufferers by stimulating certain areas within the brainstem.[33] Similarly, positron emission tomography (PET) scan studies have shown activation of brain stem regions during spontaneous migraine episodes.[34] Dysfunction of these migraine "generators" results in an alteration in sensory and vascular responses.[35]

Vasodilatation induces activation of the trigeminal sensory nerves, which release vasoactive peptides and induce further vasodilatation. Thus, a circular cascade is initiated.[36]

Individuals with a genetic propensity for migraine experience a headache when exposed to appropriate triggers. These triggers, such as stress or hormonal changes, stimulate the "migraine generator" within the brain stem. This leads to the stimulation of vasodilatation and extravasation through the walls of the intracranial blood vessels. This results in pain and also stimulates the release of factors that cause further vascular dilatation. A cycle is thus created, which results in an ongoing headache.

The pathogenesis of the aura in migraine is also unclear. The hypothesis, as initially described by Leao in 1944,[37] that a spreading wave of neuronal depolarization is followed by a wave of neuronal suppression across the surface of the brain is still the most widely accepted. Woods and colleagues have shown a similar bilateral hypoperfusion starting in the occipital lobes and spreading across the cortex during a migraine headache.[38] The aura may subsequently affect the trigeminal ganglia in the brain stem[39] and may thus influence the evolution of the headache.

Although currently these theories seem plausible, it is essential to acknowledge that the pathogenesis of migraine, as well as the pain experienced in many other types of headache, remains obscure. Conclusive evidence on this topic is currently beyond our reach.

Essentially no research has been carried out on the pathogenesis of episodic tension-type headaches in childhood.

CLASSIFICATION AND ETIOLOGY

Evaluation of the temporal profile of headache results in an easily applied clinical classification. Many children will experience more than one headache type, and it is important to analyze each type individually (Table 13–1).

Acute Headache

Acute headache usually has a recognizable etiology, such as infection, acute illness, or intoxication. In a review of 53,988 children who presented to an emergency department, 696 had a chief complaint of headache.[40] Among a random sample of 288 of these patients, the most common diagnoses were viral illness (39.2 percent), sinusitis (16 percent), migraine (15.6 percent), post-traumatic headache (6.6 percent), streptococcal pharyngitis (4.9 percent), and tension-type headache (4.5 percent). There were no cases of tumor or bacterial meningitis.[40]

Table 13–1 Clinical Classification of Pediatric Headaches

ACUTE	CHRONIC NONPROGRESSIVE
Inflammatory	**Chronic daily headache**
Meningitis	Chronic tension-type headache
Encephalitis	Transformed migraine
Dental	New persistent daily headache
Sinusitis	Hemicrania continua
	Comorbid headache
Toxins	
Carbon monoxide	**Others**
Alcohol	Ocular
	Post-traumatic
Others	Psychogenic
Ocular	
Post-traumatic	
Psychogenic	
Temporomandibular joint dysfunction	
Fever	
Seizure	
Hypertension	
Hypoxia	
ACUTE RECURRENT	CHRONIC PROGRESSIVE
Vascular	**Increased intracranial pressure**
Migraine	Tumor
	Cerebral edema
Tension-type	Hydrocephalus
	Pseudotumor cerebri
Others	Abscess
Ocular	Intracranial hemorrhage
Temporomandibular joint dysfunction	Post–lumbar puncture
Arteriovenous malformation	
	Others
	Hypertension

Acute Recurrent Headache

Acute recurrent headache comprises both migraine and tension-type headache. Without a definitive diagnostic test, the diagnosis of migraine depends on clinical criteria, which have not received universal acceptance.

Distinction between migraine and tension-type headache has presented a dilemma to physicians and researchers alike. Cluster-analysis studies of symptom complexes have failed to identify any reliable clusters that resemble currently proposed diagnostic criteria.[41,42] A "headache continuum," rather than a dichotomous approach to migraine and tension-type headache, has recently been suggested.[43]

In 1955, Vahlquist proposed the presence of aura, nausea, unilateral pain, and positive family history as criteria for migraine.[44] In 1988, the IHS proposed a new classification of headaches[45] (Table 13–2). These criteria largely dichotomize headaches into migraine or tension-type. Subsequently, there has been considerable dispute regarding the applicability of the IHS criteria to children.[46–48]

Table 13–2 Migraine Diagnostic Criteria

IHS Criteria[45]	*IHS-R (revised) Criteria[49]**
Pediatric Migraine without Aura	**Pediatric Migraine without Aura**
A. At least five attacks fulfilling B to D	A. At least five attacks fulfilling B to D
B. Headache attacks lasting 2 to 48 hours	B. Headache attack lasting 1 hour to 48 hours
C. Headache has at least two of the following: 1. Unilateral location 2. Pulsating quality 3. Moderate to severe intensity 4. Aggravation by routine physical activity	C. Headache has at least two of the following: 1. Unilateral location 2. Pulsating quality 3. Moderate to severe intensity 4. Aggravation by routine physical activity
D. During headache, at least one of the following: 1. Nausea and/or vomiting 2. Photophobia and phonophobia	D. During headache, at least 1 of the following: 1. Nausea and/or vomiting 2. Photophobia and/or phonophobia
Pediatric Migraine with Aura	**Pediatric Migraine with Aura**
(Idiopathic recurring disorder, headache usually lasts 2 to 48 hours in patients less than 15 years of age)	(Idiopathic recurring disorder, headache usually lasts 1 to 48 hours)
A. At least two attacks fulfilling B	A. At least two attacks fulfilling B
B. At least three of the following: 1. One or more fully reversible aura symptoms indicating focal cortical and/or brainstem dysfunction 2. At least one aura developing gradually over 4 minutes or two or more symptoms occurring in succession 3. No auras lasting more than 60 minutes 4. Headache follows aura with a free interval of less than 60 minutes	B. At least three of the following: 1. One or more fully reversible aura symptoms indicating focal cortical and/or brain stem dysfunction 2. At least one aura developing gradually over 4 minutes or two or more symptoms occurring in succession 3. No auras lasting more than 60 minutes 4. Headache follows aura with a free interval of less than 60 minutes

*for children under age 15
With permission from[45,49]

Pediatric migraine headaches are often of shorter duration than the 2-hour minimum required by the IHS criteria. Similarly, pediatric migraine is often bilateral, in contrast to unilateral adult migraine. Photophobia and phonophobia are more common in children than in adults, but the quality of the headache in children is often difficult to establish. In 1995, Winner and colleagues proposed revisions to the IHS criteria[49] (see Table 13–2). For migraine with aura, they suggested reducing the required duration of headaches from 2 to 48 hours to 1 to 48 hours. In a multicenter prospective study, these revised IHS criteria revealed a diagnostic rate of 93 percent compared with the 66 percent with the unrevised IHS criteria.[50]

The role of genetics in migraine is unclear. Although 72 to 89 percent of children with migraine have a positive family history, the relative contributions of genetics and other factors have not been established.[51] For children with tension-type headache, 47 percent have a positive family history.[14] In adults with chronic tension-type headache, first-degree relatives have a 3.2 relative risk of developing a similar headache.[52]

Chronic Progressive Headache

Children with headaches that are becoming more severe or are associated with other neurologic features are more likely to have a sinister etiology (Table 13–3).

Table 13–3 IHS Classification of Migraine[45]

1.1   Migraine without aura
1.2   Migraine with aura
    1.2.1   Migraine with typical aura
    1.2.2   Migraine with prolonged aura
    1.2.3   Familial hemiplegic migraine
    1.2.4   Basilar migraine
    1.2.5   Migraine aura without headache
    1.2.6   Migraine with acute onset headache
1.3   Ophthalmoplegic migraine
1.4   Retinal Migraine
1.5   Childhood periodic syndromes that are precursors to or associated with migraines
    1.5.1   Paroxysmal vertigo of childhood
    1.5.2   Alternating hemiplegia of childhood
1.6   Complications of migraine
    1.6.1   Status migrainosus
    1.6.2   Migrainous infarction
1.7   Migrainous disorder not fulfilling the above criteria

With permission from Headache Classification Committee of the International Headache Society. Classification and diagnostic criteria for headache disorders, cranial neuralgias and facial pain. Cephalgia 1988;8(Suppl 7):1–96.

Chronic Nonprogressive Headache

Chronic daily headache, with almost daily or persistent headaches, has recently been proposed as an alternative diagnostic category.[53] For children, five subtypes exist: (1) transformed migraine, (2) chronic tension-type headache, (3) new daily persistent headache, (4) hemicrania continua, and (5) "comorbid headache."[20]

- Patients with transformed migraine have met criteria for migraine in the past but have had daily headaches for more than 1 month, with increasing headache frequency and decreasing migraine symptoms.
- The criteria for chronic tension-type headache are outlined in Table 13–4.
- New daily persistent headache presents with constant headache for more than 2 weeks, without previous headaches.
- Hemicrania continua is typified by steady unilateral nonparoxysmal headache over the frontal region, which has a frequency in excess of 15 days monthly for more than 1 month. Indomethacin is usually effective in treating hemicrania continua.[54]
- Comorbid headache is concurrent daily tension-type headache with intermittent migraine headache.

A recent prospective clinic-based classification study of chronic daily headache showed that 40 percent had comorbid headache, 35 percent had new daily persistent headaches, 15 percent had transformed migraine, 5 percent had chronic tension-type headache, and 5 percent were unclassified.[20]

CLINICAL FEATURES AND DIAGNOSIS

The diagnosis of headache in childhood is almost always dependent on the clinical history. Where possible, the history should be taken directly from the child and from the child's caretaker. However, care must be taken, given the suggestibility of younger children. Children exposed to information about the prevalence of headache are more likely to complain of headache.[55] The value of a focused psychosocial history, particularly in adolescents, cannot be overemphasized. Academic, social, and family stressors should be explored, and, when appropriate, a history of depressive symptoms or previous physical or sexual abuse should

Table 13–4 IHS Classification of Tension-Type Headache[45]

2.1 Episodic Tension-Type Headache
  A At least 10 previous headache episodes fulfilling B to D
     Number of days with such headache <180/year (<15/month)
  B Headache lasting from 30 minutes to 7 days
  C At least two of the following:
     1. Pressing/tightening (nonpulsating) quality
     2. Mild or moderate intensity (may inhibit but does not prohibit daily activity)
     3. Bilateral location
     4. No aggravation by walking up stairs or similar routine physical activity
  D Both of the following:
     1. No nausea or vomiting (anorexia may occur)
     2. Photophobia and phonophobia are absent, or one but not the other is present

2.2 Chronic Tension-Type Headache
  A Average headache frequency >15 days/month, 180/year for 6 months fulfilling B to D
  B At least two of the following:
     1. Pressing/tightening quality
     2. Mild or moderate severity (may inhibit but does not prohibit daily activity)
  C Both of the following:
     1. No vomiting
     2. No more than one of the following: nausea, photophobia, or phonophobia

2.3 Headache of the Tension-Type Not Fulfilling the above Criteria
     Headache which is believed to be a form of tension-type headache but which does not quite
     meet the operational diagnostic criteria for any of the forms of tension-type headache

With permission from Headache Classification Committee of the International Headache Society. Classification and diagnostic criteria for headache disorders, cranial neuralgias and facial pain. Cephalgia 1988;8(Suppl 7):1–96.

be sought. Coping skills of the family and the child are important, as reactions by both the child and the caretakers can positively or negatively reinforce subsequent recurrences.

The neurologic examination is normal in the vast majority of cases. Abnormalities should be anticipated on the basis of the prior history. Emphasis should be placed on the funduscopic examination (papilledema), palpation of the sinuses (sinusitis), examination of the teeth and gums (dental abscess), and cranial auscultation (vascular malformation).

Acute Headache

Headache is a frequent accompaniment of febrile illness in childhood.[8] Infections with *Mycoplasma pneumoniae*[56] and *Salmonella*[57] may be associated with headache.

Headache due to meningitis is usually frontal or generalized, with radiation down the spine.[31] Other features, such as lethargy, meningismus, and fever, usually point to the seriousness of the condition. Encephalitis and Lyme disease may also present with headache.[58]

Sinusitis may account for 10 percent of chronic childhood headache.[59] When headache is due to sinusitis, resolution should occur with appropriate therapy.[59] In maxillary sinusitis, the pain may spread to the teeth and forehead.[31] Frontal sinusitis does not occur in young children but may present in adolescents, with pain above the eyes or forehead, radiating to the vertex.[31] Infection of the ethmoid sinuses results in retroorbital pain, while spenoid sinusitis is associated with occipital pain.

Significant head trauma is associated with headache in 29 percent of cases.[60]

Benign intracranial hypertension (pseudotumor cerebri) is characterized by the clinical triad of headache, papilledema, and visual disturbances. The cerebrospinal fluid (CSF) pressure is greater than 200 mm water, in the absence of demonstrable pathology. The headache is usually frontal, throbbing, and is aggravated by maneuvers that further elevate intracranial pressure. The patient may perceive a "swishing" sound in the ears.

Headache secondary to decreased CSF pressure occurs following leakage of CSF through dural tears, usually following lumbar puncture. The pain is aggravated when the patient assumes the upright position and is alleviated by the supine position. The pain may be frontal, occipital, or generalized and is often associated with nausea, dizziness, and vomiting.[61] The incidence of headache following the use of a 22-gauge needle was 5.6 percent compared with 9.3 percent after use of a 25-gauge needle.[62]

Acute Recurrent Headache

Migraine without aura accounts for 60 to 80 percent of all migraine.[47,63] Prodermal symptoms, such as hypoactivity, hyperactivity, irritability, food craving, or yawning, are reported by up to 75 percent of children with migraine.[64] Facial pallor is common before the onset of the headache. Most children, even those as young as 4 years of age, will describe their headache if given a series of choices. The quality is usually described as pounding, throbbing, or pulsating, but as many as 25 percent report sharp or pressing pain located "all over the head."[64] The headache is typically located over the frontal or temporal regions. In children, unilateral headache is less common, and even in adults, bilateral pain is reported by 30 to 40 percent of patients.[65]

The duration of migraine in children is less than 2 hours in 11 to 81 percent and less than 1 hour in 8 to 25 percent.[1,4,66,67] It very rarely occurs more than once or twice a week, and more than 8 to 10 headaches per month should suggest an alternative diagnosis.[68] Children with migraine are not more anxious or stressed than their friends,[69] but they are more likely to have headaches precipitated by fear, anxiety, or eating ice cream than are children with tension-type headaches.[14] The child will usually seek a quiet darkened room because of photophobia and phonophobia. Migraineurs complain more of abdominal and other pain along with their headache.[14] Nausea, vomiting, and abdominal discomfort may be the most disabling features. The severity of the headache is significant, however, and more than half will cry during an attack,[9] 69 percent record a maximum intensity on a five-faces scale, and 96 percent need bed rest.[70] Three quarters of children desire sleep during their headache.[71]

Migraine with aura is reported by 14 to 30 percent of children with migraine. Visual features are most common, the three most frequent manifestations being binocular visual impairment with scotoma (77 percent), distortion or hallucinations (16 percent), and monocular visual impairment or scotoma (7 percent).[72] The visual phenomena associated with migraine may be more complex, as in the "Alice-in Wonderland" phenomenon (described below). Visual aura may also occur in children with tension-type headache.[73] Complicated "migraine-like" episodes may occur following cranial irradiation and chemotherapy.[74]

Familial hemiplegic migraine (FHM) is characterized by (1) the features of migraine with aura, (2) hemiplegia, which may be prolonged, and (3) at least one first-degree relative with identical attacks.[45] This type of headache is due to an ion-channel abnormality and has been localized to chromosomes 19[75,76] and 1[77] in some families. In those without a family history, it is important to rule out other causes of acute hemiplegia, such as other vascular disorders and cardiac or mitochondrial disease.[78]

Basilar migraine, also called vertebrobasilar or Bickerstaff's migraine, accounts for 3 to 19 percent of all migraine.[63,79,80] This syndrome is characterized by brain stem symptoms such as vertigo, ataxia, or diplopia. It is prudent to consider alternative explanations such as posterior fossa tumors or dysgenetic lesions (eg, Arnold-Chiari malformation or Dandy-Walker deformity). More than 33 percent of patients have their first attack during the second decade, and in this group, the female:male ratio is 3:1.[81] The headache is usually occipital, and precipitants can be identified by as many as 70 percent.[81]

Ophthalmoplegic migraine is a challenging clinical phenomenon, which may be associated with minimal headache. It is characterized by ptosis, mydriasis, and ocular deviation. Older children may describe blurring of vision or diplopia, while younger patients may indicate their difficulties by rubbing their eyes.[82,83] The ophthalmic symptoms may occur after the headache is established.[82,83] The oculomotor nerve is most frequently involved, with pupil involvement in only 33 percent of cases, suggesting an ischemic rather than a compressive basis.[84] It has also been suggested that ophthalmoplegic migraine may be an inflammatory process, similar to the Tolosa-Hunt syndrome.[85]

Retinal (ocular or ophthalmic) migraine is characterized by sudden episodes of monocular visual loss that lasts seconds to minutes. The visual loss consists of either monocular black or gray "outs" or bright, blinding visual loss (photopsia), and the headache is usually retro-orbital and ipsilateral to the visual loss.[86]

The *Alice-in-Wonderland* and *"rushes"* phenomena are found in migraine patients but may occur independently of headache. They represent sensory misperceptions. In the Alice-in-Wonderland phenomenon, objects appear either enlarged (macropsia) or diminished in size (micropsia).[87] Children with the rushes phenomenon report a sensation that things are moving either faster or slower than reality.[88] In both situations, the patients are aware that their perceptions are false.

Confusional migraine is typified by episodes of agitation, restlessness, and combative disorientation.[89,90]

Episodic Tension-type Headache

The severity of tension-type headache is almost always described as mild or moderate,[4,14,66,91] which may be an important discriminator.[92] The headache is frequently bilateral and non-pulsatile or "pressing" in nature.[4,66] The duration tends to be shorter than that of migraine, and occasionally headaches can be brief (<30 minutes).[66] This headache is seldom aggravated by physical activities.[66,91] Nausea, phonophobia, and photophobia may be present in one-third of children with tension-type headache.[66] They often experience additional somatic complaints,[16] which are more frequent in association with social stress.[93]

Evidence for the link with tension is unclear. Among Finnish 8 to 9-year-olds, those with nonmigrainous headache were more likely to report bullying or stress at school or moderate to poor relationships with other children.[15] Children, aged 8 to 15 years, with more than one headache per month reported more stress and psychological symptomatology.[16] Headache diagnosis in this group was episodic tension-type (28 percent), chronic tension-type (30 percent), migraine coexisting with tension-type headache (29 percent), and migraine (13 percent).

Children with tension-type headache reported more anxiety than did children with migraine.[94] This anxiety was more related to issues of separation or death than to school problems, which seemed of more concern for the children with migraine.[94]

Depression has been associated with chronic daily headache in adolescents.[95] This depression has been associated with personal loss preceding the onset of headache by up to 12 months.[96]

Cluster Headaches

Cluster headaches may rarely occur in children and are typically described as a severe unilateral periorbital pain.[97] They are associated with lacrimation, rhinorrhea, and nasal stuffiness.

Indomethacin-Responsive Headache

There are four relatively common indomethacin-responsive headache syndromes. Three are described below. The fourth, hemicrania continua, is discussed above under chronic non-progressive headaches.

Exertional headaches may be precipitated by any form of exertion. They can occur during or after an activity and may be associated with nausea and vomiting.[98] The pain is described as being hit with a hammer and can be either generalized or localized. It can last from 15 minutes to 12 hours. Indomethacin is effective in up to 86 percent (level II).[99]

Cyclic migraine occurs several times per week in cycles, averaging every 6 weeks (range 2 to 20 weeks).[98] This headache also tends to respond to indomethacin (level III).

Chronic paroxysmal hemicrania is characterized by multiple, daily attacks of unilateral severe headache, lasting 5 to 30 minutes.[98] The syndrome is more common in females but is uncommon in children.[100] This headache is exquisitely responsive to indomethacin within 2 days of initiating therapy (level III).[98]

Ice Cream Headache

This headache is brief (less than 5 minutes), with frontal pain that occurs with the ingestion of cold food or drink. Ice cream headache occurs in 93 percent of migraine patients compared with 31 percent of controls.[101]

Ice-Pick Headache

This is a momentary stabbing pain in the distribution of the first division of the trigeminal nerve.[45] It is unusual in the pediatric population, but when it occurs, it is responsive to indomethacin.[98] The pain is so brief that prophylaxis is seldom necessary (level III).

Chronic Progressive Headache

Any process that increases intracranial pressure can cause headache, although lesions such as tumors, hydrocephalus, or Arnold-Chiari malformations are unusual causes of childhood headache.[103] Among children with headache secondary to tumors, characteristics that should raise concern include vomiting, early morning awakening by the headache, and increasing frequency or severity of the headache.[104] Among children with tumor-related headache, 94 percent have neurologic and/or ocular signs at the time of diagnosis.[104] These abnormal signs were present within 2 weeks of the onset of headache in 55 percent and within 4 months in 88 percent.[104]

Chronic Nonprogressive Headache

See discussion above on chronic daily headache. Temporomandibular joint (TMJ) dysfunction is an uncommon cause of headache in childhood. It is most likely in the presence of demonstrable joint abnormality. The pain is seldom severe and tends to be located around the joint with referral to the middle of the face and temporal or frontal regions of the head. Chewing usually aggravates TMJ-related pain. Most children with chronic nonprogressive headache have stress as the underlying precipitant. Analgesic-induced headache is well recognized in adults and may occur in children who are taking regular doses of simple analgesics such as acetaminophen or ibuprofen.[102]

INVESTIGATIONS

Headache diagnosis depends on pattern recognition of clinical syndromes. In young children, such clinical details may be difficult to obtain. Diaries are valuable in establishing headache characteristics, duration, and associated features.[105] Laboratory investigations, however, are seldom informative. Electroencephalography (EEG) is of minimal value in the study of children with headaches. In a retrospective study of the value of EEG in 257 children with headache, 12 percent had epileptic activity, and 8.6 percent had diffuse or focal slowing of background EEG activity.[106] Although those with migraine were more likely to have EEG findings, there was no correlation between EEG abnormalities and imaging studies or clinical course.[106] Changes in EEG, suggestive of benign epilepsy with centrotemporal

(Rolandic) spikes have been reported in 9 percent of children with migraine.[107] For these reasons, routine use of EEG is not recommended for children with headaches. Similarly, computed tomography (CT)[108,109] and magnetic resonance imaging (MRI)[110] scans are of minimal help in managing the average child with headache. Other laboratory investigations are also of little value. Abnormalities of visual-evoked potentials, which may be rectified with magnesium therapy, have been described but are not of clinical value at this stage.[111] It is currently prudent to restrict laboratory investigations to children whose headaches do not fit one of the recognized headache syndrome patterns or those who have evidence of neurologic dysfunction by history or on examination.

TREATMENT

The treatment of childhood headaches should be based on the severity of the headache and its associated disability. It is not necessary to treat all headaches. Once a decision to treat is made, the consequences of the child's pain and its relief must be evaluated in the context of rewards, secondary gain, and parental anxiety.[112] Furthermore, the study of any headache intervention in childhood must be interpreted in the context of a placebo response rate of up to 40 percent.[113] Although there are few well-designed studies of headache therapy in childhood, a recent meta-analysis of interventions in pediatric migraine has indicated some promising trends.[114] There is evidence to suggest that in children, nonpharmacologic interventions are equally effective to treat migraine or tension-type headache[115] (level I).

Headache treatment should be divided into abortive therapy and prophylactic management.

Abortive Therapy

Rest and basic analgesia are the cornerstones of headache therapy for most children (level III, recommendation B).[116] Psychological factors may play an important role in the patient's approach to abortive pharmacotherapy. A minor headache, which is thought of as a serious problem by the child and family, may lead to the perception of the child as being vulnerable.[117] Negative attitudes toward over-the-counter (OTC) medication may lead to the use of inadequate doses of medication when the headache is established.[117] The resultant subtherapeutic response further strengthens the belief that the medication is ineffective.[118] Parents and children should be encouraged to take adequate doses of medication early in the course of the headache episode, as early abortive therapy may be helpful and later therapy is often ineffective (level III, recommendation B).[117] Adolescents, particularly females, have been found to self-medicate with OTC analgesics, often without parental knowledge[118]

A recent study has shown *ibuprofen* to be more effective than *acetaminophen* in the acute treatment of migraine in childhood.[119] In this study, 88 children, aged 4 to 15.8 years, had three headaches treated in random order with single oral doses of 15 mg/kg acetaminophen, 10 mg/kg ibuprofen, and placebo. Ibuprofen was twice as likely as acetaminophen to abort migraine within 2 hours. Compared with the placebo, reduction in headache severity by at least 2 grades was reached twice as often with acetaminophen and three times as often with ibuprofen (level I, recommendation A).[119]

The use of *aspirin* is avoided in children because of a purported risk of Reye's syndrome, although there are no recent data available to support this ongoing belief (level III, recommendation D).

In adults, *caffeine* has been demonstrated to be a valuable adjuvant to acetaminophen or acetaminophen/aspirin in six randomized, double-blind, cross-over studies, involving more than 2,500 tension-type headache sufferers (level I, recommendation A).[120] Its role as an adjuvant for pediatric tension-type headache is unclear, and concerns about caffeine withdrawal may limit its use.

Medication should be discontinued in those with chronic daily headache who are analgesic users because of the possibility of analgesic withdrawal headaches after chronic use.[103,122]

Ergotamines

Ergotamines produce a powerful vasoconstrictive effect by a direct effect on the serotonin receptors and by α-adrenergic blockade. *Ergotamine* is frequently used in adults. One double-blind cross-over study of ergotamine and placebo tablets and inhalers was attempted.[47] This study of 111 children lasted 7 years, but statistical analysis was precluded by a dropout rate of 66 percent. Among the 38 children who completed all four treatments, none of the therapies seemed superior to the others (level II, recommendation D).[47]

Dihydroergotamine (DHE) is an ergot derivative with similar action to ergotamine tartrate but with fewer adverse effects. The adverse effects associated with DHE include nausea and vomiting (which can be anticipated in approximately 10 percent of patients), weakness, muscle pains, and tingling of the hands and feet. All ergot preparations should be avoided by patients with cardiovascular disease. Dihydroergotamine causes less peripheral vasoconstriction and less nausea than does ergotamine. When given with an antiemetic, DHE is effective in treating migraine associated with vomiting in adults.[122] Intravenous DHE, with metoclopramide, was helpful in children in an open-label retrospective review (level III, recommendation C).[123] When used in older children and adolescents, an initial IV or IM dose of 0.5 to 0.75 mg has been suggested.[124] Weight-based doses have not been established for children. If the headache persists, a second dose of 0.5 mg may be administered after an hour (level III, recommendation B).[125] A study of oral DHE in 12 children showed benefit, although 2 of 5 who became headache-free had a recurrence (level III, recommendation C).[125] There are no data available on the use of nasal DHE in children.

Lisuride is an ergot derivative, which acts on the serotonin and dopamine receptors at both peripheral and central level.[126] In an open trial, it appeared to have some effect in children with migraine (level III, recommendation C).[127]

New Serotonin (5-HT) Agonists

The introduction of newer prophylactic antimigraine therapy is based on the recognition of several subtypes of 5-HT (serotonin) receptors. These are currently subdivided into subtypes $5-HT_1$ through $5-HT_7$.

Activation of $5-HT_{1B}$ receptors results in selective constriction of excessively dilated intracranial vessels. Agonists with the $5-HT_{1B/1D}$ effect work on receptors on both the blood vessel walls and by preventing the release of substance P and CGRP from sensory nerves.[127,128]

In a double-blind, placebo-controlled, cross-over study, oral *sumatriptan* was not found to be better than placebo in treating migraine in children (level I, recommendation D).[129] Two open-label studies of subcutaneous sumatriptan did indicate benefit (level III, recommendation C).[130,131]

In an open-label study, *zolmitriptan* produced headache relief at 2 hours in 88 percent of adolescents aged 12 to 17 years following a dose of 2.5 mg and in 69 percent following a dose of 5 mg (level III, recommendation C). The half-life of zolmitriptan was significantly shorter in adolescents than in adults.[133]

There are no other evidence-based data to support specific therapy for acute headache treatment in children. Recommendations based on clinical experience, but without supporting data, are presented in Table 13–5.

Prophylactic Therapy

Nonpharmacologic Methods

Many children respond to simple nonpharmacologic approaches. The use of a headache diary to identify headache precipitants can have long-term value (level III, recommendation B).[134]

Table 13–5 Management of Childhood Headaches

Condition	Intervention	Quality of Evidence (level)	Recommendation
	Nonpharmacologic		
Migraine and	Reassurance	III	B
Tension-type headache	Precipitant identification and avoidance through headache diary	III	B
	Restriction diet	III	D
	Regulation of sleep	III	B
	Behavioral therapies	II	B
	Abortive		
	Ibuprofen 10 mg/kg/dose early in headache course	I	A
	Acetaminophen 15 mg/kg/dose	III	B
	Naproxen sodium 2.5 to 5 mg/kg/dose	III	B
	Ergotamines	II	D
	Dihydroergotamine (DHE) 0.5 to 1 mg IV or IM	III	C
	Sumatriptan 3 to 6 mg SC for adolescents	III	C
	Zolmitriptan	III	C
	Prophylactic		
	Flunarizine	I	A
	Cyproheptadine 0.25 to 1.5 mg/kg	III	C
	Propranolol 2-4 mg/kg	I	D
	Nimodipine	I	E
	Valproate	III	C
	Amitriptyline 0.1 mg/kg QHS, increase Q2 weeks to 0.5 to 2 mg/kg	III	C
	Methysergide	III	D
	Metoclopramide 0.1 mg/kg/dose, ≤10 mg	III	C
	Clonidine	I	E

In children under 6 years of age, the parents may have to assume the major responsibility for the diary. Children aged 7 to 10 years should be more accountable, and older patients should have exclusive responsibility for tracking precipitants. Common sources of stress include conflict with family or peers, excitement, physical stress, learning problems, and sleep difficulties (level III). Positive stress (excitement) may be as important as excessive or insufficient sleep and hunger. We have found that specific foods are seldom of significance, and the use of a food avoidance diet is seldom beneficial (level III, recommendation D).[134]

The use of psychotherapy and family therapy for children whose headaches are associated with family stress has not been scientifically studied.[117] Such therapy is expensive from psychological, financial, and time perspectives (level III, recommendation D).

Biofeedback and relaxation training have been shown to diminish the frequency of attacks in children more than in adults.[135,136] Relaxation and cognitive therapies help in the treatment of pediatric migraine[116,137–139] and tension-type headache,[140] although the studies did not use control groups who were given only attention (level II, recommendation B). In general, these techniques are most helpful in relatively mature children over the age of 9 years.[136] In a meta-analysis, progressive muscle relaxation, with or without thermal biofeedback, appeared more effective than pharmacologic interventions.[115]

Children can learn hypnosis,[141] which, along with temperature biofeedback, may be of value in treating childhood migraine.[142] In a study of 28 children aged 6 to 12 years, they were randomized to propranolol 3 mg/kd/d or placebo for 3 months and were then crossed over for a further 3 months.[143] Patients were then taught to, and did use, self-hypnosis for 3 months. The mean number of headaches was 13.3 for the placebo period, 14.9 for the propranolol period, and 5.8 during the self-hypnosis period[144] (level I, recommendation A). Behavioral therapies, which require feedback from procedures such as electromyography (EMG), are unattractive to most families (level III, recommendation D).

Pharmacotherapy

Cyproheptidine has been popular for treating pediatric headache (level III, recommendation C). This drug was originally thought to act on serotonin, but recent evidence suggests its primary mode of action as a calcium channel blocker.[144] There are no controlled studies of its use in childhood headache. One uncontrolled pilot study treated 19 children, aged 6 to 16 years, for 3 to 6 months.[145] Four had no further headaches, 13 improved, and 2 did not benefit. Weight gain and drowsiness were experienced by 8 patients each. The doses used were 0.25 mg/kg/d (maximum 2 to 16 mg/d) with ranges of 12 mg/d for 2 to 6-year-olds, 16 mg/d for 7 to 14-year-olds and 32 mg/d for older patients.[124] Side effects include sedation and appetite stimulation.

Beta-adrenergic receptor blockers   The mechanism of action of β-blockers in migraine is poorly understood. There appears to be no correlation between efficacy and β-receptor selectivity. Three controlled studies on the use of propranolol in pediatric headache have been published. One study of 28 children revealed a prophylactic effect at doses of approximately 3 mg/kg/d.[147] A further double-blind, cross-over, placebo-controlled study of 39 children failed to show any benefit from propranolol.[147] As noted above, propranolol was also ineffective in a study of propranolol, placebo, and self-hypnosis.[143] As the positive study was the oldest and had the fewest patients, propranolol cannot be recommended as valuable prophylaxis (level I, recommendation D). The use of β-blockers is contraindicated in those with asthma, congestive heart failure, and renal insufficiency, and in diabetic children who are being treated with insulin, as it may induce hypoglycemia.

Calcium channel antagonists.   Despite initial enthusiasm regarding the potential value of these agents in treating migraine, they have become less popular in the treatment of adult headaches. In children, two double-blind, placebo-controlled, cross-over studies indicated that *flunarizine* was effective in reducing the frequency and duration of childhood migraine (level I, recommendation A).[149,150] In a further study, flunarizine was compared with low dose aspirin.[150] Flunarizine reduced headache frequency significantly in 71 percent of patients but was not significantly better than aspirin. In one double-blind, placebo-controlled, cross-over trial with 30 children, there was no significant benefit from *nimodipine* over placebo.[151] Patients did better in the first arm of the study, irrespective of the medication used (level I, recommendation E). *Timolol* was also shown to be no more effective than placebo in a double-blind, cross-over study (level I, recommendation E).[152]

Valproate has been proposed as an effective therapy for migraine, but there are no studies in children.[153] In view of its potential adverse effects, it would seem prudent to avoid valproate in children with headache, until further data become available (level III, recommendation C).

Antidepressants. Although *amitriptyline hydrochloride* (Elavil) and other antidepressants have been used in children, there are no available studies to show their effectiveness (level III, recommendation C).

Antiserotoninergics Methysergide has been used to treat adult migraine since 1959 but has not been studied in children. The potentially serious adverse effect of retroperitoneal fibrosis precludes its use in children (level III, recommendation D).[154]

Isometheptene, a mild vasoconstrictor, in combination with acetaminophen and the mild sedating agent dicloralphenazone, has been shown to be effective in aborting migraine in adults.[155] Similar effectiveness has not been studied in children (level III, recommendation C).

Phenothiazines and *metoclopramide* are beneficial in adults with migraine and prominent vomiting.[156,157] Studies are not available to allow recommendations on the use of these agents in the pediatric population (level III, recommendation C). Anecdotally, they may be clinically effective. Metoclopramide may be given as an oral dose of 5 to 10 mg (up to 1 mg/kg). Side effects include sedation, dizziness, and confusion. When dystonia occurs, *diphenhydramine*, up to 5 mg/kg per 24 hours, should be given.

Clonidine has been shown to be ineffective in two studies (level I, recommendation E).[158,159]

PROGNOSIS

Bille found that of his initial cohort of children with migraine, 62 percent were headache-free for more than 2 years as young adults, but after 30 years only 40 percent continued to be free of their migraine headaches.[1] In a follow-up study after 9 to 14 years, Hinrichs and Keith found that 80 percent were completely headache-free or improved.[160] We followed up 77 patients after 10 years and found that 72.5 percent still had headaches, although 81.3 percent reported that their headaches were improved.[135] Migraine, therefore, is a life-long illness for many patients. The prognosis of most acute headaches is limited to the acute illness. The prognosis for those with chronic progressive headache is dependent on the underlying condition. The prognosis for childhood tension-type headache is at this time unclear.

SUMMARY

Although headaches affect almost 75 percent of children by their teen years, there are few evidence-based data available to guide our management of these patients. Evidence is accumulating on the pathogenesis of migraine, but the diagnosis continues to depend on clinical criteria that were primarily designed for use in adults. Traditional prophylactic medication choices have often failed to prove effective, when rigorously studied. Proof of effectiveness in adults does not necessarily indicate similar value in the pediatric population. The management of childhood headaches should be primarily a combination of nonpharmacologic and early abortive therapy. Nonpharmacologic methods include identification and avoidance of precipitants or self-hypnosis. The best abortive medication appears to be ibuprofen.[120] Further study is needed to establish the optimal approach to these patients.

REFERENCES

1. Bille B. Migraine in school children. Acta Paediatr 1962;51(Suppl 136):1–151.

2. Sillanpää M, Antilla P. Increasing prevalence of headache in 7-year-old schoolchildren. Headache 1996;36:466–70.

3. deLissovoy G, Lazarus SS. The economic cost of migraine: present state of knowledge. Neurology 1994;44:S56–62.

4. Wober-Bingol C, Wober C, Karwautz A, et al. Diagnosis of headache in childhood and adolescence: a study of 437 patients. Cephalgia 1995;15:13–21.

5. Zuckerman B, Stevenson J, Bailey V. Stomachaches and headaches in a community sample of preschool children. Pediatrics 1987;79:677–82.

6. Sillanpää M, Piekkala P. Prevalence of migraine and other headaches in early puberty. Scand J Prim Health Care 1984;2:27–32.

7. Rothner AD. Headaches in children: a review. Headache 1978;18:169–75.

8. Kandt RS, Levine RM. Headache and acute illness in children. J Child Neurol 1987;2:22–7.

9. Mortimer MJ, Kay J, Jaron A. Epidemiology of headache and childhood migraine in an urban general practice using ad hoc, Vahlquist and IHS criteria. Dev Med Child Neurol 1992;34:1095–101.

10. Silanpää M. Prevalence of migraine and other headache in Finnish children starting school. Headache 1976;15:288–90.

11. Stewart WF, Simon D, Schechter A, Lipton RB. Population variation in migraine prevalence: a meta-analysis. J Clin Epidemiol 1995;48:269–80.

12. Chu ML, Shinnar S. Headaches in children younger than 7 years of age. Arch Neurol 1992;49:79–82.

13. Aysun S, Yetuk M. Clinical experience on headache in children: analysis of 92 cases. J Child Neurol 1998;13(5):202–10.

14. Aromaa M, Sillanpää ML, Rautava P, Helenius H. Childhood headache at school entry: a controlled clinical study. Neurology 1998;50:1729–36.

15. Mesähonkala L, Sillanpää M, Tuominen J. Social environment and headache in 8- to 9-year-old children: a follow-up study. Headache 1998;38:222–8.

16. Carlsson J, Larsson B, Mark A. Psychosocial functioning in schoolchildren with recurrent headaches. Headache 1996;36:77–82.

17. Wober-Bingol C, Wober C, Wagner-Ennsgraber C, et al. IHS criteria for migraine and tension-type headache in children and adolescents. Headache 1996;36:231–8.

18. Scheller JM. The history, epidemiology and classification of headaches in childhood. Semin Pediatr Neurol 1995;2:102–8.

19. Gordon K, Dooley J, Camfield P. Pediatric idiopathic intracranial hypertension: descriptive epidemiology [abstract]. Pediatr Neurol 1994;10:9.

20. Gladstein J, Holden EW. Chronic daily headache in children and adolescents: a 2-year prospective study. Headache 1996;36:349–51.

21. Abu-Arefeh I, Russell G. Prevalence of headache and migraine in school children. Br Med J 1994;309:765–9.

22. Sillanpää M, Piekkala P, Kero P. Prevalence of headache at preschool age in an unselected child population. Cephalgia 1991;11:239–42.

23. Mortimer MJ, Kay J, Jaron A. Childhood migraine in general practice: clinical features and characteristics. Cephalgia 1992;12:238–43.

24. Metsähonkala L, Sillanpää M, Tuominen J. Use of health services in chilhood migraine. Headache 1996;36:423–8.

25. Lewis DW, Middlebrook MT, Mehallick L, et al. Pediatric headaches: what do the children want? Headache 1996;36:224–30.

26. Collin C, Hockaday JM, Waters WE. Headache and school absence. Arch Dis Child 1985;60:245–7.

27. Stang PE, Osterhaus JT. Impact of migraine in the United States: data from the National Health Interview Survey. Headache 1993;33:29–35.

28. Holden EW, Gladstein J, Trulsen M, Wall B. Chronic daily headache in children and adolescents. Headache 1994;34:508–14.

29. Goadsby P. Mechanisms of migraine pain. Presented at the American Association for the study of Headache course, Scottsdale, Arizona. November 1998.

30. Uddman R, Edvinsson L, Ekman R, et al. Innervation of the feline cerebral vasculature by nerve fibers containing calcitonin gene-related peptide: trigeminal origin and co-existence with substance P. Neurosci Lett 1985;62:131–6.

31. Gladstein J. Headaches: the pediatrician's perspective. Semin Pediatr Neurol 1995;2:119–26.

32. Nichols FT, Mawad M, Mohr JP, et al. Focal headache during balloon inflation in the vertebral and basilar arteries. Headache 1993;33:87–9.

33. Raskin NH, Hosobuchi Y, Lamb S. Headache may arise from perturbation of brain. Headache 1987;27:416–20.

34. Weiller C, May A, Limmroth V, et al. Brain stem activation in spontaneous human migraine attacks. Nature Med 1995;1:658–60.

35. Goadsby PJ, Zagami AS, Lambert GA. Neural processing of craniovascular pain: a synthesis of the central structures involved in migraine. Headache 1991;31:365–71.

36. Edvinsson L, Goadsby PJ. Neuropeptides in migraine and cluster headaches. Cephalgia 1994;14:320–7.

37. Leao AAP. Spreading depression of activity in cerebral cortex. J Neurphysiol 1994;7:379–90.

38. Woods RP, Iacoboni M, Mazziotta JC. Bilateral spreading cerebral hypoperfusion during spontaneous migraine headache. N Engl J Med 1994;331:1689–92.

39. Moskowitz MA, Nozaki K, Kraig P. Neocortical spreading depression provokes the expression of c-fos protein-like immunoreactivity with trigeminal nucleus caudalis via trigeminovascular mechanisms. J Neurosci 1993;13:1167–77.

40. Burton LJ, Quinn B, Pratt-Cheney JL, Pourani M. Headache etiology in a pediatric emergency department. Ped Emerg Care 1997;13:1–4.

41. Viswanathan V, Bridges SJ, Whitehouse W, Newton RW. Childhood headaches: discrete entities or continuum? Dev Med Child Neurol 1998;40:544–50.

42. Rossi LN, Cortinovis I, Bellettini G, et al. Diagnostic criteria for migraine and psychogenic headache in children. Dev Med Child Neurol 1992;34:516–23.

43. Rapoport AM, Sheftell FD. Headache disorders: a management guide for practitioners. Philadelphia, PA: W.B. Saunders Company; 1996.

44. Vahlquist B. Migraine in children. Int Arch Allergy Immunol 1955;7:348–55.

45. Headache Classification Committee of the International Headache Society. Classification and diagnostic criteria for headache disorders, cranial neuralgias and facial pain. Cephalgia 1988;8(Suppl 7):1–96.

46. Gladstein J, Holden EW, Peralta L, Raven M. Diagnoses and symptom patterns in children presenting to a pediatric headache clinic. Headache 1993;33:497–500.

47. Congdon PJ, Forsythe WI. Migraine in childhood: a review. Clin Pediatr 1979;18:353–9.

48. Seshia SS, Wolstein JR, Adams C, et al. International Headache Society criteria and childhood headache. Dev Med Child Neurol 1994;36:419–28.

49. Winner P, Martinez W, Mate L, Bello L. Classification of pediatric migraine: proposed revisions to the IHS criteria. Headache 1995;35:407–10.

50. Winner P, Wasiewski W, Gladstein J, Linder S, for the Pediatric Headache Committee of the American Association for the Study of Headache. Multicenter prospective evaluation of proposed pediatric migraine revisions to the IHS criteria. Headache 1997;37:545–8.

51. Hockaday JM, Barlow CF. Headache in children. In: Olesen J, Tfelt-Hansen P, Welch KMA, editors. The headaches. New York: Raven; 1993. p. 795–808.

52. Ostergaard S, Russell MB, Bendtsen L, Olesen J. Comparison of first degree relatives and spouses of people with chronic tension headache. Br Med J 1997;314:1092–3.

53. Solomon S, Lipton RB, Neuman LC. Evaluation of chronic daily headache: comparison to criteria for chronic tension-type headache. Cephalgia 1992;12:365–8.

54. Sjaastad O, Spierings ELH. "Hemicrania continua": another headache absolutely responsive to indomethacin. Cephalgia 1984;4:65–70.

55. Passchier J, Hunfeld JA, Jelicic M, Verhage F. Suggestibility and headache reports in schoolchildren: a problem in epidemiology. Headache 1993;33:73–5.

56. Jensen PS, Halber MD, Putman Ce. *Mycoplasma pneumoniae*. Crit Rev Diagn Imaging 1980;12:385–415.

57. Buchwald DS, Blaser MJ. A review of salmonellosis: II. Duration of excretion following infection with non-typhi salmonella. Rev Infect Dis 1984;6:345–56.

58. Belman AL, Iyer M, Coyle PK, Dattwyler R. Neurologic manifestations in children with North American Lyme disease. Neurology 1993;43:2609–14.

59. Faleck H, Rothner AD, Erenberg G, Cruse RP. Headache and subacute sinusitis in children and adolescents. Headache 1988;28:96–8.

60. Lanser JB, Jennekens-Schinkel A, Peters AC. Headache after closed head injury in children. Headache 1988;28:176–9.

61. Vandam LD, Dripps RD. Long-term follow-up of patients who received 10,098 spinal anesthetics. JAMA 1956;161:586–91.

62. Lynch J, Arthelger S, Krings-Ernst I, et al. Whitecare 2-gauge pencil-point needle for spinal anesthesia. A controlled trial in 300 young orthopedic patients. Anesth Intens Care 1992;20:322–5.

63. Jay GW, Tomasi LG. Pediatric headaches: a one year retrospective analysis. Headache 1981;21:5–9.

64. Lee LH, Olness KN. Clinical and demographic characteristics of migraine in urban children. Headache 1997;37:269–76.

65. Lance JW, Anthony M. Some clinical aspects of migraine: a prospective study of 500 patients. Arch Neurol 1966;15:356–61.

66. Gallai V, Sarchielli P, Carboni F, et al., on behalf of the Juvenile Headache Collaborative Study Group. Applicability of the 1988 IHS criteria to headache patients under the age of 18 years attending 21 Italian headache clinics. Headache 1995;35:146–53.

67. Metsähonkala, Sillanpää M. Migraine in children: an evaluation of the IHS criteria. Cephalgia 1994;14:285–90.

68. Rothner AD. Classification, pathogenesis, evaluation and management of headaches in children and adolescents. Curr Opin Pediatr 1992;4:946–56.

69. Cooper PJ, Bawden HN, Camfield PR, Camfield CS. Anxiety and life events in children with migraine. Pediatrics 1987;79:999–1004.

70. Hämääinen ML, Hoppu K, Santavouri P. Pain and disability in migraine or other recurrent headaches as reported by children. Eur J Neurol 1996;3:528–32.

71. Massiou H. What is lacking in the treatment of pediatric and adolescent migrane? Cephalgia 1997;17(Suppl 17):21–4.

72. Hachinski VS, Porchawka J, Steele JC. Visual symptoms in the migraine syndrome. Neurology 1973;23:570–9.

73. Linet MS, Ziegler DK, Stewart WF. Headaches preceded by visual aura among adolescent and young adults. Arch Neurol 1992;49:512–6.

74. Shuper A, Packer RJ, Vezina LG, et al. Complicated migraine-like episodes in children following cranial irradiation and chemotherapy. Neurology 1995;45:1837–40.

75. Yim GK, Nordli DR, Kandji AG, et al. Familial hemiplegic migraine: autosomal dominant condition linked to chromosome 19. Pediatr Neurol 1994;11:140.

76. Joutel A, Bousser MG, Biousse V, et al. A gene for familial hemiplegic migraine maps to chromosome 19. Nat Genet 1993;5:40–5.

77. Ducros A, Joutel A, Vahedi K, et al. Mapping of a second locus for familial hemiplegic migraine to 1q21-q23 and evidence of further heterogeneity. Ann Neurol 1997;42:885–90.

78. Klopstock T, May A, Siebel P, et al. Mitochondrial in migraine with aura. Neurology 1996;46:1735–8.

79. Bickerstaff ER. Basilar artery migraine. Lancet 1961;1:15–7.

80. Golden GS, French JH. Basilar artery migraine in young children. Pediatrics 1975;56:722–6.

81. Sturzenegger MH, Meienberg O. Basilar artery migraine: a follow-up study of 82 cases. Headache 1985;25:408–15.

82. Friedman AP, Harter DP, Merritt HH. Ophthalmoplegic migraine. Arch Neurol 1962;7:320–7.

83. Robertson WC, Schnitzler ER. Ophthalmoplegic migraine in infancy. Pediatrics 1978;61:886–8.

84. Vijayan N. Ophthalmoplegic migraine: ischemic or compressive neuropathy? Headache 1980;20:300–4.

85. Gordon N. Ophthalmoplegia in childhood. Dev Med Child Neurol 1994;36:370–4.

86. Carroll D. Retinal migraine. Headache 1970;10:9–13.

87. Golden GS. The Alice-in-Wonderland syndrome in juvenile migraine. Pediatrics 1979;63:517–9.

88. Dooley J, Gordon K, Camfield P. "The rushes." A migraine variant with hallucinations of time. Clin Pediatr 1990;29:536–8.

89. Shaabat A. Confusional migraine in childhood. Ped Neurol 1996;15:23–5.

90. Gascon G, Barlow C. Juvenile migraine presenting as acute confusional states. Pediatrics 1970;45:628–35.

91. Roh JK, Kim JS, Ahn YO. Epidemiologic and clinical characteristics of migraine and tension-type headache in Korea. Headache 1998;38:356–65.

92. Wober-Bingol C, Wober C, Wagner-Enssgraber C, et al. IHS criteria for migraine and tension-type headache in children and adolescents. Headache 1966;36:231–8.

93. Alfven G. The covariation of common psychosomatic symptoms among children from socio-economically differing residential areas. An epidemiological study. Acta Paediatr 1993;82:484–7.

94. Moscato D, Rivaroli P. Psychological characteristics of juvenile headache: differences between tension headache and migraine. Int J Clin Pharmacol Res 1997;17:117–21.

95. Kaiser RS. Depression in adolescent headache patients. Headache 1992;32:340–4.

96. Kaiser RS, Primavera JP. Failure to mourn as a possible contributory factor to headache onset in adolescence. Headache 1993;33:69–72.

97. Maytal J, Lipton RB, Solomon S, Shinnar S. Childhood onset cluster headaches. Headache 1992;32:275–9.

98. Rothner AD. Miscellaneous headache syndromes in children and adolescents. Semin Pediatr Neurol 1995;2:159–64.

99. Diamons S. Prolonged benign exertional headache: its clinical characteristics and response in indomethacin. Headache 1982;22:96–8.

100. Broeske D, Lenn NJ, Cantos E. Chronic paroxysmal hemicrania in a young child: possible relation to ipsilateral occipital inarction. J Clin Neurol 1993;8:235–6.

101. Raskin NH, Knittle SC. Ice cream headache and orthostatic symptoms in patients with migraine. Headache 1976;16:222–5.

102. Symon DN. Twelve cases of analgesic headache. Arch Dis Child 1998;78:555–6.

103. Cohen BH. Headaches as a symptom of neurological disease. Semin Pediatr Neurol 1995;2:144–50.

104. Honig PJ, Charney EB. Children with brain tumor headaches. Am J Dis Child 1982;136:121–4.

105. Metsähonkala L, Sillanpää M, Tuominen J. Headache diary in the diagnosis of childhood migraine. Headache 1997;37:240–4.

106. Kramer U, Nevo Y, Neufeld MY, Harel S. The value of EEG in children with chronic headaches. Brain Develop 1994;16:304–8.

107. Kinast M, Lueders H, Rothner AD, Erenberg G. Benign focal epileptiform discharges in childhood migraine. Neurology 1982;32:1309–11.

108. Dooley JM, Camfield PR, O'Neill M, Vohra A. The value of CT scans for children with headaches. Can J Neurol Sci 1990;17:309–10.

109. Maytal J, Bienkowski RS, Patel M, Eviatar L. The value of brain imaging in children with headaches. Pediatrics 1995;96:413–6.

110. McAbee GN, Siegel SE, Kadakia S, et al. Value of MRI in pediatric migraine. Headache 1993;33:143–4.

111. Aloisi P, Marrelli A, Porto C, et al. Visual evoked potentials and serum magnesium levels in juvenile migraine patients. Headache 1997;37:383–5.

112. Kain ZN, Rimar S. Management of chronic pain in children. Pediatr Rev 1995;16:218–22.

113. Battistella PA, Ruffilli ZR, Moro R, et al. A placebo-controlled crossover trial of nimodipine in pediatric migraine. Headache 1990;30:264–8.

114. Hermann C, Kim M, Blanchard EB. Behavioral and prophylactic pharmacological intervention studies of pediatric migraine: an exploratory meta-analysis. Pain 1995;60:239–55.

115. Haddock CK, Rowan AB, Andrasik F, et al. Home-based behavioral treatments for chronic benign headache: a meta-analysis of controlled trials. Cephalgia 1997;17:113–8.

116. Welborn CA. Pediatric migraine. Emerg Med Clinics N Am, 1997;15:625–36.

117. McGrath PJ, Reid JR. Behavioral treatment of pediatric headache. Pediatric Ann 1995;24:486–91.

118. Chambers CT, Reid GJ, McGrath PJ, Finley GA. Self-administration of over-the-counter medication for pain among adolescents. Arch Pediatr Adolesc Med 1997;151:449–55.

119. Hämääinen ML, Hoppu K, Valkeila E, Santavouri P. Ibuprofen or acetaminophen for the acute treatment of migraine in children: a double-blind, randomized placebo-controlled crossover study. Neurology 1997;48:103–7.

120. Migliardi JR, Armellino JJ, Friedman M, et al. Caffeine as an analgesic adjuvant in tension headache. Clin Pharmacol Ther 1994;56:576–86.

121. Matthew N, Kurman R, Perez F. Drug-induced refractory headache—clinical features and management. Headache 1990;30:634–8.

122. Callaham M, Raskin NH. A controlled study of dihydroergotamine in the treatment of acute migraine headache. Headache 1986;26:168–71.

123. Linder SL. Treatment of childhood headache with dihydroergotamine mesylate. Headache 1994;34:578–80.

124. Graf WD, Riback PS. Pharmacologic treatment of recurrent pediatric headache. Pediatric Ann 1995;24:477–84.

125. Hämääinen ML, Hoppu K, Santavouri PR. Oral dihydroergotamine for therapy-resistant migraine attacks in children. Pediatr Neurol 1997;16:114–7.

126. Del-Bene E, Poggioni M, Michelacci S. Lisuride as a migraine prophylactic in children: an open clinical trial. Int J Clin Pharmacol Res 1983;3:137–41.

127. Buzzi MG, Moskowitz MA. The antimigraine drug, sumatriptan (GR43175), selectively blocks neurogenic plasma extravasation from blood vessels in the dura mater. Br J Pharmacol 1990;99:202–6.

128. Hoskin KL, Kaube H, Goadsby PJ. Sumatriptan can inhibit trigeminal afferents by an exclusively neural mechanism. Brain 1996;119:1419–28.

129. Hämääinen ML, Hoppu K, Santavouri P. Sumatriptan for migraine attacks in children: a randomized placebo-controlled study. Do children with migraine respond to oral sumatriptan differently from adults? Neurology 1997;48:1100–3.

130. MacDonald JT. Treatment of juvenile migraine with subcutaneous sumatriptan. Headache 1994;34:581–2.

131. Linder SL. Subcutaneous sumatriptan in the clinical setting: the first 50 consecutive patients with acute migraine in a pediatric neurology office practice. Headache 1996;36:419–22.

132. Dowson AJ, Fletcher PE, Millson DS. Efficacy and tolerability of Zolmig in adolescent migraine [abstract]. Cephalgia 1998;18:406–7.

133. Dixon R, Kemp J, Engelman K, Ruckle JL. A comparison of the pharmacokinetics and tolerability profile of zolmitriptan in adolescents and adults. Eur J Neurol 1998;5:S54.

134. Dooley J, Bagnell A. The prognosis and treatment of headaches in children—a ten year follow-up. Can J Neurol Sci 1995;22:47–9.

135. Fentress DW, Masek BJ, Mehegan JE, Benson H. Biofeedback and relaxation-response training in the treatment of pediatric migraine. Dev Med Child Neurol 1986;28:139–46.

136. Duckro PN, Cantwell-Simmons E. A review of studies evaluating biofeedback and relaxation training in the management of pediatric headache. Headache 1989;29:428–33.

137. Richter I, McGrath PJ, Humphreys PJ, et al. Cognitive and relaxation treatment of pediatric migraine. Pain 1986;25:195–203.

138. Allen KD, McKeen LR. Home-based multicomponent treatment of pediatric migraine. Headache 1991;31:467–72.

139. Burke EJ, Andrasik F. Home vs. clinic-based biofeedback treatment for pediatric migraine: results of treatment through one-year follow-up. Headache 1989;29:434–40.

140. Haddock CK, Rowan AB, Andrasik F, et al. Home-based behavioral treatments for chronic benign headache: a meta-analysis of controlled trials. Cephalgia 1997;17:113–8.

141. Olness K. Hypnotherapy: a cyberphysiologic strategy in pain management. Ped Clin N Am 1989;36:873–84.

142. Kapelis L. Hypnosis in a behavior therapy framework for the treatment of migraine in children. Austral J Clin Exper Hypnosis 1984;12:123–6.

143. Olness K, MacDonald JT, Uden DL. Comparison of self-hypnosis and propanolol in the treatment of juvenile classic migraine. Pediatrics 1987;79:593–7.

144. Peroutka SJ, Allen GS. The calcium antagonist properties of cyproheptadine: implications for antimigraine action. Neurology 1984;34:304–9.

145. Bille B, Ludvigsson J, Sanner G. Prophylaxis of migraine in children. Headache 1977;17:61–3.

146. Ludvigsson J. Propanolol used in prophylaxis of migraine in children. Acta Neurol Scand 1974;50:109–15.

147. Forsythe WI, Gilles D, Sills MA. Propanolol (Inderal) in the treatment of childhood migraine. Dev Med Child Neurol 1984;26:737–41.

148. Sorge F, Marano E. Flunarizine v. placebo in childhood migraine: a double-blind study. Cephalgia 1985;5(Suppl 2):145–8.

149. Sorge F, DeSimone R, Marano E, et al. Flunarizine in prophylaxis of childhood migraine: a double-blind, placebo-controlled, crossover study. Cephalgia 1988;8:1–6.

150. Pothman R. Calcium-antagonist flunarizine vs. low-dose acetysalicylic acid in childhood migraine: a double-blind study. Cephalgia 1987;7(Supl 6):385–6.

151. Battistella PA, Ruffilli R, Moro R, et al. A placebo-controlled crossover trial of nimodipine in pediatric migraine. Headache 1990;30:264–8.

152. Noronha MJ. Double-blind randomized crossover trial of timolol in migraine prophylaxis in children. Cephalgia 1985;5(Suppl 3):174–5.

153. Jensen R, Brinck T, Olesen J. Sodium valproate has a prophylactic effect in migraine with aura: a triple blind, placebo-controlled crossover study. Neurology 1994;44:647–51.

154. Igarashi M, May WN, Golden GS. Pharmacologic treatment of childhood migraine. J Pediatr 1992;120:653–7.

155. Diamond S, Medina JL. Isometheptene: a nonergot drug in the treatment of migraine. Headache 1975;15:211–3.

156. Jones J, Sklar D, Dougherty J, White W. Randomized double-blind trial of intravenous prochlorperazine for the treatment of acute headache. JAMA 1989;261:1174–6.

157. Tek DS, McClellan DS, Olshaker JS, et al. A prospective, double-blind study of metoclopramide hydrochloride for the control of migraine in the emergency department. Ann Emerg Med 1990;19:1083–7.

158. Sillanpää M. Clonidine prophylaxis of childhood migraine and other vascular headache. A double-blind study of 57 children. Headache 1977;17:28–31.

159. Sills M, Congdon P, Forsythe I. Clonidine and childhood migraine: a pilot and double-blind study. Dev Med Child Neurol 1982;24:837–41.

160. Hinrichs WL, Keith HM. Migraine in childhood: a follow-up report. Mayo Clin Proc 1965;40:593–6.

CHAPTER 14

Injury Prevention: Effectiveness of Primary Care Interventions

Lynne J. Warda, MD, FRCPC

The purpose of this chapter is to summarize the literature examining the effectiveness of primary care interventions in the area of injury prevention. This summary includes interventions that have been introduced in pediatric primary care clinics and by primary care pediatricians in hospital settings, such as the newborn nursery and the emergency department. The basis for this summary is a review of the published, English-language literature, including both randomized and nonrandomized studies identified using MEDLINE (1966 to 1998), two recent systematic reviews,[1,2] and a local injury prevention bibliographic database. The reader may consult recent comprehensive reviews for discussion of the effectiveness of population- and community-based injury prevention interventions.[3–7]

DISEASE BURDEN

"The following and many similar headlines startle parent and physicians daily: "Girl dead, boy blinded by antifreeze;" "Three small children perish in home fire;" and "Boy, two, dies in two-story fall." To the physician, who today can usually successfully treat his child patients for such serious illnesses as meningitis, erythroblastosis fetalis and dehydration, it is particularly frustrating to be faced with the death or serious injury of one of these children from an accident; yet except for the first year of life accidents are the single greatest cause of death during childhood."

Robert J Haggerty N Engl J Med 1959;260:1322

Although injury rates have steadily declined since the 1950s, injuries remain the leading cause of death in children and adolescents 1 to 19 years of age.[8,9] In 1995, in the United States, there were more than 147,000 deaths, 2.6 million hospital admissions, and 37 million emergency department visits due to injury.[8] The burden of illness due to injury is similar in other developed countries.[10] Injury deaths represent only the tip of the iceberg. Using these 1995 data, one can construct an "injury pyramid" (Figure 14–1); for every death in 1995, there were 18 admissions to hospital, 252 emergency room visits, and an estimated 442 physicians' office visits.

Injury death rates peak in childhood and old age and are higher for males than females at all ages.[8] Unintentional injury accounts for the majority (80 to 90 percent) of injury deaths in childhood, although intentional injuries increase dramatically in adolescence. For children less than 15 years of age, 80 percent of injury deaths are caused by motor vehicles, fire and burns, drowning, suffocation, and firearms. Leading causes of injury death differ for infants, young children, and older children, as would be expected, given physical, mental, and behavioral developmental stages. Similarly, injury prevention strategies evolve through childhood according to developmental stages, and have changed surprisingly little since the 1950s (Table 14–1).[11]

INJURY PREVENTION

Injury control strategies address three levels of prevention. *Primary* prevention strategies reduce or eliminate the injury exposure. Examples include child-resistant closures, speed

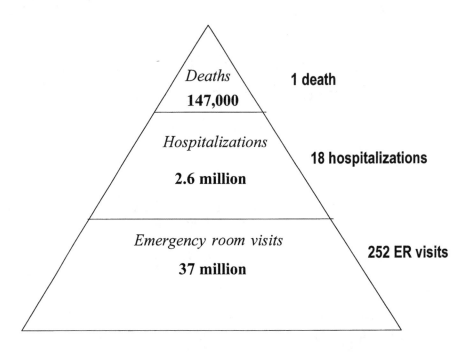

Figure 14–1 Injury pyramid of mortality and morbidity. Data for United States, 1995. With permission from National Center for Health Statistics. Health, United States, 1996–7 and Injury Chartbook. Hyattsville, Maryland; 1997.

Table 14–1 Injury Risks and Precautions at Various Ages

Typical Injury	Normal Behavior Characteristics	Precautions
Infant less than 1 year		
Suffocation	Puts everything in mouth	Keep small objects and poisons out of reach
Motor vehicle injuries	Is dependent on others for safety	Always use a car safety seat
Falls	Rolls over about 4 mo of age; creeps, stands and may walk between 6 and 12 mo	Do not leave alone on tables, beds, keep crib sides up
Burns	Is helpless to leave source of burn	Keep electric cords and appliances away; do not leave in house alone; test water in bath
Drowning	Is helpless in water	Do not leave alone in bath
2nd year		
Falls	Is able to walk; can go up and down stairs	Keep screens on windows and gate at stairs
Burns	Reaches for any utensils on stove or table	Keep handles of pots and pans on stove out of reach and hot foods away from edge of table; keep electric cords out of reach; cover unused electric outlets; do not leave alone in house

(continued)

Table 14–1 Injury Risks and Precautions at Various Ages   *(continued)*

Typical Injury	Normal Behavior Characteristics	Precautions
Drowning	Is helpless in water	Keep in enclosed space when outdoors or not in company of adults
Poisonings	Has great curiosity; puts everything in mouth	Keep medicines, household compounds and small, sharp objects out of reach
2 to 4 years Falls	Is able to open doors; can run and climb, can throw ball, ride tricycle	Keep doors locked where danger of falls: cellar, screens on windows; teach risks of throwing sharp objects
Drowning	Most unable to swim	Supervise closely when near open water; beware of buckets and bathtubs
Poisonings	Investigates closets and drawers	Keep medicines, household compounds and small, sharp objects out of reach
Burns and cuts	Has immature judgment	Keep knives and electric equipment out of reach
Firearms	Plays with mechanical gadgets	Keep firearms locked up
Motor vehicle injuries	Has immature judgment	Teach safety in street and driveway
5 to 9 years Motor vehicle injuries Bicycle accidents	Is daring and adventurous Control more advanced over large than small muscles	Teach traffic and bicycle safety
Drowning		Encourage but do not push swimming skills
Burns Firearms		Keep firearms locked up
Falls	Loyalty to group makes him willing to follow leaders	Build self-esteem
10 to 14 years Motor vehicle injuries	Need for strenuous physical activity	Teach rules of pedestrian and traffic safety; prepare for driving by setting a good example
Drowning Burns Falls	Plays in hazardous places Need for approval by agemates leads to daring or hazardous feats	Provide safe and acceptable facilities for recreation and social activities

Adapted from Shaffer T. Symposium on clinical advances: accident prevention. Pediatr Clin N Am 1954;1:421–32.

limits, and swimming pool fences. *Secondary* prevention strategies reduce or eliminate injuries once the exposure has occurred. Examples include bicycle helmets and seat belts. *Tertiary* prevention strategies attempt to reduce the severity of an injury once it has occurred. Examples include high-quality first-response systems, emergency medical treatment, and rehabilitation of injuries. Injury prevention strategies may be classified as passive or active. Active strategies involve action by the injury victim, such as fastening a seat belt. Passive strategies do not require specific action by the injury victim, for example, automobile air bags. Passive interventions commonly involve product design modifications and environmental changes and are more effective than active interventions because their activation is independent of human behavior.

Injuries result from the interaction of numerous factors related to the injured person and his or her environment. For example, in cycling injuries, factors related to the cyclist, the bicycle, and the environment contribute to the event and to the severity of injury. William Haddon developed a model for injury event analysis, on the basis of a matrix of "phases" (preinjury, injury, postinjury) and "factors" (host, agent, environment).[12,13] In the bicycle injury prevention matrix, the host is the cyclist, and the agent is the bicycle (Table 14–2). Before, during, or after the injury event, one can alter cyclist, bicycle, or environmental factors to potentially prevent injury or reduce the severity of injury. By applying Haddon's matrix to injury problems, a comprehensive approach to preventing future injury can be developed.

QUALITY OF EVIDENCE

There is a growing body of literature examining the effectiveness of injury prevention strategies. As with other areas of medicine, high-quality evidence is essential for decision making and priority setting. The best quality evidence is obtained from well-designed and well-executed randomized controlled trials, followed by controlled nonrandomized studies. The choice of outcome measures is equally important. The most persuasive evidence is obtained

Table 14–2 Haddon's Matrix Applied to Bicycle Injury Prevention

	Cyclist	Bicycle	Physical Environment	Sociocultural Environment
Pre-event	Reflective clothing Rider training Supervision Avoid hazards Route planning	Bicycle fit Bicycle maintainance Bicycle visibility eg, reflective tape or paint	Road design Road maintenance Traffic flow Bicycle paths, well-designed and lit	Driver awareness Risk attitudes Cycling attitudes Traffic legislation Helmet legislation
Event	Helmet use Protective clothing Falling technique	Bicycle design eg. padding, crash-friendly handlebars	Safety in the fall zone eg, crash-friendly signposts, curbs, car bumpers	Lower traffic speed
Post event	Cyclist visibility (to prevent other collisions) First aid skills and knowledge Learn and share from mistakes	Bicycle visibility Assess damage and correct prior to riding again	Safe zone for victim stabilization (to avoid further injury) Phones in public places Report hazards	First aid training of the general public Rapid EMS response Accessibility of high quality trauma care

EMS=emergency medical service

from studies measuring injury outcomes—injuries and injury severity. More commonly measured outcomes include injury knowledge and injury-related behaviors. However, increase in knowledge does not necessarily lead to behavior change, and improvements in safety behaviors may not lead to a change in injury occurrence. Therefore, morbidity and mortality data rank higher as outcome measures than behavior measures, which rank higher than measures of knowledge. This "hierarchy of outcome measures" is demonstrated in Figure 14–2. Due to the difficulties inherent in measuring injury as an outcome, behaviors known to be associated with a decreased risk of injury are often measured, such as smoke detector use, lowering hot water temperature, and bike helmet use.

Age-appropriate injury prevention counseling for children and adolescents has been widely recommended as an essential aspect of routine medical care.[14] The remainder of this chapter will summarize the evidence to support this recommendation.

ROAD SAFETY

Motor vehicle injuries are the leading cause of death in children and adolescents 1 to 14 years of age.[8] In 1995, motor vehicle–related deaths accounted for 18 percent of all deaths and 37 percent of all injury deaths in this age group in the United States. The majority of victims (55 to 65 percent) were occupants. Prevention of motor vehicle injuries includes adopting effective road-engineering strategies, updating and enforcing vehicle safety standards, designing and evaluating new occupant protection strategies such as air bags, supporting and enforcing relevant legislation, and changing driver and occupant behavior, particularly with respect to the correct use of seat belts and child restraints. These measures are reviewed elsewhere.[5,15] This discussion will be limited to summarizing the evidence regarding child restraint interventions in the primary-care setting. Child pedestrian injury prevention interventions have not been evaluated in the ambulatory setting; other interventions are reviewed elsewhere.[16,17]

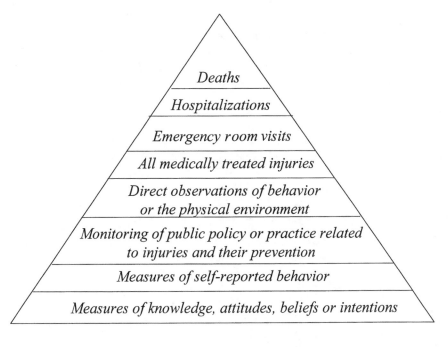

Figure 14–2 Hierarchy of injury outcome measures. Adapted from The National Committee for Injury Prevention and Control. Injury prevention: meeting the challenge. New York: Oxford University Press; 1989.

CHILD RESTRAINT FOR INFANTS AND TODDLERS

There is good evidence supporting parent counseling by pediatricians to increase child restraint for infants and toddlers. The 11 intervention studies evaluating the effectiveness of child restraint counseling for infants and toddlers are summarized in Table 14–3. Six were randomized controlled trials. These interventions included counseling at prenatal,[18–20] newborn,[20–22] and postnatal well-child visits.[20,22–28] Some interventions included demonstration of car seat use, and some included access to a car seat loan program. All included educating parents about the risks of infant injury in motor vehicles and the benefits of using a car seat and involved pediatricians to deliver or reinforce safety messages. Some interventions emphasized education regarding correct car seat use. Two studies examined the effectiveness of comprehensive injury prevention counseling using the Framingham Safety Surveys and were reinforced by concurrent community-based initiatives.[26,28] All but two of these studies demonstrated a positive effect of counseling on car seat use. The two studies showing no effect both documented high baseline car seat use, which may have decreased the potential for counseling to show an effect.[18,22]

There are, however, a number of limitations to these studies. First, follow-up observation periods were short in some studies, and the positive effect of counseling may decrease over time. An early increase in car seat use may not be sustained beyond the 4 to 6-week follow-up period. Second, follow-up was incomplete in some studies. Third, results from two studies were potentially confounded by concurrent community interventions.[26,28] Finally, the study periods range from the early 1970s to the early 1990s, with only two studies occurring after 1985; therefore, their generalizability to the late 1990s may be limited. Educational issues in the 1970s and early 1980s centered largely around nonuse of car seats, when child restraint laws were new or under development. While the majority of parents now own and use car seats, the issue of most importance now is teaching correct use.[29,30] Modern car seats are surprisingly complex and difficult to use correctly; accordingly, assessment of correct use now requires specialized training, available in Canada from the Canadian Automobile Association (CAA) or the Infant and Toddler Association, and in the United States through SafeKids. Car seat inspection services using certified inspectors are now available in many regions in North America; referral of families using car seats to these inspection sites should be incorporated into car seat counseling. Physicians should also inform parents of local legislation on child restraint in counseling sessions and, where possible, advocate strict enforcement of existing legislation by local law enforcement authorities.

Table 14–3 Summary of Child Restraint Counseling in Primary-Care Settings

Age Group	Intervention	Quality of Evidence	Recommendation
Infants and toddlers	Counseling at prenatal and neonatal visits regarding car seat use	I	A
	Counseling at well-child visits regarding child restraint use	I	A
	Counseling against front seat riding	I	A
Older children	Counseling at well-child visits regarding child restraint use	I	B
	Counseling at all visits regarding seat belt use	II-1	B

CHILD RESTRAINT FOR OLDER CHILDREN

There is conflicting evidence supporting parent counseling regarding child restraint for children older than 5 years of age. The three intervention studies evaluating the effectiveness of child restraint counseling for children of this age group are summarized in Table 14–3. One was a randomized controlled trial. These interventions included counseling at well-child visits[31,32] and at all office visits.[33] Two studies included children of all ages[32,33] and one examined children 5 to 19 years of age.[31] The randomized controlled trial demonstrated no effect of counseling, which consisted of a pamphlet, verbal instructions, and a slide-tape show. In this study, high baseline use may have limited the potential of the intervention to show an effect, and the authors also comment that the short follow-up period (2 weeks) "was insufficient to allow for all the desired changes to occur," including purchasing and installing an approved car seat. Parents' intent to buy or use a car seat was not measured.[32] The remaining two studies demonstrated positive results. One study documented a dramatic increase in the group receiving an intensive educational intervention; however, the outcome interval is not specified, and the results are limited by the use of a self-report measure.[33] The remaining study documented an increase in seat belt use immediately following counseling; however, there was no difference between groups 1 year later.[31] In this study, parents' seat belt use was highly correlated with their children's use, and routine seat belt counseling was significantly correlated with observed use.

BICYCLE INJURY PREVENTION

Every year, there are approximately 1,000 deaths, 23,000 hospitalizations, and 580,000 emergency room visits in the United States as a result of bicycle injuries. Almost 40 percent of deaths and two-thirds of emergency room visits occur in children less than 15 years of age. Males are at greater risk of injury at all ages, and the highest rates are for boys 10 to 14 years of age.[34] Prevention of bicycle injuries includes adapting the environment for improved cycling safety, educating cyclists and other road users, improving cycling and road safety skills of young cyclists, and encouraging correct and consistent helmet use by all cyclists (see Table 14–2). Interventions to improve bicycle safety taking place in the primary-care setting are summarized here. The effectiveness of community-based and legislative interventions is summarized elsewhere.[35]

There is conflicting evidence supporting counseling in the primary-care setting regarding bicycle helmet use for children. The three intervention studies evaluating the effectiveness of bicycle helmet counseling for children are summarized in Table 14–4. All were randomized controlled trials. These interventions include counseling, following a bicycle injury, in the emergency department[36] as well as in primary-care settings[36,37] and included children 5 to 18 years of age,[38] 6 to 12 years of age,[37] and children of all ages.[36]

In the first of two similar randomized controlled studies conducted by Cushman and colleagues, parents of 334 children treated in the emergency department for bicycle injuries

Table 14–4 Summary of Bicycle Helmet Counseling in Primary-Care Settings

Intervention	Quality of Evidence	Recommendation
Bicycle helmet counseling in the emergency department following a bicycle injury	I	C
Bicycle helmet counseling at routine office visits	I	C
Providing subsidized helmets (rather than free helmets) in addition to counseling	I	A

were randomly assigned to receive counseling about the risks of cycling and the benefits of helmets and were also given pamphlets about bicycle safety and helmets. Almost 90 percent of the participants were successfully contacted by telephone 2 to 3 weeks later. Among the intervention group, 9.3 percent had purchased a helmet, compared with 8.1 percent of the control group. The high proportion of control parents having purchased a helmet was thought to be due to either the "testing" effect of the survey or to the postinjury motivation to buy a helmet. The testing effect the authors describe may have been a Hawthorne effect, where subjects alter their behavior due to participation in a study, or a form of contamination, where the control group also received "counseling" about bicycle helmet use by completing the survey.[36] A similar study was then conducted in children presenting to their family physician or pediatrician for routine ambulatory care. The patients were randomly assigned to receive helmet promotion counseling and pamphlets. When parents were contacted 2 to 3 weeks later, 7.2 percent of the intervention group had purchased helmets, compared with 7.0 percent of the control group. The surprising number of control families having purchased a helmet within 2 to 3 weeks of the office visit may have been due to the testing effect of the survey or due to the concurrent community-based promotion of helmets.[38] The authors discuss the possibility that the families responding positively to the intervention, and perhaps to the survey itself, were "innovators" or "early adapters," who were "ready" to buy a helmet and needed little persuasion to do so.

The third randomized controlled trial was designed to determine whether a $5.00 copayment for a helmet would affect helmet use, when compared with providing helmets free of charge, for children between 6 and 12 years of age who reported riding bicycles but not owning a helmet.[37] Families were also counseled regarding the benefits of wearing a helmet and correct helmet use. Although the copayment and free helmet groups did not differ, both reported high and consistent helmet use (>70 percent) at follow-up. The authors comment that counseling alone for children not owning a helmet, has not been effective in increasing helmet use in other studies; therefore, providing a helmet free of charge or for a nominal fee in conjunction with counseling may have a significant effect on increasing helmet use in some populations.

HOME SAFETY

Between 1970 and 1984, in the United States, there was an average of 3,200 deaths every year due to injury in the home among children less than 15 years of age, accounting for over 25 percent of childhood injury deaths. The leading causes of such injury deaths in this age group are fires and burns, drowning, and suffocation.[39] The studies examining home safety counseling are summarized in this section, grouped by category of injury-type: prevention of burns, prevention of poisoning, prevention of falls, and general household safety.

Prevention of Burns

Fires and burns are the third leading cause of injury death for children 1 to 14 years of age in the United States, following motor vehicle crashes and drownings.[8,10] Death rates are highest for children 1 to 4 years of age and are higher for boys than girls in this age group. Over 90 percent of fire and burn deaths among children are accidental.

Prevention of residential fire injury includes fire prevention strategies; fire detection and extinguishing strategies; fire escape strategies; and first aid, medical treatment, and rehabilitation strategies. Fire prevention strategies may include reduction or modification of ignition sources, such as the "fire-safe" cigarette and child-proof lighter; improving fire safety behaviors in the home, such as smoking habits and storage of hazardous materials; and teaching children fire safety behaviors, such as not playing with matches and lighters. Fire detection and extinguishing measures include smoke alarm use and routine testing, sprinkler systems, and use of fire extinguishers. Fire escape strategies include building code enforcement and development of escape plans by families. Prevention of scalds may be achieved by reducing hot water temperatures in the home to less than 54.4°C (130°F), routinely testing bath water temperature, and increasing safe behaviors in the kitchen, bathroom, and laundry areas.

There is good evidence supporting parent counseling by pediatricians regarding burn prevention for infants and toddlers. The 10 intervention studies evaluating the effectiveness of burn prevention counseling[26–28,40–46] are summarized in Table 14–5. Six were randomized controlled trials. The interventions all included counseling at well-child visits, and some included providing parents with written materials, coupons for safety devices, offers to purchase low-cost safety devices, and free safety devices. Three studies examined the effectiveness of comprehensive injury prevention counseling using the Framingham Safety Surveys and were reinforced by concurrent community-based initiatives.[26,28,40] All but two of these studies demonstrated a positive effect of counseling on burn prevention practices and/or knowledge. Eight of the ten studies evaluated burn safety measures using an actual home visit, and the majority of positive outcomes were observed behaviors and objective and reproducible measures such as outlet cover or smoke alarm use. However, it was not clear in many cases whether the observations were blinded, and follow-up was incomplete in some studies. None of these studies used fire- or burn-related injuries as an outcome measure.

Prevention of Poisoning

Children less than 6 years of age are at greatest risk of serious injury due to poisoning. Poisoning deaths in children have decreased dramatically since the early 1960s, which is thought to be due, in part, to the introduction of child-proof packaging, intensive public education efforts, and the introduction of regional poison control centers.[47,48] The most common ingestants causing death in this age group are medications.[47] Preventive strategies include routine use of child-proof packaging for potential poisons, proper storage of medications and other hazardous household products, and prompt and appropriate treatment of poisoning, guided by the regional poison control system.

There is good evidence supporting poison prevention counseling by pediatricians. The 10 intervention studies evaluating the effectiveness of poisoning-related counseling[26–28,40–44,49,50] are summarized in Table 14–6. Five were randomized controlled trials. The interventions all included counseling at well-child visits for children less than 5 years of age. Some interventions included written materials, and several provided free ipecac.[49,51] Three studies examined the effectiveness of comprehensive injury prevention counseling using the Framingham Safety Surveys and were reinforced by concurrent community-based initiatives.[26,28,40] All but three of these studies demonstrated a positive effect of counseling on poisoning safety practices or knowl-

Table 14–5 Summary of Burn Prevention Counseling in Primary-Care Settings

Type of Burn Injury	Intervention	Quality of Evidence	Recommendation
House fire injury	Counseling regarding smoke alarm use Counseling regarding home fire safety	I	A
Electrical injury	Counseling regarding outlet cover use Counseling regarding electrical safety	I	A
Scald injury	Counseling regarding hot water temperature Counseling regarding scald prevention	I	A

Note: Free or low-cost safety devices and concurrent community interventions may enhance effectiveness.

Table 14–6   Summary of Poisoning Safety Counseling in Primary-Care Settings

Intervention	Quality of Evidence	Recommendation
Counseling regarding use of cupboard locks	I	A
Counseling regarding storage of hazardous products	I	A
Counseling regarding first aid for poisoning	I	A

Note: Free or low-cost safety devices and concurrent community interventions may enhance effectiveness.

edge. Five of the ten studies evaluated poisoning safety measures using home visits; however, the three studies of poisoning-focused rather than multitopic counseling used self-report measures only.[28,50,51] Although counseling regarding home use of ipecac was effective, it should be noted that ipecac is not recommended as a routine treatment for poisoning.[52]

Prevention of Falls

Children less than 5 years of age are at greatest risk for death due to falls; in 1986, in the United States, there were 117 deaths in children in this age group due to falls. Deaths in children less than 1 year of age are more likely due to falling from a modest height, such as from a bed, while deaths in children 1 to 2 years of age are more likely due to falling from a building or down the stairs.[41] Preventive measures for falls include counseling regarding the use of window and stair guards, appropriate supervision of infants and toddlers, and counseling parents regarding the potential hazards associated with baby walkers.

There is good evidence supporting fall prevention counseling by pediatricians. The six intervention studies evaluating the effectiveness of fall-related counseling[26–28,42,43,53] are summarized in Table 14–7. Three were randomized controlled trials. The interventions all included counseling at well-child visits for children less than 5 years of age. Some interventions included written materials, and several provided free or low-cost safety devices. Two studies examined the effectiveness of comprehensive injury prevention counseling using the Framingham Safety Surveys and were reinforced by concurrent community-based initiatives.[26,28] All but two of these studies demonstrated a positive effect of counseling on fall-related safety practices and/or knowledge. Three of the six studies evaluated fall-related safety measures using home visits; however, the single study of fall-focused rather than multitopic counseling used self-report measures only.[53]

General Household Safety

There is good evidence supporting parent counseling by pediatricians regarding general household safety for infants and toddlers. Three of the six studies examining general house-

Table 14–7 Summary of Fall Prevention Counseling in Primary-Care Settings

Intervention	Quality of Evidence	Recommendation
Counseling regarding use of window catches	I	A
Counseling regarding the reduction of fall-related hazards in the home	I	A

Note: Free or low-cost safety devices and concurrent community interventions may enhance effectiveness.

hold safety counseling[26–28,40,42,43] were randomized controlled trials.[27,42,43] The interventions all included counseling at well-child visits for children less than 5 years of age. Some interventions included written materials, coupons for safety devices, offers to purchase low-cost safety devices, and free safety devices. Three studies examined the effectiveness of comprehensive injury prevention counseling using the Framingham Safety Surveys and were reinforced by concurrent community-based initiatives.[26,28,40] All but one of these studies demonstrated a positive effect of counseling on home safety practices or knowledge. Four of the six studies evaluated home safety measures using home visits, and the majority of positive outcomes were observed behaviors and objective and reproducible measures such as the absence of hazards or presence of safety devices. However, it was not clear in many cases whether the observations were blinded, and follow-up was incomplete in some studies.

SUMMARY AND CONCLUSION

Summary of the Evidence

A summary of the evidence for injury prevention counseling is presented in Table 14–8. It should be noted, however, that although seat belt and bicycle helmet counseling are not supported by the published literature reviewed here, these activities are strongly recommended by expert groups. Two recent systematic reviews of the literature examining injury preven-

Table 14–8 Summary of Evidence for Injury Prevention Counseling

	Key Messages	Classification of Recommendations
Road safety		
Child restraint use for infants and toddlers	• Use an age-appropriate car seat for every ride • Encourage correct car seat use, inspection	A
Child restraint use for older children	• Use a seat belt for every ride • Encourage seat belt use by parent for every ride	B
Bicycle injury prevention	• Use a helmet for every ride • Encourage correct use and fit	C
Home safety		
Prevention of burns	• Install smoke detectors on every level and near all sleeping areas • Replace batteries twice every year; test function every month • Reduce hot water temperature to less than 54.4°C (130°F)	A
Prevention of poisoning	• Keep medicines and household toxic products out of reach • Use child-proof closures, whenever possible • Contact physician or poison control center for treatment information	A
Prevention of falls	• Use stair gates and window guards • Do not use baby walkers	A

tion counseling in pediatric primary care both concluded that there is a positive effect of counseling on safety behavior.[1,2] Klassen also documented a trend for simple behaviors such as reducing hot water temperature to be more effective than more complex or multiple behaviors.[2] The overall quality of evidence, however, could be improved significantly. Although 13 of the studies reviewed here were randomized controlled trials, all were flawed in one aspect or another. Common issues included lack of blinded outcome assessment, incomplete follow-up, and choice of indirect outcome measures such as safety behaviors rather than injury occurrence. Many of the studies in this series were published over 20 years ago. Although the counseling *process* may remain unchanged, the *content* has changed for some areas. For example, ipecac is not recommended as routine treatment of poisoning,[43] and car seat counseling has become more complex, given the large number of options available in the current market. There remain many unanswered research questions, the most important of which is to determine which elements of these interventions are most effective. Future evaluations must address these issues to strengthen and clarify the existing evidence.

While there is evidence to support injury prevention counseling, there is no evidence to support recommendations regarding the actual content or sequence of age-appropriate injury prevention counseling sessions. When asked to identify counseling priorities and specific preventive strategies, 23 injury prevention experts in the United States agreed in many respects but failed to reach an overall consensus.[54] Current recommendations are based on the epidemiology of injury in childhood and what is known about the effectiveness of interventions and are proposed by expert panels. For example, the American Academy of Pediatrics (AAP) recommends certain specific topics for injury prevention counseling for infants and toddlers, school-aged children, and adolescents.[14] Furthermore, the AAP markets The Injury Prevention Program (TIPP) to assist pediatricians in implementing office-based injury prevention counseling. This program includes an age-appropriate counseling schedule, information sheets, and safety surveys that are based on the Framingham Safety Surveys to help physicians target their teaching according to specific needs of the family. Although TIPP has not been formally evaluated as a counseling tool, there is some evidence that counseling using TIPP may be cost effective,[55] and pediatric residents familiar with TIPP may include more injury prevention topics and may be more likely to include certain topics when counseling parents.[56] However, further evaluation is required before any specific counseling program can be recommended.

Implications for Primary Care Pediatrics

A number of practical points arise from the literature that may have implications for introducing or improving injury prevention counseling in the pediatric primary care setting:

- *Effective counseling is not time consuming.* The time required for the study interventions was typically quite short, lasting several minutes. For example, a 1-minute focused educational message, a pamphlet, and an offer to buy a smoke detector at cost was effective in increasing smoke detector purchase and use.[41] Multitopic counseling using the Framingham Safety Survey required a mean counseling time of 3 minutes 17 seconds.[40]
- *Routine counseling is well received by physicians and parents.*[40]
- *Face-to-face interaction with the physician is an important component.* For example, a pediatrician's "brief and casual discussion" about seat belts was associated with increased seat belt installation, whereas a personal letter from the pediatrician was not successful in changing behaviour.[33]
- *Reinforcement of messages over time increases counseling effectiveness.*[31]
- *Simple, single interventions may be more effective than complex or multiple interventions.*[31,51]

- *Measures to reduce the cost of safety devices may improve compliance.* Free items have been used successfully, and items available at the office at low cost have also been successful.[41,42] Coupons may be less useful. For bicycle helmets, a small copayment was acceptable to parents and would allow a greater number of children in need to benefit.[37]

In summary, there is evidence to support injury prevention counseling in the pediatric primary-care setting. Future research is required to strengthen the existing evidence and to identify the most effective counseling strategies.

REFERENCES

1. Bass JL, Christoffel KK, Widome M, et al. Childhood injury prevention counseling in primary care settings: a critical review of the literature. Pediatrics 1993;92(4):544–50.

2. Klassen TP. The effectiveness of injury control interventions. M.Sc.: McMaster University; 1995.

3. Dowswell T, Towner E, Simpson G, Jarvis S. Preventing childhood unintentional injuries—what works? A literature review. Injury Prevention 1996;2(2):140–9.

4. Dannenberg AL, Fowler CJ. Evaluation of interventions to prevent injuries: an overview. Injury Prevention 1998;4(2):141–7.

5. Rivara FP, Grossman DC, Cummings P. Injury prevention: first of two parts. N Engl J Med 1997;337(8):543–8.

6. Rivara FP, Grossman DC, Cummings P. Injury prevention: second of two parts. N Engl J Med 1997;337(9):613–8.

7. Munro J, Coleman P, Nicholl J, et al. Can we prevent accidental injury to adolescents? A systematic review of the evidence. Injury Prevention 1995;1(4):249–55.

8. National Center for Health Statistics. Health, United States, 1996-7 and Injury Chartbook. Hyattsville, Maryland; 1997.

9. Health Canada. For the safety of Canadian children and youth: from injury data to preventive measures. Ottawa, Canada; 1997.

10. Fingerhut L, Cox C, Warner M. International comparative analysis of injury mortality: findings from the ICE on injury statistics. Hyattsville, Maryland: National Centre for Health Statistics; 1998.

11. Shaffer T. Symposium on clinical advances: accident prevention. Pediatr Clin N Am 1954;1:421–32.

12. Haddon WJ. A note concerning accident theory and research with special reference to motor-vehicle accidents. Ann N Y Acad Sci 1963;197:635–46.

13. Haddon WJ. A logical framework for categorizing highway safety phenomena and activity. J Trauma 1972;12:193–207.

14. American Academy of Pediatrics Committee on Injury and Poison Prevention. Office-based counseling for injury prevention. Pediatrics 1994;94(4):566–7.

15. Sabey B. Engineering safety on the road. Injury Prevention 1995;1(3):182–6.

16. Preston B. Cost effective ways to make walking safer for children and adolescents. Injury Prevention 1995;1(3):187–90.

17. Wazana A, Krueger P, Raina P, Chambers L. A review of risk factors for child pedestrian injuries: are they modifiable? Injury Prevention 1997;3(4):295–304.

18. Serwint JR, Wilson MEH, Vogelhut JW, et al. A randomized controlled trial of prenatal pediatric visits for urban, low-income families. Pediatrics 1996;98(6):1069–75.

19. Kanthor HA. Car safety for infants: effectiveness of prenatal counseling. Pediatrics 1976;58(3):320–2.

20. Berger LR, Saunders S, Armitage K, Schauer L. Promoting the use of car safety devices for infants: an intensive health education approach. Pediatrics 1984;74(1):16–9.

21. Christophersen ER, Sullivan MA. Increasing the protection of newborn infants in cars. Pediatrics 1982;70:21–5.

22. Christophersen ER, Sosland-Edelman D, LeClaire S. Evaluation of two comprehensive infant car seat loaner programs with 1-year follow-up. Pediatrics 1985;76(1):36–42.

23. Reisenger KS, Williams AF, Wells JK, et al. Effect of pediatricians' counseling on infant restraint use. Pediatrics 1981;67(2):201–6.

24. Scherz RG. Restraint systems for the prevention of injury to children in automobile accidents. Am J Pub Health 1976;66(5):451–6.

25. Liberato CP, Eriacho B, Schmiesing J, Krump M. SafeSmart Safety Seat Intervention Project: a successful program for the medically-indigent. Patient Edu Counsel 1989;13:161–70.

26. Bass JL, Mehta KA, Ostrovsky M. Childhood injury prevention in a suburban Massachusetts population. Pub Health Rep 1991;106(4):437–42.

27. Kelly B, Sein C, McCarthy P. Safety education in a pediatric primary care setting. Pediatrics 1987;79(5):818–24.

28. Guyer B, Gallagher S, Chang B-H, et al. Prevention of childhood injuries: evaluation of the Statewide Childhood Injury Prevention Program (SCIPP). Am J Pub Health 1989;79:1521–7.

29. Bull MJ, Stroup KB, Gerhart S. Misuse of car safety seats. Pediatrics 1988;81(1):98–101.

30. Campbell H, Macdonald S, Richardson P. High levels of incorrect use of car seat belts and child restraints in Fife—an important and under-recognised road safety issue. Injury Prevention 1997;3:17–22.

31. Macknin ML, Gustafson C, Gassman J, Barich D. Office education by pediatricians to increase seat belt use. Am J Dis Child 1987;141:1305–7.

32. Miller JR, Pless IB. Child automobile restraints: evaluation of health education. Pediatrics 1977;59(6):907–11.

33. Bass LW, Wilson TR. The pediatrician's influence in private practice measured by a controlled seat belt study. Pediatrics 1964;33:700–4.

34. Baker S, Li G, Fowler C, Dannenberg A. Injuries to bicyclists: a national perspective. Baltimore, Maryland: The Johns Hopkins University Injury Prevention Center; 1993.

35. Graitcer PL, Kellerman AL, Christoffel T. A review of educational and legislative strategies to promote bicycle helmets. Injury Prevention 1995;1(2):122–9.

36. Cushman R, Down J, MacMillan N, Waclawik H. Helmet promotion in the emergency room following a bicycle injury: a randomized trial. Pediatrics 1991;88(1):43–7.

37. Kim AN, Rivara FP, Koepsell TD. Does sharing the cost of a bicycle helmet promote helmet use? Injury Prevention 1997;3:38–42.

38. Cushman R, James W, Waclawik H. Physicians promoting bicycle helmets for children: a randomized trial. Am J Pub Health 1991;81(8):1044–6.

39. National Center for Injury Prevention and Control. Home and leisure injuries in the United States: a compendium of articles from the Morbidity and Mortality Weekly Report, 1985-1995. Atlanta, Georgia: Centers for Disease Control and Prevention; 1996.

40. Bass JL, Mehta KA, Ostrovsky M, Halperin SF. Educating parents about injury prevention. Pediatr Clin N Am 1985;32(1):233–41.

41. Miller RE, Reisenger KS, Blatter MM, Wucher F. Pediatric counseling and subsequent use of smoke detectors. Am J Pub Health 1982;72(4):392–3.

42. Clamp M, Kendrick D. A randomised controlled trial of general practitioner safety advice for families with children under 5 years. Br Med J 1998;316:1576–9.

43. Dershewitz RA, Williamson JW. Prevention of childhood household injuries: a controlled clinical trial. Am J Pub Health 1977;67(12):1148–53.

44. Dershewitz RA. Will mothers use free household safety devices? Am J Dis Child 1979;133:61–4.

45. Thomas KA, Hassanein RS, Christophersen ER. Evaluation of group well-child care for improving burn prevention practices in the home. Pediatrics 1984;74(5):879–82.

46. Katcher M, Landry G, Shapiro M. Liquid-crystal thermometer use in pediatricians' office counseling about tap water burn prevention. Pediatrics 1989;83:766–71.

47. Baker SP, O'Neill B, Ginsburg MJ, Li G. The injury fact book. 2nd ed. New York: Oxford University Press; 1992.

48. National Committee for Injury Prevention and Control. Injury prevention: meeting the challenge. New York: Oxford University Press; 1989.

49. Dershewitz RA, Posner MK, Paichel W. The effectiveness of health education on home use of ipecac. Clin Pediatr 1983;22:268–70.

50. Alpert JJ, Levine MD, Kosa J. Public knowledge of ipecac syrup in the management of accidental poisonings. J Pediatr 1967;71(6):890–4.

51. Woolf A, Lewander W, Filippone G, Lovejoy F. Prevention of childhood poisonings: efficacy of an educational program carried out in an emergency clinic. Pediatrics 1987;80(3):359–63.

52. American Academy of Clinical Toxicology, European Association of Poisons Centers and Clinical Toxicologists. Poison statement: Ipecac syrup. Clin Toxicol 1997;35(7):699–709.

53. Kravitz H, Grove M. Prevention of accidental falls in infancy by counseling mothers. Illinois Med J 1973;144:570–3.

54. Cohen LR, Runyan CW, Downs SM, Bowling JM. Pediatric injury prevention counseling priorities. Pediatrics 1997;99(5):704–10.

55. Miller TR, Galbraith M. Injury prevention counseling by pediatricians: a benefit-cost comparison. Pediatrics 1995;96(1):1–4.

56. Wright MS. Pediatric injury prevention: preparing residents for patient counseling. Arch Pediatr Adolesc Med 1997;151:1039–43.

CHAPTER 15

Fever

Amir Shanon, MD, MPA

————

Fever is defined as body temperature above the normal range. Normal body temperatures vary throughout the day, following a regular cycle ranging from 36° C to 37.8° C. The lowest body temperature occurs in the early morning hours (2:00 to 4:00 am), and the highest temperature occurs in the late afternoon. The difference between the lowest and highest temperatures may be as much as 0.5°C. Body temperature may also increase as a result of too much clothing or strenuous exercise, especially during hot weather.

Variations in temperature also depend on the body site where temperature is measured. A rectal temperature ≥ 38.0°C as well as an oral temperature ≥ 37.5°C indicates the presence of fever.

Wunderlich,[1] regarded as the first scientist who gave 37°C its special meaning for normal body temperature, described the diurnal variations of body temperature and alerted clinicians to the fact that "normal body temperature" is actually a temperature range rather than a specific temperature.

Fever is a symptom, not a disease. For a long time, fever has been recognized as a cardinal sign of disease; often, it is the only sign of a disease found on physical examination. Fever is the normal response to various viral and bacterial infections.

Fever can be regarded as a risk factor for bacterial infections; however, distinguishing viral and bacterial infections and evaluation of the severity of illness on the basis of fever characteristics (pattern, degree) alone, are difficult.

Fever is common during childhood illnesses. Some investigators claim that fever is an integral part of the immunologic function and of the defense mechanisms and therefore should not be treated. Opinions differ regarding whether patients are better off with or without fever, whether fever is "good or bad." Once it is decided that fever has to be treated, other concerns come into play, as it has been shown that parents' lack of knowledge of antipyretic medication and of accuracy and correctness of dosing is alarming. According to one study,[2] only 67 percent of parents accurately measured the amount of medication to be given to their children; 43 percent gave the correct amount, and only 30 percent accurately measured and gave the correct dose to their children.

Antipyretic medication is not expected to affect the course of the disease causing the fever and is usually given due to concern for the comfort of the child. Antipyretic drug use is widespread, and it is therefore important to make sure that those given to children are safe and efficacious.

Although fever, in itself, is harmless, parents' fear of fever, also termed "fever phobia," is common. Fever phobia is the cause for many unnecessary visits to the physician and improper use of fever medications and other methods used to bring the temperature down at all costs. Optimal management of the febrile child—combining the findings from the history, physical examination, and laboratory tests—has not been clearly defined yet and should be tailored on an individual basis.

FEVER PHOBIA

Schmitt[3] first described the concept of parental fever phobia and demonstrated a high prevalence of unrealistic fears of fever in parents of febrile children. Schmitt surveyed parents of

81 children about their understanding of fever. The survey was carried out in a hospital-based pediatric clinic. Most parents were worried about low-grade fever, and 85 percent of them gave antipyretic medicine for temperatures of 38.9°C and 56 percent treated temperatures of 37 to 37.8°C with antipyretics. Ninety-four percent of parents believed that fever could cause side effects, including dehydration, brain damage, blindness, convulsions, coma, and death; 52 percent believed that fever of 40°C or less could cause serious neurologic consequences. Many of the children were not acutely ill at the time of the visit, and yet 63 percent of the parents "worried lots" about possible harmful effects from fever and 36 percent "worried some."

Fifty-seven percent of the families surveyed had one child; 14 percent of all families had only one child younger than 6 months of age, and hence their past experience with febrile illnesses might have been limited. In addition, Schmitt's findings were based on a largely indigent, inner-city population. A later study[4] found similar attitudes prevailing among middle- and upper-middle class parents as well. This prospective study surveyed parents of 202 febrile children, 6 months to 6 years old, who visited a private pediatric group practice for a chief complaint of fever. Parents' knowledge, attitudes, and fears concerning fever and its treatment were studied. Forty-eight percent of the parents considered temperatures less than 38°C to be fever; 43 percent felt temperature less than 40°C could be dangerous to the child; 15 percent believed that if left untreated, temperature could rise to 42°C or higher. The dangers feared by the parents included death (11 percent), permanent brain damage or stroke (27 percent), and febrile seizures or loss of consciousness (48 percent). Twenty-one percent of the parents advocated treatment of temperatures less than 38°C and 97 percent advocated treatment of temperatures less than 40°C.

Parents of young infants had a higher threshold for what they considered a fever. These views were not related to the age of the responding parent or the presence of other children in the household. Most attitudes did not indicate an association with socioeconomic status, although parents of higher socioeconomic status were significantly more concerned about the risk of brain damage and seizures as sequelae of fever than were parents of lower socioeconomic status. It was suggested that undue parental anxiety about the dangers of fever might lead to excessive use of antipyretic medication.

The overall number of parents surveyed in these two studies was relatively small, both studies took place in the 1980s, and similar studies have not been repeated since. Fever, however, is still a common cause for visits to the doctor, partly, we assume, because fever phobia still exists. The authors of these surveys advocated education of parents by caregivers as a solution to the "fever phobia" phenomenon. The role of education in the management of this and other pediatric issues is controversial.

In one study, 151 pediatricians, with a median of 10 years in practice in primary or episodic care in subspecialties or in both disciplines, were surveyed.[5] Sixty-five percent agreed that an elevated body temperature in and of itself could become dangerous to a child, while 28 percent disagreed with this statement. Of the pediatricians who believed fever could be dangerous, 60 percent cited temperatures of ≥ 104°F as significant. Seizures were cited as the most frequent complication of fever (58 percent). Other complications included dehydration (23 percent), brain damage (10 percent), and obtundation (9 percent). When asked about "the most serious complication" of fever, 26 percent added death to the list. Just over 9 percent of respondents treated fever of less than 101°F, while 89 percent routinely treated fever between 101 and 102°F. Seventy-one percent recommended treatment to bring down the fever for the comfort of the child, and 88 percent agreed that a child with fever who is sleeping should be left undisturbed. Eighty percent of the respondents always or often tried to educate parents and children about fever.

One might question whether the findings presented in this study could be extrapolated to other pediatric centers or other pediatricians. The sample size was relatively small, only

64 percent of the surveyed pediatricians answered the questionnaire, and, as suggested by the authors themselves, certain responders might have misinterpreted some of the questions. The findings of this study do suggest, however, that fever phobia may be due in part to the incomplete and mixed messages pediatricians convey to parents.

In conclusion, there is fair evidence that parents and caregivers are overconcerned about fever. Whether fever phobia does or does not exist depends, at least to some extent, on the answer to the question: "Is fever good or bad?"

IS FEVER GOOD OR BAD?

Mackowiack in his review article[6] mentions that fever has been defined "as a state of elevated core temperature." The elevated core temperature is often, but not necessarily, part of the defensive response of multicellular organisms (host) to the invasion of live microorganisms or inanimate matter recognized as pathogenic or alien by the host. During fever, the host behaves as if its thermoregulatory "set point" is elevated.[7]

There are substantial data indicating the potentiating and inhibitory effects of the febrile response on resistance to infection. However, there is no consensus about the appropriate clinical situations, if any, in which fever or its mediators should be suppressed.

Fever has a long phylogenetic history, and data illustrating its beneficial effects originate from several studies. Mammals, reptiles, amphibians, and fish have been shown to manifest fever in response to challenge with microorganisms. Furthermore, enhanced resistance of animals to infection with increased body temperature within the physiologic range has been demonstrated. Suppression of the febrile response results in a substantial increase in mortality.[8–10]

Like animal data, clinical data include evidence of the beneficial effects of fever and the adverse effects of antipyretics on the outcome of infections. In a retrospective analysis of 218 patients with gram-negative bacteremia, Byrant and colleagues reported a positive correlation between elevated temperature on the day of bacteremia and survival. Mortality rate was higher in those patients who did not develop fever.[11] In an examination of factors influencing the prognosis of spontaneous bacterial peritonitis, Weinstein and colleagues[12] identified a positive correlation between a temperature reading of more than 38° C and survival. The author concluded that body temperature elevation indicated better function of host defense mechanisms that, when present, add to a person's ability to withstand the infection process.

Doran and colleagues[13] in a randomized, double-blind, placebo-controlled trial, found that children with chickenpox who are treated with acetaminophen had a longer time (1.1 days) to total crusting of lesions than placebo-treated control subjects. The number of days until complete resolution of the varicella lesions was virtually identical in the two groups. On day 2, children in the treated group were more active compared with those in the placebo group. On the other hand, they had more itching on day 4.

There was no difference between groups in any of the scaled symptoms (itching, activity, appetite, or overall condition) when symptoms were analyzed for trends over time. It should be stressed, however, that many of the children studied were not febrile during their illness and that the validity of the study results depended on the accuracy of the parent's diaries.

Stanely and colleagues[14] reported that adults infected with rhinovirus exhibit longer duration of nasal shedding when they receive aspirin than when given placebo. Graham and colleagues[15] in a double-blind, randomized, placebo-controlled study, intranasally challenged 60 healthy volunteers with rhinovirus. They were then randomized to one of four treatment arms: aspirin, acetaminophen, ibuprofen, or placebo. Use of aspirin and acetaminophen was associated with suppression of serum neutralizing antibody response and with increased nasal symptoms and signs. The effect of ibuprofen on antibody level was weaker and did not differ significantly from that of placebo. Aspirin, acetaminophen, and ibuprofen did not significantly increase virus shedding in comparison with placebo, although the duration of shedding in the aspirin and acetaminophen groups tended to be slightly longer.

It should be stressed that both studies included volunteers who were challenged with the virus, and it was not clear whether they were febrile at all. The effect of the antipyretic medication in the studied population might be different, compared with patients who suffer from a "natural" viral disease.

The data in these studies could be interpreted in different ways and do not necessarily prove a causal relationship between fever and improved prognosis during infection. However, they do constitute strong circumstantial evidence that fever is an adaptive response in most situations. There is good evidence that fever has a significant role in modulating the immunologic system during an infection; however, proof of beneficial or adverse effects of fever and/or antipyretic medication on the outcome of infections has yet to be established.

Accepting the notion that antipyretics have no real effect on the illness,[16] the treatment of febrile children with antipyretics should be reserved for those who have the greatest need for relief. The main indication for prescribing an antipyretic medication is not to reduce the temperature but to relieve the child's discomfort and thereby, anxiety in the parents. We should treat the child, not the thermometer. A febrile child who is uncomfortable, irritable, and anorectic could benefit from antipyretic treatment.[16]

ASSESSMENT SCALES TO MEASURE SEVERITY OF ILLNESS

How can we assess whether a child having fever is critically ill or not? Physicians who care for acutely ill children recognize the characteristic called "toxicity" on the basis of their clinical impression that the child "looks sick" or "acts sick." Although decisions regarding the management of the febrile child are frequently based on this clinical judgment about severity of illness, few attempts have been made to quantify toxicity or severity of illness in a consistent and reproducible manner.

Two investigators have created different scales, which were meant to detect serious illnesses in pediatric patients and to demonstrate the association between a febrile child's appearance and the presence or absence of serious illness.

Nelson[17] studied 1,106 consecutive patients with nontraumatic complaints presenting to a pediatric emergency room. The patients had 97 different diagnoses. The five best predictors of clinical severity of acute pediatric illness were respiratory effort, skin color, activity or level of consciousness, temperature, and the functional status variable of playing. Each variable received two points, a score of 10 was designated not sick and 7 or fewer points as very sick. The score was validated by comparing it with the physician's assessment of the patients' condition as rated on the linear analogue scale— no or mild illness, moderate illness, or severe illness.

According to the physicians, 551 children had no or mild illnesses. An index score of 8 or higher correctly identified 522 of these children giving the index a sensitivity of 94.7 percent for this diagnosis. Of the 81 children with clinically severe illnesses, 57 (70.4 percent), had a score of 7 or less, and 75 (92.6 percent) had a score of 9 or less.

The author stated that the index was meant to be used to triage patients in an emergency room setting. It was meant to be used as a screening device rather than as a substitute for evaluation by a health professional. Objective measures such as laboratory tests and, specifically, the ultimate outcome of the illness were not used to validate the index.

Waskerwitz[18] later used the index, studying 292 febrile children under the age of 2 years, with initial temperatures of 39.5°C or higher. The physicians' assessment was based on the functional status examination reported by Nelson,[17] which was used to organize the information obtained from the parents regarding the child's eating, drinking, sleeping, and play activities. After this information and the remaining history were elicited, the physician performed a physical examination, listed the initial diagnosis, and determined whether bacteremia existed, using an arbitrary scoring system. Physicians of different levels of pediatric training performed the scoring; 5.8 percent of the patients had bacteremia.

The physicians' assessment was the most useful factor in predicting bacteremia—predictive value 14 percent, specificity 83 percent, sensitivity 47 percent. The physicians' assessment reliably separated those patients at risk and identified all patients with serious complications. The evaluation process, however, was cumbersome and not easy to reproduce.

McCarthy and colleagues, in a series of studies,[19,20] developed a different scale. The scale was later used[21] to study the occurrence and positive predictive value of the history and physical examination findings suggestive of serious illnesses in ill-appearing and well-appearing febrile children. One hundred and three consecutive children aged 24 months and less with fever ≥ 38.3°C were studied. The children were evaluated by using the scale. Two attending physicians and a resident took the history. The physical examination was performed by one of the attending physicians and the resident. The history and physical examination were scored as to whether they did or did not suggest a serious illness. Serious illness was defined as the presence of a positive laboratory test.

This study investigated the interaction between a febrile child's appearance, history, and physical examination findings and the presence of serious illness. The study answered the following two questions: (1) Do ill-appearing febrile children more frequently have a history and physical examination findings that suggest a serious illness than well-appearing children? (2) Do ill-appearing febrile children with abnormal history and physical examination findings more often have a serious illness as defined by a positive laboratory test than well-appearing febrile children with abnormal findings?

The scale included the following parameters: (1) quality of cry: strong, whimpering, or weak; (2) reaction to parent stimulation: is content or cries briefly then stops, cries off and on, or cries continuously; (3) state variation: if awake stays awake; if asleep and stimulated, wakes up quickly; awakes with prolonged stimulation; or will not rouse; (4) color; (5) hydration; (6) response (talk, smile) to social overtures. Each parameter was scored 1 point when normal, 3 points when there was a moderate impairment, and 5 points when there was a severe impairment. If a child had a score greater than 10, he was defined as ill-appearing, and if the score was 10 or less, the child was said to be well-appearing.

For the purpose of the study, a serious illness was defined as an illness associated with one or more of the following abnormal laboratory results: a bacterial pathogen isolated from the cerebrospinal fluid (CSF), blood, urine, stool, deep soft tissue or pleura, an infiltrate seen on chest radiography, abnormal values of serum electrolytes, or hypoxemia during lower respiratory tract infection. The patients were followed up until the illness resolved.

The results of this study indicated that an ill-appearing febrile child with abnormal physical findings almost always has a serious illness (79 percent). Conversely, the well-appearing child with abnormal findings on physical examination has an underlying serious illness much less frequently (25 percent).

These studies originated in the late 1980s, and unlike Apgar and other similar scores, scales evaluating "toxicity" in the child, as such, have not become a routine in the daily work of pediatricians. Nevertheless, evaluation of "toxicity" is paramount in the assessment and management of the febrile ill-appearing child. In practice, physicians use their clinical judgment without attributing to it a specific score. The management of the febrile child is beyond the scope of this chapter; however, it is important to note that this issue is still debated and controversial. Practice guidelines for the management of infants and children have been developed[22] and also have been criticized.[23]

Clinical impression of toxicity is integrated into the practice guidelines as one component among others; however, specific scales or specific parameters from observational scales are not. The more important components of the practice guidelines include the findings on physical examination and, most of all, the results of laboratory tests. The management of the child depends on a combination of the findings and results of all these.

The management of the febrile child is influenced by the child's age, the management being more aggressive in neonates and infants 3 to 36 months of age. For many years, the prevailing policy in most academic centers was routine hospitalization of febrile neonates and antibiotic treatment following a complete sepsis work-up (obtaining CSF, blood, and urine cultures), pending their results. This attitude was based on a number of facts: first, the risk of bacteremia was higher in the younger age groups; second, clinical evaluation alone was not sufficient in predicting severity of disease; and third, the degree and pattern of fever could not distinguish between the mildly ill and the severely ill patients.

The management of 2 to 3-month-old infants as well as those under 2 years of age was, and still is, debated. While some authors favor aggressive management, namely, blood cultures and commencing parenteral antibiotic treatment pending their results, others favor the observant and expectant attitude, taking into account the fact that the hospitalization and treatment of these children carry their own risks.[24]

Febrile children can be separated into two groups—the low-risk and the high-risk groups. Close follow-up is always the mainstay of the management of all febrile children; however, those belonging to the low-risk group can be managed on an ambulatory basis, with or without antibiotic treatment.

Economic considerations have become a major factor influencing decision making concerning the management of patients. Another important factor that should be accounted for is the development of resistance to antibiotics. Resistance to antibiotics is on the rise, whereas the introduction of new antibiotics lags behind. It is also important to note that since the introduction of the Haemophilus type b vaccine, the incidence of bacteremia has dramatically decreased.[25]

Considering all the pros and cons, we believe that the risks of hospitalization and increased resistance to antibiotics due to the overuse of antibiotics outweigh the 1.6 percent risk of bacteremia. The observant and expectant attitude in the management of the febrile child is, therefore, justified. Each child should be evaluated and managed on an individual basis, taking into account factors such as availability of follow-up and knowledge of the caregivers. Good evidence to support one attitude over another is still lacking, and the issue, therefore, remains unsettled.

BEST MEDICATIONS AND METHODS FOR REDUCTION OF TEMPERATURE

Since it was advised not to prescribe aspirin routinely for children under 12 years of age because of a possible association with Reye's Syndrome, there are two other main options: acetaminophen and ibuprofen. Confidence in acetaminophen results from its longstanding use. Ibuprofen has been available since 1990 as an antipyretic, although it is not recommended for use for children under two years of age because of insufficient clinical experience. As ibuprofen belongs to the group of nonsteroidal anti-inflammatory agents, it might have adverse effects on the gastrointestinal and renal systems and might be unhelpful in asthmatic patients.

The safety and efficacy of acetaminophen and ibuprofen, by themselves or in comparison with one another or with placebo, have been looked into in numerous clinical studies. Overall, these studies support the use of each medication, and one can therefore conclude that both are safe and efficacious. It is important, however, to note that the variety of outcome measures and the use of different dosages of both medications complicate the comparison among these studies. Factors adding to the difficulty in comparing these medications include different settings— patients admitted to hospital wards in some cases and outpatients in others; variations in the ages of children enrolled in the studies; and variability of the underlying disease.

Accumulating evidence from studies comparing the use of single doses of both acetaminophen and ibuprofen in the treatment of febrile children supports the use of both medications. Randomized controlled studies[26,27] found both medications to be effective at dosages ranging from 10 to 15 mg/kg for acetaminophen and from 5 to 10 mg/kg for ibuprofen. In our view, however, the more important studies are those comparing the longterm effects and safety of ibuprofen and acetaminophen, when multiple doses of both medications are used in the treatment of febrile children.

Three studies addressed this question. The first study[28] took place in pediatric wards and included 150 patients, aged 2 months to 12 years, suffering from different common pediatric illnesses. This was a double-blind, parallel-group, randomized study using multiple doses of antipyretic medicines. Children having axillary temperatures higher than 37.5°C were treated with antipyretic medication. Outcome measures included palatability of the medication, changes in irritability and clinical condition, reduction of fever, overall efficacy at the end of the treatment, and the number and nature of encountered adverse effects. Ibuprofen 20 mg/kg/24h and acetaminophen 50 mg/kg/24h were given.

It was concluded that ibuprofen suspension was as effective, palatable, and well tolerated as acetaminophen in the treatment of fever in young children. Adverse effects presumably caused by ibuprofen included urticarial rash, vomiting, and abdominal pain. Adverse effects presumably caused by acetaminophen included sore throat, nose bleed, and purpuric rash at the site of the blood pressure cuff. No significant difference was found between the two medications. Most adverse events were mild in nature and had a doubtful or no relationship to therapy.

The second study[29] compared ibuprofen given in three different doses (2.5 mg/kg, 5 mg/kg, and 10 mg/kg) with acetaminophen given at a dosage of 15 mg/kg, for 24 to 48 hours. This too was a prospective, randomized, double-blind, parallel-group study using multiple doses of both medications. A control group was not included since it was believed it was ethically unjustifiable.

The study took place in a pediatric ward and included 64 children, aged 6 months to 11 years. These children had fever higher than 39°C (measured orally or rectally), lasting less than 48 hours. Fever was due to an infectious illness. Multiple doses of ibuprofen and acetaminophen were given at 6-hour intervals. Outcome measures included fever reduction and the number and nature of adverse effects.

It was found that the first doses of ibuprofen (10 mg/kg) and acetaminophen (15 mg/kg) were more effective in reducing fever than ibuprofen given a dosage of 2.5mg/kg and 5 mg/kg, when these were first given. From the second dose and up, however, all four were equally effective. As far as adverse effects were concerned, ibuprofen caused sweating and gastrointestinal upset, while acetaminophen caused hypothermia, abdominal pain, agitation, and nervousness. All adverse effects were, at most, of moderate nature. It was concluded that ibuprofen 10 mg/kg and acetaminophen 15 mg/kg were equally effective and equally well tolerated.

The third study,[30] a multicenter, double-blind, randomized, parallel-group study, included 151 patients, aged 6 months to 5 years, with fever greater than 38°C. All children suffered from an infectious disease, were hospitalized, and were treated with antibiotics (amoxycillin or augmentin).

Fever was treated with ibuprofen 7.5 mg/kg or acetaminophen 10 mg/kg. The second dose was given regardless of the degree of hyperthermia, and the subsequent doses were given at 6-hour intervals if the temperature was above 37.8°C. The temperature was measured rectally with a mercury thermometer.

During the first 72 hours, 9 patients who were treated with ibuprofen suffered adverse effects (5 gastrointestinal symptoms, 3 skin reactions, 1 case of epistaxis). Five of the patients treated with acetaminophen suffered adverse effects (2 gastrointestinal symptoms, 2 skin reactions, 1 epistaxis).

Table 15–1 Summary of Interventions for Treating a Febrile Child

Condition	Intervention	Quality of Evidence	Recommendations
Febrile uncomfortable child with presumed viral infection	Antipyretics	I	A
Febrile uncomfortable child	Sponging with tepid water	I	C
Febrile child	Assessment scale	II-2	B

In the percentage of temperature reduction at 4 hours, ibuprofen was superior. Acceptability of medication was higher in the acetaminophen group; however, there was no statistically significant difference between the two medications, and both were equally efficacious.

According to these and other studies, there is good evidence to support the recommendation that acetaminophen and ibuprofen are equally effective and safe and that, therefore, both drugs have an established place in managing febrile children.

TEPID SPONGE BATHING

The efficacy of tepid sponge bathing in reducing fever in young children has been studied in a number of randomized controlled studies. The efficacy of tepid water sponging in reducing temperature was compared with the use of acetaminophen alone[31–33] or with the use of the three antipyretic medications: aspirin, acetaminophen, and ibuprofen.[34]

During the first 30 minutes of intervention, sponging was found to be more effective than antipyretic medication in reducing body temperature; however, after 60 minutes, the effects of each medication became superior to sponging with tepid water. Furthermore, subjects in the sponging study group had significantly higher discomfort scores.[32] When using tepid water sponging alone, the possibility of rebound temperature increase 30 to 60 minutes after the bath could be anticipated.

In conclusion, tepid water sponging, when given in combination with antipyretic medication, during the first 30 minutes of intervention, may be superior to treatment with antipyretic medication alone. Tepid water sponging can cause discomfort and therefore should be reserved for the extremely uncomfortable child who has a very high temperature.

A summary of interventions for treating a febrile child is provided in Table 15–1.

REFERENCES

1. Wunderlich CA. On the temperature in diseases: a manual of medical thermometry. London: The New Sydenham Society; 1871:5.

2. Weinkle DA. Over the counter medications. Do parents give what they intend to give? Arch Pediatr Adolesc Med 1997;151:654–6.

3. Schmitt BD. Fever phobia. Misconceptions of parents about fevers. Am J Dis Child 1980;134:176–81.

4. Kramer MS, Naimark L, Leduc DG. Parental fever phobia and its correlates. Pediatrics 1985;75:1110–3.

5. May A, Bauchner H. Fever phobia: the pediatrician's contribution. Pediatrics 1992;90:851–4.

6. Mackowiack PA. Concepts of fever. Arch Intern Med 1998;158:1870–81.

7. Kluger MJ. Fever revisited. Pediatrics 1992; 90:846–9.

8. Kluger MJ, Ringler DH, Anver MR. Fever and survival. Science 1975;188:166–8.

9. Berenheim HA, Kluger MJ. Fever: effects of drug induced antipyresis on survival. Science 1976;193:237–9.

10. Covert JR, Reynolds WW. Survival value of fever in fish. Nature 1977;267:43–5.

11. Byrant RE, Hood AF, Koenig MG. Factors affecting mortality of gram negative rod bacteremia. Arch Intern Med. 1971;127:120–8.

12. Weinstein MR, Iannini PB, Staton CW, Eichoff TC. Spontaneous bacterial peritonitis: a review of 28 cases with emphasis on improved survival and factors influencing prognosis. Am J Med 1978;64:592–8.

13. Doran TF, DeAngelis C, Baumgardner RA, et al. Acetaminophen: more harm than good for chicken pox? J Pediatr 1989;114:1045–8.

14. Stanely ED, Jackson GG, Panusarn C, et al. Increased viral shedding with aspirin treatment of rhinovirus infection. JAMA 1975;231:1248–51.

15. Graham MH, Burrel CJ, Douglas RM, et al. Adverse effects of aspirin, acetaminophen, and ibuprofen on immune function, viral shedding, and clinical status in rhinovirus infected volunteers. J Infect Dis 1990;162:1277–82.

16. Kramer MS, Naimark LE, Brauer RR, et al. Risks and benefits of paracetamol antipyresis in young children with fever of presumed viral origin. Lancet 1991;337:591–4.

17. Nelson KM. An index of severity for acute pediatric illness. Am J Pediatr Health 1980:70:804–7.

18. Waskerwitz S, Berkelhamer JE. Outpatient bacteremia: clinical findings in children under two years with initial temperature of 39.5° C or higher. J Pediatr 1981;99:231–3.

19. McCarthy PL, Jekel JF, Stashwick CA, et al. Further definition of history and observation variables in assessing febrile children. Pediatrics 1981;67:687–93.

20. McCarthy PL, Sharpe MR, Spiesel SZ, et al. Observation scales to identify serious illness in febrile children. Pediatrics 1982;70:802–9.

21. McCarthy PL, Lembo RM, Baron MA, et al. Predictive value of abnormal physical examination findings in ill-appearing and well-appearing febrile children. Pediatrics 1985;76:167–72.

22. Baraff LJ, Bass JW, Fleisher GR, et al. Practice guidelines for the management of infants and children 0 –36 months of age with fever without source. Pediatrics 1993;92:1–12.

23. Kramer MS, Shapiro ED. Management of the young febrile child: a commentary on recent practice guidelines. Pediatrics 1997;100:128–34.

24. DeAngelis C, Joffe A, Willis E, Wilson M. Hospitalization and outpatient treatment of young, febrile infants. Am J Dis child 1983;137:1150–2.

25. Lee GM, Harper MB. Risk of bacteremia for febrile young children in the post *Haemophilus influenza* type b era. Arch Pediatr Adolesc Med 1998; 152:624–8.

26. Autret E, Reboul-Marty J, Henry-Launois B, et al. Evaluation of ibuprofen versus aspirin and paracetamol on efficacy and comfort in children with fever. Eur J Clin Pharmacol 1997;51:367–71.

27. Vauzelle-Kervroedan F, L'Athis P, Parinte-Khayat A, et al. Equivalent antipyretic activity of ibuprofen and paracetamol in febrile children. J Pediatr 1997;131(5):683–7.

28. McIntyre J. Comparing efficacy and tolerability of ibuprofen and paracetamol in fever. Arch Dis Child 1996;74(2):164–7.

29. Walson PD, Galetta G, Chomilo F, et al. Comparison of multidose ibuprofen and acetaminophen therapy in febrile children. Arch Pediatr Adolesc Med 1992;626–32.

30. Autert E, Breart G, Jonville AP, et al. Comparative efficacy and tolerance of ibuprofen syrup and acetaminophen syrup in children with pyrexia associated with infectious diseases and treated with antibiotics. Eur J Clin Pharmacol 1994;46:197–201.

31. Steele RW, Tanaka PT, Lara RP, Bass JW. Evaluation of sponging and of oral antipyretic therapy to reduce fever. J Ped 1970;77:824–9.

32. Sharber J. The efficacy of tepid sponge bathing to reduce fever in young children. Am J Emerg Med 1997;15(2):188-92.

33. Agbolosu NB, Cuevas LE, Milligan P, et al. Efficacy of tepid sponging versus paracetamol in reducing temperature in febrile children. Ann Trop Pediatr 1997;17(3):283-8.

34. Aksoylar S, Aksit S, Caglayan S, et al. Evaluation of sponging and antipyretics medication to reduce body temperature in febrile children. Acta Pediatr Jpn 1997;39(2):215-7.

CHAPTER 16

Screening for Anemia in Infants and Toddlers

Michael E.K. Moffatt, MD, FRCPC

ANEMIA IN INFANTS

Anemia is a state in which the quantity or quality of circulating red cells is reduced below the normal level.[1] Anemia is usually defined by measuring the concentration of hemoglobin in the blood. Defining normal levels for small children has been difficult, but consensus around several cut-off points has now been achieved.[2–4] Babies are born with a high hemoglobin level, often greater than 180 mL, but the value falls rapidly as fetal hemoglobin is converted to the adult type. The low point is reached between 2 and 4 months of age (110 g/L). Thereafter, it rises slowly throughout childhood, reaching adult levels after puberty. The normal range for children between 6 months and 2 years of age is between 110 and 130 g/L. Most authors agree with the World Health Organization standard of 110 g/L as the lower limit for children after the age of 6 months.

Anemia can be due to a wide array of causes. Deficiencies of hemopoietic factors, namely, iron, folate, and vitamin B_{12} are the most common, but for practical purposes, in the developed countries, only iron is a significant cause in children. Genetic causes of hemolytic anemia are the next largest group, followed by infectious causes (malaria being prominent in some tropical countries), and causes of increased blood loss.

An extensive review of population studies worldwide up to the early 1980s[1] estimated the prevalence of anemia for preschool children to be 10 percent in the developed countries, and on average 51 percent in the developing countries, with a wide range. Some examples of more recent studies show a decline in the prevalence in a middle-class population of children 9 to 23 months of age in Minneapolis from 6.2 percent in the early 1970s to 2.7 percent by 1986;[5] in Ottawa, a prevalence in infants, across a wide range of social class, of 3.6 percent in 1990;[6] a declining prevalence in Italian infants from 5.2 percent in 1983 to 1.3 percent in 1992;[7] in Sydney, Australia, a prevalence in toddlers of 1.2 percent in 1996.[8] Thus, the prevalence of anemia seems to be decreasing in the affluent parts of the developed countries. By contrast, there was still a rate of 21.2 percent in an inner city Boston population of 1-year-old infants in 1998[9] and 25 percent in the poorest districts of Montreal in 1991,[10] although the latter results are somewhat inflated due to the use of a cut-off point of 115 g/L. In a slum in India,[11] the prevalence was 76 percent, about two-thirds being iron deficiency anemia (IDA) and most of the rest due to deficiencies of folate and vitamin B_{12}. The gap in rates between the affluent and less affluent children is relevant when discussing issues of screening.

For practical purposes, iron deficiency is really the only cause of anemia that merits consideration of screening by means of hemoglobin measurement. It is, by far, the most common cause. In populations where genetic hemolytic anemias such as sickle cell disease or thalassemia are common, screening methods can be directly aimed at the diagnosis of interest, and it can be done at birth. The proportion of anemic children with iron deficiency also appeared to be falling in the middle-class population studied by Yip.[5]

SCREENING AND CASE FINDING

Screening implies systematically approaching the general public and offering a test at a time when they are not specifically seeking health advice. *Case finding* is done when a test is administered in the process of an office visit for some other purpose. The recommendation that each child have a hemoglobin between 6 and 12 months of age[12] is usually made in the doctor's office and falls into the category of case finding. There are several criteria that must be met before such an activity becomes worthwhile. First, the diagnostic test must be sufficiently accurate to identify the disease at an early stage before irreparable damage has been done. Second, the disease must have some significant consequences. Third, the disease must be treatable in an easily acceptable manner. Fourth, the screening must lead to early treatment and better outcomes rather than to treatment of the disease at the time when it has become symptomatic and would be diagnosed anyway.

In the case if IDA, there are a number of these points that remain in doubt with respect to current methods of testing and treatment. The process of becoming iron deficient is a lengthy one. Term infants are born with sufficient iron stores to maintain their iron status for about 4 months. After that, they must take adequate amounts of absorbable iron in their diets to avoid becoming iron deficient. Three stages of iron deficiency have been identified. First, the bone marrow stores become depleted. Subsequently, erythropoiesis is affected so that red blood cells become smaller, and the concentration of hemoglobin in the cells decreases. Finally, the hemoglobin level begins to fall. These stages may progress over months, depending on how much iron the infant consumes. The hemoglobin measurement is only useful in the third stage, and less severe iron deficiency may have existed for months.

The hemoglobin test is also not highly sensitive for the diagnosis of IDA. One study,[13] where the outcome was based on response to therapy, found a sensitivity of 66 percent and a specificity of 65 percent. Alternative tests include serum ferritin and free erythrocyte protoporphyrin (FEP). Ferritin has good sensitivity (86 percent) and specificity (92 percent), compared with bone marrow as the gold standard.[14] Unfortunately, it is an expensive test that is not widely accessible. Free erythrocyte protoporphyrin has some merit as another potential screening test that could detect IDA in the second stage.[15] It is inexpensive but is not widely used, partly due to the fact that it is elevated in other disease conditions, most notably lead poisoning. Values >0.9 mg/L are considered indicative of IDA. Levels >1.6 g/L overlap with those in children with lead poisoning.

The red blood cell indices are not useful as a screening tool. As IDA develops, microcytosis occurs and the amount of hemoglobin per red cell decreases. This results in changes in mean corpuscular volume (MCV), mean cell hemoglobin concentration (MCHC), and red cell distribution width (RDW). These indices are automatically measured in many laboratories that use Coulter counters. The lower limit of MCV for children 9 to 12 months is 70 fl. MCHC lower than 30 percent and RDW >13.5 are both indicative of IDA. However, the sensitivity and specificity are less than those of hemoglobin measurement. Taken together with hemoglobin measurement, they can be helpful, particularly as supporting evidence that a low hemoglobin level is due to IDA, but no one has advocated them as screening tests by themselves.

HOW HARMFUL IS IRON DEFICIENCY?

This is the crucial question in relation to recommendations around case finding or regular testing for IDA. While there are obvious complications such as heart failure in severe IDA, this type of problem is now very rare in the developed countries. It has been suggested that stroke may be another complication of IDA,[16] but it is also a rare occurrence, and the evidence for a causal association with iron is weak. The main focus and justification for concern is the possible, more subtle developmental effects of IDA. Since iron is involved in many enzyme processes in the developing brain, the idea is biologically plausible, and there is some animal evidence to support the claim.[17] Apart from iatrogenic disease, this is one of the rare times when there is a possibility of the highest level of evidence about causation—randomized controlled trials. While it is not ethically acceptable to make children iron deficient, there are several trials that provide solid evidence that iron-fortified formula milk can prevent IDA in most children.[18–20] There are many populations in both the developed and the developing countries that do not have easy access to iron-fortified formula milk. It is, therefore, ethical to provide an additional formula to some children who normally would not receive it and monitor their developmental progress. This has been done in at least three such studies.[18,20,21] One study found a lasting effect[18] on both psychological and motor developments, another a transient effect on motor development only,[20] and the third no effect over a 2-month period.[2]

Prevention studies are sometimes criticized for the fact that the IDA developing in control groups may not be very severe. An alternative experimental approach is to randomly assign children with IDA to treatment or placebo.[22–26] Such studies are currently on tenuous ethical ground because of the concern over the question of infant development. For ethical reasons, treatment according to assigned groups was often continued only for a very short time period when these studies were being done in the 1980s. Three of these studies showed a difference; in one study, iron was administered parenterally[22] and two studies had the longest duration of treatment.[25,26] The two short-term oral iron studies[23,24] showed no effect. There has yet to be a formal systematic review published on the topic, and at this point, the evidence remains unclear. The studies are listed in Table 16–1.

There has been quite consistent literature from cohort and case-control studies, which has confirmed an association between IDA and developmental delay.[27–34] Unfortunately, this type of evidence is unsatisfactory, even though some studies[29,34] have tried to control for the effects of social deprivation and poverty in the analysis. For this evidence (level II), it becomes impossible to separate subtle developmental effects of parenting practices and living conditions from the potential effects of IDA. Although closely associated with poor living conditions, the iron deficiency may still be an epiphenomenon, while the "cause" of the developmental delay may be the social conditions. Thus, this substantial body of literature has to be viewed with skepticism, and definitive knowledge of the developmental consequences of IDA will have to await further randomized controlled trials. However, on balance, there are more positive than negative experimental studies. There seems a reasonably strong possibility that iron deficiency does cause developmental delays, and treatment is effective and relatively innocuous.

TARGET FOR CASE FINDING

In middle-class populations in the developed countries, the prevalence of IDA has fallen to the point where aggressive case finding makes little sense. If, for example, the sensitivity and specificity of the hemoglobin test is only about 65 percent and the prevalence of anemia is 2 percent, then less than 1 in 20 positive tests will mean anemia is present (positive predictive value). Even when the prevalence rises to 10 percent, the positive predictive value is only 1 in 6. These numbers can be improved by using multiple tests (for example, the red blood cell indices) or by using a more expensive test like serum ferritin. The cost of one ferritin test is about the same as that of iron-fortified formula milk for a month and is many times greater than that of a course of oral iron.

It makes sense to test children who live in poor circumstances, particularly in the inner city areas of major urban centers and in rural areas with low income and education levels. Another marker that has been identified is children who are behind in their immunizations. Boutry and Needleman have recently shown that a simple dietary history in an urban core population of children over the age of 15 months has a moderately good specificity (79 per-

Table 16–1 Randomized Trials Assessing the Effect of Preventing or Treating IDA on Infant Development

Author	Year	Conclusion	Duration	Comments
Treatment Studies				
Oski[22]	1978	Intramuscular iron resulted in improvements in Bayley scores, 7 to 10 days later	1 week	Blinding unclear. Small sample. Statistical significance of results questionable
Lozoff[23]	1982	No difference in Bayley PDI or MDI after oral iron	1 week	
Lozoff[24]	1987	No difference in Bayley PDI or MDI	1 week	Guatemalan children with significant anemia
Aukett[25]	1986	Improvement in developmental score using DDST	2 months	Conclusion criticized because of inappropriate dichotomization of continuous data and the use of a screening test as an outcome measure
Idjradinata[26]	1993	Infants with IDA treated with iron. Bayley scores improved	4 months	Infants 12 to 18 mo
Prevention Studies				
Moffatt	1994	Bayley Psychomotor Index declined more in infants assigned to non–iron fortified formula at 9 and 12 months, but not at 15 months. Mental development showed no change in either group	Birth to 15 months	Significant losses to follow-up over time in this cohort
Lozoff	1996	No difference in Bayley scores of previously breast-fed infants between 6 and 12 months treated with oral iron or placebo	2 months	
Williams	1999	Differences in Griffith's scale score and personal social subscale in infants treated with iron-fortified formula versus cow's milk	Supplementation from 6 to 18 months. Followed to 24 months	Differences apparent at 24 months

PDI = Psychomotor Development Index; MDI = Mental Development Index; DDST = Denver Developmental Screening Test; IDA = iron deficiency anemia cent).[35] Dietary deficiency was defined as (1) less than five servings each of meat, grains, vegetables, and fruit per week; (2) more than 16 oz of milk per day; or (3) daily intake of fatty snacks, sweets, or more than 16 oz of soft drink. In their study, it was unnecessary to test children who did not have this history, thus excluding three-quarters of the children from the study. Whether this can be applied to younger children under the age of 1 year has not been tested, but it makes sense to target the testing at children who have not been getting iron-containing milk and are not breast fed. If useful, it could reduce the amount of testing needed even in situations of poverty. Other high-risk children are those born prematurely or with low birth weight.

TREATMENT OF IRON DEFICIENCY ANEMIA

When a child is documented to have IDA, treatment usually consists of 5 to 6 mg of elemental iron per kilogram per day in the form of ferrous sulfate. It is usually given in the form of drops. It should not be given with milk. Vitamin C increases the absorption of iron, and therefore a small amount of fruit juice is recommended as a "chaser." Lozoff documented excellent hematologic response to iron treatment in both American and Guatemalan children.[23,24,34] However, it is notably difficult to obtain compliance with iron therapy in inner city populations, and a great deal of family education effort is required. Recently,[36] it has been shown that iron adds little to the hematologic response in children who are already on iron-fortified formula milk. Children with IDA who are receiving whole milk should be switched to iron-fortified formula milk.

PREVENTION OF IRON DEFICIENCY ANEMIA: ALTERNATIVES TO CASE FINDING AND SCREENING

Primary prevention of IDA makes more sense than case finding. We have strong evidence (level II-2) that breast feeding protects against IDA at least until 4 months of age[37–39] and

Table 16–2 Summary of Recommendations

Condition	Intervention	Level of Evidence	Recommendation
Iron deficiency	Hemoglobin screening/case finding	III	High risk groups only at 9 to 12 months—LBW, poverty, underimmunized, children on whole milk with no iron added. Poor evidence as yet (C)
Developmental delay prevention	Prevention of iron deficiency	I	Conflicting results. Balance appears to be in favor of a causal relationship. Fair evidence to make prevention of IDA a priority (B)
Iron deficiency	Prevention by breast-feeding	III[6,37–39,45,46]	Breast-feeding should be encouraged for all infants for at least 6 months (B). If weaning occurs, the use of follow-on formula containing iron is recommended (B)
Iron deficiency	Prevention by iron-fortified formula	I[18–20,42–44]	All formula-fed infants for 12 mo

probably much longer in exclusively breast-fed infants,[40,41] since other foods seem to interfere with bioavailability of breast milk iron. Promotion of breast-feeding is recommended for this and other reasons.

Iron-fortified infant formula milk also reduces the incidence of IDA, compared with unfortified formula milk or cow's milk. The evidence here comes from well-conducted double-blind randomized controlled trials (level I) mainly in high-risk populations.[20,42,43] The effect is almost universally positive. Only one study found no difference,[44] and this may be attributed to a decreasing intake of milk in both groups. The fact that very few children in either group developed IDA suggests that this was not a truly high-risk group. Iron-fortified formula milk is recommended at least until 1year of age and is especially valuable in high-risk groups. When formula feeding is initiated at birth or in the first few months, a formula containing 8 or 12.7 g/L iron is usually recommended. In the follow-on formula for infants who have been breast-fed for 6 months, the amount of iron in the formula need not be very high, as Walter[43] has shown in his study in Chile, where a concentration of 2.3 mg/L was almost as good as one with 12.7 g/L. Infants who are weaned from breast milk before a year of age should be given a follow-on formula containing iron rather than plain cow's milk.

The summary of recommendations for interventions for IDA is provided in Table 16–2.

REFERENCES

1. DeMaeyer E, Adiels-Tegman M. The prevalence of anaemia in the world. World Health Stat Quart 1985;38:302–16.

2. Yip R. Age-related changes in laboratory values used in the diagnosis of anemia and iron deficiency. Am J Clin Nutr 1984;39:427–36.

3. Dallman PR, Siimes M, Stekel A. Percentile curves for hemoglobin and red cell volumes in infancy and childhood. J Pediatr 1979;94:26–31.

4. Saarinen V, Siimes M. Developmental changes in red blood cell counts and indices in infants after exclusion of iron deficiency by laboratory criteria and continuous iron supplementation. J Pediatr 1978;92:412–6.

5. Yip R, Walsh KM, Godlfarb MG, Binkin NJ. Declining prevalence of anemia in childhood in a middle-class setting: a pediatric success story? Pediatrics 1987;80:330–4.

6. Green-Finestone L, Feldman W, Heick H, Luke B. Prevalence and risk factors of iron deficiency anemia among infants in Ottawa-Carleton . Can Diet Assoc J 1991;52:20–3.

7. Salvioli GP, Faldella G, Alessandroni R, et al. Iron nutrition and iron status changes in Italian infants in the last decade. Ann 1st Super Sanita 1995;31:455–9.

8. Karr M, Alperstein G, Causer J, et al. Iron status and anaemia in preschool children in Sydney. Aust NZ J Public Health 1996;20:618–22.

9. Adams WG, Geva J, Coffman J, et al. Anemia and elevated lead levels in underimmunized inner-city children. Pediatrics 1998;101:E6.

10. Lehmann F, Gray-Donald K, Mongeon M, DiTommaso S. Iron deficiency anemia in 1-year-old children of disadvantaged families in Montreal. Can Med Assoc J 1992;146:1571–7.

11. Gomber S, Kumar S, Rusia U, et al. Prevalence and etiology of nutritional anaemias in early childhood in an urban slum. Ind J Med Res 1998;107:269–73.

12. Guidelines for Health Appraisal III. 3rd ed. Evanston, Illinois; American Academy of Pediatrics; 1997.

13. Freire WB. Hemoglobin as a predictor of response to iron therapy and its use in screening and prevalence estimates. Am J Clin Nutr 1989;50:1442–9.

14. Reibo E. Diagnosis of iron deficiency. Scand J Hematol 1985 (Suppl);43:5–39.

15. Yip R, Schwartz S, Deinard A. Screening for iron deficiency with the erythrocyte protoporphyrin tests. Pediatrics 1983;72:214–9.

16. Hartfield DS, Lowry NJ, Keene DL, Yager JY. Iron deficiency: a cause of stroke in infants and children. Pediatr Neurol 1997;16:50–3.

17. Lozoff B, Brittenham GM. Behavioral aspects of iron deficiency. Prog Hematol 1986;14:23–53.

18. Williams J, Wolff A, Daly A, et al. Iron supplemented formula milk related to reduction in psychomotor decline in infants from inner city areas: randomised study [process citation]. Br Med J 1999;318:693–8.

19. Daly A, MacDonald A, Aukett A, et al. Prevention of anaemia in inner city toddlers by an iron supplemented cows' milk formula. Arch Dis Child 1996;75:9–16.

20. Moffatt MEK, Lonstaffe S, Besant J, Dureski C. Prevention of iron deficiency and psychomotor decline in high risk infants through the use of iron-fortified infant formula: a randomized clinical trial. J Pediatr 1994;125:527–34.

21. Lozoff B, DeAndraca I, Walter T, Pino P. Does preventing iron deficiency anemia improve developmental scores? Pediatr Res 1996;39:136A–136A.

22. Oski FA, Honig AS. The effects of therapy on the developmental scores of iron-deficient infants. J Pediatr 1978;92:21–5.

23. Lozoff B, Brittenham GM, Wolff AW. The effects of short-term oral iron therapy on developmental deficits in iron-deficient anemic children. J Pediatr 1982;100:351–7.

24. Lozoff B, Brittenham GM, Wolff AW. Iron deficiency and iron therapy effects on infant developmental test performance. J Pediatr 1987;79:981–95.

25. Aukett MA, Parkes YA, Scott PH, Wharton BA. Treatment with iron increases weight gain and psychomotor development. Arch Dis Child 1986;61:849–57.

26. Idjradinata P, Pollitt E. Reversal of developmental delays in iron-deficient anaemic infants treated with iron [see comments]. Lancet 1993;341:1–4.

27. Deinard AS, List A, Lindren B, et al. Cognitive deficits in iron-deficient and iron-deficient anemic infants. J Pediatr 1986;108:681–9.

28. Domergues JP, Archambaud MP, Ducot B, et al. Iron deficiency and psychomotor development tests. Arch Fr Pediatr 1989;46:487–90.

29. Walter T, DeAndraca I, Chadud P, Perales CG. Iron deficiency anemia: adverse effects on infant development. Pediatrics 1989;84:7–17.

30. Lozoff B, Jiminez E, Wolff AW. Long-term developmental outcome of infants with iron deficiency. N Engl J Med 1991;325:687–94.

31. Oski FA, Honig AS, Helu B, Howantz P. Effect of iron therapy on behavior and performance in nonanemic, iron-deficient infants. Pediatrics 1983;71:877–80.

32. Lozoff B, Wolff AW, Urritia JJ, Viteri FE. Abnormal behavior and low developmental test scores in iron-deficient anemic infants. J Dev Behav Pediatr 1985;6:69–75.

33. Walter K, Kovalskys J, Stekel A. Effect of mild iron deficiency on mental developmental scores. J Pediatr 1983;102:519–22.

34. Lozoff B, Wolff AW, Jimenez E. Iron-deficiency anemia and infant development: effects of extended oral iron therapy. J Pediatr 1996;129:382–9.

35. Boutry M, Needlman R. Use of diet history in the screening of iron deficiency. Pediatrics 1996;98:1138–42.

36. Irigoyen M, Davidson LL, Carriero D, Seaman C. Randomized, placebo-controlled trial of iron supplementation in infants with low hemoglobin levels fed iron-fortified formula [erratum in Pediatrics 1992;90(3):474]. Pediatrics 1991;88:320–6.

37. Saarinen UM. Need for iron supplementation in infants on prolonged breast feeding. J Pediatr 1978;93:177–80.

38. Saarinen UM, Siimes M. Iron absorption from breast milk, cow's milk and iron-supplemented formula: an opportunistic use of changes in total body iron determined by hemoglobin, ferritin and body weight in 132 infants. Pediatr Res 1979;13:143–7.

39. Garry PJ, Owen GM, Hooper EM, Gilbert BA. Iron absorption from human milk and formula with and without iron supplementation. Pediatr Res 1981;15:822–8.

40. Pisacane A, De Vizia B, Valiante A, et al. Iron status in breast-fed infants. J Pediatr 1995;127:429–31.

41. Siimes MA, Salmenpera L, Perheentupa J. Exclusive breast-feeding for 9 months: risk of iron deficiency. J Pediatr 1984;104:196–9.

42. Gilld DG, Vincent S, Segal DS. Follow-on formula in the prevention of iron deficiency: a multicenter study. Acta Paediatr 1997;86:683–9.

43. Walter T, Pino P, Pizarro F, Lozoff B. Prevention of iron-deficiency anemia: comparison of high- and low-iron formulas in term healthy infants after six months of life. J Pediatr 1998;132:635–40.

44. Stevens D, Nelson A. The effect of iron in formula milk after 6 months of age. Arch Dis Child 1995;73:216–20.

CHAPTER 17

Urinary Tract Problems in Primary Care

Paul T. Dick, MDCM, MSc, FRCPC

The urinary tract system, including the kidneys, collecting system, bladder, and urethra, is the focus for numerous complaints and problems in childhood. A great variety of relatively rare conditions, such as severe developmental anomalies and glomerular diseases, involve secondary- or tertiary-care expertise or consultation. However, there are a few very common problems and issues that are often handled in primary-care practices. These include urinary tract infections (UTIs), nocturnal enuresis, and neonatal male circumcision.

URINARY TRACT INFECTIONS

Epidemiology

Diagnosis and management of urinary tract infections are probably the most common urinary tract issues that currently confront primary care practitioners as an acute-care problem. Urinary tract infections are considered one of the most common bacterial infections observed in childhood, rivaled only by ear, throat, and minor skin infections. However, there are few sound or recent population-based studies to provide reliable age-specific incidence rates of symptomatic UTIs and the natural history of UTIs.

Using a computerized registry of nine outpatient clinics and a childrens' hospital that provides virtually all the care for sick children in the city of Goteburg, Sweden, Marild and Jodal were able to estimate retrospectively the incidence rate of first UTIs with the census population as a denominator. They estimate that up to 1.8 percent of males and 6.6 percent of females were diagnosed with a symptomatic urinary tract infection by the time they reach 6 years of age. However, the incidence of urinary tract infections is not constant within this age group. There is fair evidence of a peak in incidence in the first year of life for males, with the rate of infections being equal between infant males and females at 7.7 and 9.7 per year per 1,000 children at risk (ie, no prior infection), respectively. However, the incidence rate in females peaks in early childhood. It declined slowly to 2 to 5 per year per 1,000 children at risk aged 3 to 6 years. The incidence rate for males declined more rapidly and to less than 1 per year per 1,000 for males older than a year of age. The incidence of UTIs in males is affected by the circumcision status, with an incidence rate of hospitalization in the first year of 7.0 per 1,000 in uncircumcised males compared with 1.9 per 1,000 in males circumcised in the neonatal period.[2]

Many children with a first urinary tract infection will go on to develop recurrent urinary tract infections. However, no sound population-based, age- and sex-specific rates of recurrence have been published. The best estimates come from descriptive studies that suggest that up to 32 percent of male and 40 percent of female children with a first UTI may subsequently experience one or more additional urinary tract infections.[3] The risk of recurrence is highest within the year following an infection. A small group of children go on to experience repeated UTIs. Descriptive studies suggest that children with underlying neurologic, and urologic abnormalities (such as vesicoureteral reflux) and voiding dysfunction are at a greater risk of recurrence.

Etiology

The organisms involved in UTIs in children come from a fairly narrow spectrum of organisms that normally colonize the perineum and gastrointestinal tract. In over 85 percent of cases, the organism involved is *Escherichia coli*. Other organisms include *Proteus* species, *Klebsiella* species, and *Enterococcus faecalis*. A detailed review of the etiology and the pathophysiology of UTIs in children is beyond the scope of this chapter. The bulk of epidemiology and pathophysiology research supports the general belief that UTIs in children are the result of a variety of factors, including bacterial virulence factors and host factors.[4] Both fimbrial and bacterial adhesin molecules facilitate the ability of fecal coliforms, in particular the P-fimbriae of *Escherichia coli*, to adhere to mucosal surfaces including the uroepithelium. In addition, the organisms responsible for infection appear to be able to multiply rapidly, despite the high osmolality and the concentration of urea in urine. Also, uropathogenic strains of *Escherichia coli* have features enabling them to resist lysis, avoid phagocytosis, and cause direct uroendothelial damage. Using these advantages, it appears that these uropathogenic organisms are able to colonize and ascend the urinary tract of affected hosts.

A variety of host factors have been postulated as accounting for a given individual's susceptibility to UTI. In general, these can be classified into three broad categories on the basis of their association with (1) bacterial virulence factors, (2) urinary tract anatomy, and (3) voiding physiology. Over time, there has been a tug of war over some of these concepts, with anatomy dominating in the first few decades of the past half century and virulence factors and voiding dysfunction receiving more attention in the most recent decade. Unfortunately, while there are many pathophysiology and descriptive studies seeking to address these risk factors, there are no sound estimates of the risk that all these factors confer at a population or primary-care practice level.

Bacterial Virulence

It is postulated that exposure to uropathogenic strains of organisms, the status of host receptors for attachment, and reduced immune protection or microbial competition account for much of the risk of UTIs.[4] There is some fair evidence from a case-control study that the infants of mothers who had bacteruria during pregnancy have up to four times the risk of UTI as those infants of nonbacteruric mothers.[5] There is also some evidence that breast-feeding and transfer of maternal IgA immunity may have a protective effect.[6] The role of *E. coli* receptor presence and density in the propensity to developing UTIs and pyelonephritis requires more research, as does the role of altered host flora secondary to antibiotic use.

Urinary Tract Anatomy

For decades, much of the focus for the etiology of UTIs has been on anatomic abnormalities and variations. However, there is currently only good quality epidemiologic evidence for two of these risk factors: sex and circumcision status. Published data on incidence rates of UTI consistently demonstrate that female children have approximately a 2- to 4-fold increased incidence of UTI compared with male children.[1] It is postulated that a number of anatomic differences account for this increased risk, including a shorter urethral segment and the susceptibility of the female periurethral mucosal membrane to heavy colonization with uropathogens. Several cohort studies have demonstrated a statistically significant reduction in the rate of UTIs amongst circumcised male infants.[2] More recent studies have generated modest relative risk reduction (3- to 4-fold) estimates for circumcised males.[2,7] These do not agree with the high relative risk reduction estimates (ie, over 10- to 40-fold) that were reported by Wiswell and others in the 1970s and 1980s.[96]

It has been postulated for decades that anatomic abnormalities associated with obstruction, urinary stasis, incomplete bladder emptying, and interference with the one-way valve function of the ureterovesicular junction create a significantly increased risk for UTI in children. However, there is poor epidemiologic evidence that underlying anomalies, such as vesi-coureteral reflux, are independently responsible for an increased risk of UTIs. Yet, there are many descriptive studies demonstrating vesicoureteral reflux in up to a third of children and obstructive lesions in up to 4 percent of selected children with their first UTI.[8] The observed frequency of anatomic abnormalities in these studies of children with UTIs appear to be greater than that of these conditions in the general child population.[9,10] In addition, case series of asymptomatic infants and children with vesicoureteral reflux diagnosed through antenatal ultrasonography or through screening because of siblings with reflux have been reported to have a risk of UTI of 15 percent.[11,12] This rate is higher than that expected for the corresponding general population but also suggests that the majority of children with reflux do not develop UTIs. These observations, together with the experiences of specialists fol-lowing up children with reflux and reflux nephropathy, continue to suggest that there is an association between anatomic abnormalities and UTI. However, the importance of these anomalies in all but a select population of children may well have been overstated in the past, and the exact relationship of these abnormalities in the etiology of urinary tract infections, including their interaction with voiding dysfunction and bacterial virulence factors, still awaits elucidation.

Voiding Physiology

The strong relationship between bacteriuria and/or recurrent symptomatic UTIs with the neuropathic bladder dysfunction associated with cerebral palsy and spina bifida has been widely recognized. With the advent and availability of urodynamic techniques for investi-gating voiding disturbances, there has been increased attention on the role of voiding phys-iology in the etiology of childhood UTIs in neurologically intact children. It has been postulated that urethral reflux and increased residual urine may be among the mechanisms by which UTIs are caused by voiding dysfunction. A number of descriptive studies have demonstrated the presence of abnormal urodynamic voiding patterns in referred children with chronic voiding problems associated with UTIs, recurrent UTIs, vesicoureteral reflux, and covert bacteriuria (ie, bacteriuria associated with some abnormalities in voiding habits, but no fever or dysuria).[13-15] The abnormalities described included bladder hypercontractil-ity/instability, sphincter dysynergia, reduced bladder capacity, and/or increased residual urine. The majority of these children also had corresponding histories of subacute or chronic voiding problems, including incontinence, enuresis, frequency, and urgency. While apparent abnormalities in urodynamics have been observed in infants hospitalized with their first UTI, it is not clear exactly when voiding abnormalities appear in the natural history of UTIs and when and whether they represent the cause and/or effect of UTIs.

Clinical Presentation

Children with UTIs present to a variety of clinical service settings. Though the majority of literature on childhood UTIs is based on children presenting to hospital emergency depart-ments or hospital-based clinics, a significant proportion of children do present to primary-care practice settings. However, the pattern of presentation has not been widely studied at a population level. In one retrospective population-based study, Marild and Jodal observed that 84 percent of children under 2 years of age were diagnosed with their first UTI at the hospital.[1] Of children 2 to 6 years of age, only 52 percent were diagnosed at the hospital. It is not known if these results are a fair representation of the situation in other communities.

Common Symptoms of Urinary Tract Infection

Children with UTIs present with a broad spectrum of signs and symptoms. In part, this is due to the fact that UTIs present at all ages. The specific signs of frequency and costoverte-bral angle tenderness and the symptoms of dysuria and flank pain that are readily elicited from a 6-year-old may not be evident on an assessment of a 6-month-old. Accordingly, it is difficult to rely on a stereotypical presentation for suspicion of UTI. Although fever is often observed with UTIs in children, it is insensitive as a lone criterion for suspecting a urinary tract infection. Fever was not reported with 56 percent of females and 40 percent of males with their first infection.[1] These same data indicate that the proportion of children with non-febrile first UTIs was 24 percent and 26 percent for males and females age less than 2 years, respectively. However, nonfebrile infections accounted for 71 percent and 74 percent of first UTIs for females and males, respectively, in children 2 to 6 years of age.

Craig and colleagues report the symptoms and signs from a consecutive sample of children presenting with UTIs to a pediatric emergency department that provides primary-care services to a large population of inner-city of children.[16] Of this sample, 77 percent of children were less than 2 years of age with the remainder being 2 to 5 years of age. A history of fever was obtained in 79 percent, but only 59 percent had fever at the time of presentation. Other nonspecific signs reported were irritability, anorexia, malaise or lethargy, vomiting, and diarrhea in approximately 50 to 20 percent respectively. The more specific symptoms of dysuria and abdominal pain and signs of frequency and abnormal-smelling urine were each only noted in approximately 10 to 15 percent of these cases.

Covert Urinary Tract Infection in Febrile Children

A number of descriptive studies demonstrate the importance of recognizing the prevalence of covert UTI in young children presenting to the emergency room with fever and no specific or definite signs of a focus of infection. In a prospective study of 442 febrile infants less than 8 weeks of age, 7.5 percent had positive urine cultures.[17] In recent samples including children up to 1 year of age (and in one study, females up to 2 years of age), the prevalence of catheter specimen–confirmed bacteriuria has been reported to be 3 to 5 percent.[18,19] The prevalence of bacteriuria in a prospectively evaluated consecutive sample of 664 children aged up to 5 years (excluding children with complaints of dysuria) was 1.7 percent. However, in those febrile children older than 1 year of age without dysuria, the prevalence of bacteriuria was only 0.5 percent versus 3.7 percent in those less than a year of age. Taken together, these results suggest that covert urinary tract infection is predominantly a problem in infants and toddlers less than 1 to 2 years of age. There are no adequate studies describing the prevalence of covert febrile UTIs in children within a more general primary-care practice context or in older children.

Signs of Renal Insufficiency, Urinary Tract Anomalies, and Failure to Thrive

Case series and case reports also indicate that children may present with chronic symptoms and/or failure to thrive, secondary to chronic UTI and nephropathy or associated problems. This includes children presenting with signs and/or symptoms of significant underlying urinary tract anomalies, such as abdominal masses representing bilateral hydronephrosis, and/or an abnormal urinary stream consistent with posterior urethral valves. In many cases, the associated renal injury appears to be due largely to congenital dysplasia and/or obstructive nephropathy rather than due to infection itself. Fortunately, the frequency of serious covert renal injury and urologic anomalies in children presenting with UTIs appears to be extremely low. It is probable that this risk is made even smaller in areas with widespread use of prenatal ultrasonography, which can detect some of the more severe urologic anomalies in utero. There are no studies that provide an accurate estimate of the prevalence of such serious presentations in primary care.

Asymptomatic Bacteriuria

There is good evidence that a small proportion of school-aged girls have asymptomatic bacteriuria at any given point in time. In a classic study 40 years ago, Kunin and colleagues demonstrated a point prevalence of catheter specimen–confirmed bacteriuria of 1.2 percent in girls 6 to 10 years of age using a school-based sampling approach.[20] These children were not identified as symptomatic at the time of sampling, but some had a history of recurrent symptomatic urinary tract infections. Only one-third of these children had evidence of pyuria. Of note, Kunin did not detect confirmed bacteriuria in any of the school-aged boys sampled. Asymptomatic bacteriuria has also been noted in infants. One study detected bacteriuria in 1.8 percent and 0.5 percent of female and male infants under 2 years of age, respectively.[21] Another study of newborns revealed asymptomatic bacteriuria in 0.9 percent and 2.5 percent of females and males, respectively. These infants did well with a very low rate of conversion to symptomatic infection or other problems on follow-up over 5 years.[21,22]

Diagnosis

Definition

It is difficult to specify absolute criteria for defining UTI in terms of urine culture results because no clear gold standard reference is available. Culture counts for urine specimens are recognized as a continuous logarithmic distribution. Though urine from the bladder and the collecting system is theoretically sterile, there may often be some degree of bacterial contamination while obtaining the specimen. Accordingly, this ambiguity indicates that culture results should not be interpreted in an arbitrary fashion. For specimens obtained by urethral catheterization, a colony count of $\geq 50 \times 10^6$ CFU/L appears to correspond to a transition between contamination and clinical bacteriuria. In a study of 2,181 catheter urine specimens from children less than 2 years of age, colony counts in the category of 10 to 49×10^6 CFU/L and lower were associated with a dropping proportion of urine specimens with elevated WBC count (≥ 10 WBC/mm^3) on microscopy and were more likely to yield mixed organisms or gram-positive organisms consistent with contamination.[23]

For suprapubic aspiration specimens, the expectation and observation of contamination is less than with other methods. Experts have suggested that any colony growth of uropathogenic organisms is clinical bacteriuria. Regardless, interpreting apparently minimal growth ($<100 \times 10^3$ CFU/L) is difficult.[24] As contamination is more common with clean-catch and bag urine specimens, the counts usually used for interpretation are higher than those used for catheter and aspiration specimens. Single uropathogen counts of $\geq 100 \times 10^6$ CFU/L are widely interpreted as positive. However, even counts of this magnitude can represent contamination. Conversely, counts in the range of 10 to 49×10^6 CFU/L may represent clinical bacteriuria, even though contamination commonly results in counts within this range.

Obtaining Specimens

Several options are available for collecting urine specimens in children. Children older than 2 years can usually be coached to provide clean-catch urine or even a midstream specimen in a sterile bottle. In young children and infants, where urination on request is not possible, four options remain: (1) to collect a bag specimen, (2) to try and catch a spontaneously voided urine with a clean catch into a sterile specimen, (3) to acquire a specimen using urethral catheterization, and (4) suprapubic aspiration of urine directly from the bladder. Catheterization and aspiration are widely considered the gold standard methods but are relatively invasive, and success is operator dependent. In addition, these techniques have a resource cost for the practitioner in terms of time and, to a lesser extent, equipment. Alternatively, urine sampling using a urine specimen bag or by spontaneous clean catch does not have these constraints for the professional or any invasiveness for the patient.

The disadvantage of the spontaneous urine clean catch is that it only works with young infants, who will lie still and void spontaneously. It requires parents to sit and watch and be prepared for the opportunity to catch the urine in a sterile container. When it can be obtained, evidence suggests that the false-positive culture contamination rate is very low (0 out of 85 specimens).[25,26]

Fixing a bag to the perineum with the bag's opening surrounding the urethral meatus is the simplest way of collecting urine. In one study involving circumcised males, the false-positive rate was reported to be low (0 out of 90).[27] However, urine obtained by bag (or other sterile containers fixed to the perineum) have been reported to have false-positive culture contamination rates from 6 to 16 percent with newborns.[28,29] There is a lack of studies on the accuracy of bag urine specimens in older children. The false positives associated with bags are problematic considering that the prevalence of UTIs in the setting in which they are needed is approximately 5 percent. The positive predictive value in these circumstances would be less than 50 percent. Proceeding with management on the basis of a culture result with this range of positive predictive value may be risky, as these values are more likely to be associated with unnecessary intervention including recall, therapy, imaging, and admission.

Considering the current problems with bag urine specimen accuracy, its use can probably only be justified in a narrow set of circumstances. It may be useful as a preliminary test in a low-risk, well population for ruling out UTI. If the culture is negative, there is no further need for investigation. If, however, the specimen is positive, a more accurate method of urine specimen collection would be required to confirm the diagnosis. While some have advocated using a second bag collection or using special techniques in collection to enhance the accuracy, these approaches have not undergone the necessary evaluation.

Urinalysis

Urinalysis is frequently used as a preliminary or adjunct test for the diagnosis of UTI in children. There is evidence that skillful microscopy for detection of bacteria and leukocytes is an efficacious preliminary diagnostic test for UTIs. Urinalysis dipsticks have less accuracy than skillful microscopy but still may have some use in preliminary assessment where skillful microscopy is not available. Using midstream urine, catheter urine, or suprapubic aspiration urine cultures as reference standards, Lohr and colleagues evaluated the diagnostic characteristic of urine dipstick leukocyte esterase and nitrate strips and urine microscopy for diagnosis of UTI in children being investigated for UTI.[30] The culture criteria for UTI were $>0.1 \times 10^6$, $>1 \times 10^6$, and $>10 \times 10^6$ CFU/L, respectively, for suprapubic, catheter, and midstream specimens. The most sensitive component of urinalysis was the visualization of bacteria (sensitivity 99 percent, specificity 71 percent) in a spun urine specimen (Table 17–1.). The most specific component was the nitrite strip (100 percent). The leukocyte esterase strip was reported as having only moderately good sensitivity (79 percent) and specificity (71 percent). A more recent study of children with suspected UTI, using the same reference criteria, reported somewhat better results with the Ames Multistix strip for leukocyte esterase (sensitivity 89 percent, specificity 78 percent).[31] Enhanced urinalysis using unspun urine and a hemocytometer counting chamber has been proposed as the most accurate form of urinalysis for diagnosing UTIs. In comparison with a reference value of $\geq 50 \times 10^6$ CFU/L, the finding of either >10 WBC per mm^3 or any bacteria on 10 fields had a sensitivity of 96 percent and specificity of 93 percent.[23]

Indications for Investigation

When children present with specific signs and symptoms of UTI, including dysuria, frequency, costovertebral angle or flank pain, and tenderness, the need for investigation is clear. Likewise, urine culture and urinalysis are a recognized part of the investigative work-up for children with failure to thrive and findings suggesting renal insufficiency or urologic anomalies. The major challenge in setting indications for the investigation of UTI is in the approach to young children with fever. As a large proportion of children with UTIs present in this fashion, and fever is one of the most common reasons prompting parents to seek med-

Table 17–1 Diagnostic Characteristics of Urine Microscopy and Dipstick for Diagnosis of UTIs in Children.

Method	Criteria	Sensitivity(%)	Specificity(%)
10 mL spun 6 min at 1,800 rpm	>5 WBC/HPF	80	84
10 mL spun 6 min at 1,800 rpm	Any bacteria/HPF	99	71
Leukocyte esterase Ames Multistix	Trace - large	79	72
Nitrite Ames Multistix	Positive	37	100
Combination	As above	100	60

With permission from Lohr J, Portilla M, Geuder T, et al. Making a presumptive diagnosis of urinary tract infection by using a urinalysis performed in an on-site laboratory. J Pediatr 1993; 22-5.
WBC = whole blood count, HPF = ?

ical advice for their children, decisions on how to manage this group will have significant implications on the effectiveness of detection and on the utilization rate of investigations.

A number of studies, including cross-sectional observational designs and a decision analysis, have been carried out to help identify which young children with fever should be investigated for covert UTI.[18,19,32] These studies provide data for risk ratio and likelihood ratio estimates for a number of clinical features of children less than 2 years of age presenting to an emergency department with fever (Table 17–2.). Though the likelihood ratios are of moderate or minimal magnitude (ie, they are all <5 and >0.2), they can be used for estimating the posterior probabilities for children for a given prevalence estimate. For example, consider the case of an 8-month-old Caucasian female presenting to the emergency department with fever, who is assessed as having no obvious focus of infection, has a high fever, and is looking ill. With a UTI prevalence estimate of 4 percent in children less than 2 years of age presenting to the emergency department with fever, the probability of UTI can be calculated using statistical analysis and is around 32 percent. These methods consider the likelihood ratios for age, race, absence of an alternate focus of infection, the toxic appearance, and the level of fever. By contrast, analysis provides a probability of less than 1 percent in the case of a well-looking 2-month-old circumcised male with low-grade fever and signs of an upper respiratory infection (URI).

While calculations using likelihood ratios are useful for demonstrating the effect of clinical features on the probability of UTIs, the ratios generated in these circumstances are not always easy to use in clinical settings for two reasons. First, none of the likelihood ratios are large. One cannot easily select only one or two features that would operate effectively in clinical practice. Second, there are a number of relatively common features with similar likelihood ratios. This means that in many cases, the effect of the ratios will average out and not result in a posterior probability that is clearly different from the prior probability.

Considering the potential harms and costs of unnecessary testing and missed diagnoses, Kramer and colleagues carried out a decision analysis to identify the best strategies for selecting children for UTI investigation.[32] They concluded that there are no strategies that are clear winners. All strategies that optimized the reduction in morbidity from UTIs were associated with high ratios of children tested and false-positive diagnoses. It was suggested that the strategy of combined urinalysis and urine culture in young children with a fever ≥ 39°C is most reasonable. This particular strategy would seem to prevent approximately 90 percent of preventable UTI morbidity, as would the strategy of testing all febrile children, with urinalysis and urine culture having to be performed only on half the number of children.

Table 17–2 Risk Factors for UTI in Young Children Presenting with a Fever.

Risk Factor	OR/RR for UTI	Study
Fever ≥ 39°C	1.8	Hoberman, 1993 [19]
	2.3* (F)	Shaw, 1998 [18]
	7.0[†]	Kramer, 1994 [32]
No obvious source	2.1*	Hoberman, 1993 [19]
	4.0* (M)	Shaw, 1998 [18]
	2.8[†]	Kramer, 1994 [32]
Female gender	3.5*	Hoberman, 1993 [19]
	1.7[†]	Kramer, 1994 [32]
Caucasian race	1.8	Hoberman, 1993 [19]
	5.6* (F)	Shaw, 1998 [18]
Age	1.2 <2m	Hoberman, 1993 [19]
	3.0* <12m (F)	Shaw, 1998 [18]
Circumcision	7.0* M	Shaw, 1998 [18]
	(3.0 to 20) (M)	Multiple sources [2,7,96]
Toxicity/ill-appearing	2.2* (F)	Shaw, 1998 [18]

*statistically significant.
[†]This data was cited as unpublished data.[32]
F = female; M = male

Currently, there are no studies available that have effectively evaluated the contrasting strategies for testing febrile children for UTIs. As Kramer and colleagues acknowledge, there are important questions that remain about the trade-offs to be made in selecting children without specific signs and symptoms for investigation of UTIs.[32] Do all children have an equivalent risk of UTI morbidity and sequelae? Or, do milder infections (ie, looking well, no high fever and rigors) and/or bacteriuria associated with fever in the context of an another focus really pose a significant risk of sequelae if undiagnosed at first presentation? Furthermore, how do parents and children value the immediate inconvenience of testing, with the attendant false positives and distress from urinary catheterization, as compared with the remote risks of serious health status sequelae? What about the setting of primary care practices where the prevalence and spectrum of UTI may differ from that of the emergency department? The data and persisting questions clearly indicate that there is no good evidence to support a dogmatic single management strategy for testing febrile children in all settings. In health-care settings where large numbers of sick, febrile infants are seen without a continuous therapeutic relationship between physician and family, a more conservative strategy with a lower threshold for testing may be justified (Table 17–3.). Alternatively, in primary-care practices with a milder spectrum of illness and possibly lower prevalence of UTIs, a more selective approach using the clinical features may be warranted, with careful instructions to parents and follow-up to investigate children with deterioration or persistent fever. Reason dictates that caution should be exercised in all settings to ensure immediate identification of UTIs in young infants (less than 6 months of age), children who appear ill, and those who present with prolonged fever or symptoms.

Therapy

In the acute setting, the therapy of UTIs is relatively straightforward. Failure to respond promptly to an appropriate antibiotic is rare. Current choices for empiric therapy with oral

Table 17–3 Possible Strategies for Selecting UTI Investigations for Children Less Than 2 Years of Age Presenting with Fever.

Category of Criteria	Basic Requirement	More Cautious Alternative	More Selective Alternative
Temperature at presentation	≥ 40°C without focus	≥ 39°C	≥ 39°C
Age (months)	< 3 to 6		
Demographics		*or* Caucasian female, or uncircumcised male	*and* Caucasian female, or uncircumcised male
Duration (days)	> 3 without alternative focus		
Signs and symptoms	Toxicity, specific UTI signs, significant pain	*or* Ill-appearing, or no alternative focus	*and/or* Ill-appearing, or no alternative focus
Previous history	Previous UTIs, immune defect, urologic anomaly, neuropathic bladder		

*Investigation is easy to justify for the basic requirement category. For a conservative approach, all children less than 2 years of age presenting with a fever of ≥ 39° or any other criteria would be selected for investigation (in addition to the basic requirement). For a more selective approach, a combination of fever ≥ 39° with other criteria from the selective alternative could be used (in addition to the basic requirement).

therapy include trimethoprim-sulfamethoxazole or a cephalosporin (eg, cefixime, cefprozil, cephalexin) and with parenteral therapy include second- or third-generation cephalosporins or the combination of ampicillin with an aminoglycoside.[33]

Choice of route of administration and duration of therapy are more complex. Children who are assessed as toxic and dehydrated, or are expected to have difficulty with oral hydration should obviously receive antibiotics at least initially by the intravenous route. However, there is currently no peer-reviewed published evidence to indicate that children with UTIs (with or without suggestive signs of pyelonephritis) require parenteral antibiotics and hospitalization on a routine basis. It may be prudent to initiate therapy using the parental route in young infants less than 3 to 6 months of age considering the increasingly frequent observation of bacteremia and metastatic infection as age decreases.[17,34-37] In addition, children with evidence of complicated UTI and clinical findings suggesting underlying obstruction or renal insufficiency or UTI due to prolonged, refractory, or relapsing infection may deserve more intensive therapy. Several large case series suggest that children who present with a more severe, prolonged infection and/or delayed diagnosis have a greater risk of scarring.[38-40] More caution may also be warranted in children less than 2 years of age considering some case series reports that renal scarring is more likely with UTIs in this age group and that scarring has more of an effect on renal growth and glomerular function at this age than in older children.[41-43] It should, however, be noted that other series have failed to show some of these associations between clinical attributes and risk of scarring.[44]

More clarity is needed for determining when intravenous antimicrobial therapy is warranted or not warranted. A study that involved randomizing infants 1 to 24 months of age with febrile UTIs to initial intravenous therapy versus oral therapy with cefixime is in the process of being presented and published.[45] Renal scarring at 6 months was reported to have occurred in 9.8 percent of children treated orally compared with 7.2 percent of children receiving parenteral therapy initially. This difference was not statistically significant, and according to the authors, these results recommend that oral therapy can be used safely and effectively in children this age.

There is good evidence that short-course antibiotic therapy is not as effective in treating UTIs in children. Fifteen randomized controlled trials have been performed comparing single-or short-course therapy with conventional therapy.[45] Twelve of these fail to detect a difference in outcomes, but all have significant methodologic problems, including a lack of power. The three studies that have sufficient sample size and constitute the best available evidence clearly demonstrate a statistically significant increase in treatment failures and relapsed infection with therapy less than 7 days in duration.[46-48]

Children who have significant renal anomalies, such as reflux, or have developed a pattern of recurrent UTIs are often prescribed 6-month or longer prophylactic antibiotic therapy to reduce the risk of recurrences. There is good evidence from two randomized controlled trials using low-dose therapy with co-trimoxazole or nitrofurantoin that the rate of recurrent UTIs is significantly decreased compared with placebo in children with UTIs and no urologic anomalies and in girls with at least three prior UTIs.[49,50] The optimal duration of prophylactic therapy for different circumstances has not been clearly identified in the literature.

Diagnostic Imaging

Children with complicated UTIs not responding well to therapy or who have clinical signs suggesting an unusually severe infection or an underlying problem warrant further investigation with ultrasonography to rule out obstruction and potentially cystourethrography to detect reflux, as well as Dimercaptosuccinic acid radionucleotide (DMSA) scan to assess renal parenchymal damage or abnormalities. However, there is no strong evidence to support the routine use of these imaging modalities in investigating children with their first, unremarkable UTI.[8] The prevalence of underlying anomalies, especially vesicoureteral reflux, the potential increased risk of scarring, and renal compromise in young children with UTIs are, at best, fair evidence for recommending diagnostic imaging with ultrasonography and voiding cystourethrography in children less than 2 year of age.[33]

Screening and Treating Asymptomatic Bacteriuria

There is evidence that treatment of asymptomatic bacteriuria is unnecessary in children without a history of recurrent UTIs or other significant renal or urologic problems. There is evidence from RCTs that antimicrobial treatment of school girls with asymptomatic bacteriuria in this age group has no significant effect on renal scarring as measured by intravenous pyelography.[51-53] There have not been any studies evaluating treatment of asymptomatic bacteriuria in infants.

PRIMARY NOCTURNAL ENURESIS

Epidemiology

Bed-wetting is a frequently encountered childhood problem that primary-care physicians caring for children will be often asked about. Unlike acute childhood illnesses or chronic problems with some sort of identifiable onset (such as recurrent abdominal pain), bed-wetting usually emerges slowly as a problem with children who fail to progress in the expected transition to reliable night-time dryness by 6 years of age. This primary nocturnal enuresis must be kept distinct from secondary nocturnal enuresis, which is defined as nocturnal enuresis occuring in a child who has previously consistently maintained night-time dryness.

Primary nocturnal enuresis should also be distinguished from day-time enuresis, though the two may occur together. Both day-time enuresis and secondary enuresis require significantly more attention to the possibility of underlying problems, such as urinary tract infections, diabetes, or neurologic disturbances.

In a random sample of 3,206 7-year-old Finnish children, the overall prevalence of enuresis was 9.8 percent.[54] The prevalence of nocturnal enuresis alone was 6.4 percent, with a prevalence of day-time enuresis and mixed enuresis of 1.8 and 1.6 percent, respectively. The authors identified two distinct groups: cases with mixed day and night enuresis, which was more associated with neurologic damage or developmental delay, and cases with nocturnal enuresis alone, seemingly related to maturational issues. Differences in definitions and sampling may significantly affect the rates of enuresis reported by studies. However, despite this, there is consistency in some of the associations noted, most notably the association with age. In a Rochester survey study, nocturnal enuresis was reported in 33 percent of 5-year-olds, 18 percent of 8-year-olds, 7 percent of 11-year-olds, and 0.7% of 17-year-olds.[55] In a United Kingdom study, nocturnal enuresis was reported with 4.7 percent of children 11 to 12 years old and 1.1 percent of children 15 to 16 years of age.[56] Not only is nocturnal enuresis more frequent in boys, but the decline with age also appears later for boys, prompting the suggestion that the criteria for diagnosis should by raised to 8 years for boys, compared with 6 for girls.[57]

Therapy

In affected children, the only negative effect of primary nocturnal enuresis is on their mental health. Children who were still wetting their beds after the age of 10 years appeared to have a detectable increased risk of conduct, attention, and anxiety problems compared with children who were dry before age 5 years in a birth cohort of 1,265 urban New Zealand children followed up for 15 years.[58] This increased risk was small, and there was no association with other psychiatric problems. However, it is not entirely clear whether this is a causal association or whether children with behavioral problems are more likely to have primary nocturnal enuresis. There is scant good evidence regarding the effect of therapy on the mental health outcomes of children with primary nocturnal enuresis. One randomized controlled trial of conditioning therapy with alarm versus a 3-month waiting period failed to demonstrate any statistically significant differences in behavior, anxiety, or locus of control in children 8 to 14 years of age.[59] However, there were significant improvements in self-concept in those receiving therapy compared with those in the waiting period.

There is currently no evidence that routine, early (ie, at or before 6 years of age) medical intervention benefits children with primary nocturnal enuresis. Therefore, the need for treatment in the management of primary nocturnal enuresis is generally dictated by the extent of concern and the desire for treatment expressed by the child and family, not by the age of the child. Thus, for many younger children with primary nocturnal enuresis, an adequate explanation of the condition, reassurance, and encouraging ownership by the child can be an important clinical option while awaiting spontaneous improvement in the enuresis.

Tricyclic Antidepressant Therapy

There is an extensive body of literature on the medical treatment of primary nocturnal enuresis. Within this literature is some fairly consistent evidence of efficacy for three specific therapies. There are a number of small placebo-controlled cross-over trials evaluating the effect of tricyclic antidepressants on the number of nights with enuresis.[60-70] Methodologic problems with small sample sizes and different outcome definitions account for some of the differences in results from these trials. While not all show a statistically significant benefit, they do provide evidence of efficacy in reducing episodes of nocturnal enuresis. However, it does appear that this effect persists, for the most part, only while the child is taking the mediation. In a well-designed, multicenter, randomized, double-blind, parallel-treatment trial involving 80 children 5 to 13 years of age, imipramine (25 mg each evening) for 30 days was compared with placebo and a quadricyclic antidepressant, mianserin.[70] At baseline, all groups had, on average, two dry nights a week. By the end of the 5-week course of therapy, the children in the imipramine group had an average of five dry nights a week compared with three dry nights per week in the other two groups. However, after 4 weeks off all therapy, the difference between the groups had disappeared with all three groups having 3 to 3.5 dry nights per week. Thus, although 72 percent of children experienced a definite improvement while taking imipramine, this was lost in almost half the cases following discontinuation. Tricyclic antidepressants appear to be relatively free of side effects when taken at this dosage level. However, the potentially disastrous consequences that could ensue from an overdose of these medications must be kept in mind.

Desmopressin Therapy

Desmopressin is another medical treatment for primary nocturnal enuresis that has been evaluated for efficacy. Moffat and colleagues have provided an excellent evidence-based systematic review of the literature regarding desmopressin therapy for enuresis.[71] They were able to identify 18 randomized controlled clinical trials (11 cross-over trials and 7 parallel group trials). As per the studies involving tricyclic antidepressants, collective interpretation of these studies is hampered somewhat by different designs and differing outcome definitions. Nevertheless, there is good evidence that desmopressin (20 micrograms) administered by nasal spray nightly is efficacious in reducing nocturnal enuresis. However, the proportion of children experiencing a reduction in enuresis ranged from 10 to 91 percent in these studies, and only approximately 25 percent achieved short-term dryness for a period of consecutive days. A number of these studies indicate that the effect is most noticeable in children over 9 years of age.[72-74] Most studies with follow-up also demonstrate a loss of efficacy after the course of therapy has been completed,[72,75-78] and there appears to be relatively little additional benefit associated with increased dosing (40 micrograms nightly).[77,79] Anecdotal reports in the literature suggest that therapy with desmopressin can put children at risk for hyponatremia and seizures. Fortunately, this event appears to be rare.

Classic Conditioning with Urine Sensing Alarms

While a variety of different types of behavioral conditioning approaches have been suggested and studied, most of the evidence supports classic conditioning with a urine-sensitive alarm as the most efficacious behavioral technique for treating primary nocturnal enuresis.[80-83] Not all studies of classic conditioning with an alarm have demonstrated efficacy.[84] However, a number of well-designed, parallel-group, randomized controlled trials demonstrate clinically and statistically significant improvements in enuresis with use of these approaches for up to 3 months compared with placebo.[76,80,82,85] Lynch demonstrated that 50 percent of children achieved 14 consecutive dry nights with this approach. It appears that this effect is evident regardless of the specific device,[81] whether it is a mat sensor or a small sensor attached to the garment in the perineal region.[86]

Selection of Therapy

In contrast to desmopressin or the tricyclic antidepressants, conditioning with urine-sensing alarms appears to result in a more durable amelioration of enuresis. Wille compared desmopressin and alarm in a 3-month parallel-group randomized controlled trial with continuation of therapy for a further 3 months in the event of relapse.[76] In this study, the alarm approach resulted in significant improvement in 86 percent of children compared with 70 percent improvement in the desmopressin group (not statistically significant). Those receiving desmopressin therapy were significantly drier in the first week; however, relapses subsequently occurred in 40 percent, versus only 5 percent in the alarm group. In a large case series with a minimum of 1-year follow-up, families were provided with a choice of therapies, including observation.[87] Of the 79 who chose the alarm, 63 percent were continent with, at most, one enuresis episode per month at 6 months follow-up, and 53 percent were still continent at 12 months. The median duration of alarm use was 4 months. Of the 88 and 44 who chose 6 months of treatment with desmopressin and imipramine, respectively, continence was reported as 68 percent and 36 percent at 6 months but only 10 percent and 16 percent at 12 months. For comparison, 16 percent of those followed up with observation alone were continent at 12 months. These results are consistent with the notion that desmopressin and the tricyclic antidepressants are able to provide short-term improvement during the course of therapy but no real acceleration in the development of permanent continence.

Two randomized controlled trials suggest that the combination of desmopressin and alarm conditioning is superior to either alone.[85,88] In each case, the combination approach resulted in an additional benefit of one more dry night per week compared with desmopressin or alarm alone during the intervention period. However, in both cases, the treatment course was brief, and there was no prolonged follow-up to determine the duration of this effect.

The available evidence provides good support for treatment recommendation for children with primary nocturnal enuresis. While there is no evidence to support routine early intervention beyond observation and reassurance, there is evidence to support the use of a urine-sensing alarm device with children over 6 years of age who identify enuresis as a significant problem and desire more than observation. There is also evidence that desmopressin and tricyclic antidepressants can play a role as efficacious therapy for achieving short-term goals in reducing enuresis. This could be important for children who need to improve continence for short periods of time, such as during camping, or who have not had success with using an alarm and wish to try another therapy. There is currently no strong evidence to support the routine use of combined therapy.

Circumcision

Epidemiology

Circumcision of neonatal males has become an extremely common procedure in North America during the 20th century. The variety of reasons used to justify neonatal male circumcision include religious ritual, physical conformity within families, hygiene, and/or preventive health intervention. The National Center for Health Statistics has estimated that 64 percent of males born in the United States were circumcised during 1995.[89] In Ontario, Canada 30 percent of male infants born in 1995 were circumcised in the neonatal period according to the hospital discharge abstract records.[90]

Though neonatal male circumcisions have been quite popular during much of the century, the evidence regarding the potential health benefit of routine neonatal circumcision has accumulated only quite recently. Furthermore, there has been an ongoing debate regarding the health effects and medical value of circumcision. In this context of widespread practice within the North American society and the number of health effects often attributed to circumcision, the literature is usually oriented around circumcision and its effects rather than around the specific health conditions that circumcision is purported to prevent or ameliorate. This approach has been taken by numerous professional bodies, who have produced statements or guidelines on neonatal male circumcision.[89-91]

Phimosis, Paraphimosis, and Balanitis

A number of childhood penile problems are encountered in primary-care practice and emergency departments. Phimosis has been described in up to 4 percent of uncircumcised male children.[92-94] In younger children, the frequency of prepucial adhesions and inability to retract the prepuce is higher, supporting the notion that gradual reduction in adhesions and phimosis represents a developmental process.[93] It is in older children and adolescents that phimosis becomes a problem because of painful erections and risk of paraphimosis. Chronic balanitis and inflammation of the prepuce may result in a more severe secondary phimosis caused by scarring.

While circumcision eliminates phimosis and paraphimosis, there is a paucity of evidence regarding the overall magnitude of the benefit of routine circumcision in the prevention of these problems. It does not appear that circumcision completely abolishes penile problems or that the reduction in problems is of adequate significance to justify the procedure. While the rate of penile problems (predominantly balanitis) is higher in uncircumcised boys, a New Zealand study suggests a higher risk of penile problems (mainly meatal ulcers) in the circumcised group in the first year of life, with the risk reversing by the third year of life, mainly due to balanitis and inflammation in the uncircumcised group.[95] In another study, the reported rate of balanitis and inflammation were reported by parents to be approximately two-fold higher in uncircumcised males, but in general, these problems were considered to be mild.[93] There are no controlled trials or rigorous case-control or cohort studies available to clearly demonstrate the magnitude of benefit or importance of routine circumcision for the prevention of penile problems. There is also no good quality evidence that circumcision either substantially improves or reduces sexual function.

Urinary Tract Infection

There is consistent evidence that neonatal male circumcision reduces the risk of being diagnosed with a urinary tract infection early in childhood. While studies conducted earlier in the latter half of the 20th century suggested higher risk reduction with circumcision,[96] more recent cohort and case-control studies suggest a relative risk for UTI of 3- to 7-fold among uncircumcised male infants.[2,7,17,35] In a population-based cohort study, the risk of hospitalization for UTI in the first year of life was 1 in 140 in uncircumcised males versus 1 in 530 in circumcised children.[2] Thus, although the relative risk reduction is significant, it is estimated that 195 newborn males need to be circumcised to prevent a single hospitalization for UTI.

An assumption is often made that the reduction in infection risk from circumcision will result in a proportional reduction in potential long-term outcomes, such as hypertension and renal failure. Direct evidence of this relationship is not currently available, given the rarity of these outcomes and the long follow-up time required for these manifestations to appear. There do seem to be some differences between UTIs in uncircumcised males and those in circumcised males. Ruston and Majd have noted that the prevalence of vesicoureteral reflux in males less than 6 months of age (93 percent uncircumcised) was significantly lower than in males 6 months of age or older (50 percent circumcised).[97] On the other hand, the prevalence of renal defects on DMSA scan was significantly higher in the younger children. However, it is not clear whether these differences mean that uncircumcised males with UTIs have a different rate of rare long-term outcomes than circumcised males.

Cancer of the Penis

Squamous cell carcinoma of the penis has an age-adjusted annual incidence of approximately 1 in 100,000 males in the developed countries.[98,99] While case series have suggested a link between circumcision status and carcinoma of the penis, only one study provides a reasonable estimate of this increased risk. A case-control study of men with carcinoma of the penis reported that uncircumcised men had 3.2 times the risk of carcinoma.[100] However, it has been suggested that much of the increased risk in uncircumcised men is due to phimosis, a factor consistently identified as increasing the risk in several studies.[100-102] In addition, these studies also indicate that genital warts, multiple partners, and smoking are risk factors for carcinoma. It has been suggested that good hygiene will reduce the risk of carcinoma secondary to phimosis and that the rate of carcinoma can be reduced in some populations without circumcision.[99]

Human Immunodeficiency Virus

There is a growing body of evidence that circumcision may confer some protection against the risk of acquiring human immundeficiency virus (HIV) through sexual contact.[103-108] The body of literature in this area has been recently reviewed.[109-110] The majority of these studies were cross-sectional. Two studies, which were prospective case-control analyses, indicated a positive relationship between uncircumcised status and risk of HIV infection. Overall, studies suggesting a protective effect of circumcision reported relative risk estimates of 1.5 to 8.4 for HIV acquisition in uncircumcised males.[110] However, these studies have been criticized for failing to adjust for confounders, misclassification problems, and other methodologic problems.[109] Furthermore, behavioral factors play a far greater role in the acquisition of infection. There is no direct evidence regarding the effectiveness and relative importance of neonatal male circumcision as an infection control measure in populations with prevalent HIV infection.

Harms of Circumcision

The complication rate for neonatal male circumcision appears to be in the range of 0.2 to 0.6 percent according to two large series.[111,112] Bleeding and infection are the most common complications, but most of these are minor. Anecdotal reports of more severe complications include poor cosmesis, cysts, invasive infection and sepsis (meningitis), and major surgical problems such as fistula, amputation, and necrosis. There are no studies with a large enough sample or population to provide good estimates of the rates of these outcomes.

While neonatal pain inflicted during procedures such as circumcision has been discounted as an important problem for much of this century, there is now a conclusive body of evidence that neonates experience pain. There is even the suggestion that the experience of the procedural pain of circumcision may influence the response to a painful procedure (immunization) later in infancy.[113] While it is beyond the scope of this chapter to describe this evidence or to compare circumcision procedures or analgesic techniques, there is good evidence that analgesia reduces pain significantly and is safe.[89]

Balancing Benefits and Harms of Circumcision

Overall, there is insufficient evidence to justify a recommendation of routine neonatal male circumcision. There is fair evidence from case-control or cohort studies that uncircumcised status is associated with increased risk of urinary tract infection and squamous cell carcinoma of the penis. However, it does not appear that this translates into evidence of a substantial reduction in important health outcomes to justify a recommendation in favor of routine circumcision. A recent cost-utility analysis suggested that circumcision results in an average life expectancy improvement of 14 hours, with a net discounted lifetime cost of $102.[114] Assuming that there is no risk of carcinoma following circumcision, another decision analysis has suggested that circumcision results in an increased life expectancy of 105 quality-adjusted days and excess expected lifetime cost of $25.35.[115] Even with optimistic estimates of the effect of circumcision on life-shortening outcomes, this incremental benefit in life expectancy is small. This supports the notion that the decision to circumcise is really a "toss up" (ie, there is no clear "winning" strategy). This falls short of the clear evidence for benefit needed to recommend a major health intervention. This has been recognized by professional bodies,[89,91] which have not recommended routine circumcision but encourage unbiased disclosure of the potential benefits and harms to parents.

Table 17–4 Urinary Tract Problems in Primary Care: Summary of Recommendations and Evidence

	Intervention	Strength of Evidence	Recommendation
Suspect UTI			
Children with specific (dysuria, urine abnormalities, suprapubic or flank pain, prior history of urinary tract anomalies) and/or persistent unexplained nonspecific (eg, failure to thrive, abdominal pain, fever) signs and symptoms consistent with UTI.	Assess for UTI If diagnosed with a UTI, treat with antimicrobial therapy.	UTIs are prevalent in children (Level III ecological studies)	A
Young females (ie, less than 2 years of age), young uncircumcised males, and circumcised infant males with an unexplained febrile illness	Assess for UTI	Young females, young uncircumcised males, and circumcised infant males with an unexplained febrile illness have an increased risk of UTI (level II prospective cross-sectional studies) Assessment of young children with a febrile illness and temperature over 39° C would seem to result in the prevention of 90 percent of the preventable long-term morbidity secondary to UTIs in this group (Level III decision analysis)	B
UTI Diagnosis			
Children who are over 2 months of age and not ill-looking, but at risk for UTI	Perform dipstick and/or microscopy urinalysis for a presumptive diagnosis of UTI to; 1. direct the use of empiric antimicrobial therapy pending culture results in children over	A positive leukocyte esterase/nitrite dipstick examination or a positive spun urine microscopy for any bacteria or >5 WBC per HPF has moderately high sensitivity (80 to 90 percent) and moderate specificity (70	B

(continued)

Table 17–4 Urinary Tract Problems in Primary Care: Summary of Recommendations and Evidence *(continued)*

	Intervention	Strength of Evidence	Recommendation
	2 months of age who do not appear toxic; and 2. determine the likelihood of UTI and necessity for invasive urine specimen sampling in children who are not ill enough to warrant immediate antimicrobial therapy	to 80 percent) for UTI (Level II prospective cross-sectional study) Any bacteria in 10 fields or >10 WBC per mm^3 in unspun urine examined by cytometer counting chamber has high (>90%) sensitivity and specificity for UTI (Level II prospective cross-sectional study)	
Children who are less than 2 months of age or are unable to provide a clean-catch or mid-stream urine specimen, who 1. are ill enough to warrant immediate antimicrobial therapy, or 2. have a high likelihood of UTI (eg, specific symptoms and signs, positive urinalysis, or bag urine culture)	Urine culture by supra-pubic aspiration or urethral catheterization, not by bag collection	Culture of urine specimens obtained by urethral catheterization is highly accurate in diagnosing UTI (Level II prospective cross-sectional studies) Culture of urine specimens obtained by bag collection have a high sensitivity for diagnosing UTIs, but a low specificity and predictive value in diagnosing UTI compared with urethral catheterization or suprapubic aspiration (Level III descriptive studies)	B
Children who are unable to produce a clean catch and without specific symptoms of UTI who are not ill enough to warrant immediate antimicrobial therapy	Urine culture from a bag collection	A negative culture from a bag urine specimen has a high negative predictive value for UTI (Level III descriptive studies)	C

(continued)

Table 17–4 Urinary Tract Problems in Primary Care: Summary of Recommendations and Evidence *(continued)*

	Intervention	Strength of Evidence	Recommendation
UTI Therapy			
Children with diagnosed UTIs	Treat with antimicrobial therapy	UTIs can result in renal scarring and contribute to long-term health status outcomes (Level III case series)	A
	Treatment duration should be a minimum of seven days	Antimicrobials are effective treatment for UTIs (Level III unequivocal results from uncontrolled studies); therapy with courses of antimicrobials for less than 7 days are associated with higher rates of early recurrence (Level I randomized controlled trial [RCT])	A
Children older than three months of age with UTI, providing they are not sick-looking or toxic, are well hydrated, and ingest the medication without vomiting	Administer antimicrobial by oral route	There is no published evidence indicating that routine parenteral therapy results in better outcomes than selective use; results presented from one RCT indicate no difference in outcomes with febrile infants 2 months to 2 years of age (Level I, RCT is pending publication*)	B*
Children with recurrent UTIs or with vesicoureteral reflux or other significant urologic anomalies	Administer low dose antimicrobials for prophylaxis for a minimum of 6 months	There is good evidence that recurrent UTIs are reduced by prophylactic therapy (Level I RCT)	A
Children with asymptomatic bacteruria and no history of recurrent UTIs	Antimicrobial therapy	Treatment of asymptomatic bacteruria does not result in better outcomes (Level I RCT)	E
UTI Diagnostic Imaging			
Children with a first, uncomplicated symptomatic UTI	Routine imaging with DMSA scan, VCUG, and/or US during or following the infection	There is little evidence that routine imaging of children with a first uncomplicated UTI improves outcome (Level III descriptive studies)	C

(continued)

Table 17–4 Urinary Tract Problems in Primary Care: Summary of Recommendations and Evidence *(continued)*

	Intervention	Strength of Evidence	Recom- mendation
Children less than 2 years of age with symptomatic UTIs or children with UTIs involving failure to thrive, specific signs of underlying uro- logic problem, toxicity, delayed resolution, or recur- rent infection	Imaging with US or DMSA scan during or immediately following infection	Significant urologic anomalies and renal damage are more common and severe in young infants or in children with a complicated course or recurrent infections (Level III large case series)	B
	Imaging with contrast or radionucleotide VCUG during or following the acute infection		B
Neonatal Male Circumcision			
Healthy newborn male infants	Routine circumcision	Fair evidence exists of some health benefits to neonatal male circumcision (eg, reduced risk of infections and penile problems); the degree of certainty and magnitude of the benefit versus harms of circum- cision are insufficient for recommending a pre- ventive intervention of this nature (Level II case-control and other analytic studies)	C
Primary Nocturnal Enuresis			
Children 6 years of age or older with primary nocturnal enuresis, which is perceived as a problem by the child	Classic conditioning therapy with urine sensing alarm	Good evidence that alarm therapy significantly and durably accelerates the development of nocturnal continence (Level I RCT)	A
Children 6 years of age or older with poor re- sponse to alarm ther- apy and/orhave indica- tions for more im- mediate or temporary nocturnal continence (eg, to reduce barriers to trips, etc.)	Intranasal desmopressin or oral tricyclic antidepressant therapy	Good evidence that both tricyclic antidepressants and desmopressin can quickly and significantly improve nocturnal con- tinence; however, this effect is not as durable as alarm therapy and is largely lost following ces- sation of medication (Level I RCT and Level II non- randomized controlled trial)	A

WBC = whole blood count; HPF = ?
DMSA = Dimercaptosaccinic acid radionucleotide scan; VCUG = voiding cystourethrogram
US = ultrasonography

REFERENCES

1. Marild S, Jodal U. Incidence rate of first-time symptomatic urinary tract infection in children under 6 years of age. Acta Paediatr Scand 1998;87:549–52.

2. To T, Agha M, Dick P, Feldman W. Cohort study on circumcision of newborn boys and subsequent risk of urinary tract infection. Lancet 1998;352:1813–6.

3. Winberg J, Andersen H, Bergstrom T, et al. Epidemiology of symptomatic urinary tract infection in childhood. Acta Paediatr Scand 1974;252:3–20.

4. Roberts JA. Factors predisposing to urinary tract infections in children. Pediatr Nephrol 1996;10(4):517–22.

5. Patrick MJ. Influence of maternal renal infection on the fetus and infant. Arch Dis Child 1967;42(222):208–13.

6. Pisacane A, Graziano L, Zona G. Breastfeeding and urinary tract infection. Lancet 1990;335:50.

7. Craig J, Knight J, Sureshkumar P, et al. Effect of circumcision on incidence of urinary tract infection in preschool boys. J Pediatr 1996;128:23–7.

8. Dick P, Feldman W. Routine diagnostic imaging for childhood urinary tract infections: a systematic overview. J Pediatr 1996;128:15–22.

9. Sheih CP, Liu MB, Hung CS, et al. Renal abnormalities in schoolchildren. Pediatrics 1989;84:1086–90.

10. Steinhart J, Kuhn J, Eisenberg B, et al. Ultrasound screening of healthy infants for urinary tract abnormalities. Pediatrics 1988;82:609–14.

11. Burge DM, Griffiths MD, Malone PS, Atwell JD. Fetal vesicoureteral reflux: outcome following conservative postnatal management. J Urol 1992;148(5 Pt 2):1743–5.

12. Noe HN. The long-term results of prospective sibling reflux screening. J Urol 1992;148(5 Pt 2):1739–42.

13. Hansson S, Hjalmas K, Jodal U, Sixt R. Lower urinary tract dysfunction in girls with untreated asymptomatic or covert bacteriuria. J Urol 1990;143(2):333–5.

14. Koff SA, Murtagh DS. The uninhibited bladder in children: effect of treatment on recurrence of urinary infection and on vesicoureteral reflux resolution. J Urol 1983;130(6):1138–41.

15. Koff SA, Wagner TT, Jayanthi VR. The relationship among dysfunctional elimination syndromes, primary vesicoureteral reflux and urinary tract infections in children. J Urol 1998;160(3 Pt 2):1019–22.

16. Craig J, Irwig L, Knight J, et al. Symptomatic urinary tract infection in preschool Australian children. J Paediatr Child Health 1998;34:154–9.

17. Crain E, Gershel J. Urinary tract infections in febrile infants younger than 8 weeks of age. Pediatrics 1990;86:363–7.

18. Shaw K, Gorelick M, McGowan K, et al. Prevalence of urinary tract infection in febrile young children in the emergency department. Pediatrics 1998;102:16–24.

19. Hoberman A, Chao HP, Keller D, et al. Prevalence of urinary tract infection in febrile infants. J Pediatr 1993;123:17–23.

20. Kunin C, Southall I, Paquin A. Epidemiology of urinary-tract infections—A pilot study of 3057 school children. N Engl J Med 1960;263:817–23.

21. Siegel SR, Siegel B, Sokoloff BZ, Kanter MH. Urinary infection in infants and preschool children. Five-year follow-up. Am J Dis Child 1980;134(4):369–72.

22. Wettergren B, Hellstrom M, Stokland E. Six year follow-up of infants with bacteriuria on screening. Br Med J 1990;301:845–8.

23. Hoberman A, Wald ER, Penchansky L, et al. Enhanced urinalysis as a screening test for urinary tract infection [see comments]. Pediatrics 1993;91(6):1196–9.

24. Hellerstein S. Recurrent urinary tract infections in children. Pediatr Inf Dis 1982;1(4):271–81.

25. Boehm JJ, Haynes JL. Bacteriology of "midstream catch" urines. Studies in newborn infants. Am J Dis Child 1966;111(4):366–9.

26. Pryles C. Percutaneous bladder aspiration and other methods of urine collection for bacteriologic study. Pediatrics 1965;36:128–31.

27. Schlager T, Dunn M, Dudley S, Lohr J. Bacterial contamination rate of urine collected in a urine bag from healthy non-toilet trained male infants. J Pediatr 1990;116:738–9.

28. Schlager T, Hendley J, Dudley S. Explanation for false-positive urine cultures obtained by bag techniques. Arch Pediatr Adolesc Med 1995;149:170–3.

29. McCarthy J, Pryles C. Clean voided and catheter neonatal urine specimens. Arch Dis Child 1963:473–7.

30. Lohr J, Portilla M, Geuder T, et al. Making a presumptive diagnosis of urinary tract infection by using a urinalysis performed in an on-site laboratory. J Pediatr 1993;122:22–5.

31. Webb K, Patten C, McLean L. A comparison of the filtracheck-UTI and dipstick urinalysis in the diagnosis of pediatric urinary tract infections. Ambulatory Pediatric Association Annual Meeting, Washington, May 5, 1997.

32. Kramer M, Tange S, Drummond K, Mills E. Urine testing in young febrile children: a risk-benefit analysis. J Pediatr 1994;125:6–13.

33. Anonymous. American Academy of Pediatrics. Practice parameter: the diagnosis, treatment, and evaluation of the initial urinary tract infection in febrile infants and young children. Pediatrics 1999;103:843–52.

34. Wiswell T, Smith F, Bass J. Decreased incidence of urinary tract infections in circumcised male infants. Pediatrics 1985;75:901–3.

35. Herzog L. Urinary tract infections and circumcision: a case control study. Am J Dis Child 1989;143:348–50.

36. Bachur R, Caputo G. Bacteremia and meningitis among infants with urinary tract infections. Pediatr Emerg Care 1995;11:280–4.

37. Ginsburg C, McCracken G. Urinary tract infection in young infants. Pediatrics 1982;69:409–12.

38. Smellie JM, Ransley PG, Normand IC, et al. Development of new renal scars: a collaborative study. Br Med J (Clinical Research Ed.) 1985;290(6486):1957–60.

39. Winter A, Hardy B, Alton D, et al. Acquired renal scars in children. J Urol 1983;129:1190–4.

40. Anonymous. South Bedfordshire Practitioners' Group. - Development of renal scars in children: missed opportunities in management. Br Med J 1990;301:1082–4.

41. Winberg J, Bollgren I, Lakkenius G. Clinical pyelonephritis and local renal scarring: a selected review of pathogenesis, prevention, and prognosis. Pediatr Clin North Am 1982;29:801–14.

42. Stokland E, Hellstrom M, Jacobsson B, et al. Renal damage one year after first urinary tract infection: role of dimercaptosuccinic acid scintigraphy. J Pediatr 1996;129:815–20.

43. Berg U, Johansson S. Age as a main determinant of renal functional damage in urinary tract infection. Arch Dis Child 1983;58:963–9.

44. Benador D, Benador N, Slosman D, et al. Are younger children at highest risk of renal sequelae after pyelonephritis? Lancet 1997;349:17–9.

45. Hoberman A, Wald E, Hickey R, et al. Oral versus initial intravenous therapy for urinary tract infections in young febrile children. San Fransisco, CA: Pediatric Academic Societies Meeting; May 4, 1999.

46. Avner E, Ingelfinger J, Herrin J, et al. Single-dose amoxicillin therapy of uncomplicated pediatric urinary tract infections. J Pediatr 1983;102:623–7.

47. McCracken G, Ginsburg C, Namasonthi V, et al. Evaluation of short term antibiotic therapy in children with uncomplicated urinary tract infection. Pediatrics 1981;67:796–801.

48. Moffatt M, Embree J, Grimm P, Law B. Short-course antibiotic therapy for urinary tract infections in children. Am J Dis Child 1988;142:57–61.

49. Smellie J, Katz G, Gruneberg R. Controlled trial of prophylactic treatment in childhood urinary-tract infection. Lancet 1978:175–8.

50. Lohr J, Nunley D, Howards S, Ford R. Prevention of recurrent urinary tract infections in girls. Pediatrics 1977;59:4.

51. Savage D, Howie G, Adler K. Controlled trial of therapy in covert bacteriuria in childhood. Lancet 1975;1:358–61.

52. Lindberg U. Asymptomatic bacteriuria in school girls. V. The clinical course and response to treatment. Acta Paediatr Scand 1975;64:718–24.

53. Hanson E, Hansson S, Jodal U. Trimethoprim-sulphadiazine prophylaxis in children with vesico-ureteric reflux. Scand J Infect Dis 1989;21:201–4.

54. Järvelin M, Huttunen N, Seppänen J, et al. Screening of urinary tract abnormalities among day and nightwetting children. Scand J Urol Nephrol 1990;24:181–9.

55. Byrd R, Weitzman M, Lanphear N, Auinger P. Bed-wetting in US children: epidemiology and related behavior problems. Pediatrics 1996;98:414–9.

56. Swithinbank L, Carr J, Abrams P. Longitudinal study of urinary symptoms in children. Scand J Urol Nephrol 1994;163(Suppl):67–73.

57. Verhulst F, van der Lee J, Akkerhuis G, et al. The prevalence of nocturnal enuresis: do DSM III criteria need to be changed? A brief research report. J Child Psychol Psychiatr Allied Discipl 1985;26(6):989–93.

58. Fergusson D, Horwood L. Nocturnal enuresis and behavioral problems in adolescence: a 15-year longitudinal study. Pediatrics 1994;94:662–8.

59. Moffat M, Kato C, Pless I. Improvements in self-concept after treatment of nocturnal enuresis: randomized controlled trial. J Pediatr 1987;110:647–52.

60. Petersen KE, Andersen OO. Treatment of nocturnal enuresis with imipramine and related preparations. A double blind trial with a placebo. Acta Paediatr Scand 1971;60(2):244.

61. Mishra PC, Agarwal VK, Rahman H. Therapeutic trial of amitryptyline in the treatment of nocturnal enuresis—a controlled study. Ind Pediatr 1980;17(3):279–85.

62. Meadow R, Berg I. Controlled trial of imipramine in diurnal enuresis. Arch Dis Child 1982;57(9):714–6.

63. Martin GI. Imipramine pamoate in the treatment of childhood enuresis. A double-blind study. Am J Dis Child 1971;122(1):42–7.

64. Lines DR. A double-blind trial of amitriptyline in enuretic children. Med J Austral 1968;2(7):307–8.

65. Laybourne PCJ, Roach NE, Ebbesson B, Edwards S. Double-blind study of the use of imipramine (Tofranil) in enuresis. Psychosomatics 1968;9(5):282–5.

66. Lake B. Controlled trial of nortriptyline in childhood enuresis. Med J Austral 1968;2(14):582–5.

67. Kardash S, Hillman ES, Werry J. Efficacy of imipramine in childhood enuresis: a double-blind control study with placebo. Can Med Assoc J 1968;99(6):263–6.

68. Agarwala S, Heycock JB. A controlled trial of imipramine ('Tofranil') in the treatment of childhood enuresis. Br J Clin Pract 1968;22(7):296–8.

69. Forsythe WI, Merrett JD. A controlled trial of imipramine ('Tofranil') and nortriptyline ('Allegron') in the treatment of enuresis. Br J Clin Pract 1969;23(5):210–5.

70. Smellie J, McGrigor V, Meadow S, et al. Nocturnal enuresis: a placebo controlled trial of two antidepressant drugs. Arch Dis Child 1996;75.

71. Moffatt M, Harlos S, Kirshen A, Burd L. Desmopressin acetate and nocturnal enuresis: how much do we know? Pediatrics 1993;92:420–5.

72. Aladjem M, Wohl R, Boichis H, et al. Desmopressin in nocturnal enuresis. Arch Dis Child 1982;57(2):137–40.

73. Pedersen P, Hejl M, Kjoller S. Desamino-D-arginine vasopressin in childhood nocturnal enuresis. J Urol 1985;133:65–6.

74. Post EM, Richman RA, Blackett PR, et al. Desmopressin response of enuretic children. Effects of age and frequency of enuresis. Am J Dis Child 1983;137(10):962–3.

75. Terho P. Desmopressin in nocturnal enuresis. J Urol 1991;145:818–20.

76. Wille S. Comparison of desmopressin and enuresis alarm for nocturnal enuresis. Arch Dis Child 1986;61(1):30–3.

77. Miller K, Klauber G. Desmopressin acetate in children with severe primary nocturnal enuresis. Clin Ther 1990;12:357–66.

78. Pedersen PS, Hejl M, Kjoller SS. Desamino-D-arginine vasopressin in childhood nocturnal enuresis. J Urol 1985;133(1):65–6.

79. Janknegt A, Smans A. Treatment with desmopressin in severe nocturnal enuresis in childhood. J Urol 1990;66:535–7.

80. Wagner WG, Matthews R. The treatment of nocturnal enuresis: a controlled comparison of two models of urine alarm. J Dev Behav Pediatr 1985;6(1):22–6.

81. Rappaport L. Prognostic factors for alarm treatment. Scandi J Urol Nephrol 1997;183(Suppl):55–7;discussion 57–8.

82. Lynch NT, Grunert BK, Vasudevan SV, Severson RA. Enuresis: comparison of two treatments. Arch Phys Med Rehab 1984;65(2):98–100.

83. El-Anany FG, Maghraby HA, Shaker SE, Abdel-Moneim AM. Primary nocturnal enuresis: a new approach to conditioning treatment. Urology 1993;53:405–8.

84. Elinder G, Soback S. Effect of Uristop on primary nocturnal enuresis. A prospective randomized double-blind study. Acta Paediatr Scand 1985;74(4):574–8.

85. Sukhai R, Harris A. Combined therapy of enuresis alarm and desmopressin in the treatment of nocturnal enuresis. Eur J Pediatr 1989;148:465–7.

86. Fordham KE, Meadow SR. Controlled trial of standard pad and bell alarm against mini alarm for nocturnal enuresis. Arch Dis Child 1989;64(5):651–6.

87. Monda J, Husmann D. Primary nocturnal enuresis: a comparison among observation, imipramine, desmopressin acetate and bed-wetting alarm systems. J Urol 1995;154:745–8.

88. Bradbury M. Combination therapy for nocturnal enuresis with desmopressin and an alarm device. Scand J Urol Nephrol 1997;183(Suppl):61–3.

89. Anonymous. American Academy of Pediatrics, Task Force on Circumcision. Circumcision Policy Statement. Pediatrics 1999;103:686–93.

90. To T, Feldman W, Dick P, Tran M. Pediatric health services utilization: circumcision. In: Goel V, Williams J, Anderson G, et al, editors. Patterns of health care in Ontario: the ICES practice atlas. Ottawa: Canadian Medical Association;1996. p. 294–7.

91. Anonymous. Fetus and Newborn Committee, Canadian Pediatric Society. Neonatal circumcision revisited. Can Med Assoc J 1996;154:769–80.

92. Fergusson D, Lawton, JM., Shannon, FT. Neonatal circumcision and penile problems: an 8-year longitudinal study. Pediatrics 1988;81:537–41.

93. Herzog L, Alvarez S. The frequency of foreskin problems in uncircumcised children. Am J Dis Child 1986;140:254–256.

94. Oster J. Further fate of the foreskin: incidence of preputial adhesions, phimosis, and smegma among Danish schoolboys. Arch Dis Child 1968;43:200–3.

95. Fergusson D, Horwood L, Shannon F. Factors related to the age of attainment of nocturnal bladder control: an 8-year longitudinal study. Pediatrics 1986;78:884–90.

96. Wiswell T, Hachey W. Urinary tract infections and the uncircumcised state: an update. Clin Pediatr 1993;32.

97. Rushton H, Majd M. Pyelonephritis in male infants: how important is the foreskin? J Urol 1992;148:733–6.

98. Young J, Percy C, Asine A. Surveillance, epidemiology, and end results, incidence and mortality data 1973-77. Natl Cancer Inst Monogr 1981;57:17.

99. Frisch M, Frus S, Kjaer S, Melbye M. Falling incidence of penile cancer in an uncircumcised population (Denmark 1943-90). Br Med J 1995;311:1471.

100. Maden C, Sherman K, Beckmann A, et al. History of circumcision, medical conditions, and sexual activity and risk of penile cancer. J Natl Cancer Inst 1993;85:19–24.

101. Hellberg D, Valentin J, Eklund T, Milsson S. Penile cancer: is there an epidemiological role for smoking and sexual behavior? Br Med J 1987;295:1306–8.

102. Brinton L, Li J, Rong S, et al. Risk factors for penile cancer: results from a case-control study in China. Intl J Cancer 1991;47:504–9.

103. Seed J, Allen S, Mertens T. Male circumcision, sexually transmitted disease, and risk of HIV. J AIDS Hum Retrovirol 1995;8:83–90.

104. Tyndall M, Ronald R, Agoki E, et al. Increased risk of infection with human immunodeficiency virus type 1 among uncircumcised men presenting with genital ulcer disease in Kenya. Clin Infect Dis 1996;23:449–53.

105. Kreiss J, Hopkins S. The association between circumcision and human immunodeficiency virus infection among homosexual men. J Infect Dis 1993;168:1404–08.

106. Pepin J, Quigley M, Todd J. Association between HIV-2 infection and genital ulcer diseases among male sexually transmitted disease patients in Gambia. AIDS 1992;6:489–93.

107. Simonsen J, Cameron D, Gakinya N. Human immunodeficiency virus infection among men with sexually transmitted diseases: experience from a center in Africa. N Engl J Med 1988;319:274–8.

108. Bwayo J, Plummer F, Omau M. Human immunodeficiency virus infection in long-distance truck drivers in East Africa. Arch Intern Med 1994;154:1291–6.

109. Moses S, Plummer F, Bradley J, et al. The association between the lack of male circumcision and the risk for HIV infection: a review of the epidemiological data. Sex Trans Dis 1994;21:201–10.

110. De Vincenzi I, Mertens T. Male circumcision: a role in HIV prevention? [editorial]. AIDS 1994;8:153–60.

111. Gee S, Ansell J. Neonatal circumcision: a ten-year overview with comparison of Gomco clamp and Plastibell device. Pediatrics 1976;58:824–7.

112. Harkavy K. The circumcision debate. Pediatrics 1987;79:649–50.

113. Taddio A, Katz J, Ilersich A, Karen G. Effect of neonatal circumcision on pain response during subsequent routine vaccination. Lancet 1997;349:599–603.

114. Ganiats T, Humphrey J, Taras H. Routine neonatal circumcision: a cost-utility analysis. Med Decision Making 1991;11:282–93.

115. Lawler F, Bisonni R, Holtgrave D. Circumcision: a decision analysis of its medical value. Fam Med 1991;23:587–93.

CHAPTER 18

Allergy

Adelle Roberta Atkinson, RN, BSc, MD, FRCPC, FAAP

Allergic diseases are an extremely common cause of both acute and chronic illness in children. They are among the most common reasons why a child is brought to the attention of a primary-care practitioner.[1] This translates into a great deal of morbidity and burden of illness on society. The purpose of this chapter is to discuss the major allergens within the realm of pediatric allergy as well as the approach to the diagnosis and management of immunoglobulin E (IgE) -mediated hypersensitivity within those allergenic groups. The emphasis is on the evidence available for diagnostic tests and treatment strategies to aid the practitioner in making informed clinical decisions. Controversies which affect the primary-care practitioner are also discussed.

The allergies important in pediatrics include food, drug, and environmental allergies. Each of these areas will be introduced in the following section with special attention paid to areas of controversy.

FOOD ALLERGY

Hippocrates is credited with one of the first written accounts of an IgE-mediated (urticarial) reaction to food, specifically milk.[2] In 1921, Prausnitz and Kustner elucidated that the phenomenon responsible for an "allergic" reaction was present in serum and could be transferred to a nonsensitive individual.[2] With the introduction of the double-blind, placebo-controlled oral food challenge in 1976, the study of food allergy began its scientific journey.[3]

Adverse reactions to food include toxic and nontoxic reactions. Toxic reactions can occur in anyone, with the reaction being a direct result of the properties of the food ingested, for example, toxins secreted by *Salmonella*. Nontoxic reactions depend specifically on the susceptibility of the host and can be immune mediated (allergy) or non–immune mediated (intolerance). Intolerances account for the majority of adverse food reactions; however, it is the IgE-mediated immune response that will be the focus of this section.[2] Immunoglobulin E-mediated responses to food hypersensitivity take the form of cutaneous eruptions (urticaria/angioedema, atopic dermatitis), respiratory symptoms (rhinoconjunctivitis, asthma), very specific gastrointestinal complaints (oral allergy syndrome, allergic eosinophilic gastroenteritis), and anaphylaxis.[4]

Surveys of both children and adults reveal that approximately 25 percent of the population believe they have a food allergy.[4] The prevalence of true food allergy, however, is far less and quoted by Sampson to be approximately 5 percent of children less than 3 years of age and 1.5 percent of the general population.[4] What is also clear is that children with atopic dermatitis have a higher incidence of food allergy than the general population, and the more severe their dermatitis, the greater is the chance that they have a food allergy.[2]

The most common food allergens include cow's milk, chicken egg, legumes (specifically peanuts and soyabeans), tree nuts (almonds, Brazil nuts, cashew nuts, filberts, hickory nuts, pecan, pine nuts, pistachios, and walnuts), fish, crustaceans (lobster and shrimp), mollusk (mussels and scallops), and cereal grains.[2]

The Peanut

The peanut deserves special mention as it is one of the most allergenic foods in children.[2] The peanut is a member of the legume family and therefore not related to other nuts. Allergic reactions to peanuts can be life threatening. Therefore, patients with this allergy must take great care in avoiding eating peanuts and all products potentially containing peanuts. However, even when one is extremely careful, there is unfortunately a great deal of accidental exposure especially in foods such as baked goods, in which the allergen can be hidden.[5]

It has always been believed that unlike some other food allergies, allergy to peanuts is not outgrown. In a longitudinal study by Bock in 1989, a group of patients who were positive to peanuts by history and skin prick test accidentally ingested it up to 14 years after testing. None tolerated it.[6] More recent work by Hourihane in 1998 has shown that there may be some patients with very few other allergies who do, in fact, lose their peanut allergy over time. This study was in a case-control format, and the patient numbers were small with only 15 in each group.[7] The concept of losing sensitivity to peanuts is intriguing and further study in this area will be of great value.

The peanut is ubiquitous in our society. Therefore, allergy to this seemingly innocuous legume is worthy of serious and ongoing study.

Egg Hypersensitivity and Administration of the MMR Vaccine

There has been ongoing controversy and concern over the years about the safety of administering the MMR vaccine to children with documented hypersensitivity to egg protein. Given that the incidence of egg allergy in the pediatric population is reported to be approximately 0.5 percent,[8] there is the potential for a significant number of children to have their vaccination either delayed or omitted.

There are numerous good studies in the literature showing the safety of administering the MMR vaccine to egg-allergic children.[8–10] Freigang and colleagues, in 1994, published one of the largest studies on the administration of the MMR vaccine to 500 egg-allergic children. Early on in the study, they abandoned skin testing (after 120 patients) as it did not appear to have any relationship to the final reaction to the immunization.[9] There was no anaphylaxis described in any patients and only 5 patients had minor local reactions to the vaccination.[9] In 1995, James and colleagues published another study combining all the experience of giving the MMR vaccine to egg-allergic children described in the literature since 1963. The results showed that 99.75 percent of children who are allergic to eggs and have a positive skin test can receive the vaccine in the usual way without any severe anaphylactic reactions.[8]

On the basis of good evidence, the National Advisory Committee on Immunization has changed the recommendations in the fifth edition of the Canadian Immunization Guide. They are as follows:

1. Given that the Yellow Fever and influenza vaccines are prepared from viruses grown in embryonated eggs, they should not be given unless the risk of the disease outweighs the small risk of a systemic hypersensitivity reaction.
2. Egg allergy is no longer considered a contraindication to immunization with MMR. Children with a history of egg allergy may be immunized in the routine manner without prior testing. As an additional measure of safety, however, it may be prudent to observe them for 30 minutes after immunization for any signs of an allergic reaction.
3. A previous anaphylactic reaction to a vaccine containing measles-mumps-rubella is an absolute contraindication to receiving the vaccine a subsequent time.
4. If an individual who has had a prior anaphylactic reaction to a vaccine requires reimmunization, yellow fever or influenza vaccine prepared in embryonated chicken eggs the American Academy of Pediatrics "Report of the Committee on Infectious Diseases" also

agrees and recommends that the MMR can be administered to children with a history of egg allergy.[10a] It is also recommended that if an individual has a history of anaphylactic hypersensitivity to hen's eggs, skin testing and a graded challenge can be considered. If a graded challenge is to be conducted it should be done in an appropriately equipped facility by skilled personnel who are both familiar with the procedure itself and the treatment of anaphylaxis.[11]

Clearly, the institution of these guidelines, which are based on good evidence, will begin to ensure an increase in immunization rates in our population. They will also result in a decrease in morbidity and discomfort in the patient caused by unnecessary testing and graded immunizations and decrease in parental anxiety (see also Chapter 3 on immunization).

PENICILLIN ALLERGY AND CROSS-REACTIONS

Penicillin was discovered by Fleming in 1928[12] and since that time has become the most widely prescribed antibiotic in the world.[13]

Of great concern is the number of children with a history of "hypersensitivity" to penicillin. Not only is the medication inexpensive, but it also has a quite favorable side-effect profile, when compared with other antimicrobials. Cutaneous reactions and gastrointestinal symptoms are not uncommon in connection with penicillin use and are often interpreted as allergic reactions.[14] This leads to a significant number of children being referred to both hospital and community allergists for evaluation of their sensitivity.

Penicillin is highly immunogenic and considered to be the most common drug causing allergic reactions.[15] The prevalence of penicillin allergy in the general population is quoted as being between 1 and 10 percent.[15] The prevalence of adverse reactions to cephalosporins ranges from 1 to 10 percent also.[16] These figures are based on reporting and therefore may turn out to be overestimates of the prevalence, when confirmed via skin testing and oral challenges.

There is ongoing concern on the part of physicians treating patients with "hypersensitivity" to penicillin about its cross-reactivity with cephalopsorins. This concern has the potential to further reduce the antibiotic choices for given infections. The concern has stemmed from the fact that both penicillin and cephalosporins contain a beta-lactam ring.[12] Earlier in-vitro studies demonstrated antigenic cross-reactivity with little information on the clinical relevence;[12] some authors felt that these studies, in fact, overestimated the risk.[17]

As early as 1967, there appeared in the literature published accounts of patients who were penicillin allergic and, when given a cephalosporin they had not encountered previously, had a type I hypersensitivity reaction.[18,19] Most of these early reports were in the form of case reports. The generally accepted rate of cross-reactivity in the literature has varied between 6 and 15 percent.[20] There have not been any randomized controlled trials (RCTs) to further define this percentage, and one study has reported that it is, in fact, safe to administer cephalosporin antibiotics to penicillin-allergic patients.[16] Unfortunately, this particular study used published reports and postmarketing data from pharmaceutical corporations as the basis for the analysis.[16] Solley and colleagues prospectively studied patients with a history of penicillin allergy and both negative and positive skin tests. The group with negative skin tests had a 1.3 percent reaction rate (well within the average quoted for cephalosporin reactions alone), and there were no reactions in the positive skin test group.[21]

Given that there have been no RCTs prospectively comparing the incidence of IgE-mediated reactions to cephalosporins in penicillin-allergic patients virus non–penicillin-allergic patients, it is difficult to determine how concerned one should be when considering administation of cephalosporins to penicillin-allergic patients. Although the percentage may be much lower than is the current teaching, until there is better evidence, one must be cautious when considering prescribing cephalosporin antibiotics to penicillin-allergic patients.

Environmental Allergy

Environmental allergies may be manifested clinically as rhinitis, conjunctivitis, or asthma exacerbations. These allergies may be perennial, with or without seasonal exacerbations, or only seasonal.[22] They are IgE-mediated reactions to a variety of aeroallergens. Typical seasonal allergens are pollens and molds, while typical perennial aeroallergens include dust mites, molds, animal allergens, and certain occupational allergens.[22]

In the United States, the most common indoor allergens are dust mite feces, cockroach (both the insect's body and feces contain the allergen), and cat dander. The most common outdoor allergens are pollens and fungal spores.[23]

Rhinitis is defined as inflammation of the membranes lining the nose. It is characterized by nasal congestion, rhinorrhea, sneezing, itching of the nose, and/or postnasal drainage.[23] Allergic rhinitis is believed to affect 20 to 40 million people in the United States. Up to 40 percent of children may be affected, with the greater percentage of males.[22] Given the large numbers of patients affected in the population, the morbidity and burden of illness are marked in terms of costs to the health-care system as well as time away from work.[22]

Diagnosis of Immediate Hypersensitivity

The diagnosis of IgE-mediated reactions to the various allergens described above begins with a thorough history, including very specific questions about each of the potential allergens, timing, and a description of the clinical symptoms. Previous trials of therapy should also be documented.[24] A very important detail that may be overlooked is to investigate the extent to which the symptoms interfere with the patient's life.[24] After a complete physical examination, it is time to decide which tests, if any, will aid in the diagnosis. Allergy testing does not diagnose allergic disease but rather determines the presence or absence of allergen-specific IgE antibodies.[1] These results combined with the clinical presentation aid the physician in diagnosing allergic disease.

To properly study a diagnostic tool, there must be a gold standard to which the test can be compared. Ideally, this standard should be able to induce typical signs and symptoms and be reproducible. It must also be done in a double-blind, placebo-controlled fashion.[1] This is possible in some areas of allergy such as food allergy but is more challenging in other areas such as environmental allergies.[1]

Skin Prick Testing

Skin tests have been used as the major diagnostic tool in allergy since 1865, when they were first introduced by Blackley.[25] There have been some modifications over the years, and it is believed that they may provide important information that can corroborate clinical suspicion of a specific allergy. They are simple and time efficient, which explains their global use by trained allergists.[25]

Skin prick testing was described in 1924 by Lewis and Grant and became widely used in the 1970s.[25] It involves the placement of a small drop of extract as well as a small drop of both saline and histamine controls on the volar surface of the forearm or the back. A sterile lancet is then used to break the epidermis. Each allergen must be placed 2 cm apart. The area is then observed for clinical reaction for 15 to 20 minutes.[26] For a reaction to be considered positive, there must be a wheal that is at least 3 mm larger than the negative control.[26]

Skin prick testing is believed to be the most specific screening method to detect the presence of IgE antibodies in patients with a clinical history of reaction to allergen exposure.[26] Skin prick testing has been demonstrated to be highly reproducible when both inter- and intravariations were calculated, using histamine dihydrochloride.[27] Although the presence of a positive skin prick test does not necessarily correlate with the presence of clinical symptoms, there may be a higher incidence of clinically significant allergy with larger reactions.[26] This mode of testing is used in the area of food allergy, environmental allergy, drug allergy, and latex allergy.

Testing for Penicillin Allergy

Penicillin allergy has been studied extensively. In 1992, the results of a collaborative clinical trial conducted by the National Institute of Allergy and Infectious Diseases were published. The usefulness of four penicillin allergen skin tests in the prediction of IgE-mediated reactions following administration of penicillin was assessed.[28] This study demonstrated the high negative predictive value (NPV) of a negative skin test, which has been reproduced elsewhere.[28-30] The NPV of skin testing to the major and minor determinants of penicillin in patients with a positive history was in the order of 98 to 99 percent. However, as the majority of patients who had positive skin tests did not go on to receive oral penicillin, the positive predictive value (PPV) is unknown. The specificity of the test is also quite high, in the order of 99 percent, in this defined group of patients, but again, the sensitivity could not be determined from this data. Despite this lack of data, there are those who believe that the PPV of a skin prick test is high.[30] This assumption is based on the observation made in a number of studies that patients with positive skin tests who were given penicillin, either deliberately or inadvertently, did show a clinical reaction 40 to 100 percent of the time.[21,29,30] These numbers are small and observed incidentally. However, to determine the PPV of positive skin prick testing to penicillin, further careful studies need to be carried out in a systematic fashion. Until these studies are done, the PPV of this test is unclear. A further question to be studied lies in the area of negative skin tests. Given the high NPV of a negative test, should one proceed to an oral challenge or feel safe in giving a proper course of treatment on the basis of the test alone? Pichichero and Pichichero outline that skin testing without an oral challenge may allow room for non–IgE-mediated adverse reactions to be missed.[31] These authors also described that pediatrician-diagnosed adverse reactions to a variety of antibiotics accurately predicted IgE sensitivity only 34 percent of the time.[31] In other words, 66 percent of the physician-diagnosed "penicillin allergic" patients were, in fact, not allergic, as confirmed by negative skin testing and oral challenge.[31] The false-positive diagnosis rate may have been even higher as none of the 34 percent of patients with a positive skin test were challenged with oral penicillin.

The NPV of skin prick testing for the major and minor determinants of penicillin is high as is the specificity in patients with a history of an adverse reaction to penicillin. However, given the concern of missing a non–IgE-mediated reaction by omitting the oral challenge component, it would appear prudent to take this next step despite this reliability. With respect to the PPV, further work is required to make this determination. If it is, in fact, low, should we change our approach and go directly to an oral challenge in the area of penicillin allergy?

Testing for Food Allergy

Skin prick testing is widely used in the clinical evaluation of food allergy. Positive results indicate the possibility that the patient may have a clinical reaction to that particular food. The PPV, however, is less than 50 percent, while the NPV is greater than 95 percent in a trial that studied children with atopic dermatitis.[32-34] These values were determined through comparison with the "gold standard" in the diagnosis of food allergy, the double-blind, placebo-controlled food challenge (DBPCFC).[33] Thus, the skin prick test is a way to rule out an IgE-mediated food allergy but is only suggestive of clinical food allergy in the case of a positive test.[32] One must also remember that there are no standardized allergens in this area.[35] Therefore, a variety of extracts as well as fresh foods are often used in the test.

Using peanut allergy as an example, one can understand from Sampson's study that the NPV and the sensitivity are 100 percent.[33] However, the specificity and PPV of this allergen are 58 percent and 44 percent, respectively.[32] This false-positive rate carries with it a set of consequences. Should the false-positive skin test not be challenged orally, in a patient with no history of a clinical reaction, the patient becomes labeled as peanut allergic. This increases anxiety in the family; with some foods, this may cause nutritional deficiencies and put the patient at risk for eating disorders. Other family members are also affected by the restrictions. Travel and staying with friends become real issues. With this in mind, and the fact that skin testing has the potential to be costly to the health-care system, it would be interesting to consider whether there is a role for the DBPCFC to be used more frequently, even as first line in certain situations.

Given the complexity of the use and interpretation of skin prick tests, they must be employed judiciously by a trained allergist.

Testing for Environmental Allergy

In the area of environmental allergy, skin prick testing may not be required in the initial evaluation. The current recommendations by the Joint Task Force (representing the American Academy of Allergy, Asthma and Immunology, the American College of Allergy, Asthma and Immunology and the Joint Council on Allergy, Asthma, and Immunology) for the Diagnosis and Management of Rhinitis include that an initial therapeutic trial of pharmacologic therapy may be used for nonsevere rhinitis prior to referral and skin testing.[24] The recommendations by the same Joint Task Force for the use of skin testing are as follows. Skin testing has a role in delineating an allergic component to a patient's symptoms. It may also have a role in the development of immunotherapy as third-line therapy in difficult-to-treat patients by identifying specific allergens.[22] Although there may be a high NPV in this skin prick testing, it is not clear how a positive test correlates with the presence or absence or severity of clinical symptoms.

Ownby discusses the difficulty in evaluating skin tests for inhalant allergies, as reproducing natural exposure is very difficult.[1] Reddy and colleagues in 1978 concluded that skin prick testing correlated well with nasal provocation in patients with a history of allergic rhinitis.[36] Unfortunately, nasal provocation as well as radioallergosorbent test (RAST) and leukocyte histamine release assays were used as the gold standard and these have not been proved to accurately reproduce naturally occurring phenomena.[36] Cavanaugh and colleagues compared skin testing with bronchial provocation testing and found a reasonable correlation. However, they did acknowledge that to determine the significance of any allergic diagnostic test, one needed an absolute reference point, and neither of these techniques has proved to be that point.[37] Skin testing for environmental allergies must be viewed as an aid in the diagnosis. It must correlate with symptoms and signs. To properly assign diagnostic value to skin testing for inhalant allergies, further research is needed in the area of developing a gold standard that is reproducible.

Intracutaneous Testing

Intracutaneous testing goes one step further in skin testing and is described as being used to increase the sensitivity of skin prick testing in certain situations. This test is often performed after a negative skin prick test, especially if there is concern about drugs and venoms, to increase the sensitivity.[25] Intracutaneous tests are performed by injecting a measured amount of a standardized extract into the dermal layer, causing a wheal. The tests are then evaluated in a similar fashion as the prick testing.

Intracutaneous testing has been described as a method to increase the sensitivity of certain diagnostic evaluations.[25] It has been postulated that in patients who have low levels of clinical sensitivity, the skin prick test may, in fact, be falsely negative, while an intracutaneous test may identify these patients.[25] As discussed previously, the NPV of the skin prick test is high; therefore, further research would be required to elucidate whether or not this extra step would, in fact, improve the overall accuracy of skin testing. One could argue that proceeding to a challenge may be more scientifically sound. In the area of food allergy, Bock found as early as 1978, that the intradermal skin test did not have a greater PPV than the skin prick test, when compared with the gold standard.[38] In fact, there is some evidence to suggest that it may have quite a high false-positive rate, as a number of children in this study who were skin prick negative and intradermal positive went on to have a negative DBPCFC.[38] Sampson believes that the use of intradermal skin tests in the diagnosis of food allergy is inappropriate until such time as studies demonstrate that the sensitivity, specificity, PPV, and NPV are greater than skin prick testing, when compared with the DBPCFC.[39] Intradermal testing is widely used in the area of penicillin and venom allergies. The PPV of this test has not been studied in detail. The NPV can be considered similar to that of the skin prick test.

Double-Blind, Placebo-Controlled Food Challenge

The DBPCFC, which is felt to be the gold standard in the diagnosis of food allergy, involves the administration, in a blinded fashion, of increasing amounts of the food in question. Once the patient has tolerated 10 g of lyophilized food, an open feeding study under observation is performed for confirmation.[32] The diagnostic accuracy is felt to be very good; however, there are the occasional false-negative reactions, when the patient does not receive enough of the challenge substance or the lyophilization process alters the allergenic properties of the food, such as in the case of fish.[32] This method of ruling out (or in) food allergy minimizes the number of foods being eliminated from the diet.[40]

As with food allergy, the most reliable method for proving or disproving penicillin allergy is to perform an oral challenge in a controlled setting. These challenges are routinely performed after negative skin tests; however, they have not been studied systematically in a large number of patients with positive skin tests.

Radioallergosorbent Test

The in-vitro RAST has been used extensively over the years. In 1983, Sampson published a study that examined the sensitivity and specificity of RAST as compared with skin prick testing and the gold standard DBPCFC. Similar to skin prick testing, RAST was found to have a very high NPV (82 to 100 percent), while the PPV was low, between 25 and 75 percent.[33] It is clear from this study that the two tests together are no more valuable than either test alone.[33] The skin prick test is more sensitive than RAST.

Other Diagnostic Tests

There are currently a number of tests that are either unproven or inappropriate in the diagnostic work-up of allergic disease. First, there are the tests that are incapable of any measurement.[26] These include the cytotoxic test, provocation-neutralization, electrodermal diagnosis and applied kinesiology, reaginic pulse test, and tissue chemistry.[26] There is a further group of tests that do have some validity, but not in the diagnosis of allergy. These include allergen-specific IgG, circulating immune complexes to foods, immunoglobulins, complement, and lymphocyte counts.[26]

TREATMENT

General Principles

The mainstay of allergy management is avoidance. This is more difficult in some allergies than others. With food allergy, elimination diets have their potential adverse effects. Malnutrition and eating disorders may ensue.[4] Patients must also be taught to be diligent about scrutinizing food labels and to be careful about the possibility of hidden allergens.[4] Avoidance is simpler with penicillin allergy, in which case there are other alternatives that can be used. The patient and family must be diligent about informing health care workers about the allergy, and conversely health-care workers must be diligent about questioning patients about their allergy history. Avoidance is much more difficult with environmental allergy, as one can only manipulate and control the environment to a certain extent.

Food Allergy

The only proven therapy for food allergy is elimination of the offending allergen from the diet of the affected individual.[2] Similar to prescribing pharmacotherapy, prescribing an elimination diet in a child must be done with caution and follow-up. Depending on the allergen, restricting the diet of any child is fraught with the possibility of creating problems such as malnutrition and possibly eating disorders.[2] Patients and parents must be taught to scrutinize the labels of foods for potential allergens.

Some medications have been used in food-allergic patients, such as H_1 and H_2 antagonists, corticosteroids, ketotifen, and prostaglandin synthetase inhibitors.[2] Their efficacy has been found to be minimal and their side effects unacceptable.[2]

There is still no role for immunotherapy in the management of food allergy.[2]

Given that most children will outgrow their allergies to certain foods, it is important that they be re-evaluated at the appropriate time for a possibile oral challenge. Milk allergy is often outgrown by 3 years of age, and it may then be possible to re-introduce it into a child's diet.[2]

Penicillin Allergy

Avoidance of penicillin in the current era of medicine is relatively straightforward, given the number of choices for an alternative. However, there are situations in which penicillin must be used.

If a patient cannot avoid penicillin, and has a confirmed IgE and clinical reaction to the drug, desensitization can be accomplished. This process must be done according to published guidelines in an intensive care setting. It must be done each time penicillin is required. Desensitization is achieved by administering increasing doses of drug every 20 to 30 minutes. When a full therapeutic dose has been tolerated, the treatment can begin.[41] It is of note that a large number of these patients will have a mild allergic reaction during the desensitization and therapeutic phases.[41]

Environmental Allergy

Environmental Control

The management of environmental allergies rests in three major areas: environmental control, pharmacologic therapy, and immunotherapy.

The Joint Task Force developed Practice Parameters for the Diagnosis and Management of Rhinitis in 1998 describing five categories of environmental triggers for allergic rhinitis: pollens, molds, house dust mites, animals, and insect allergens.[22]

Avoidance is more difficult with outdoor allergens than with indoor allergens.[42] Environmental control begins by reducing pollen exposure.[22] Windows and doors should be kept closed and air conditioning used, if possible. Solomon and colleagues have shown that even single-unit air conditioners used in one room significantly decrease pollen and spore counts, when compared both with control rooms and with the outside.[43] Decreasing extended periods of time outside during the high pollen season is also of value.[22]

The major source of allergen in house dust is the fecal residue of the dust mite. As the major food source of the dust mite is exfoliated human skin scale, these mites survive in such areas as bedding, fabric covered furniture, soft toys, and carpeting.[22] They replicate in humid environments. Dust mite–sensitive individuals should avoid carpets as much as possible. Mattresses, box springs, and pillows should be encased in allergen-proof enclosures.[22] Bed-linen should be washed frequently in water greater than 130°F.[22]

The major cat allergen is *Fel d* I and is found on cat skin/dander and saliva as well as urine. The major dog allergen is *Can f* I, also found in dog skin/dander and saliva.[22] Avoidance clearly remains the most effective way of dealing with animal sensitivity. A HEPA or electrostatic air purifier may reduce airborne allergens to a certain extent.[22]

Pharmacologic Therapy

Oral antihistamines. Histamine is the major chemical mediator of inflammation producing the symptoms of allergic rhinitis.[22] It causes increased vascular permeability and dilatation of blood vessels and stimulates sensory nerve endings, causing glandular secretion. Therefore, one of the mainstays of allergy therapy has been oral antihistamines. These drugs are antagonists of histamine at the H_1-receptor site. Their peak concentration is within 2 to 3 hours.[22] Oral antihistamines have repeatedly been shown to decrease the symptoms of allergic rhinitis. In a double-blind, randomized, placebo-controlled, multicenter trial, brompheniramine, a first-generation antihistamine, was shown to significantly reduce the symptoms of allergic rhinitis, when compared with terfenadine, a second-generation antihistamine, and with placebo.[44] However, it has also been shown repeatedly that first generation antihistamines (eg, diphenhydramine, hydroxyzine) cause somnolence and central nervous system (CNS) depression.[22,44] In most states of the United States, persons taking these drugs are considered "under the influence of drugs."[22] Incidentally, terfenadine was removed from the market in the United States in 1998 as there was concern that it may cause prolongation of the QTc interval and cardiac dysrhythmias.[22]

The CNS depression is a significant adverse reaction to the first-generation antihistamines. Of concern in pediatrics is the effect this will have on children's ability to concentrate in the classroom. However, if children are not treated with medication, they may be symptomatic in the classroom, which can also interfere with concentration. A study by Vuurman and colleagues looked at the effect of allergic rhinitis on learning by comparing four groups. One group was treated with a first-generation antihistamine, the second with a second-generation antihistamine, the third with placebo, and the fourth were normal controls without seasonal allergic rhinitis. Although the study was not blinded, the results provide food for thought. The normal controls' average learning performance was superior to the other three groups. Within the atopic children, those treated with the second-generation antihistamine had the highest scores while those treated with the first-generation antihistamine had the lowest scores.[45] Shanon and colleagues also compared first-generation (chlorpheniramine) and second-generation (astemizole) antihistamines. This study was done as a prospective, randomized, double-blind, cross-over study.[46] Using a number of objective measures of attention, auditory and visual memory, and motor coordination as well as evaluation of physical side effects, this study demonstrated that there were no clinically important adverse effects with either drug. The objective testing suggests that school performance with either medication should not be a problem.[46]

Because of their inability to penetrate the CNS well, the second-generation antihistamines (cetirizine, loratadine) have been marketed as producing decreased side effects such as somnolence or drowsiness. This has been demonstrated both objectively and subjectively.[44,47] However, most studies have shown that this class of antihistamines is not more effective in treating allergic rhinitis and in some cases is less effective than the first-generation group.[22,44,46]

Nasal antihistamines. Nasal antihistamines are recommended in the "practice parameters for the diagnosis and management of rhinitis" (Joint Task Force on Practice Parameters in Allergy, Asthma, and Immunology)[22] as first-line therapy for allergic rhinitis. In a double-blind, randomized, placebo-controlled, multicenter trial azelastine nasal spray was shown to be efficacious in the treatment of seasonal allergic rhinitis, when compared with placebo.[48,49] Both these studies were performed in adults and in children 12 years and over.

Oral decongestants. Oral decongestants are alpha-adrenergic agents (pseudoephedrine, phenylephrine and phenylpropanolamine). They cause nasal vasoconstriction.[22] Oral decongestants have been shown in double-blind, randomized, placebo-controlled studies to improve the symptoms of rhinitis, when compared with placebo.[50] Their side-effect profile, however, includes insomnia, anorexia, and excessive nervousness.[22] There is also evidence that a combination medication including a decongestant and an antihistamine improves rhinitis symptoms, not only when compared with placebo but also with either medication alone.[51]

Corticosteroids. Nasal corticosteroids, through their anti-inflammatory effects, are effective in controlling the major symptoms of allergic rhinitis which are sneezing, itching, nasal blockage, and rhinorrhea.[22] Welsh and colleagues in 1987 compared two nasal corticosteroids, cromolyn, and placebo. All groups were randomized, but only beclomethasone and placebo were double blinded, the other two being single blinded presumably due to different dosing regimens. They found that all treatments were superior to placebo, with the corticosteroids also being superior to cromolyn.[52] The most common side effect of nasal corticosteroids is nasal irritation.[22] Indeed, there are case reports in the literature of actual nasal perforation, both in adults and in children, with prolonged use and possibly incorrect administration.[53]

One of the advantages of nasal versus systemic steroids is the decreased amount of systemic absorption and therefore side effects. A multicenter, double-blind, parallel-group, dose-tolerance, placebo-controlled trial studying fluticasone propionate aqueous nasal spray showed that it was favorable over placebo in two respects. There was a significant decrease in clinical symptoms as well as normal cortisol concentrations, normal adrenocorticotropic hormone (ACTH) stimulation indices, and normal urinary free cortisol levels, which were not significantly different from the placebo group.[54] This is believed by the authors to indicate that there is very little systemic absorption of this therapy. Indeed, there may be greater absorption by some of the other nasal corticosteroids.[54]

Given that nasal corticosteroids have been shown in good studies to be effective in the treatment of allergic rhinitis, one must differentiate within this group. In 1993, van As and colleagues compared fluticasone propionate and beclomethasone dipropionate in a multicenter, double-blind, randomized, placebo-controlled study. Once-daily fluticasone was shown to be as effective as twice-daily beclomethasone.[55] There is also good evidence that fluticasone is less absorbed systemically than beclomethasone.[54] There are no reported adverse systemic effects associated with fluticasone with doses up to 1,600 µg daily for 4 weeks.[55] An important factor to keep in mind is that most studies evaluating nasal corticosteroids have included children 12 years and older. Once-daily therapy may have some benefit in terms of compliance.

Oral corticosteroids are not indicated for the treatment of chronic rhinitis. The "practice parameters for the diagnosis and management of rhinitis" acknowledge that they may have a role in severe cases that are unresponsive to other therapies, if used in short bursts only.[22] There are no controlled trials evaluating the effectiveness of this therapy, and given its very limited role in the treatment of this condition, some authors believe that it will be unlikely that any will be carried out.[56]

Intranasal cromolyn. Cromolyn sodium inhibits the degranulation of mast cells once they have been sensitized, thus decreasing release of the mediators of inflammation.[22] Given that it prevents the allergic event, it must be given prophylactically. Studies done in the early 1970s suggest that it may have a protective effect by decreasing nasal symptoms.[57,58] The "practice parameters" suggest that it may be useful and should be considered in very young children and pregnancy.[22]

Intranasal anticholinergics.   The most extensively studied intranasal anticholinergic agent is ipratropium bromide. It is a quaternary amine that minimally crosses the nasal and gastrointestinal membranes, exerting its effects locally on the nasal mucosa.[22] In a double-blind, multicenter, randomized, placebo-controlled study, ipratropium bromide was shown to significantly improve symptomatology, especially the duration and severity of rhinorrhea.[59]

Oral antileukotriene agents.   These agents may cause some improvement in the symptoms of allergic rhinitis. This is an area that requires further study.[22]

Immunotherapy: Clinical Practice Guidelines

In May of 1995, the Canadian Society of Allergy and Clinical Immunology published evidence-based clinical practice guidelines for the use of allergen immunotherapy.[60] These guidelines are to be used by practitioners for patients in whom allergen avoidance and drug therapy have been unsuccessful.

Clinical practice guidelines gather, appraise, and combine evidence.[61] They attempt to address the issues relevant to a clinical decision and, on the basis of evidence, make recommendations intended to guide clinical practice.[61] Based on criteria for interpreting clinical practice guidelines, the guidelines put forth by the Canadian Society of Allergy and Clinical Immunology working group are clearly well founded. The objectives were stated clearly. The recommendations were based on good evidence and were clinically appropriate.

Whether immunotherapy is indicated in a specific patient context should be decided only after careful identification of the factors that cause the specific symptoms. The reaction must be IgE-mediated. First-line therapy includes avoidance of allergens, if possible. Second-line therapy involves H_1-receptor antagonists, decongestants, and corticosteroids.

"The Clinical Practice Guidelines" recommend that immunotherapy be considered as third-line therapy for patients with a history of IgE-mediated systemic reactions to Hymenoptera venom, allergic rhinitis, and may be useful in patients with asthma exacerbated by environmental factors. The guidelines go on to suggest that for a beneficial response, patients must be treated with high doses versus low-dose therapy. Standardized allergens should be used in increasing concentrations over months and then maintenance therapy for 4 to 5 years. Modified allergenic extracts for short-term preseasonal therapy are not recommended.[60]

The working group of the Canadian Society of Allergy and Clinical Immunology reviewed in detail the effectiveness of treating each specific indication for immunotherapy. The efficacy of this treatment in the context of allergic rhinitis is supported by a number of well-designed, double-blind, placebo-controlled studies. However, greater than 90 percent of patients respond to avoidance and drug management and do not require immunotherapy.[61]

Support for recommending immunotherapy for asthma is not as clear. Many studies were not carried out under ideal conditions. However, some well-designed, double-blind, placebo-controlled studies have demonstrated its efficacy. Given the lack of clear evidence, the guidelines recommend consideration of immunotherapy with a standardized allergen for poorly controlled allergic asthma only after allergen avoidance and appropriate pharmacotherapy have been given a proper trial.[60]

Venom immunotherapy for yellow jackets, yellow hornets, white-faced hornets, wasps, and honeybees is reported to be more than 95 percent protective in patients with previous anaphylaxis. The current recommendation is for insect venom to be injected every 4 to 6 weeks. This should be continued for 5 years.[60]

Immunotherapy is contraindicated in the following circumstances: non–IgE-mediated allergy, IgE-dependent allergy to foods, patients whose only symptoms are urticaria or atopic dermatitis, coexisting autoimmune disease, severe uncontrolled asthma, less than 5 years of age, previous failed trial of immunotherapy, no reduction of symptoms after 2 years of injections, and injections given for more than 5 years.[60]

The use of sublingual-swallow immunotherapy was shown by Clavel and colleagues in a recent double-blind, placebo-controlled, multicenter trial to significantly reduce the need for oral corticosteroids and other adjuvant therapy for allergic rhinitis.[62] Forty of the 120 patients studied were children. Given that the indications for the immunotherapy described above include those patients who have failed environmental control and medical management, a third-line type of therapy that did not involve an injection would be desirable in children. Further work in this area is required in the pediatric population, with clinically significant outcomes defined well.

In June of 1997, Nelson and colleagues published a study examining the efficacy of immunotherapy for desensitization to peanuts. The study looked at 12 patients in total with allergy to peanuts. Half the patients were given the immunotherapy, and half were controls. The study was not randomized. Skin testing, peanut-specific IgE and IgG, and DBPCFC were performed in all patients. The results showed that there may be an increased tolerance to oral peanuts in the study patients. However, systemic reactions were reported in almost all study patients.[63] This area requires more work and is not recommended as standard of care.

Other Treatment Methods

There are a number of other treatment methods with which the practitioner may have contact. The following examples are unproven methods for the treatment of IgE-mediated allergy: neutralization therapy, acupuncture, homeopathy, detoxification, autogenous urine therapy, and enzyme-potentiated immunotherapy.[64]

A summary of the treatment of food, drug, and environment allergies is provided in Table 18–1.

ANAPHYLAXIS

Anaphylaxis, which means the opposite of protection, was a term first coined by Portier and Richet in 1902.[65] It is now known that it is a pathologic phenomenon that occurs on

Table 18–1 Treatment of Food, Drug, and Environmental Allergies

Condition	Intervention	Quality of Evidence	Recommendation
Food allergy	Avoidance	Level I	A
	Oral medication	Level II-3	E
	Immunotherapy	Level III	D
Penicillin allergy	Avoidance	Level I	A
	Desensitization	Level II-3	A
Environmental allergy	Environmental control	Level II-1	A
	Oral antihistamines	Level I	A
	Nasal antihistamines	Level I	A
	Oral decongestants	Level I	A
	Nasal corticosteroids	Level I	A
	Oral corticosteroids	Level III	C
	Intranasal cromolyn	Level II-1	B
	Intranasal anticholinergics	Level I	A
	Antileukotriene agents	Level III	C
	Immunotherapy	Level I	A

subsequent re-exposure to a particular antigen, causing an overwhelming immune response.[66]

Although the number of patients presenting with anaphylaxis appears to be increasing, the actual incidence is difficult to determine.[66] This is, in part, due to the fact that a universally accepted definition does not yet exist.[67] A widely accepted working definition is that it is comprised of severe involvement of respiratory function and/or hypotension,[67] as well as other clinical features such as skin involvement and gastrointestinal symptoms.[68]

An anaphylactic reaction results from exposure to a specific allergen in a patient with specific IgE antibodies. The result is activation of mast cells and release of the mediators of inflammation.[67] It can be difficult to distinguish this type of reaction from an anaphylactoid reaction that results in the activation of mast cells and release of the same mediators with no relationship to IgE.[67]

Etiology

The most common cause of anaphylaxis is food allergy. In North America, the most common offenders are peanuts and shellfish.[68] *Hymenoptera* are often the stinging insects causing anaphylaxis. This group includes the yellow jacket, yellow hornet, white-faced hornet, wasp, and honeybee.[68] Other causes of anaphylaxis include medications (antibiotics, acetylsalicylic acid, and nonsteroidal anti-inflammatory drugs), exercise, vaccines, immunotherapy, and latex.[67,68] Over the past 10 years, natural rubber latex has become an important allergen. Stretchable rubber products such as gloves are usually implicated. High-risk groups include patients with spina bifida and/or genitourinary abnormalities, hospital workers, workers in the latex industry, and atopic individuals.[68]

Clinical Features

As no universally accepted definition exists, the clinical features are difficult to elucidate. However, the features often associated with anaphylaxis are quite specific to the route of administration of the offending allergen. When the allergen is injectable—such as in immunotherapy, intravenous antibiotics, or anesthetic agents—often the reaction will be composed of systemic hypotension and shock. If the allergen is absorbed transmucosally, there will often be lip, facial, and laryngeal edema, associated with respiratory difficulty.[67] Most often, there is itching, flushing, urticaria, and angioedema of the skin. Even this finding is not absolute, as there have been a number of reports that describe anaphylaxis in children and the absence of skin manifestations.[68] Upper respiratory tract symptoms may include rhinorrhea, sneezing, itching, swelling of the tongue and laryngeal areas, and congestion. Signs of lower respiratory tract involvement may include wheezing, chest tightness, shortness of breath, and cough. Hypotension, palpitations, and dysrhythmias may also be present. From a gastrointestinal perspective, nausea, vomiting, cramping, and diarrhea have been described. A subjective feeling of anxiety and impending doom has been described.[68]

Investigations

Elevation of serum tryptase has been considered a marker for anaphylaxis. It is released from mast cells, in both anaphylactic and anaphylactoid reactions. Given that it is not always raised in severe reactions and must be measured within a very specific time period, its usefulness requires further study.[67] Anaphylaxis is a clinical diagnosis. Currently, very few, if any, laboratory tests aid in the diagnosis.

Clinical Course

Anaphylactic reactions are most commonly uniphasic but can be biphasic or protracted. In uniphasic reactions, the symptoms occur quickly and respond to therapy with no further sequelae. The biphasic reaction occurs in approximately 15 to 30 percent of cases. With this type of reaction, the initial set of symptoms resolve, and there is a period of quiescence. The symptoms then return typically 4 to 8 hours later. Therefore, an appropriate observation period is warranted.[68] Those patients with moderate reactions should be observed for 12 hours, and those who have had severe respiratory distress or hypotension should be observed for a minimum of 24 hours.[68]

Diagnosis

The evaluation of a patient with a history of anaphylaxis relies on a comprehensive history and physical examination, followed by referral to an allergist/immunologist. "The Practice Parameters" on the diagnosis and management of anaphylaxis make this recommendation, as these specialists have the required training to evaluate patients with this potentially life-threatening condition and to coordinate testing, if appropriate.[69] The follow-up, including possible challenges in the future, counseling and therapeutic options are within the realm of this subspecialty.[69]

Skin testing (discussed earlier) is appropriate in certain situations.[69] It should be performed by a trained allergist who is familiar with the testing and its interpretation.

Management

Given the severity and life-threatening potential of anaphylactic reactions, the cornerstone of management is prevention.[69] A thorough history for drug allergy should be taken in every patient. Oral antibiotics should be used whenever possible due to their decreased potential to cause anaphylaxis when compared with intravenous antibiotics.[65] Patients should wear MedicAlert bracelets or necklaces and should carry identification. Patients with anaphylactic histories should always carry a kit for self-injection of epinephrine.[65] Appropriate school personnel should be informed of a susceptible child's condition and educated on how to administer the epinephrine.

In the situation of an acute anaphylactic reaction, emergency assessment including airway, breathing, and circulation must be done and treatment instituted immediately. Epinephrine is the most important medication to consider in the acute situation.[70] It has potent effects that counteract the detrimental effects of mediator release.[71] Delays in the administration of this medication by as much as 30 minutes are believed to have caused fatalities.[68,72] A position statement on the use of epinephrine in the treatment of anaphylaxis clearly outlines that both the lay and professional people must be educated such that epinephrine is available and administered in a timely fashion in case of anaphylaxis.[73]

Epinephrine has been quoted in numerous sources as the first-line therapy for anaphylaxis.[74] It has been described as being efficacious in numerous clinical reports. It is difficult to study different doses and routes of epinephrine administration for the treatment of anaphylaxis in a controlled fashion, given the severity of the condition. Thus, it is difficult to challenge the dosages and routes that are widely accepted in the literature.

The recommended dosage for children currently quoted in "The Practice Parameters" from 1998 is 0.01 mg/kg up to a maximum of 0.5 mg per dose of a 1:1000 (wt/vol) solution given subcutaneously or intramuscularly.[69] This is in keeping with the most recent recommendations from the Canadian Immunization Guide.[75] Recently, Simons and colleagues compared the subcutaneous route with the intramuscular route of epinephrine injection. In this randomized, single-blind, single-dose study, 17 children with a history of systemic anaphylaxis were given either 0.01 mL/kg of epinephrine subcutaneously or 0.3 mg intramuscularly.[74] Higher plasma levels were achieved more quickly via the intramuscular route.[74] Although this intuitively appears superior, the clinical significance has yet to be determined.

Intravenous epinephrine is also widely recommended in the literature as therapy for the critically ill patient; however, it must be used with caution in a highly monitored situation.[68–70]

Table 18–2 Treatment of Anaphylaxis

Condition	Intervention	Quality of Evidence	Recommendation
Anaphylaxis	• Prevention: avoidance, Medic-alert bracelet, carrying self-injecting epinephrine	Level I	A
	• Epinephrine	Level II-3	A
	-Antihistamine	Level I	A
	-Steroids	Level III	B

Diphenhydramine 1 to 2 mg/kg or 25 to 50 mg/dose is recommended by "The Practice Parameters" and others for its antihistamine effects.[68,69,75] Steroids may also be administered; however, their efficacy in preventing a late-phase reaction has not been fully established.[69]

Throughout the pharmacotherapy for an anaphylactic reaction, the patient should be supported with respect to airway stability and cardiorespiratory status. Airway support in the form of an airway or intubation may be required. Blood pressure support in the form of fluid boluses and inotropic support may be required.

Depending on the severity of the anaphylactic reaction, careful observation is necessary.[69] On complete recovery, the patient must be referred to the appropriate specialist for follow-up, counseling and a discussion of therapeutic options.[69] An epinephrine self-administration kit and MedicAlert bracelet/necklace should be prescribed.

A summary of the treatment of anaphylaxis is provided in Table 18–2.

REFERENCES

1. Ownby DR. Allergy testing: In vivo versus in vitro. Pediatr Clin N Am 1988;35(5):995–1009.

2. Sampson HA. Adverse reactions to foods. In: Middleton Jr E, Reed CE, Ellis EF, et al, editors. Allergy: principles and practice. Mosby, St. Louis, Missouri 1998;p.1162–82.

3. May CD. Objective clinical and laboratory studies of immediate hypersensitivity reactions to food in asthmatic children. J Allergy Clin Immunol 1976;58:500–15.

4. Sampson HA. Food allergy. JAMA 1997;278:1888–94.

5. Hourihane JO, Bedwani SJ, Dean TP, Warner JO. Randomised, double-blind, crossover challenge study of allergenicity of peanut oils in subjects allergic to peanuts. Br Med J 1997;314:1084–8.

6. Bock SA, Atkins FM. The natural history of peanut allergy. J Allergy Clin Immunol 1989;83:900–4.

7. Hourihane JO, Roberts SA, Warner JO. Resolution of peanut allergy: case-control study. Br Med J 1998;316:1271–5.

8. James JM, Burks AW, Roberson PK, Sampson HA. Safe administration of the measles vaccine to children allergic to eggs. N Engl J Med 1995;332:1262–6.

9. Freigang B, Jadavji TP, Freigang DW. Lack of adverse reactions to measles, mumps, and rubella vaccine in egg-allergic children. Ann Allergy 1994;73:486–8.

10. Fasano MB, Wood RA, Cooke SK, et al. Egg hypersensitivity and adverse reactions to measles, mumps, and rubella vaccine. J Pediatr 1992;120:878-81.

10a. American Academy of Pediatrics. Active and passive immunization. In: Peter G, editor. 1997 Red Book: Report of the Committee on Infectious Diseases. 24th edition. Elk Grove Village, IL: American Academy of Pediatrics, 1997:32–3.

11. Canadian immunization guide, 5th Ed. Canadian Medical Association, 1998;p.7–8.

12. Suresh A, Reisman RE. Risk of administering cephalosporin antibiotics to patients with histories of penicillin allergy. Ann Allergy Asthma Immunol 1995;74:167–70.

13. Weiss ME, Adkinson NF. Immediate hypersensitivity reactions to penicillin and related antibiotics. Clin Allergy 1988;18:515–40.

14. Graff-Lonnevig V, Hedlin G, Lindfors A. Penicillin allergy—a rare pediatric condition? Arch Dis Child 1988;63:1342–6.

15. Sussman GL, Davis K, Kohler PF. Penicillin allergy: a practical approach to management. Can Med Assoc J 1986;134:1353–6.

16. Anne S, Reisman RE. Risk of administering cephalosporin antibiotics to patients with histories of penicillin allergy. Ann Allergy Asthma Immunol 1995;74:167–70.

17. Blanca M, Fernandez J, Miranda A, et al. Cross-reactivity between penicillins and cephalosporins: clinical and immunologic studies. J Allergy Clin Immunol 1989;83:381–5.

18. Editorial. Cross-allergenicity of penicillins and cephalosporins. JAMA 1967;199(7):495–6.

19. Grieco MH. Cross-allergenicity of the penicillins and the cephalosporins. Arch Intern Med 1967;119:141–6.

20. Miller MM. Cross-reactivity of cephalosporins with penicillin. Ann Allergy 1996;137(Supp 6):542.

21. Solley GO, Gleich GJ, van Dellen RG, et al. Penicillin allergy: clinical experience with a battery of skin-test reagents. J Allergy Clin Immunol 1982;69:238–44.

22. Dykewicz MS, Fineman S. Diagnosis and management of rhinitis: complete guidelines of the Joint Task Force on Practice Parameters in Allergy, Asthma, and Immunology. Ann Allergy Asthma Immunol 1998;81:478–518.

23. O'Riordan TG, Smaldone GC. Aerosols. In: Middleton Jr E, Reed CE, Ellis EF, et al, editors. Allergy: principles and practice 1998;p.532–43.

24. Dykewicz MS, Fineman S, Skoner DP, et al. Joint task force algorithm and annotations for diagnosis and management of rhinitis. Ann Allergy Asthma Immunol 1998;81:469–73.

25. Demoly P, Michel F, Bousquet J. In vivo methods for study of allergy skin tests, techniques, and interpretation. In: Middleton Jr E, Reed CE, Ellis EF, et al, editors. Allergy: principles and practice. 1998;p.430–9.

26. Bernstein IL, Storms WW. Practice parameters for allergy diagnostic testing. Joint Task Force on Practice Parameters for the Diagnosis and Treatment of Asthma. The American Academy of Allergy, Asthma and Immunology and American College of Allergy, Asthma and Immunology. Ann Allergy Asthma Immunol 1995;75:543–625.

27. Taudorf E, Malling HJ, Laursen LC, et al. Reproducibility of histamine skin prick test. Inter- and intravariation using histamine dihydrochloride 1, 5, and 10 mg/mL. Allergy 1985;40(5):344–9.

28. Sogn DD, Evans R III, Shephard GM, et al. Results of the National Institute of Allergy and Infectious Diseases Collaborative Clinical Trial to test the predictive value of skin testing with major and minor penicillin derivatives in hospitalized adults. Arch Intern Med 1992;152:1025–32.

29. Chandra RK, Joglekar SA, Tomas E. Penicillin allergy: anti-penicillin IgE antibodies and immediate hypersensitivity skin reactions employing major and minor determinants of penicillin. Arch Dis Child 1980;55:857–60.

30. Ressler C, Mendelson LM. Skin test for diagnosis of penicillin allergy—current status. Ann Allergy 1987;59:167–70.

31. Pichichero ME, Pichichero DM. Diagnosis of penicillin, amoxicillin, and cephalosporin allergy: reliability of examination assessed by skin testing and oral challenge. J Pediatr 1998;132(1):137–43.

32. Burks AW, Sampson HA. Diagnostic approaches to the patient with suspected food allergies. J Pediatr 1992;121:S64–71.

33. Sampson HA, Albergo R. Comparison of results of skin tests, RAST, and double-blind, placebo-controlled food challenges in children with atopic dermatitis. J Allergy Clin Immunol 1984;74:26–33.

34. Sampson HA. Comparative study of commercial food antigen extracts for the diagnosis of food hypersensitivity. J Allergy Clin Immunol 1988;82:718–26.

35. Dreborg S. Skin tests in the diagnosis of food allergy. Pediatr Allergy Immunol 1995;6(Suppl 8):38–43.

36. Reddy PM, Nagaya H, Pascual HC, et al. Reappraisal of intracutaneous tests in the diagnosis of reaginic allergy. J Allergy Clin Immunology 1978;61(1):36–41.

37. Cavanaugh MJ, Bronsky EA, Buckley JM. Clinical value of bronchial provocation testing in childhood asthma. J Allergy Clin Immunology 1977;59(1):41–7.

38. Bock SA, Lee WY, Regigio L, et al. Appraisal of skin tests with food extracts for diagnosis of food hypersensitivity. Clin Allergy 1978;8:559–64.

39. Sampson HA, Rosen JP, Selcow JE, et al. Intradermal skin tests in the diagnostic evaluation of food allergy. J Allergy Clin Immunol 1996;(Sept 98[3]):714–5.

40. Leihas JL, McCaskill CC, Sampson HA. Food allergy challenges: guidelines and implications. J Am Dietetic Assoc 1987;87:604–8.

41. Adkinson NF. Drug allergy. In: Middleton Jr E, Reed CE, Ellis EF, et al, editors. Allergy: principles and practice 1998;p.1212–24.

42. Druce HM. Allergic and nonallergic rhinitis. In: Middleton Jr E, Reed CE, Ellis EF, et al, editors. Allergy: principles and practice 1998;p.1005–16.

43. Solomon WR, Burge HA, Boise JR. Exclusion of particulate allergens by window air conditioners. J Allergy Clin Immunol 1980;65:305–8.

44. Klein GL, Littlejohn T III, Lockhart EA, Farey SA. Brompheninrmine, terfenadine, and placebo in allergic rhinitis. Ann Allergy Asthma Immunol 1996;77:365–70.

45. Vuurman EF, van Veggel LM, Witerwijk MM, et al. Seasonal allergic rhinitis and antihistamine effects on children's learning. Ann Allergy 1993;71:121–6.

46. Shanon A, Feldman W, Leikin L, et al. Comparison of CNS adverse effects between astemizole and chlorpheniramine in children: a randomized, double-blind study. Dev Pharmacol Ther 1993;20:239–46.

47. Simons FE, Reggin JD, Roberts FR, Simons KJ. Benefit-risk ratio of the antihistamines (H_1-receptor antagonists) terfenadine and chlorpheniramine in children. J Pediatr 1994;124:979–83.

48. Ratner PH, Findlay SR, Hampel F Jr, et al. A double-blind, controlled trial to assess the safety and efficacy of azelastine nasal spray in seasonal allergic rhinitis. J Allergy Clin Immunol 1994;94:818–25.

49. LaForce C, Dockhorn RJ, Prenner BM, et al. Safety and efficacy of azelastine nasal spray (Astelin NS) for seasonal allergic rhinitis: a 4-week comparative multicenter trial. Ann Allergy Asthma Immunol 1996;76:181–8.

50. Erffmeyer JE, McKenna WR, Lieberman PL, et al. Efficacy of phenylephrine-phenyl-propanolamine in the treatment of rhinitis. South Med J 1982;75:562–4.

51. Falliers CJ, Redding MA. Controlled comparison of a new antihistamine-decongestant combination to its individual components. Ann Allergy 1980;45:75–80.

52. Welsh PW, Stricker WE, Chu CP, et al. Efficacy of beclomethasone nasal solution, flunisolide, and cromolyn in relieving symptoms of ragweed allergy. Mayo Clin Proc 1987;62:125–34.

53. LaForce C, Davis V. Nasal septal perforation in patients using intranasal beclomethasone dipropionate (BDP). J Allergy Clin Immunol 1985;75:186.

54. van As A, Bronsky EA, Grossman J, et al. Dose tolerance study of fluticasone propionate aqueous nasal spray in patients with seasonal allergic rhinitis. Ann Allergy 1991;67:156–62.

55. van As A, Bronsky EA, Dockhorn RJ, et al. Once daily fluticasone propionate is as effective for perennial allergic rhinitis as twice daily beclomethasone diproprionate. J Allergy Clin Immunol 1993;91:1146–54.

56. Siegel SC. Topical intranasal corticosteroid therapy in rhinitis. J Allergy Clin Immunol 1988;81:984–91.

57. Taylor G, Shivalkar PR. Disodium cromoglycate: laboratory studies and clinical trial in allergic rhinitis. Clin Allergy 1971;1:189–98.

58. Pelikan Z, Snoek WJ, Booij-Noord H, et al. Protective effect of disodium cromoglycate on the allergen provocation of the nasal mucosa. Ann Allergy 1970;28:548–53.

59. Meltzer EO, Orge; JA. Bronsky EA, et al. Ipratropium bromide aqueous nasal spray for patients with perennial allergic rhinitis: a study of its effect on their symptoms, quality of life, and nasal cytology. J Allergy Clin Immunol 1992;90:242–9.

60. Canadian Society of Allergy and Clinical Immunology: guidelines for the use of allergen immunotherapy. Can Med Assoc J 1995;152(9):1413–9.

61. Hayward RSA, Wilson MC, Tunis SR, et al, for the Evidence-Based Medicine Working Group. User's guides to the medical literature VIII. How to use clinical practice guidelines A. Are the Recommendations Valid? JAMA 1995;274(7):570–4.

62. Clavel R, Bousquet J, Andre C. Clinical efficacy of sublingual-swallow immunotherapy: a double-blind, placebo-controlled trial of a standardized five-grass-pollen extract in rhinitis. Allergy 1998;53:493–8.

63. Nelson HS, Lahr J, Rule R, et al. Treatment of anaphylactic sensitivity to peanuts by immunotherapy with injections of aqueous peanut extract. J Allergy Clin Immunol 1997;99:744–51.

64. Terr AI. Unconventional theories and unproved methods in allergy. In: Middleton Jr E, Reed CE, Ellis EF, et al, editors. Allergy: principles and practice 1998;p.1235–49.

65. Lieberman P. Anaphylaxis and anaphylactoid reactions. In: Middleton Jr E, Reed CE, Ellis EF, et al, editors. Allergy: principles and practice 1998;p.1079–92.

66. Stewart AG, Ewan PW. The incidence, etiology and management of anaphylaxis presenting to an accident and emergency department. Quart J Med 1996;89:859–64.

67. Ewan PW. ABC of allergies. Br Med J 1998;316:1442–5.

68. Vadas P, Gold M, Graham C. Diagnosis and emergency management of anaphylaxis. Allergy 1998;(Sept):11–5.

69. Nicklas. The diagnosis and management of anaphylaxis. Joint Task Force on Practice Parameters, American Academy of Allergy, Asthma and Immunology, American College of Allergy, Asthma, and Immunology, and the Joint Council of Allergy, Asthma and Immunology. J Allergy Clin Immunol 1998;101(6 Pt 2):S465–528.

70. Gavalas M, Sadana A, Metcalf F. Guidelines for the management of anaphylaxis in the emergency department. J Accident Emerg Med 1998;15:96–8.

71. Rinke CM. Epinephrine for treatment of anaphylactic shock. JAMA 1984;251:2118–22.

72. Sampson HA, Mendelson L, Rosen JP, et al. Fatal and near-fatal anaphylactic reaction to food in children and adolescents. N Engl J Med 1992;327(6):380–4.

73. AAAI Board of Directors. The use of epinephrine in the treatment of anaphylaxis [position statement]. J Allergy Clin Immunol 1994;94:666–8.

74. Simons FE, Roberts JR, Gu X, Simons KJ. Epinephrine absorption in children with a history of anaphylaxis. J Allergy Clin Immunol 1998;101:33–7.

75. Anonymous. Anaphylaxis: statement on initial management in non-hospital settings. Can Med Assoc J 1996;154:1519–22.

CHAPTER 19

Musculoskeletal Disorders

Brian Feldman, MD, MSc, FRCPC

Musculoskeletal disorders are highly prevalent and a source of major health impact. In population surveys, about 30 percent of adults report that they have musculoskeletal disease. This is a major cause of morbidity and health-care utilization.[1]

Children, too, often seek health-care consultation because of painful musculoskeletal conditions and, more rarely, because of autoimmune diseases. The first section of this chapter considers the epidemiology of rheumatic conditions in childhood and looks at the frequency of these diseases and what is known about risk factors. The second section of the chapter examines common diagnostic tests and strategies used to manage these conditions. The final section reviews the evidence and makes recommendations for therapy for the major rheumatic illnesses of childhood.

EPIDEMIOLOGY OF RHEUMATIC DISEASE IN CHILDREN AND ADOLESCENTS

For the most part, the conditions that will be discussed in this chapter are relatively common, chronic, and usually nonfatal childhood disorders. Our understanding of the frequency and determinants of these disorders comes primarily from two sources. Recently, several large registry studies have reported the frequency of referrals to subspecialty care for children with a variety of rheumatic illnesses. Also, a number of large population-based epidemiologic studies have been published, detailing the incidence and prevalence of musculoskeletal disorders in children.

Nonarticular Rheumatism

There are a variety of painful musculoskeletal conditions that are not caused by inflammation in the tissues or by autoimmunity. These conditions have been grouped under the label "nonarticular rheumatism" (or sometimes "soft-tissue rheumatism"). Many of the most common painful conditions of childhood fall under this category. These illnesses are usually characterized by aches and pains. As a group, they present frequently to primary-care providers and make up a large part of the case load of pediatric rheumatologists. The most common forms of nonarticular rheumatism that affect children are growing pain, the hypermobility/juvenile episodic arthralgia syndrome, fibromyalgia, and backache.

Growing Pain

The clinical syndrome of growing pain presents in a very typical fashion. The condition affects school-aged or preschool children. It presents as late-day or evening limb pains—often very severe—which may awaken the child at night. These pains are recurrent and intermittent. The pain is usually diffusely located, often in the thighs or calves, and not usually located directly at a joint. Growing pain is most often in the lower extremities and more often bilateral than unilateral. Many parents give the history that their child's pain is worse after a very active day. The pain is always relieved by rubbing, a warm bath, or a mild analgesic. After an episode, the child goes to sleep and the child wakes up normally the next day with no pain and no limp.

Children with growing pain often seek the advice of a physician. Growing pain is the 15th most common diagnosis made by pediatric rheumatologists participating in the United

States disease registry (which collects data from 38 centers). Growing pain accounts for about 2 percent of patients seen at these centers.[2] Likewise, this diagnosis accounts for just over 2 percent of diagnoses made by Canadian pediatric rheumatology registry participants[3] and for almost 4 percent of diagnoses in a study of New England referral centers.[4]

Pediatric rheumatologists are probably only referred the most severe cases, and so this experience is likely just the tip of the iceberg. In one study, pediatricians and family practitioners both reported that about 1 percent of their patient visits are for growing pain. Only about 4 or 5 percent of these children were referred on to subspecialty care.[5]

Unfortunately, for this condition, population epidemiology is scarce. It is reported that between 4 and 34 percent of children get growing pain. The likely prevalence is somewhere in between. One Danish survey of over 2,000 school children showed a prevalence of growing pain of about 12 percent for boys and 18 percent for girls.[6] In the Danish study, growing pain was almost as common as headache and more common than recurrent abdominal pain. Another study, a random survey of 10 percent of all Aberdeen school children (aged 5 to 15 years) found fewer children with growing pain—almost 3 percent—but used a stricter definition.[7] Even if only 3 percent of children get growing pain, it is clearly a very common problem and one which most physicians who deal with children will come in contact with.

Hypermobility/Juvenile Episodic Arthralgia

Juvenile episodic arthralgia is the name given to a benign pain syndrome commonly affecting children who are "double jointed." Unlike the pain from inflammatory arthritis—which is accentuated first thing in the morning, and after periods of rest – the pain in juvenile episodic arthralgia is worse after activity. The pain is usually localized to specific joints and often comes on after prolonged walking or playing. Sometimes, especially in young musicians and typists, the upper limbs are affected. Rarely, mild and transient joint effusions are reported.

Juvenile episodic arthralgia is related to local or general hypermobility. Although this pain syndrome can be seen in children with Ehlers-Danlos or Marfan syndrome, most affected children will have benign hypermobility unrelated to a genetic problem of connective tissue formation. Benign hypermobility is thought to be an autosomal dominant inherited disorder; in clinical practice, one parent will usually have a history of being double jointed.

Although it is a time-honored association, there has been some recent controversy as to whether hypermobility causes arthralgia or is just sometimes coincidentally seen. A recent Finnish study examined grade 3 and grade 5 students from all but two elementary schools in Lahti. The students were examined and given a questionnaire about pain. Just over 8 percent of the girls and 7 percent of the boys were identified as being at least moderately hypermobile. In both the hypermobile children and control children with no hypermobility, about 30 percent had musculoskeletal pain at least once a week. The study's authors concluded that both hypermobility and pain are normal and common in preadolescents. They further concluded that the two were causally unrelated.[8] This study may not be definitive. The students studied were young and may not have been able to reliably fill in pain questionnaires. This may have accounted for the very high frequency of pain and for the lack of a relationship to joint hypermobility.

An Israeli study, in which 429 elementary students from one public school in Beer Sheva were followed up, reached the opposite conclusion. The children were diagnosed with joint hypermobility, using a common set of criteria. Hypermobility was diagnosed if a child was able to perform three or more of the following:

1. Hyperextension of the fingers so that they were parallel to the forearms
2. Apposition of the thumbs to the surface of the forearms
3. Hyperextension of the elbows >10°
4. Hyperextension of the knees >10°
5. Flexion of the trunk, with knees straight and the palms of the hands touching the floor

Both the hypermobile children and a random sample of age- and sex-matched non hypermobile children were followed up for 1 year, with monthly parental pain question-naires. Altogether, 12 percent of the students were hypermobile (18 percent of the girls and 8 percent of the boys). Juvenile episodic arthralgia was seen much more often in the hyper-mobile children—40 percent of the hypermobile children versus 17 percent of the control children.[9] Most likely, hypermobility is related to episodic, activity-related joint pains.

The hypermobility/juvenile episodic arthralgia syndrome is the fourth most common diagnosis encountered by pediatric rheumatologists (4 to 5 percent of all new patients seen).[2,3,10]

Fibromyalgia and Chronic Fatigue Syndrome

Chronic fatigue syndrome and fibromyalgia (FM) are similar conditions with a high degree of overlap.[11] These two disorders likely represent part of a spectrum of pain and fatigue dis-orders. It has been suggested that—like the old story of the blind men and the elephant—the same disorder is called fibromyalgia by the rheumatologist, irritable bowel syndrome by the gastroenterologist, migraine headache syndrome by the neurologist, and chronic fatigue syndrome by the generalist. These disorders are mostly distinguishable by their dominant symptoms. Children who present to rheumatologists mostly present with pain as the dom-inant syndrome, so in this chapter we will consider this group of disorders under the term "fibromyalgia."

Fibromyalgia is a common disorder in young adults and teenagers. It presents as diffuse pain and fatigue. Very commonly, there are concomitant symptoms, namely, paresthesias, headache, irritable bowel complaints, dizzyness, and profound all-over morning stiffness. Fibromyalgia may be associated with marked functional impairment, even though there are remarkably few pathologic findings on examination.

The study of fibromyalgia has been simplified since the American College of Rheuma-tology (ACR) proposed diagnostic criteria in 1990 (see below).[12] It is not a new syndrome. There appear to be biblical references to fibromyalgia, and both Charles Darwin and Florence Nightingale had it. Through the ages, though, it has taken on different names such as "neurasthenia" and "fibrositis."[13]

The most appealing explanation for the pathogenesis of fibromyalgia is that it is a sleep disorder. Harvey Moldofsky and others, since the 1970s, have recognized and described a highly typical sleep disorder that occurs in most patients with fibromyalgia. This disorder is characterized by an alpha wave EEG pattern seen during non-REM sleep.[14] The sleep disor-der may account for one of the highly typical symptoms of fibromyalgia—unrestorative sleep (described by patients as "waking up still tired"). Supporting this, normal volunteers, espe-cially those with poor physical fitness, develop the symptoms and signs of fibromyalgia when deprived of non-REM sleep.

An attractive hypothesis is that this sleep disorder is either inherited or induced by trauma or infection. Inheritance is suggested by the finding that over 70 percent of patients with fibromyalgia have a mother with similar complaints (compared with none in a group of asymptomatic controls).[15] In clinical practice, patients often present after an episode of trauma or infection. This sleep disorder then leads to pain, pain leads to worse sleep, which leads to more pain, thus creating a vicious cycle.

Although the prevalence of fibromyalgia in children is lower than that in adult women, it is still very common. In one Israeli study, children from a single school were consecutively screened for fibromyalgia. Twenty-one of 338 (6.2 percent) had fibromyalgia diagnosed by the ACR criteria. These children were between the ages of 9 and 15 years. As in adults, fibromyalgia was much more common in females.[16]

A Mexican study found a lower prevalence. In this study, 548 students (all aged between 9 and 15 years) from one primary and two secondary schools were screened. Only 7, all girls, fulfilled the ACR criteria for fibromyalgia, suggesting an estimated prevalence of 1.2 percent.[17]

Fibromyalgia accounts for about 2 percent of new patients reported to the American pediatric rheumatology registry[2] and almost 4 percent reported to the Canadian registry.[3]

Backache

Standard orthopedic and subspecialty textbooks generally suggest that backache in children is rare, and therefore, when it occurs, it is always a cause for concern. In fact, backache is probably rare in very young children under the age of 5, but in school-aged children and adolescents, it is quite common.[18]

Backache in older children and adults has similar causes and associations. They are as follows:

1. Mechanical, including postural, injury and overuse
2. Infectious/inflammatory conditions such as diskitis, vertebral osteomyelitis, and, very rarely, juvenile ankylosing spondylitis
3. Neoplastic, benign and malignant
4. Developmental, including spondylolysis/spondylolisthesis and Scheuermann's disease
5. Very rarely, conversion reaction

Mechanical causes are, by far, the most prevalent. Children who suffer from back pain seem to fall into two categories: athletic kids, who develop strains and sprains from strenuous sports;[19] and those who are "couch potatoes," watch a lot of television, smoke, and have weak trunk muscles.[20,21]

Back pain is highly prevalent. In one Swiss study, 615 secondary students (all students from two high schools were studied) answered a validated pain questionnaire. These children reported a lifetime prevalence of back pain of 74 percent; 4 percent reported almost continuous back pain. In total, 14 percent of these secondary school students had sought medical care for back pain.[22] Similarly, an Icelandic national random sample of 2,173 children in grades 6 and 10 showed a 44 percent overall prevalence of back pain; a little over 20 percent of the children reported at least weekly pain. Just over 7 percent had sought medical care.[23] Back pain accounts for between 1 and 5 percent of referrals to pediatric rheumatologists.[2,3,10]

Juvenile Arthritis

The term juvenile arthritis (JA) will be used in this chapter as a general term to label many different types of childhood arthritis. There is some confusion in the terminology used worldwide to describe these conditions. North American criteria consider idiopathic juvenile rheumatoid arthritis separately from arthritis associated with psoriasis, arthritis associated with inflammatory bowel disease, and juvenile ankylosing spondylitis, whereas European criteria include all these together under the umbrella term "Juvenile Chronic Arthritis" (see below).

It is difficult to know the true prevalence and incidence of JA because of differences among studies in classification criteria, racial background, and referral source. Using meta-analytic techniques, Oen and Cheang calculated weighted average prevalences from all studies reported between 1977 and 1995.[24] They found that studies using population-based methods reported the highest prevalence (132/100,000 children), whereas community (practitioner) -based studies found a lower prevalence of 26/100,000. The prevalence was lowest for referral clinic–based studies (12/100,000). Prevalence estimates also varied depending on where the studies were carried out. North American studies found a higher prevalence (32/100,000) than did European studies (8/100,000).

Most of the population-based studies of JA did not apply strict criteria and did not verify cases and therefore may have overestimated the prevalence. However, a more recent population-based Australian study, in which cases were verified by rheumatologic examination, found a very high prevalence of 400/100,000. In this study, a number of undiagnosed cases were discovered.[25] This points out the importance of using population estimates rather than referral-based estimates and suggests that JA is at least as common as other chronic diseases such as diabetes and cystic fibrosis.

Racial factors in JA have not been well studied. It appears that of North American and European Caucasian children, the large majority have the pauciarticular (or oligoarticular) subtype (see below). This is not true for other racial groups in which the polyarticular form is more common. Some American aboriginal groups have a much higher frequency of spondylitic forms of arthritis.[24]

Environmental etiologic factors have been suggested by the cyclic incidence of JA. For instance, a study of the population served by the Mayo clinic showed peaks in incidence in 1967, 1975, and 1987.[26] Seasonality, too, has been found in the systemic onset form of JA (see below) in some areas but not in others. This might be indicative of infectious or other environmental agents.[27]

Systemic Lupus Erythematosus

Systemic lupus erythematosus (SLE) is an inflammatory disease characterized by a widespread vasculopathy (that potentially affects many organ systems) and polyserositis. The pathologic findings seem to be due to the presence of a number of autoreactive antibodies that bind to self-antigens and lead to inflammatory damage. It is, perhaps, the prototypical autoimmune disease.

Whereas JA seems to be a unique form of arthritis, different from adult arthritis with few exceptions, most childhood SLE is very similar to the adult disease. Most affected children are really young women post-pubertal; the age at onset just happens to be under 18 years. Early onset, in some cases, goes along with more severe disease and a higher rate of certain complications (like nephritis) than seen in adult-onset SLE.

Childhood-onset SLE is quite rare. Incidence figures derived from specialty clinics are likely to be underestimates. This is because children with SLE are looked after by a wide variety of practitioners, including pediatric nephrologists, adult nephrologists, adult rheumatologists, general pediatricians, and pediatric rheumatologists. Also, some cases remain undiagnosed in the community. Random screening of 3,500 women from a Birmingham general practice found a prevalence of 2/1,000 women, higher than usually reported. This higher prevalence was due to the investigators identifying undiagnosed cases (3 of 7 cases had not yet been diagnosed).[28]

The Canadian pediatric rheumatology registry study produced a minimum incidence rate of about 0.36/100,000 children at risk per year.[3] In this study, SLE accounted for about 2 percent of the new diagnoses made by Canadian rheumatologists. Similar numbers were seen by American registry participants; about 2.5 percent of newly referred patients had SLE. It was the eighth most common diagnosis made.[2] A Finnish study, using national health insurance drug plan statistics, found the incidence of SLE to be higher at 0.9/100,000 children per year.[29] Even so, it would appear that SLE is quite uncommon in children.

Racial differences have been examined in SLE. The condition is more common in children with Southeast Asian, African, or Caribbean background. The United States National Center for Health Statistics data suggest that among children aged 1 to 14 years, the mortality rate from SLE among African American children is about eight times that of Caucasian children. This may represent a higher prevalence of disease, more severe disease, and/or poorer access to health care in the case of African Americans.[30]

Systemic lupus erythematosus affects girls more often than boys. Sex hormones are thought to play an important role in the pathogenesis. In those children who present before puberty, there is less of a female predominance, which supports the importance of sex hormones. However, clinical studies of very young children with SLE have not revealed differences in racial distribution, family history, or outcome.[31] This suggests that even if sex hormones are an important factor in the etiology of SLE, there are other stronger determinants of the disease.

Environmental factors are known to be important in some cases of SLE. For example, SLE can be induced by some medications and triggered by sunlight. So far, though, there have been no convincing reports of environmental toxins/pollution or other identifiable environmental agents causing lupus.[32]

Juvenile Dermatomyositis

The features of juvenile dermatomyositis (JDM), like SLE, are due to a widespread vasculopathy that is likely autoimmune in origin. The most commonly affected organs are the muscles (clinically apparent as muscle weakness) and the skin; the characteristic rash is a pathognomonic feature.

Juvenile dermatomyositis is quite a rare disease – less common than JA or SLE. The incidence of JDM in the United Kingdom has been determined recently from the British Pediatric Surveillance Unit. A postcard survey was carried out with British practitioners. Reported cases were confirmed by a more detailed questionnaire. The incidence in the United Kingdom was about two per million children per year. In this study, almost 90 percent of the identified cases were Caucasian and over 80 percent girls.[33]

A seasonal onset of JDM has been seen in some clinics. This might be the case if an infection or other seasonal environmental agent caused the disease. However, in a relatively large case-control study, using cases identified by a North American JDM registry and using both healthy and JA controls, there was no evidence of infectious or other environmental causes.[34]

Localized Scleroderma

Localized scleroderma is primarily a skin disorder. It is characterized by the development of plaques (morphea) or bands (linear scleroderma) of indurated skin. The lesions are initially inflammatory and later become fibrotic with the deposition of large amounts of abnormal collagen. The lesions often regress spontaneously; however, they may permanently affect the growth of underlying muscle, bone, or joints.

Localized scleroderma is fairly common. A population-based study from the Rochester Epidemiology Project calculated annual incidence rates (in adults and children) of about 3/100,000 population per year. In one-third of morphea cases, and two-thirds of linear scleroderma cases, the onset was before 18 years of age. The prevalence of LS by age 18 years was calculated to be 50/100,000 population.[35]

Systemic scleroderma, in contrast, is very rare in childhood. This form of scleroderma accounted for less than 0.1 percent of diagnoses made by Canadian pediatric rheumatologists[3] and 0.2 percent of diagnoses made by American pediatric rheumatologists.[2]

The factors associated with the development of either form of scleroderma have not been well studied in children.

Kawasaki Disease and Other Vasculitides

Primary vasculitis is relatively rare in childhood with the exceptions of the syndromes of Kawasaki disease (KD) and Henoch-Schönlein purpura (HSP). Rheumatologists in Canada tend to see more cases of Kawasaki disease. It accounted for about 4 percent of new diagnoses in the Canadian registry as opposed to about 1 percent for HSP.[3] The reverse is true in the United States.[2]

Henoch-Schönlein Purpura

HSP is an IgA-immune complex-mediated vasculitis. It affects the smallest vessels. The pathology is leukocytoclastic vasculitis. The most common manifestations are palpable purpura affecting primarily the lower extremities and buttocks, abdominal pain (sometimes associated with intussusception), glomerulonephritis, and arthritis. These are all manifestations of inflammation of the local capillaries. As with most types of vasculitis, virtually all other organs can be affected.

The epidemiologic features of HSP have been examined in a Danish study of hospitalized cases. All cases of HSP admitted to hospital, as determined by a central registry, were studied. The investigators found a yearly incidence of about 14 to 18 per 100,000 children under age 15 years. They found no evidence of clustering, which suggested no contagious outbreak. There was an increased frequency in winter and an increased frequency in day-care or nursery attenders, which may have been due to infectious contacts. Streptococcal bacteria have been thought to play a role in the development of HSP. However, in the Danish study, fewer than 20 percent of the identified children had evidence of current or recent streptococcal infections. On the basis of their data, the Danish group thought that a wide variety of infectious agents might trigger the illness.[36]

Kawasaki Disease

Kawasaki disease is a systemic vasculitis, mostly affecting young children, often under the age of 4 years and is almost always a self-limited disease. In most children, the disease features resemble those of measles or of scarlet fever (see below). However, KD can lead to permanent damage or death, usually through vasculitis of the coronary arteries.

Kawasaki disease is a relatively common disease with a marked variation in frequency among different nationalities. For example, a national American survey of hospital discharges between 1984 and 1987 calculated a minimal annual incidence rate of about 7.6 cases per 100,000 children under the age of 5 years.[37] However, a similar survey of Japanese hospitals found a more than 10-fold higher annual incidence, about 90/100,000 children under the age of 5 years.[38]

EVIDENCE-BASED DIAGNOSIS

Classification Criteria

The rheumatic diseases of childhood are mostly chronic, inflammatory illnesses. In general, there are no pathognomonic laboratory tests. For many of the rheumatic diseases, there is a great deal of overlap in the pathology of involved tissues. Therefore, for most of these illnesses, the diagnosis is based on signs and symptoms.

To aid in gathering homogeneous groups of patients for research, various organizations have developed classification criteria. This effort has been led by the American College of Rheumatology (ACR). In developing these criteria, regression models or classification tree–based models are used to determine the signs, symptoms, and laboratory tests that best classify patients on the basis of a "gold standard" diagnosis. The gold standard for the ACR criteria has been the diagnosis made by an expert rheumatologist.

These classification criteria were not intended to be used to make a diagnosis for an individual patient. However, when used as a diagnostic aid, they can be considered as having defined sensitivities and specificities. Some of these characteristics have been well studied.

Fibromyalgia

In 1990, the ACR developed criteria for the classification of fibromyalgia.[12] This greatly simplified the classification of this disease as previous sets of criteria were much more complex and, in some cases, divergent. The criteria set forth by the ACR are as follows:

1. widespread pain, defined as pain that involves areas
   - above and below the waist,
   - on the right and left sides, and
   - both axial and appendicular; *and*

2. at least 11 of 18 tender points by light palpation (Figure 19–1).

In adult patients, the criteria correctly classified patients, with a sensitivity of >88 percent and specificity of >81 percent compared with the expert rheumatologists' diagnosis.

Juvenile Arthritis

The classification of childhood arthritis has been the subject of some controversy. Competing sets of classification criteria, with slightly different definitions, have been proposed in North America and in Europe.[39] More recently, the International League of Associations for Rheumatology (ILAR) has developed preliminary criteria and has renamed the disorder as juvenile idiopathic arthritides (JIA).[40] These new criteria have not been tested for formal diagnostic properties and have not yet been widely endorsed. However, the new criteria do incorporate the best points of the previous systems.

To meet the ILAR criteria, arthritis must develop before the age of 16 years, it must be chronic (lasting continuously for more than 6 weeks), and it must be unexplained by other diagnoses or mechanical disorders.

Arthritis is defined as swelling within a joint or limitation of joint movement, accompanied by joint pain or tenderness. (Previous classifications have used joint warmth as being additional evidence of arthritis.)

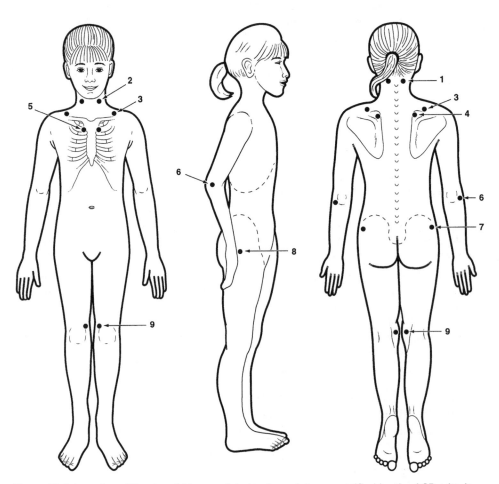

Figure 19–1 Location of 9 pairs of fibromyalgia tender points as specified by the ACR criteria.

In the ILAR criteria, onset subtypes are defined by features present within the first 6 months of disease. The new ILAR criteria feature seven subtypes. Although it is too soon to say how popular these critieria will become, the categories make sense and are similar to the previous schemes. The onset subtypes are as follows:

1. Systemic arthritis, which is defined by the presence of a spiking fever (quotidian fever) for at least 2 weeks, accompanied by at least one of these:
   * Evanescent pink rash
   * Generalized lymphadenopathy
   * Hepatomegaly or splenomegaly
   * Serositis (pericardial, pleural, or peritoneal)
2. Oligoarthritis, defined by four or fewer joints affected with arthritis in the first 6 months
3. Polyarthritis (rheumatoid factor [RF] negative), defined by the presence of five or more joints affected with arthritis in the first 6 months
4. Polyarthritis (RF positive), with five or more joints affected and a positive blood test for RF (at least twice, at least 3 months apart). (This separate category defines a group of young adults who develop what is essentially adult rheumatoid arthritis before the age of 16 years)
5. Psoriatic arthritis, that is, arthritis in a patient with psoriasis, or arthritis and at least two of the following:
   * Dactylitis (inflammatory sausage swelling of a digit)
   * Nail pitting or onycholysis
   * Family history of dermatologist confirmed psoriasis in a first-degree relative
6. Enthesitis-related arthritis, which is described below:
   * The presence of arthritis and enthesitis (Enthesitis refers to inflammation of the areas where a tendon or ligament inserts into bone. The affected areas are usually at the patella, tibial tuberosity, insertion of the Achilles tendon, or at the insertion of the plantar fascia into the heel or base of the toes.)
   * or, arthritis or enthesitis with at least two of the following:
     -Sacroiliac joint tenderness or inflammatory spinal pain
     -Presence of HLA-B27
     -Family history of a first- or second-degree relative with medically confirmed HLA-B27–related disease (eg, ankylosing spondylitis)
     -Anterior uveitis associated with pain, redness, or photophobia
     -Onset of arthritis in a boy after the age of 8 years
7. Idiopathic chronic arthritis that does not fit the above categories, or overlaps more than one category

Systemic Lupus Erythematosus

The criteria for SLE have been published by the ACR and recently updated.[41,42] These criteria, listed below, are based on 11 groups of signs, symptoms, and laboratory tests.

1. Malar (butterfly) rash
2. Discoid lupus rash
3. Photosensitive rash
4. Oral or nasal mucocutaneous ulcerations
5. Nonerosive arthritis
6. Nephritis, defined by:
   * proteinuria >0.5 g/day, *or*
   * cellular casts
7. Encephalopathy, defined by:
   * seizures, *or*
   * psychosis

8. Pleuritis or pericarditis
9. Cytopenias, defined as:
   • Coomb's positive hemolytic anemia, *or*
   • leukopenia, *or*
   • lymphopenia
10. Immunologic disorder, defined as:
    • anti-ds-DNA antibodies, *or*
    • anti-Sm antibodies, *or*
    • anti-phospholipid antibodies (determined by IgG or IgM anticardiolipin, lupus anti-coagulant, or a false-positive serologic test for syphilis)
11. Positive antinuclear antibodies (ANA)

If a patient meets 4 of these 11 criteria, they are considered to have SLE. In adult patients, this cut-off of 4 of 11 criteria correctly identifies patients, with a sensitivity of 0.96 and specificity of 0.96. Similarly, when tested in a cohort of Brazilian children with SLE and disease controls, these criteria differentiated the children with SLE with a sensitivity of 0.96 and a specificity of 1.0.[43]

Juvenile Dermatomyositis

Although the Bohan and Peter criteria for myositis have not been tested against expert opinion, they are widely accepted and are often used in diagnosing patients with JDM.[44] The criteria include the five signs and laboratory tests listed below:

1. Symmetrical weakness of the limb-girdle and anterior neck flexors
2. Muscle biopsy evidence of myositis
3. Elevation of serum muscle enzymes (CK, AST, ALT, aldolase, LD)
4. Electromyographic evidence of myopathy
5. Rash, especially an edematous, purple-coloured rash over the eyelids (heliotrope rash) and red, scaly rash over the extensor surface of the knuckles (Gottron's sign) or other joints.

To be considered as having "definite" JDM, a patient must have the rash and at least three other criteria. "Probable" JDM is diagnosed when the rash and two other criteria are present. If only the rash and one other criterion are present, a diagnosis of "possible" JDM is made.

Kawasaki Disease

The criteria used in the diagnosis of Kawasaki disease have also not been tested against any external standard, but they are well established and widely accepted.[45] These criteria are as follows:

1. Fever lasting 5 days or more, *and* 4 of the criteria listed below
2. Bilateral congestion of the bulbar conjunctivae that is nonexudative
3. Changes to the lips and oral cavity
   • dryness, redness and fissuring of the lips, or
   • strawberry tongue, or
   • diffuse reddening of the oral and pharyngeal mucosa
4. Changes to the peripheral extremities
   • reddening of the palms and soles, or
   • indurative edema, or
   • membranous desquamation of the fingertips (usually seen later in the convalescent stage)
5. Polymorphous rash of the trunk, without vesicles or crusts
6. Acute nonpurulent swelling of cervical lymph nodes, 1.5 cm or more in diameter, usually unilateral

It is important to consider mimics of KD. Children with KD appear to have an acute infectious illness. Conditions that often mimic the features of KD include streptococcal infections (like scarlet fever), drug reactions, and especially measles. Children with these conditions can sometimes meet the above criteria for KD.[46]

Serologic Tests

Serologic tests are often ordered to rule in, or rule out rheumatic disorders when children present with musculoskeletal pain, rash, or fatigue.

Rheumatoid Factor as a Case-Finding Test

Rheumatoid factor is the name given to the circulating autoantibodies directed toward a patient's own immunoglobulins (usually an IgM antibody directed against IgG antibodies). The RF-positive polyarticular subgroup of patients with JA (see above) makes up the smallest group—about 5 percent of children with arthritis. The sensitivity of the RF as a case-finding test for arthritis, therefore, is only about 0.05. However, the specificity is high in children, as there are few other situations in which young people develop an RF. In fact, the specificity may be as high as 0.98.[47] The sensitivity is too low to be helpful in case-finding, and, therefore, RF should not be measured when trying to make a diagnosis of arthritis.

However, RF does help to define a group of children (those with RF-positive polyarticular-onset JA) who may have a worse prognosis, once arthritis has been definitely diagnosed. Therefore, for patients already diagnosed with polyarticular JA, the measurement of RF is warranted.

Antinuclear Antibodies as a Case-Finding Test

Antinuclear antibodies (ANA) are autoantibodies directed against the constituents in a patient's own cell nuclei. Antinuclear antibodies are frequently present in the sera of patients with JA, SLE, JDM, LS, and other rheumatic diseases. The test, though, is limited in specificity—both in distinguishing between rheumatic diseases and in distinguishing healthy subjects from those with rheumatic disease. About 5 to 15 percent (depending on the population sampled) of healthy children have a positive ANA test.

Because of its limited specificity, the ANA is not a particularly good case-finding test. Without objective clinical evidence of arthritis or SLE, almost all positive ANA tests are likely to be false positives. When used in case-finding, the ANA test leads to a large number of unnecessary referrals to pediatric rheumatologists and likely to unnecessary anxiety in patients and families. In fact, a positive ANA test with no other evidence of disease was the third most common diagnosis made by pediatric rheumatologists participating in the American registry.[2]

Even those children who do have some signs and symptoms of rheumatic disease and a persistently positive ANA test are at a very low risk of developing an autoimmune disease over time. In a Canadian study, children with musculoskeletal pain—but no definite features of autoimmune disease such as objective arthritis, rash, or sicca syndrome—and a positive ANA test were followed up over time. None of 24 patients, followed for an average of 5 years, developed an autoimmune rheumatic disease.[48]

What is the ANA test good for? The ANA test is highly sensitive in SLE; the sensitivity is 0.99 or even higher. Therefore, a negative ANA test can be used to rule out SLE. Also, a positive ANA test may differentiate those children with JA at highest risk for uveitis (see below). This was certainly true of the older, less sensitive assays. Recent assays are more sensitive; a large majority of children with JA now test positive for ANA. The ability of the current ANA tests in predicting the risk for uveitis in those children with JA is less certain.

Specific Autoantibodies in Systemic Lupus Erythematosus

As discussed, the ANA is an extremely sensitive test in SLE, but it is not as specific. There are, however, other serologic markers that are much more specific. Anti-ds-DNA antibodies (serum autoantibodies to native double-stranded DNA) are highly specific for SLE (98 percent), but less sensitive (50 to 70 percent). Because of the high specificity, a positive anti-ds-DNA test is useful to rule in a diagnosis of SLE.[49] There are other specific autoantibodies seen in patients with SLE; the anti-Sm (anti-Smith) antibody is also useful for ruling in SLE, and a positive test fulfills one of the classification criteria (see above).

Myositis-Specific Autoantibodies in Juvenile Dermatomyositis

Recently, a number of highly specific autoantibodies have been described in adult patients with myositis. These antibodies include a group of related antibodies directed against synthetase proteins (of which anti-Jo-1 is the most common) and antibodies directed against other cellular constituents, including anti-SRP, anti-Mi2 and anti-MAS antibodies. While these antibodies may be present in the sera of highly selected children,[50] they are only infrequently seen in children with JDM.[51] Testing for these antibodies in children with straightforward JDM is not worthwhile.

EVIDENCE-BASED THERAPY FOR CHILDHOOD RHEUMATIC ILLNESSES

Nonarticular Rheumatism

Growing Pain

Growing pains are frequently seen in general and specialty practices. Almost all physicians surveyed treat their patients with some combination of reassurance, local massage, and mild analgesics.[5] While these methods seem effective, none have been formally studied, and therefore these local measures get a grade C recommendation.

Stretching has been recommended by some as a way of treating and preventing growing pain, and there is level I evidence to support this. In one study,[52] 36 children were recruited, using standard criteria, from four community practices. The patients were randomly assigned to a control group that received reassurance only or to a treatment group of patients who were given an active stretching program. The program consisted of twice-daily (morning and night) stretches as illustrated in Figure 19–2. The children in both groups had about 10 painful episodes per month at baseline. The active stretching group had almost complete resolution of painful episodes by 3 months and no further episodes by 9 months. In contrast, the control group still had two painful episodes per month at 18 months. In this study, there was no blinding. In addition, there was no "attention placebo," so the effect seen may have been due to increased time with parents rather than the stretching per se. Until these results are replicated, stretching should have a grade B recommendation.

Hypermobility/Juvenile Episodic Arthralgia

Authorities have recommended a number of treatments for children with hypermobility (level III). These treatments have included education programs to teach joint protection, physiotherapy to strengthen the mobile joints, and regular nonsteroidal anti-inflammatory drug (NSAID) treatment.[53] There are no controlled studies of any sort for the treatment of hypermobility. Since hypermobility seems to be a benign condition and one that most children seem to outgrow, treatment of this condition gets a grade C recommendation. Reassurance that the condition does not lead to disability or joint destruction seems to be the most appropriate response.

Fibromyalgia

Given what we know about the pathogenesis of FM, it would seem reasonable to direct therapy toward improving sleep quality and reversing physical deconditioning.

STRETCHING PROGRAM

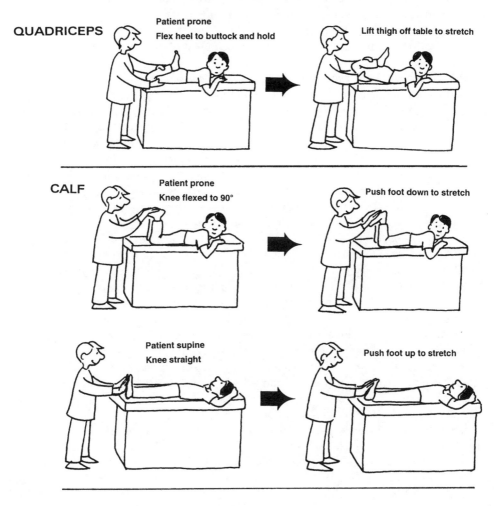

QUADRICEPS

Patient prone

Flex heel to buttock and hold

Lift thigh off table to stretch

CALF

Patient prone

Knee flexed to 90°

Push foot down to stretch

Patient supine

Knee straight

Push foot up to stretch

HAMSTRINGS

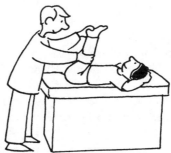

Patient supine

Lift leg by heel

Hold knee straight

Flex hip to stretch

NOTE: Hold each stretch for 15-20 seconds

Repeat each stretch 10-20 times

Alternate legs

Figure 19–2

Like many other rheumatic diseases, the therapy of FM has been systematically studied only in adults. There is some evidence that the prognosis in children with FM is more favorable than in adults; in a follow-up study of an Israeli cohort of children, 73 percent of the originally identified children no longer had FM at 30 months.[54] In contrast, most adults continue to have FM for life. Therefore, results from adult studies have to be interpreted with caution.

Neck support.   Some experts have suggested that the pain and fatigue in FM are due to referred signals, perhaps set off by irritated nerve roots, from an unsupported cervical spine during sleep. This has led to the suggestion that special support of the neck at night can improve sleep quality and ameliorate FM. There is level II-1 evidence that FM patients prefer specialized neck support pillows (the "Shape of Sleep" pillow was used in this study) to neck ruffs or standard pillows. The studied subjects tried each type of pillow for 2 weeks in a self-selected order. Despite a preference for the special neck support pillow, however, there were no significant differences in any of the sleep, function, or pain measures. This was a small study, and there was likely a high risk of a false-negative (type II) error.[55] Specialized neck support, therefore, gets a grade C recommendation.

Cognitive behavioural therapy (CBT).   Since FM is characterized by disabling pain, some have suggested that strategies designed to teach skills of pain control, skills to lessen disability, and skills designed to build confidence (ie, CBT) might help. There is level II-3 evidence that intensive inpatient behavioral programs can lessen a number of symptoms associated with FM.[56] However, the only current level I evidence suggests that, at least in the outpatient setting, the addition of CBT to standard education does not provide any benefit over standard education alone.[57] Therefore, outpatient-based CBT programs get a grade D recommendation, and inpatient intensive programs get a grade C recommendation.

Antidepressants, hypnotics, and other pharmacotherapy.   A number of RCTs have suggested that antidepressants in low doses and some hypnotics are useful in treating FM, at least in the short term. In some cases, the mechanism is thought to be related to sleep improvement. There have been no studies of children with FM.

There is level I evidence that amitriptyline in low doses improves FM symptoms in the short term; however, after a few months, placebo patients also improve to the same degree.[58] While sleep improves on amitriptyline, the mechanism of improvement in FM is not clear. At least in one study, the characteristic sleep-EEG alpha-wave abnormality (see above) did not improve in the amitriptyline-treated FM patients.[59] In addition, there is level I evidence that fluoxetine is also an effective short term therapy, and that the combination of amitriptyline and fluoxetine may be better than either alone.[60]

Several other medications have been studied in adults with FM, but their use has been limited and their role unclear even in adult patients.

Amitriptyline is usually started in a low (10 mg) night-time dose. The effect is often seen within 2 or 3 weeks. The dose may be slowly worked up in increments of 10 mg. The side effects are usually mild and patients often develop tolerance to the side effects over a few days. Amitriptyline, therefore, gets a grade B recommendation for the treatment of FM, at least in the short term.

Exercise.   There are several arguments to support the need for exercise in patients with FM. First, FM patients are deconditioned, compared with other sedentary adults. Second, exercise is a potent modulator of sleep. Finally, sleep deprivation has been shown to cause the signs and symptoms of FM in deconditioned volunteers but not in fit volunteers.

There is level I evidence that cardiorespiratory exercise improves pain in adults with FM.[61,62] However, compliance with exercise is especially poor in patients with FM. Many patients complain that exercise makes their symptoms worse for a period of time before an improvement occurs. In the study by Martin and colleagues,[61] only about half of the eligible patients completed the program. The best approach (recommendation B) would seem to be a gentle aerobic program, consisting of nonjarring exercise such as swimming or cycling. The exercise should be carried out at least three times weekly for at least 20 minutes, and preferably longer, per session. The exercise must become strenuous enough to cause the heart rate to rise and the breathing to become labored. Most FM patients will need to work into their program gradually.

Complementary therapies for FM. Although complementary/alternative health therapies are widely used in all chronic diseases, patients with FM are particularly high users. For instance, one study compared adults referred to a rheumatologist for FM with those referred for other diagnoses. Ninety-one percent of the FM patients had sought complementary health care compared with 63 percent of the other referred patients.[63] It is important, therefore, to discuss the evidence for complementary therapies in children with FM.

Bright light: the symptoms of FM are seasonal in almost half the studied adults with the disorder. This has suggested to some the possibility that FM is related to seasonal affective disorder (SAD), which is often treated with periods of daily bright light. One small RCT that employed a cross-over design has studied the use of a bright light visor in adults with FM. This study showed no difference between the time periods when patients were wearing the light visor and the time periods when the visor was covered with an opaque screen (level I). Although this study was small and the likelihood of a false negative (type II) error was high, the treatment effects were negligible.[64] It remains possible that a different method of delivering bright light would be more helpful. Therefore, bright light therapy gets a level D recommendation.

Biofeedback: biofeedback has been studied and shown to be of modest benefit (level I) in adult patients with FM. The biofeedback was obtained by using electromyographic (EMG) recordings of the trapezius muscles to monitor muscular relaxation. The effect of biofeedback, in this study, was best when combined with fitness exercise.[65] Biofeedback of this nature gets a grade B recommendation for FM in children.

Hypnotherapy: hypnosis has been used as a therapy for many types of chronic pain. There is level I evidence in adult patients that hypnosis is effective in improving the symptoms of FM. The patients in this study participated in eight, 1-hour sessions over 3 months. In addition, they were provided with an audio-tape for autohypnosis to be used on a daily basis. Control patients were given physiotherapy consisting of relaxation therapy and massage. Symptoms (using a variety of patient-report measures) were all improved in the hypnotherapy group, although the effects were small. The hypnotherapy patients had a reduced need for analgesics.[66] Therefore, hypnotherapy gets a grade B recommendation for childhood FM.

Nutritional supplements: nutritional therapies have not been exhaustively studied, not even in adults with FM. There is only one RCT, a cross-over study of Super Malic. Super Malic is a combination of malic acid and magnesium hydroxide. The study showed no effect of Super Malic (level I); however, the dose may not have been adequate. A subsequent (open label) dose-finding phase of the study did result in some subjective improvement.[67] Therefore, Super Malic gets a grade D recommendation; other nutritional supplements get a grade C recommendation.

Homeopathy: there is one study that used a rigorous (double-blind, placebo-controlled) method to investigate the use of a homeopathic medicine (R toxicodendron 6C). The treated subjects were a subgroup of adults with FM felt to have appropriate symptoms for this treatment.[68] Although the results suggested a positive effect, the analysis may have been flawed; a more rigorous statistical analysis suggested no effect.[69] Therefore, homeopathy currently gets a grade C recommendation.

Treatment of children with FM. Overall, a reasonable plan would be a combination of an aerobic exercise program, neck support pillow, and reasonable strategies for analgesic control. Those patients who do not improve may need amitriptyline, 10 mg qhs to begin with and, if necessary, increased in 10-mg increments to 60 mg. Nonresponders should further consider combination pharmacotherapy (amitriptyline and fluoxetine) and the addition of complementary therapies such as hypnotherapy and biofeedback. Intensive programs that include CBT should be further evaluated in controlled studies.

Backache

There are, apparently, no studies directed toward the treatment of childhood and adolescent mechanical back pain. The major task for the practitioner is to sort out those cases that are likely benign from those needing urgent treatment (Figure 19–3).[18]

The signs of potential "serious" illness include:

1. age <5 y,
2. fever, systemic illness,
3. neurologic symptoms or signs,
4. refusal to walk, or
5. increasing pain unrelieved by rest/immobilization.

The signs of potentially "important," although less serious, illness include:

6. pain at rest/night or pain with cough,
7. sciatica,
8. pain for >3 months,
9. family history of ankylosing spondylitis,
10. change in activity,
11. gait change,
12. decreased straight leg raise,
13. back deformity (including scoliosis),
14. back stiffness,
15. percussion tenderness,
16. bony tenderness, or
17. midline skin defect.

In the absence of these findings, conservative therapy is appropriate. Advice for the specifics of conservative treatment has come from adult studies.

Rest.   Although rest was once the mainstay of treatment, there is now level I evidence (in adults) that less rest is better than more.[70] Furthermore, there is level I evidence that suggests that no rest is at least as good as (if not better than) less rest.[71] Therefore, for children, an early return to activities and mobilization gets a grade B recommendion.

Traction.   Early studies examining traction as a treatment for adult back pain were methodologically flawed and did not provide a clear answer.[72] More recently, there is level I evidence, in adults, that traction is not effective.[73] Therefore, traction should not be used for chronic nonspecific back pain in children (recommendation D).

Back Support.   Back support devices have not been widely studied. However, back support devices seem to be widely used. One RCT (level I) compared a back support device with standard advice in adult patients.[74] The back support group used less than half the amount of analgesics and had improved vocational ability in the short-term trial. Back support strategies should be considered in children with chronic backache (recommendation B).

Education.   Education programs designed to teach correct posture, correct lifting and other back care practices are sometimes called "back school" programs. Koes, in a systematic review of RCTs, found most of the studies to be of poor methodologic quality; there was a great deal of inconsistency in the results.[75] The benefits of back school, if seen, were usually only of short duration. In a meta-analysis of 19 RCTs, it was found that back school programs were more effective if offered in the setting of a comprehensive exercise/rehabilitation

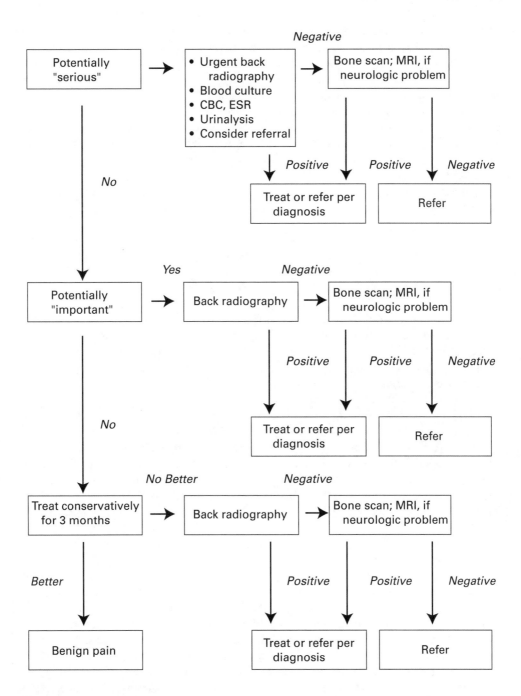

Figure 19–3   Investigation and Treatment Algorithm for Children with Backache (see text).

program.[76] Thus, although there is level I evidence in adults, the evidence is inconsistent and rates a grade C recommendation. If used, back school programs should be combined with exercise programs that are shown to be of benefit.

Exercise.   In recent years, a number of exercise programs have been designed for adult patients with back pain. The focus has been on local muscular training (trunk flexion, trunk extension, and spine flexibility) or on overall fitness exercise.

There is level I evidence in adult studies that exercise advice, by itself, does not improve pain, disability, or medical-care needs, when compared with attention placebo (sham ultrasonography).[77] However, there is strong evidence (level I) that supervised fitness exercise (fitness classes) added to exercise instruction and back school education results in significant improvements in pain and in subjective and objective function.[78] The results of supervised fitness classes have a long-term impact (at least 2 years).[79] The exercises used in these supervised fitness classes consist of circuit resistance training, light aerobics, and flexibility exercises. Therefore, the treatment of children with chronic backache should include a supervised fitness program in addition to other conservative strategies (recommendation B).

Transcutaneous electrical nerve stimulation (TENS).　This therapy has been widely used in the past for chronic backache and is still used in the management of many other chronic pain syndromes. In one Texas study, 145 adult back pain patients were randomized to four groups (exercise and sham TENS, TENS, exercise and TENS, sham TENS alone). In this study, the exercise groups improved but there was no independent effect of TENS.[80] Therefore, there is level I evidence to give a grade D recommendation that TENS should not be used in children with back pain as it is likely ineffective.

Analgesics.　A number of RCTs have been carried out to study the efficacy of analgesic agents in acute back strain in adult patients. However, there have not been any studies for children. Acetaminophen, or over-the-counter nonsteroidal anti-inflammatory drugs (NSAIDs) may be used as necessary for pain relief (recommendation C). Children should be warned to take NSAIDs with meals to avoid gastric upset. Opioid analgesics are not indicated; there is no evidence to support their use. Children who require opioid analgesia for backache should be considered for prompt referral.

Facet injections.　Facet joint injections have been widely practiced in adults under the assumption that the source of much chronic back pain is due to degenerative arthritis of the facets. This rationale is unlikely to apply to children. There is level I evidence from a Quebec City study that facet injections are ineffective. In this study, adult patients were screened so that the source of pain was most likely facet degeneration. One hundred and one patients were randomized to lumbar facet injection with corticosteroid under fluoroscopy or to saline placebo injection under double-blind conditions. There was no difference between the groups at 1 and 3 months follow-up and only a slight benefit at 6 months.[81] These data support a grade E recommendation that facet injections *not* be given in children with back pain.

Complementary therapies for backache.　Manipulation: there has been a great deal of controversy about the role of chiropractic treatment and other forms of spinal manipulation in treating acute and chronic back pain. Like many of the other interventions discussed in this chapter, manipulation has not been properly evaluated in children. There have been, however, several studies that have examined the role of manipulation in adults.

Manipulation is widely sought after by adults and children with back pain. In the United States, it is estimated that 30 percent of adults with back pain seek chiropractic care. This is almost as large as the proportion (40 percent) who seek medical (which includes osteopathic) care. Patients report a greater satisfaction with backache care received from chiropractors than with care provided by general practitioners or family doctors. This is apparently due to the greater amount of time that chiropractors spend with their patients and to patients' perception that chiropractors have greater confidence.[82]

There is accumulating level I evidence to support a small but definite benefit of chiropractic over standard medical care in the treatment of chronic back pain.[83] As chiropracty is a "hot topic," there have been several meta-analyses examining its efficacy. There is even a systematic review of the reviews. Most of the meta-analyses and reviews have been of low quality. Nine of 10 best reviews support a positive effect of manipulation.[84] However, recently, an RCT studying the cost-effectiveness (level I) showed chiropractic care was no better than physiotherapy, and there was no difference in cost.[85]

The overall benefit of chiropractic manipulation remains unclear in adults and, therefore, gets a grade C recommendation for children. Manipulation may have the same role as physiotherapy.

Acupuncture/electroacupuncture: there have been no RCTs of traditional acupuncture in back pain, not even in adult patients. There is one study of electroacupuncture. This study was done in a British general practice setting. The investigators studied an electroacupuncture unit that stimulates skin points but uses no needles. They studied 40 adults with an acute back injury, who were randomized to acetaminophen and sham acupuncture, or to acupuncture and placebo acetaminophen. The electroacupuncture treatments were done twice, for 15 minutes each time. The two treatment groups did not differ at 1 and 2 weeks (both had substantial improvement in reported pain and mobility) but at 6 weeks the electroacupuncture group was better than the acetaminophen group.[86] This is level I evidence, but the study does not really apply to children with chronic backache. Therefore, acupuncture and electroacupuncture get a grade C recommendation.

Spa Therapy: spa therapy refers to the use of a variety of treatments, including mud baths, mineral water immersion, and like therapies, in a spa setting. There is level I evidence in adults, that 3 weeks in a French spa works better than being on a waiting list, for a variety of clinically important outcomes.[87] It is unclear from this study which aspect of the spa therapy was beneficial, since there was no attention control. Spa therapy is costly, very time intensive, and has not been studied in children. Therefore, spa therapy gets a grade C recommendation.

Juvenile Arthritis

Juvenile arthritis is less common than nonarticular rheumatism; most practitioners will not have a large experience in treating JA. There have been very few controlled studies of therapy on which to base recommendations. It is usually recommended that children with arthritis receive comprehensive care in a specialized clinic setting. Comprehensive care means assessment by a specialist (most often a pediatric rheumatologist but sometimes a pediatrician or rheumatologist with expertise in JA), educational support, comprehensive rehabilitation therapy including pool therapy, splinting, orthotics, and so on. The evidence for some of these modalities is drawn from studies of adult arthritis, and so some caution must be used when applying these results to children.

Education and Family Support

Chronic illness may have a large impact on families and can lead to stress, parental depression, and marital discord, as well as to behavior and social problems in the affected child. In JA, it is less clear how often this happens; the studies are inconsistent. The most consistent finding is that children with JA participate less in school activities and have fewer friends; JA seems to lead to social isolation. In addition, it appears that family factors, such as family harmony and parental emotional well-being, may have a greater effect on arthritic children than the severity of the disease itself.[88]

Studies using qualitative methods have identified areas of educational need for families and children with JA. Within the family, educational needs include understanding the "empathy-resentment-guilt" cycle, information about the disease and prognosis, addressing the likelihood of death, and developing coping skills and social supports.[89] At the individual level, children with JA need to learn how to cope with the school environment, how to manage the pain and stiffness, and how to preserve joint function.[90]

There are no studies supporting the use of specific educational interventions in JA (level III). However, given the needs identified and the likelihood of success, an educational program dealing with factors listed above gets a grade B recommendation.

Physiotherapy and Rehabilitation in Juvenile Arthritis

Hydrotherapy. One of the mainstays of JA rehabilitation treatments is hydrotherapy. Hydrotherapy refers to exercises carried out in a warmed (often close to body temperature) therapy pool. The buoyancy of the water enables children to exercise without any jarring effects on their arthritic joints. The heat of the water allows for increased stretching of painful joints. There is only level III evidence of the effectiveness of hydrotherapy in children. In adults with active rheumatoid arthritis (RA), there is level I evidence that hydrotherapy is (marginally) better than land-based exercises and attention placebo in reducing pain and improving function.[91] Clinical experience shows that children who receive pool therapy find it immediately helpful in controlling symptoms and improving function. The question is, does the treatment help in the long run? Hydrotherapy is costly and requires the supervision of an experienced physiotherapist. Until controlled studies show its benefit in JA, hydrotherapy can be given only a grade B recommendation.

Comprehensive rehabilitation therapy. Typical rehabilitation interventions for children with very involved arthritis require a team approach. The rehabilitation team might include a physiotherapist to prescribe exercises designed to increase the range of motion and the strength of the affected joints, an occupational therapist to provide mobility and functional aids and solve problems around areas of functional difficulty, a social worker who will give emotional and vocational counseling, and a wide range of other professionals. This comprehensive care approach is often provided in an inpatient setting.

No controlled studies have evaluated the efficacy of this approach in children (level III). There have been several quasiexperimental and properly randomized controlled trials of structured rehabilitation care in adults with inflammatory arthritis, usually RA and ankylosing spondylitis. For example, there is level II-1 evidence that a single, inpatient, rehabilitation stay (of about 2 weeks) reduces pain and disease activity, and improves physical function, emotional well being, compliance, and knowledge of arthritis in adults with RA.[92] Comprehensive outpatient treatment programs may provide similar benefits to inpatient programs at a much smaller cost (level II-1).[93] Outpatient programs should, however, include supervised weekly group sessions (level I), as they lead to moderate improvements over unsupervised care, at only a modest increase in cost.[94] There is level I evidence that even sending community-based physiotherapists into RA patients' homes (for 4 hours over 6 weeks) leads to some improvements in knowledge and self-efficacy, and reduction in morning stiffness.[95]

On this basis, comprehensive rehabilitation therapy for children with JA gets a grade B recommendation.

Fitness exercise. Children with arthritis are less active than their peers and are deconditioned. Adults with RA can improve pain management, function, and arthritis control by taking part in vigorous fitness training. There is level II-3 evidence in children that an aerobic fitness training program can improve pain management and arthritis control. The program that was studied consisted of an 8-week intervention. Children exercised 3 times weekly in a progressive fashion. The exercise program was comprehensive and included a variety of aerobic exercises, strengthening using resistance, and stretching.[96] Fitness exercise gets a grade B recommendation.

Splints. Splints, especially for the hands and wrists, are often prescribed to children with arthritis of these joints. The purpose is to maintain, or improve, the range of motion. Often, these splints are worn at night. Daytime "work" splints are sometimes prescribed to reduce pain caused by activities. There is only level III evidence for the use of splints in children. There is level I evidence supporting wrist orthotics used in adults with inflammatory arthritis for the purposes of increasing function and reducing pain.[97] Referral to an orthotist should be considered for a child with JA who has limited range of motion of the wrists (recommendation B). Splinting of other joints has not been rigorously studied (level III) and therefore must be given a grade C recommendation.

Orthotics.   Orthotic devices, fitted to the child's shoes, are often prescribed for foot support. Custom orthotics can be quite expensive. There are no studies supporting this practice in children with JA (level III). There is level I evidence for adults with RA that posted orthotics are no better than placebo orthotics in relieving pain or reducing disability over a period of 3 years.[98] Until further studies are done, orthotics for the feet get a grade C recommendation in JA.

Pharmacotherapy for Juvenile Arthritis

Corticosteroid joint injections.   The use of steroid injections has completely changed the treatment of arthritis in children, especially in those with pauciarticular (oligoarticular) arthritis. In clinical practice, it is obvious that these injections are immediately and dramatically effective in reducing pain and swelling. After joint injections, joint contractures are often reduced; additionally, the reduction of inflammation improves the effectiveness of physiotherapy to increase joint range even further. In young children, especially those under 7 years, corticosteroid injections are often given under light general anesthesia.

The effect of joint injections, using long-acting corticosteroids like triamcinolone hexacetonide, can last for many months (level II-3).[99,100] The side effects are minimal, consisting of local skin atrophy (an extension effect of the corticosteroid) in fewer than 10 percent, and the radiographic appearance of small calcifications in the joint in fewer than 5 percent. These calcifications are almost never of any clinical importance.[101] The introduction of a needle into a joint may rarely lead to infection in the joint. This complication appears to be very rare. There is a theoretical concern that local corticosteroids may be a risk factor for avascular necrosis of adjacent bones.[102] This is hard to tease out, as arthritis itself, or other concomitant medications may be the cause of avascular necrosis.

There is level I evidence in adults that at least 24 hours of joint rest following corticosteroid injection leads to better outcomes over a longer period.[103] Whether long-term outcomes are improved has not yet been studied. Therefore, the early use of corticosteroid joint injections as a main therapy in oligoarticular arthritis gets a grade A recommendation, and the use of joint injections in other forms of arthritis for symptom control and relief of contractures gets a grade B recommendation. Children should be advised to rest their injected joints for 24 to 48 hours after injection (recommendation B).

Systemic Medications for Juvenile Arthritis

There is recent evidence that some members of the class of antiarthritic medications, called disease-modifying antirheumatic drugs (DMARDs), reduce the degree of joint destruction that occurs in adults with RA. This evidence and a better understanding of the long-term sequelae of arthritis have led to earlier and more aggressive use of medications in arthritis.

Nonsteroidal anti-inflammatory medications (NSAIDs).   Aspirin had been the traditional mainstay of treatment of arthritis. Several of the newer NSAIDs have been shown (level I) to reduce symptoms and inflammation in JA.[104,105] They are preferred, because of a more favorable therapeutic index and easier dosing regimens. There is little to choose between the NSAIDs.

Naproxen sodium has a longer half-life than some of the other NSAIDs that are approved for children. Since it only needs to be given twice daily and is widely available in a suspension, naproxen is often the first NSAID to be prescribed for children with JA. The use of naproxen (or one of the other NSAIDs) in the early treatment of JA gets a grade A recommendation.

It may take as long as 6 weeks to see the full anti-inflammatory effect of an NSAID medication. Not waiting 6 weeks is a common reason for the apparent failure of NSAIDs in children with JA.

Side effects of all NSAIDs include nausea and dyspepsia as well as much rarer renal and hepatic toxicity. Gastrointestinal side effects may be quite common,[106] but serious gastrointestinal side effects are rare.[107] Some patients may benefit from an antacid or a gastroprotective agent taken along with NSAIDs. There is little supportive evidence (level III evidence for misoprostol[108]) for this practice in children, and therefore, the addition of a gastroprotective agent gets a grade C recommendation.

One special side effect of naproxen is the development of photosensitive blisters (leaving shallow scars) on the face, especially in fair skinned patients. This exanthem has been called "naproxen pseudoporphyria." Patients taking naproxen should be warned about this potential side effect; aggressive use of a sunscreen is sometimes recommended (level III, recommendation C).[109]

Recently, a new class of NSAIDs has been developed. These new NSAIDs selectively inhibit cyclo-oxygenase-2 (COX-2), which is the enzyme associated with inflammation in JA but not associated with protection of the gastric mucosa. Cox-2-selective NSAIDs have the potential to be less toxic to the gastrointestinal tract. These new NSAIDs have not yet been studied in children and therefore get a grade C recommendation.

Disease-modifying antirheumatic drugs.   Methotrexate: Methotrexate is now the most widely used DMARD for both children and adults. Its use is well supported by RCTs in adults with RA. There is also level I evidence supporting the efficacy of methotrexate in children with arthritis who have disease resistant to treatment with NSAIDs.[110] In this study, carried out jointly by American and former U.S.S.R. centers, a weekly dose of 10 mg/m² was effective. Methotrexate at a dose of 5 mg/m² was no better than placebo therapy. Methotrexate, at a minimum dose of 10 mg/m² once weekly, therefore gets a grade A recommendation for the treatment of arthritis in those patients unresponsive to NSAIDs.

The current practice is to start methotrexate early in the course of disease for children with polyarticular JA. There is evidence from studies in adult RA that methotrexate can limit the progression of bone erosions that result from aggressive arthritis. Since bone erosions are also seen in the polyarticular and systemic-onset subtypes of JA, many pediatric rheumatologists feel that there is a rationale for the early use of methotrexate in these children. Methotrexate, however, does not seem to be as effective in the systemic-onset subtype of JA.[111]

Methotrexate can be given orally or parenterally (usually subcutaneously) and is given weekly. The dose is often worked up from 10 mg/m² to as high as 20 or 25 mg/m² weekly.

The major worrisome side effect is the development of liver fibrosis. Dosage adjustments are made on the basis of monthly blood tests evaluating liver transaminases and albumin (level II-3).[112]

Folic acid (usually 1 mg daily) is given to reduce the more frequent minor side effects, namely, nausea and oral chancres. There is level I evidence for the use of folic acid in adults with RA.[113] However, the effectiveness of folic acid in children is less certain. One small crossover trial found little or no effect.[114] Therefore, folic acid supplementation for methotrexate-treated patients gets a level B recommendation.

Etanercept: the production of biologic therapies has been the most provocative and anticipated new development in the therapy of arthritis. Biologics are usually recombinant molecules designed to target specific reactions in the immune system or to inhibit the function of specific cell types. The most exciting target so far is tumor necrosis factor (TNF), which is known to be activated in a variety of inflammatory states, including arthritis.

There is recent, level I evidence that blocking TNF action through the use of antibodies against TNF, or by "mopping up" circulating TNF with soluble receptors (etanercept) is remarkably effective in adults with RA.[115–117] An RCT (level I) showing the effectiveness of etanercept in JA patients who did not tolerate or failed methotrexate has just been completed[118] but has not yet been published. Etanercept gets a grade A recommendation for those patients with severe JA for whom methotrexate is not an option.

Sulfasalazine: sulfasalazine is widely used as a DMARD in the treatment of adult RA. There is now level I evidence (from a small RCT) that sulfasalazine is more effective than placebo in the treatment of JA.[119] About half those children taking sulfasalazine (in this study, the patients had polyarticular and oligoarticular JA) showed a response in a number of important disease features, compared with about 25 percent in the placebo group. However, sulfasalazine was associated with frequent side effects. Sulfasalazine gets a grade B recommendation as a DMARD for JA.

Gold: intramuscular gold was once commonly used in the treatment of childhood arthritis. It is associated, however, with a high toxicity rate. Because of the availability of more effective and safer alternatives (for example, methotrexate), gold is now rarely used in children. There is level I evidence that the oral preparation of gold (auranofin) has no effect in treating JA.[120] Therefore, intramuscular gold gets a grade C recommendation, while oral gold gets a grade E recommendation.

Hydroxychloroquine: there is level I evidence that suggests that the response of children with JA to hydroxychloroquine is unlikely to be clinically important.[121] Hydroxychloroquine, however, has recently been widely used in combination with other DMARDs in the therapy of adult RA. There may be an as yet undefined role for hydroxychloroquine as part of combination therapy for JA. Hydroxychloroquine gets a grade D recommendation as monotherapy and a grade C recommendation as part of combination therapy.

Azathioprine: azathioprine is a potentially cytotoxic agent that is rarely used in JA. There is level I evidence from a small study of 32 subjects with severe JA that the toxicity of azathioprine outweighs its benefit. Therefore, azathioprine gets a grade D recommendation.[122]

Cyclosporine: because there is still a sizeable minority of children with JA who do not respond to methotrexate, many other agents that can potentially relieve inflammation have been tried. Cyclosporine is an effective agent used in the treatment of adult RA. There is only level III evidence, however, in children, which suggests that cyclosporine may have a role in JA.[123–125] Cyclosporine, therefore gets a grade C recommendation.

Corticosteroids: appropriate doses of corticoteroids result in an undoubted and obvious clinical response (ie, reduction of pain, stiffness, and often signs of inflammation) in the short term. However, a high likelihood of serious side effects has prompted most rheumatologists to limit the use of corticosteroids in the treatment of JA as much as possible. It remains unclear whether corticosteroids have any long-term benefit. There is level I evidence that adult patients with RA develop fewer bone erosions over a 2-year period, if treated with prednisolone (7.5 mg daily) as compared with placebo.[126] A recent meta-analysis showed that the short-to medium-term effects of prednisone were the same as, or better than, other active therapies for the control of symptoms.[127] It seems reasonable to give a grade B recommendation for the short-term use of low doses of oral corticosteroids as bridging therapy in those patients with severe arthritis who require DMARDs, most of which take several months to achieve a reasonable clinical effect. Oral corticosteroids may be used to control symptoms while waiting for a DMARD to work. Corticosteroids get a grade C recommendation for longer-term use.

Oral Tolerance: oral tolerance with chicken cartilage has recently generated a lot of interest in the treatment of inflammatory arthritis. This is due to an exciting early report (level I) of a study in adults with RA.[128] Oral tolerance is based on the proposal that small, frequent exposures to the cartilage antigen can reduce an arthritic patient's immune response to their own cartilage. Oral tolerance has a theoretical advantage over other antiarthritic therapies; chicken cartilage is a natural substance with no known adverse effects.

A subsequent study of oral tolerance (level I), again in adult RA, failed to confirm a strong effect.[129] There is only level III evidence suggesting some effect in children with arthritis.[130] Therefore, oral tolerance gets a grade C recommendation.

Uveitis Screening

Children with JA are at risk of developing potentially sight-limiting uveitis. For many children with JA, this is the most worrisome aspect of their disease. The reason for concern is that the uveitis of JA is often asymptomatic and unrecognized until permanent damage has been done. Uveitis associated with JA is often easily treated; therefore, it makes sense to screen for the development of uveitis and treat it before damage occurs. Children with the oligoarticular-onset subtype, especially those with a positive ANA test, seem to be at the highest risk for uveitis.

Children with JA can present with uveitis as late as 10 years after the onset of arthritis.[131]

The American Academy of Pediatrics (AAP) has published guidelines for the frequency of ophthalmologic examinations for children with JA (level III).[132] These guidelines categorize children as being at high risk, medium risk, or low risk. High-risk children are to be screened every 3 to 4 months, medium risk children every 6 months, and low risk children every 12 months.

The AAP guidelines define high-risk children as those with oligoarticular or polyarticular onset, who are ANA positive, and have disease onset before the age of 7 years. Four years after the onset of arthritis, these patients are at medium risk, and 7 years after onset they are at low risk.

The guidelines define medium-risk children as those with oligoarticular- or polyarticular-onset disease, who are ANA negative, or have the onset of their disease after age 7 years. Four years after the onset of arthritis these children become low risk.

Children with systemic-onset arthritis are all considered to be in the low-risk category.

Although these guidelines have not been formally evaluated, the seriousness of the problem leads to a grade A recommendation.

Transition.

As children with JA grow into adulthood, they face special challenges. Children with arthritis may need special preparation to be able to work and adapt to a more independent life. Many children with JA have developed a special, long-term realtionship with their medical care providers. As they approach adulthood, these patients need to move from a more paternalistic pediatric health-care system to an adult-oriented health-care system where they have to fend for themselves. Many models of transition care have been put forward, but there is little or no research to guide decisions on choosing the best model. We have only testimonial evidence (level III) to support the different programs.[133,134] While it is clear that there is a need for transitional services, any particular model can get only a grade C recommendation.

Approach to Treatment of Juvenile Arthritis

Oligoarticular-onset JA. It is initially important, when a child presents with oligoarticular joint inflammation, to carefully make a positive diagnosis of JA. In those children (about half the children with oligoarticular JA) who present with a single swollen joint, it is especially important to rule out other causes of monoarthritis (such as tuberculosis, hemophilia in a boy, septic arthritis, or cancer). Children with JA should initially receive a 6-week trial of an NSAID and usually a referral to a physiotherapist. If the signs and symptoms of inflammation continue or if contractures develop, then a referral to a pediatric rheumatologist or to an adult rheumatologist experienced in dealing with children should be considered for joint injections and follow-up care. These children are usually at the highest risk for uveitis and should be screened as above. The prognosis in this subtype of JA is good, and families will need educational support.

Polyarticular and systemic-onset JA. Children with these more severe forms of arthritis should be referred to a comprehensive care clinic so that they can receive the multidisciplinary therapies listed above. These children should have uveitis screening, as appropriate. Children with chronic arthritis affecting several joints are highly likely to need transition care when they become adolescents.

Systemic Lupus Erythematosus and Juvenile Dermatomyositis

Childhood SLE and JDM are both rare diseases and both potentially fatal. Children with these diseases should be referred to subspecialty care. Patients with SLE should be followed up by a pediatric rheumatologist or nephrologist. Patients with JDM should be seen by a pediatric rheumatologist or neurologist. In some communities, an adult rheumatologist or a pediatrician with special expertise might be most appropriate.

There are some basic principles that are applicable to both these diseases that families need to know.

Sun Avoidance

The rash of both SLE and JDM may be photosensitive. Children with these diseases should use a strong (SPF 30 or above) waterproof sunscreen in the summer.

Diet

Many children with SLE or JDM will be treated with prednisone. There is no real evidence of the effect of diet on the side effects of prednisolone in children. To avoid excessive weight gain and fluid retention, it makes sense to limit the calories and sodium intake (recommendation B). Often a dietician can be helpful to families in planning meals for a child taking prednisone.

Medications

Since many SLE and JDM patients will be treated with prednisone, they and their families should be educated about corticosteroids. The major side effects that these children often experience include cushingoid appearance and associated appetite increase, mood changes (rarely psychosis), adrenal suppression, growth suppression, bone problems (osteoporosis and avascular necrosis), hypertension, glucose intolerance, infections, peptic ulceration, eye problems (cataracts, glaucoma), and rarely muscle weakness.[135]

Children with the more serious organ manifestations of SLE are often treated with immunosuppressive medications. This is especially true for children with central nervous system and renal SLE. There is level I evidence supporting the efficacy of cyclophosphamide in reducing the eventual need for dialysis or renal transplantation in adults with lupus nephritis. Immunosuppressive medications are associated with significant side effects (for example, the serious side effects of cyclophosphamide include fatal infections, malignancy, sterility, and hemorrhagic cystitis) and should therefore be prescribed under the care of an experienced specialist.[136]

Localized Scleroderma

Although the lesions of LS can cause local deformity, the process is most often self-limited. A variety of treatments have been advocated (level III), including corticosteroids, methotrexate, vitamin D, and ultraviolet A (UVA) light. All should be considered experimental and used under the care of a dermatologist or pediatric rheumatologist (recommendation C) until definitive studies are done.

Kawasaki Disease

Most often, the acute signs and symptoms of KD will resolve within 10 to 14 days. Untreated, however, about 20 percent of children will develop coronary artery aneurysms and about 2 percent will have a myocardial infarction. Treatment is recommended to reduce these cardiac sequelae.

There is level I evidence that high doses of intravenous immunoglobulin can largely prevent the occurrence of coronary lesions, whether given over 4 days, or as a 2 g/kg single-day treatment.[137,138] Patients usually feel better by the next day with resolution of fever and a very low (about 2 or 3 percent) frequency of coronary lesions. A single-day infusion is more cost effective than a 4-day treatment as it is associated with a shorter hospital stay.[139] Therefore, treatment of KD in the acute phase (the first 10 days of illness) with 2 g/kg of intravenous immunoglobulin (IVIG) as a single infusion gets a grade A recommendation.

The traditional treatment of KD is to combine acetylsalicylic acid (ASA) in high doses (80 to 100 mg/kg/day divided into four doses) with IVIG. When the fever has resolved for 24 to 48 hours, the dose of ASA is reduced to 3 to 5 mg/kg/day to achieve an antiplatelet effect. Low-dose ASA is continued until the subacute phase resolves, usually by 6 weeks. (The subacute stage is marked by resolution of fever, elevated acute-phase reactants, high platelet count, and peeling of the skin of the digits.) However, in a meta-analysis reviewing studies of both high- and low-dose ASA there was no difference in coronary outcomes as long as high-dose IVIG was used.[140] Therefore, high-dose ASA initially and switching to low dose after 24 to 48 hours of being afebrile, as an adjunctive therapy gets a grade B recommendation.

Because of the potential morbidity of the coronary lesions, patients should be seen in the acute phase by a pediatric cardiologist or by a cardiologist experienced with children for an echocardiographic evaluation and for follow-up.

Henoch-Schönlein Purpura

Corticosteroids

Henoch-Schönlein purpura is a self-limited disease in the vast majority of cases. Supportive therapy is all that is usually required. Corticosteroids have traditionally been considered effective for reducing the symptoms of arthritis and gastrointestinal pain in HSP, but high level evidence is lacking. There is level II-3 evidence that prednisone, 1 to 2 mg/kg/day may shorten the duration of abdominal pain to a certain extent, but by 72 hours, there is no difference in pain between children treated or untreated with corticosteroids.[141]

More recently, investigators have examined the effects of corticosteroids in preventing the development of delayed nephropathy (which may account for more than half the cases of HSP nephritis). Two studies have reached opposite conclusions. One American study (level II-2) found that exactly the same number of children treated with prednisone developed nephritis as those who were not treated.[142] Conversely, an Italian study (level II-1), in which children who did not have nephritis at presentation were treated with 2 weeks of prednisone (1 mg/kg/day) or with nothing, found that the untreated group developed nephritis more often than those who were treated.[143] In fact, nobody in the treated group developed nephritis. The number needed to treat to prevent one case of nephritis in this second study was about 9. None of the nephritis cases had persistent disease, and none developed serious renal failure; the clinical significance of this reported treatment effect is questionable.

Until better evidence is available, the use of corticosteroids in HSP gets a grade C recommendation.

Other Treatments

Factor XIII replacement was investigated in one small Japanese study (level I) after the observation was made that (1) factor XIII is decreased in the plasma of patients with active HSP, and (2) that the level of factor XIII is inversely proportional to the severity of the disease.[144] The investigators found a more rapid resolution of joint, gastrointestinal, and renal findings in the factor XIII group. This study has not been replicated; therefore, at this point, factor XIII treatment must get a grade C recommendation.

Another small study (level II-1) was done recently, comparing ranitidine (5 mg/kg) with placebo in children with HSP and gastrointestinal bleeding.[145] Gastrointestinal bleeding was diagnosed by abdominal pain and occult blood in the stools. This study found that signs and

Table 19–1 Summary of Treatments for Musculoskeletal Disorders

Condition	Treatment	Level of Evidence	Recommendation
Growing pain	Conservative meaures	III	C
	Stretching	I	B
Hypermobility	Physiotherapy	III	C
Fibromyalgia	Neck Support Pillow	II-1	C
	Cognitive behavior therapy	II-3	C
	Antidepressants	I	B
	Aerobic exercise	I	B
	Bright light	I	D
	Biofeedback	I	B
	Hypnotherapy	I	B
	Super Malic	I	D
	Homeopathy	I	C
Backache	Rest	I	D
	Traction	I	D
	Back support	I	B
	Back school	I	C
	Supervised exercise	I	B
	TENS	I	D
	Manipulation	I	C
	Acupuncture	I	C
Juvenile arthritis	Education	III	B
	Hydrotherapy	I	B
	Comprehensive team	I	B
	Fitness exercise	II-3	B (see pg. 20)
	Wrist splints	I	B
	Steroid joint injections	II-3	B (see pg. 21)
	NSAIDs	I	A
	Methotrexate	I	A
	Etanercept	I	A
	Sulfasalazine	I	B
	Hydroxychloroquine	I	D
	Cyclosporine	III	C
	Uveitis screening	III	A
SLE and JDM	Sun avoidance	III	B
	Fat/salt reduced diet	III	B
Kawasaki disease	IVIG	I	A
Henoch-Schönlein purpura	Corticosteroids	II-1	C

SLE = systemic lupus erythematosus; JDM = juvenile dermatomyositis; TENS = transcutaneous electrical nerve stimulation; NSAIDs = nonsteroidal anti-inflammatory drugs; IVIG = intravenous immunoglobulin symptoms resolved about 2 days earlier in the treated group. Until this study is repeated in a proper RCT, ranitidine should get a grade C recommendation.

CONCLUSION

The pediatric rheumatic illnesses include a spectrum of illnesses ranging from the common and benign pain syndromes to the relatively rare but serious autoimmune diseases. Although much of our data came from adult studies, it is clear that we have many successful treatments to offer our patients. A summary of the therapies for various musculoskeletal disorders in children is provided in Table 19–1.

REFERENCES

1. Badley EM, Webster GK, Rasooly I. The impact of musculoskeletal disorders in the population: are they just aches and pains? Findings from the 1990 Ontario Health Survey. J Rheumatol 1995;22(4):733–9.

2. Bowyer S, Roettcher P. Pediatric rheumatology clinic populations in the United States: results of a 3 year survey. J Rheumatol 1996;23(11):1968–74.

3. Malleson PN, Fung MY, Rosenberg AM. The incidence of pediatric rheumatic diseases: results from the Canadian Pediatric Rheumatology Association Disease Registry. J Rheumatol 1996;23(11):1981–7.

4. Denardo BA, Tucker LB, Miller LC, et al. Demography of a regional pediatric rheumatology patient population. Affiliated Children's Arthritis Centers of New England. J Rheumatol 1994;21(8):1553–61.

5. Macarthur C, Wright JG, Srivastava R, et al. Variability in physicians' reported ordering and perceived reassurance value of diagnostic tests in children with 'growing pains'. Arch Pediatr Adolesc Med 1996;150:1072–6.

6. Oster J, Nielsen A. Growing pains. A clinical investigation of a school population. Acta Paediatr Scand 1972;61(3):329–34.

7. Abu-Arafeh I, Russell G. Recurrent limb pain in schoolchildren. Arch Dis Child 1996;74:336–9.

8. Mikkelsson M, Salminen JJ, Kautiainen H. Joint hypermobility is not a contributing factor to musculoskeletal pain in pre-adolescents. J Rheumatol 1996;23(11):1963–7.

9. Gedalia A, Press J. Articular symptoms in hypermobile schoolchildren: a prospective study. J Pediatr 1991;119(6):944–6.

10. Symmons DPH, Jones M, Osborne J, et al. Pediatric rheumatology in the United Kingdom: data from the British Pediatric Rheumatology Group National Diagnostic Register. J Rheumatol 1996;23(11):1975–80.

11. Wessely S, Hotopf M, Sharpe M. Chronic fatigue and its syndromes. Oxford: Oxford University Press; 1998.

12. Wolfe F, Smythe HA, Yunus MB, et al. The American College of Rheumatology 1990 Criteria for the Classification of Fibromyalgia. Report of the Multicenter Criteria Committee. Arthritis Rheum 1990;33(2):160–72.

13. Smythe H. Fibrositis syndrome: a historical perspective. J Rheumatol 1989;16(Suppl 19):2–6.

14. Moldofsky H. Sleep-wake mechanisms in fibrositis. J Rheumatol 1989;16(Suppl 19):47–8.

15. Roizenblatt S, Tufik S, Goldenberg J, et al. Juvenile fibromyalgia: clinical and polysomnographic aspects. J Rheumatol 1997;24:579–85.

16. Buskila D, Press J, Gedalia A, et al. Assessment of nonarticular tenderness and prevalence of fibromyalgia in children. J Rheumatol 1993;20(2):368–70.

17. Clark P, Burgos-Vargas R, Medina-Palma C, et al. Prevalence of fibromyalgia in children: a clinical study of Mexican children. J Rheumatol 1998;25(10):2009–14.

18. Feldman BM, Laxer RM. Back pain in children: When is it serious? Med N Am 1991;:3125–31.

19. Newcomer K, Sinaki M. Low back pain and its relationship to back strength and physical activity in children. Acta Paediatr 1996;85:1433–9.

20. Salminen JJ, Erkintalo Tertti M, Laine M, Pentti J. Low back pain in the young—a prospective three-year follow-up study of subjects with and without low back pain. Spine 1995;20(19):2101–8.

21. Balague F, Dutoit G, Waldburger M. Low back pain in schoolchildren—an epidemiological study. Scand J Rehab Med 1988;20:175–9.

22. Balague F, Skovron ML, Nordin M, et al. Low back pain in schoolchildren—a study of familial and psychological factors. Spine 1995;20(11):1265–70.

23. Kristjansdottir G. Prevalence of self-reported back pain in school children: a study of sociodemographic differences. Eur J Pediatr 1996;155:984–6.

24. Oen KG, Cheang M. Epidemiology of chronic arthritis in childhood. Semin Arthritis Rheum 1996;26(4):575–91.

25. Manners PJ, Diepeveen DA. Prevalence of juvenile chronic arthritis in a population of 12-year-old children in urban Australia. Pediatrics 1996;98(1):84–90.

26. Peterson LS, Mason T, Nelson AM, et al. Juvenile rheumatoid arthritis in Rochester, Minnesota 1960-1993—is the epidemiology changing? Arthritis Rheum 1996;39(8):1385–90.

27. Feldman BM, Birdi N, Boone JE, et al. Seasonal onset of systemic-onset juvenile rheumatoid arthritis. J Pediatr 1996;129:513–8.

28. Johnson AE, Gordon C, Hobbs FDR, Bacon PA. Undiagnosed systemic lupus erythematosus in the community. Lancet 1996;347:367–9.

29. Kaipiainen-Seppanen O, Savolainen A. Incidence of chronic juvenile rheumatic diseases in Finland during 1980-1990. Clin Exp Rheumatol 1996;14:441–4.

30. Walsh SJ, Algert C, Gregorio DI, et al. Divergent racial trends in mortality from systemic lupus erythematosus. J Rheumatol 1995;22(9):1663–8.

31. Lehman TJA, McCurdy DK, Bernstein BH, et al. Systemic lupus erythematosus in the first decade of life. Pediatrics 1989;83(2):235–9.

32. Wallace DJ, Quismorio FP Jr. The elusive search for geographic clusters of systemic lupus erythematosus. Arthritis Rheum 1995;38(11):1564–7.

33. Symmons DPM, Sills JA, Davis SM. The incidence of juvenile dermatomyositis: results from a nation-wide study. Br J Rheumatol 1995;34(8):732–6.

34. Pachman LM, Hayford JR, Hochberg MC, et al. New-onset juvenile dermatomyositis. Arthritis Rheum 1997;40(8):1526–33.

35. Peterson LS, Nelson AM, Su WPD, et al. The epidemiology of morphea (localized scleroderma) in Olmsted County 1960-1993. J Rheumatol 1997;24:73–80.

36. Nielsen HE. Epidemiology of Henoch-Schönlein purpura. Acta Paediatr Scand 1988;77:125–31.

37. Taubert KA, Rowley AH, Shulman ST. Nationwide survey of Kawasaki disease and acute rheumatic fever. J Pediatr 1991;119(2):279–82.

38. Yanagawa H, Yashiro M, Nakamura Y, et al. Epidemiologic pictures of Kawasaki disease in Japan: from the nationwide incidence survey in 1991 and 1992. Pediatrics 1995;95:475–9.

39. Laxer RM. What's in a name: the nomenclature of juvenile arthritis. J Rheumatol 1993;20(Suppl 40):2–3.

40. Petty RA, Southwood TR, Baum J, et al. Revision of the proposed classification criteria for juvenile idiopathic arthritis: Durban, 1997. J Rheumatol 1998;25(10):1991–4.

41. Hochberg MC. Updating the American College of Rheumatology revised criteria for the classification of systemic lupus erythematosus. Arthritis Rheum 1997;40(9):1725.

42. Tan EM, Cohen AS, Fries JF, et al. The 1982 revised criteria for the classification of systemic lupus erythematosus. Arthritis Rheum 1982;25:1271–7.

43. Ferraz MB, Goldenberg J, Hilario MO, et al. Evaluation of 1982 ARA lupus criteria data set in a pediatric population. J Rheumatol 1992;19(Suppl 33):120.

44. Bohan A, Peter JB. Polymyositis and dermatomyositis (first of two parts). N Engl J Med 1975;292(2):344–7.

45. Dajani AS, Taubert KA, Gerber MA, et al. Diagnosis and therapy of Kawasaki disease in children. Circulation 1993;87(5):1776–80.

46. Burns JC, Mason WH, Glode MP, et al. Clinical and epidemiologic characteristics of patients referred for evaluation of possible Kawasaki disease. J Pediatr 1991;118:680–6.

47. Shmerling RH, Delbanco TL. The rheumatoid factor: an analysis of clinical utility. Am J Med 1991;91:528–34.

48. Cabral DA, Petty RA, Fung M, Malleson PN. Persistent antinuclear antibodies in children without identifiable inflammatory rheumatic of autoimmune disease. Pediatrics 1992;89(3):441–4.

49. Griner PF. Systemic lupus erythematosus. In: Griner PF, Panzer RJ, Greenland P, editors. Clinical diagnosis and the laboratory: logical strategies for common medical problems. Chicago: Year Book Medical Publishers; 1986; p. 504–17.

50. Rider LG, Miller FW, Targoff IN, et al. A broadened spectrum of juvenile myositis. Myositis-specific autoantibodies in children. Arthritis Rheum 1994;37(10):1534–8.

51. Feldman BM, Reichlin M, Laxer RM, et al. Clinical significance of specific autoantibodies in juvenile dermatomyositis. J Rheumatol 1996;23(10):1794–7.

52. Baxter MP, Dulberg C. "Growing pains" in childhood—a proposal for treatment. J Pediatr Orthoped 1988;8(4):402–6.

53. Gedalia A, Brewer EJJ. Joint hypermobility in pediatric practice—a review. J Rheumatol 1993;20(2):371–4.

54. Buskila D, Neumann L, Hershman E, et al. Fibromyalgia syndrome in children—an outcome study. J Rheumatol 1995;22(3):525–8.

55. Ambrogio N, Cuttiford J, Lineker S, Li L. A comparison of three types of neck support in fibromyalgia patients. Arthritis Care Res 1998;11(5):405–10.

56. White KP, Nielson WR. Cognitive behavioural treatment of fibromyalgia syndrome: a followup assessment. J Rheumatol 1995;22:717–21.

57. Vlaeyen JW, Teeken-Gruben NJ, Goossens ME, et al. Cognitive-educational treatment of fibromyalgia: a randomized clinical trial. I. Clinical effects. J Rheumatol 1996;23(7):1237–45.

58. Carette S, Bell MJ, Reynolds WJ, et al. Comparison of amitriptyline, cyclobenzaprine, and placebo in the treatment of fibromyalgia. Arthritis Rheum 1994;37(1):32–40.

59. Carette S, Oakson G, Guimont C, Steriade M. Sleep electroencephalography and the clinical response to amitriptyline in patients with fibromyalgia. Arthritis Rheum 1995;38(9):1211–7.

60. Goldenberg D, Mayskiy M, Mossey C, et al. A randomized, double-blind crossover trial of fluoxetine and amitriptyline in the treatment of fibromyalgia. Arthritis Rheum 1996;39(11):1852–9.

61. Martin L, Nutting A, MacIntosh BR, et al. An exercise program in the treatment of fibromyalgia. J Rheumatol 1996;23(6):1050–3.

62. McCain GA. Role of physical fitness training in the fibrositis/fibromyalgia syndrome. Am J Med 1986;81(3A):73–7.

63. Pioro-Boisset M, Esdaile JM, Fitzcharles M. Alternative medicine use in fibromyalgia syndrome. Arthr Care Res 1996;9(1):13–7.

64. Pearl SJ, Lue F, MacLean AW, et al. The effects of bright light treatment on the symptoms of fibromyalgia. J Rheumatol 1996;23(5):896–902.

65. Buckelew SP, Conway R, Parker J, et al. Biofeedback/relaxation training and exercise interventions for fibromyalgia: a prospective trial. Arthritis Care Res 1998;11(3):196–209.

66. Haanen HC, Hoenderdos HT, van Romunde LK, et al. Controlled trial of hypnotherapy in the treatment of refractory fibromyalgia. J Rheumatol 1991;18(1):72–5.

67. Russell IJ, Michalek JE, Flechas JD, Abraham GE. Treatment of fibromyalgia syndrome with Super Malic: a randomized, double-blind, placebo-controlled, crossover pilot study. J Rheumatol 1995;22(5):953–8.

68. Fisher P, Greenwood A, Huskisson EC, et al. Effect of homeopathic treatment on fibrositis (primary fibromyalgia). Br Med J 1989;299(6695):365–6.

69. Colquhoun D. Re-analysis of clinical trial of homeopathic treatment in fibrositis. Lancet 1990;336:441–2.

70. Atlas SJ, Volinn E. Classics from the spine literature revisited: a randomized trial of 2 versus 7 days of recommended bed rest for acute low back pain. Spine 1997;22(20):2331–7.

71. Wilkinson MJ. Does 48 hours' bed rest influence the outcome of acute low back pain? Br J Gen Practice 1995;45(398):481–4.

72. van der Heijden GJ, Beurskens AJ, Koes BW, et al. The efficacy of traction for back and neck pain: a systematic, blinded review of randomized clinical trial methods. Physical Therapy 1995;75(2):93–104.

73. Beurskens AJ, de Vet HC, Koke AJ, et al. Efficacy of traction for non-specific low back pain: A randomised clinical trial. Lancet 1995;346:1596–1600.

74. Valle-Jones JC, Walsh H, O'Hara J, et al. Controlled trial of a back support ('Lumbotrain') in patients with non-specific low back pain. Curr Med Res Opin 1992;12(9):604–13.

75. Koes BW, van Tulder MW, van der Windt WM, Bouter LM. The efficacy of back schools: a review of randomized clinical trials. J Clin Epidemiol 1994;47(8):851–62.

76. Di Fabio RP. Efficacy of comprehensive rehabilitation programs and back school for patients with low back pain: a meta-analysis. Physical Therapy 1995;75(10):865–78.

77. Faas A, Chavannes AW, van Eijk JT, Gubbels JW. A randomized, placebo-controlled trial of exercise therapy in patients with acute low back pain. Spine 1993;18(11):1388–95.

78. Frost H, Klaber Moffett JA, Moser JS, Fairbank JCT. Randomised controlled trial for evaluation of fitness programme for patients with chronic low back pain. Br Med J 1995;310:151–4.

79. Frost H, Lamb SE, Klaber Moffett JA, et al. A fitness programme for patients with chronic low back pain: 2-year follow-up of a randomised controlled trial. Pain 1998;75(2-3):273–9.

80. Deyo RA, Walsh NE, Martin DC, et al. A controlled trial of transcutaneous electrical nerve stimulation (TENS) and exercise for chronic low back pain. N Engl J Med 1990;322(23):1627–34.

81. Carette S, Marcoux S, Truchon R, et al. A controlled trial of corticosteroid injections into facet joints for chronic low back pain. N Engl J Med 1991;325(14):1002–7.

82. Cherkin DC, MacCornack FA. Patient evaluations of low back pain care from family physicians and chiropractors. West J Med 1989;150:351–5.

83. Meade TW, Dyer S, Browne W, et al. Low back pain of mechanical origin: randomised comparison of chiropractic and hospital outpatient treatment. Br Med J 1990;300:1431–7.

84. Assendelft WJ, Koes BW, Knipschild PG, Bouter LM. The relationship between methodological quality and conclusions in reviews of spinal manipulation. JAMA 1995;274(24):1942–8.

85. Skargren EI, Oberg BE, Carlsson PG, Gade M. Cost and effectiveness analysis of chiropractic and physiotherapy treatment for low back and neck pain. Six-month follow-up. Spine 1997;22(18):2167–77.

86. Hackett GI, Seddon D, Kaminski D. Electroacupuncture compared with paracetamol for acute low back pain. Practitioner 1988;232:163–4.

87. Constant F, Collin JF, Guillemin F, Boulange M. Effectiveness of spa therapy in chronic low back pain: a randomized clinical trial. J Rheumatol 1995;22(7):1315–20.

88. Reisine ST. Arthritis and the family. Arthritis Care Res 1995;8(4):265–71.

89. Konkol L, Lineberry J, Gottlieb J, et al. Impact of juvenile arthritis on families—an educational assessment. Arthritis Care Res 1989;2(2):40–8.

90. Bartholomew LK, Koenning G, Dahlquist L, Barron K. An educational needs assessment of children with juvenile rheumatoid arthritis. Arthritis Care Res 1994;7(3):136–43.

91. Hall J, Skevington SM, Maddison PJ, Chapman K. A randomized and controlled trial of hydrotherapy in rheumatoid arthritis. Arthritis Care Res 1996;9(3):206–15.

92. Spiegel JS, Spiegel TM, Ward NB, et al. Rehabilitation for rheumatoid arthritis patients. Arthritis Rheum 1986;29(5):628–37.

93. Nordstrom DCE, Konttinen YT, Solovieva S, et al. In- and out-patient rehabilitation in rheumatoid arthritis. Scand J Rheumatol 1996;25:200–6.

94. Bakker C, Hidding A, van der Linden S, van Doorslaer E. Cost effectiveness of group physical therapy compared to individualized therapy for ankylosing spondylitis. A randomized controlled trial. J Rheumatol 1994;21(2):264–8.

95. Bell MJ, Lineker SC, Wilkins AL, et al. A randomized controlled trial to evaluate the efficacy of community based physical therapy in the treatment of people with rheumatoid arthritis. J Rheumatol 1998;25(2):231–7.

96. Klepper SE. Effects of an eight-week physical conditioning program on disease signs and symptoms in children with chronic arthritis. Arthritis Care Res 1999;12(1):52–60.

97. Kjeken I, Moller G, Kvien TK. Use of commercially produced elastic wrist orthoses in chronic arthritis: a controlled study. Arthritis Care Res 1995;8(2):108–13.

98. Conrad KJ, Budiman-Mak E, Roach KE, Hedeker D. Impacts of foot orthoses on pain and disability in rheumatoid arthritics. J Clin Epidemiol 1996;49(1):1–7.

99. Padeh S, Passwell JH. Intraarticular corticosteroid injection in the management of children with chronic arthritis. Arthritis Rheum 1998;41(7):1210–4.

100. Hertzberger-ten Cate R, de Vries-van der Vlugt BCM, van Suijlekom-Smit LWA, Cats A. Intra-articular steroids in pauciarticular juvenile chronic arthritis, type 1. Eur J Pediatr 1991;150:170–2.

101. Job-Deslandre C, Menkes CJ. Complications of intra-articular injections of triamcinolone hexacetonide in chronic arthritis in children. Clin Exp Rheumatol 1990;8:413–6.

102. McCarty DJ, McCarthy G, Carrera G. Intraarticular corticosteroids possibly leading to local osteonecrosis and marrow fat induced synovitis. J Rheumatol 1991;18:1091–4.

103. Chakravarty K, Pharoah PDP, Scott DGI. A randomized controlled study of post-injection rest following intra-articular steroid therapy for knee synovitis. Br J Rheumatol 1994;33:464–8.

104. Giannini EH, Brewer EJ, Miller ML, et al. Ibuprofen suspension in the treatment of juvenile rheumatoid arthritis. Pediatric Rheumatology Collaborative Study Group. J Pediatr 1990;117(4):645–52.

105. Haapasaari J, Wuolijoki E, Ylijoki H. Treatment of juvenile rheumatoid arthritis with diclofenac sodium. Scand J Rheumatol 1983;12(4):325–30.

106. Dowd JE, Cimaz R, Fink CW. Nonsteroidal antiinflammatory drug-induced gastroduodenal injury in children. Arthritis Rheum 1995;38(9):1225–31.

107. Keenan GF, Giannini EH, Athreya BH. Clinically significant gastropathy associated with non-steroidal anti-inflammatory drug use in children with juvenile rheumatoid arthritis. J Rheumatol 1995;22:1149–51.

108. Gazarian M, Berkovitch M, Koren G, et al. Experience with misorprostol therapy for NSAID gastropathy in children. Ann Rheum Dis 1995;54:277–80.

109. Allen R, Rogers M, Humphrey I. Naproxen induced pseudoporphyria in juvenile chronic arthritis. J Rheumatol 1991;18:893–6.

110. Giannini EH, Brewer EJ, Kuzmina N, et al. Methotrexate in resistant juvenile rheumatoid arthritis. Results of the U.S.A.-U.S.S.R. double-blind, placebo-controlled trial. The Pediatric Rheumatology Collaborative Study Group and The Cooperative Children's Study Group. N Engl J Med 1992;326(16):1043–9.

111. Halle F, Prieur AM. Evaluation of methotrexate in the treatment of juvenile chronic arthritis according to the subtype. Clin Exp Rheumatol 1991;9:287–302.

112. Erickson AR, Reddy V, Vogelgesang SA, West SG. Usefulness of the American College of Rheumatology recommendations for liver biopsy in methotrexate-treated rheumatoid arthritis patients. Arthritis Rheum 1995;38(8):1115–9.

113. Ortiz Z, Shea B, Suarez-Almazor ME, et al. The efficacy of folic acid and folinic acid in reducing methotrexate gastrointestinal toxicity in rheumatoid arthritis. A meta-analysis of randomized controlled trials. J Rheumatol 1998;25:36–43.

114. Hunt PG, Rose CD, McIlvain-Simpson G, Tejani S. The effects of daily intake of folic acid on the efficacy of methotrexate therapy in children with juvenile rheumatoid arthritis. A controlled study. J Rheumatol 1997;24:2230–2.

115. Elliott MJ, Maini RN, Feldmann M, et al. Randomised double blind comparison of a chimaeric monoclonal antibody to tumour necrosis factor alpha (cA2) versus placebo in rheumatoid arthritis. Lancet 1994;344:1105–10.

116. Moreland LW, Baumgartner SW, Schiff MH, et al. Treatment of rheumatoid arthritis with a recombinant human tumor necrosis factor receptor (p75)-Fc fusion protein. N Engl J Med 1997;337:141–7.

117. Weinblatt ME, Kremer JM, Bankhurst AD, et al. A trial of etanercept, a recombinant tumor necrosis factor receptor:Fc fusion protein, in patients with rheumatoid arthritis receiving methotrexate. N Engl J Med 1999;340(4):253–9.

118. Lovell DJ, Giannini EH, Whitmore JB, et al. Safety and efficacy of tumor necrosis factor receptor p75 FC fusion protein (TNFR:FC; Enbrel) in polyarticular course juvenile arthritis. Arthritis Rheum 1998;41(Suppl 9):S130.

119. van Rossum MAJ, Fiselier TJW, Rranssen MJAM, et al. Sulfasalazine in the treatment of juvenile chronic arthritis—a randomized, double-blind, placebo-controlled, multicenter study. Arthritis Rheum 1998;41(5):808–16.

120. Giannini EH, Barron KS, Spencer CH, et al. Auranofin therapy for juvenile rheumatoid arthritis: results of the five-year open label extension trial. J Rheumatol 1991;18:1240–2.

121. Brewer EJ, Giannini EH, Kuzmina N, Alekseev L. Penicillamine and hydroxychloroquine in the treatment of severe juvenile rheumatoid arthritis. Results of the U.S.A.-U.S.S.R. double-blind placebo-controlled trial. N Engl J Med 1986;314(20):1269–76.

122. Kvien TK, Hoyerall HM, Sandstad B. Azathioprine versus placebo in patients with juvenile rheumatoid arthritis: a single center double-blind comparative study. J Rheumatol 1986;13:118–23.

123. Pistoia V, Buoncompagni A, Scribanis R, et al. Cyclosporin A in the treatment of juvenile chronic arthritis and childhood polymyositis-dermatomyositis. Results of a preliminary study. Clin Exp Rheumatol 1993;11:203–8.

124. Ostensen M, Hoyaeraal HM, Kass E. Tolerance of cyclosporine A in children with refractory juvenile rheumatoid arthritis. J Rheumatol 1988;15:1536–8.

125. Reiff A, Rawlings DJ, Shaham B, et al. Preliminary evidence for cyclosporin A as an alternative in the treatment of recalcitrant juvenile rheumatoid arthritis and juvenile dermatomyositis. J Rheumatol 1997;24:2436–43.

126. Kirwan JR. The effect of glucocorticoids on joint destruction in rheumatoid arthritis. N Engl J Med 1995;333:142–6.

127. Saag KG, Criswell LA, Sems KM, et al. Low-dose corticosteroids in rheumatoid arthritis. Arthritis Rheum 1996;39(11):1818–25.

128. Trentham DE, Dynesius-Trentham RA, Orav EJ, et al. Effects of oral administration of type II collagen on rheumatoid arthritis. Science 1993;261:1727–30.

129. Sieper J, Kary S, Sorensen H, et al. Oral type II collagen treatment in early rheumatoid arthritis. Arthritis Rheum 1996;39(1):41–51.

130. Barnett ML, Combitchi D, Trentham DE. A pilot trial of oral type II collagen in the treatment of juvenile rheumatoid arthritis. Arthritis Rheum 1996;39(4):623–8.

131. Akduman L, Kaplan HJ, Tychsen L. Prevalence of uveitis in an outpatient juvenile arthritis clinic: onset of uveitis more than a decade after onset of arthritis. J Pediatr Ophthalmol Strabismus 1997;34:101–6.

132. Anonymous. Guidelines for ophthalmologic examinations in children with juvenile rheumatoid arthritis. Pediatrics 1993;92(2):295–6.

133. White PH, Shear ES. Transition/job readiness for adolescents with juvenile arthritis and other chronic illness. J Rheumatol 1992;19(Suppl 33):23–7.

134. Chamberlain MA, Rooney CM. Young adults with arthritis: meeting their transitional needs. Br J Rheumatol 1996;35:84–90.

135. Melo-Gomes JA. Problems related to systemic glucocorticoid therapy in children. J Rheumatol 1993;20(Suppl 37):35–9.

136. Bansal VK, Beto JA. Treatment of lupus nephritis: a meta-analysis of clinical trials. Am J Kidney Dis 1997;29(2):193–9.

137. Newburger JW, Takahashi M, Beiser AS, et al. A single intravenous infusion of gamma globulin as compared with four infusions in the treatment of acute Kawasaki syndrome. N Engl J Med 1991;324:1633–9.

138. Newburger JW, Takahashi M, Burns JC, et al. The treatment of Kawasaki syndrome with intravenous gamma globulin. N Engl J Med 1986;315:341–7.

139. Klassen TP, Rowe PC, Gafni A. Economic evaluation of intravenous immune globulin therapy for Kawasaki syndrome. J Pediatr 1993;122:538–42.

140. Durongpisitkul K, Gururaj VJ, Park JM, Martin CF. The prevention of coronary artery aneurysm in Kawasaki disease: a meta-analysis of the efficacy of aspirin and immunoglobulin treatment. Pediatrics 1995;96(6):1057–61.

141. Rosenblum ND, Winter HS. Steroid effects on the course of abdominal pain in children with Henoch-Schonlein purpura. Pediatrics 1987;79(6):1018–21.

142. Saulsbury FT. Corticosteroid therapy does not prevent nephritis in Henoch-Schonlein purpura. Pediatr Nephrol 1993;7(1):69–71.

143. Mollica F, Li Volti S, Garozzo R, Russo G. Effectiveness of early prednisone treatment in preventing the development of nephropathy in anaphylactoid purpura. Eur J Pediatr 1992;151(2):140–4.

144. Fukui H, Kamitsuji H, Nagao T, et al. Clinical evaluation of a pasteurized factor XIII concentrate administration in Henoch-Schonlein purpura. Japanese Pediatric Group. Thrombosis Res 1989;56(6):667–75.

145. Narin N, Akcoral A, Aslin MI, Elmastas H. Ranitidine administration in Henoch-Schonlein vasculitis. Acta Paediatr Jap 1995;37(1):37–9.

CHAPTER 20

Common Sleep Problems in Children

Darcy L. Fehlings, MD, MSc, FRCPC
Golda Milo-Manson, MD, MHSc, FRCPC

Sleep problems in children and adolescents are common and are frequently brought to the attention of the primary care physician. Sleep problems can be divided into two general categories: insomnias (defined in this chapter to mean difficulty falling or staying asleep) and parasomnias (disorders of sleep arousal associated with behaviors that intrude on sleep). This chapter discusses the clinical features and management of common pediatric sleep problems. A critical review of the evidence supporting the management techniques is presented and the quality of this evidence discussed.

INSOMNIAS

Frequent Night Awakenings

Frequent night awakenings (NA) is one of the most common sleep problems, particularly in young children aged 6 months to 4 years. The reported prevalence rates vary according to the definition of NA from 10 percent (defined as a child who wakes up at least two times per night) to 30 percent (defined as a child who wakes up at least three times per week).[1-7] There is evidence that sleep problems persist over time. Zuckerman and colleagues[8] found in a longitudinal study that 41 percent of children who had a night awakening problem at 8 months still had a sleep problem at 3 years of age. These children were also more likely to have behavioral problems during the day, particularly tantrums. An NA pattern also affects parents whose own sleep becomes disrupted.

Several factors have been associated with frequent night awakenings. These have included a difficult temperament,[5] perinatal difficulties,[1,5] neurodevelopmental problems,[9] maternal depression, and family stress.[7,8,5] Parental responses, such as night-time feeding and cosleeping, have been considered potential risk factors.[7,10] From the child's perspective, these responses can be very soothing and can reinforce and maintain the NA.

Another variable that is widely accepted as a potential risk factor for an NA problem is the presence of nonadaptive sleep associations. Sleep associations have been well described by Ferber and represent the regular bedtime environment or conditions that are present as the child falls asleep.[11] Nonadaptive sleep associations are defined as bedtime conditions that the child cannot recreate by himself, for example, falling asleep while feeding (Table 20–1). Ferber theorized that children with nonadaptive sleep associations would have difficulty falling asleep alone after an NA. They would not settle to bed until the sleep associations were recreated by the caregiver. Research supports nonadaptive sleep associations as a risk factor for NA. Keener[12] found that children who were put to bed asleep and therefore, by definition, had nonadaptive sleep associations had more night awakenings than children put to bed awake. Adair and colleagues[13] reported that 9-month-old infants whose parents were present when the child fell asleep were significantly more likely to wake at night than infants whose parents were not present. A study evaluating the risk of sleep problems in infants discharged from neonatal intensive care units did not identify perinatal difficulties as a risk factor. Instead, they found that children whose parents stayed with them until they were asleep were more likely to wake at night.

Table 20–1 Examples of Nonadaptive Sleep Associations

Falling asleep while feeding (breastfeeding or bottle feeding)
Falling asleep while being held by a parent
Falling asleep outside the bedroom and being brought into the bedroom asleep
Falling asleep with a pacifier that the child cannot put back in his/her mouth

Difficulty Settling to Bed

Difficulty settling to bed is also a very common sleep problem. It often starts in the preschool-age child and by elementary school age (5 to 12 years) becomes the most frequently reported sleep problem with a prevalence rate of 27 percent.[14] It often correlates with the time that the child moves from a crib to a bed and therefore is not as easily contained. Developmentally, it corresponds to the time that the child is exerting his/her independence from the primary caregiver.

Delayed Sleep Phase Syndrome

Delayed sleep phase syndrome (DSPS) refers to a shifting of the biologic sleep clock forward. The child/adolescent falls asleep late and wakes up late in the morning. The human sleep clock, without external cueing, runs on an average 25-hour cycle. Therefore, it is easy to shift the bedtime later each night and then sleep in during the morning. The syndrome can often be associated with difficulty settling to bed in the preschooler but becomes even more prevalent in the adolescent. This occurs for a combination of reasons: increased autonomy of the adolescent over bedtime routines, social and school demands in the evening, and an increased sleep requirement once the youth has entered puberty. Factors such as excessive caffeine, alcohol, or drug intake also need to be considered. In the adolescent, DSPS can be associated with daytime sleepiness and poor school performance.

EVIDENCED-BASED MANAGEMENT FOR PEDIATRIC INSOMNIAS

There are two basic modalities for the management of NA, difficulty settling, and delayed sleep phase syndrome. These include behavioral management and the use of medications.

Description of Behavioral Management Techniques

Techniques for Night Awakenings

The four basic principles for treating night awakenings are:

1. Identifying nonadaptive sleep associations and guiding the parents in training the child to fall asleep alone under conditions that the child can recreate himself or herself,
2. Identifying and removing any night-time positive reinforcers (enjoyable things happening to the child during the NA),
3. Keeping morning awakening time consistent, and
4. Rewarding good sleep behavior.

At the beginning of treatment, the parents should be encouraged to list the nonadaptive sleep associations that are present and the positive reinforcers of the NA. This list can then be addressed gradually over 2 to 3 weeks. The parents should be encouraged to keep a sleep diary to monitor the child's sleep progress. There are many different approaches and variations of techniques. Practical examples of techniques that the authors have used over many years in a pediatric sleep disorders clinic are outlined below.

Structured Bedtime Routine.   Parents should be encouraged to structure a bedtime routine and keep it the same each night. Four to seven activities should be chosen and done with the child in the same order each night. The bedtime routine ideally should last approximately 20 minutes. The structure and familiarity of the routine will help to make the child feel more secure about going to bed. It also sets limits about what is allowed at bedtime.

Teaching a child in a crib to fall asleep alone.   This technique is well described in Ferber's book "Solve Your Child's Sleep Problems" and is an excellent reference book for parents.[11] After the structured bedtime routine is completed, the child should be put into the crib awake. The parent then leaves the room but is allowed to intermittently come back and reassure the "crying" child. The parent is instructed to stay in the room for 1 minute and to wait longer between checks. The parent should also increase the time between checks each subsequent night. The parent can use this routine to respond to the child during the NA to decrease the amount of parental presence, which can act as a positive reinforcer for the NA.

Teaching a child in a bed how to fall asleep alone.   The above method does not work as well for a child who is in a bed as the child often will follow the parent out of the room. A routine that works well for this age is the "chair-sitting" routine. It was first described by Richman.[15] The parent starts by sitting in a chair close to the child. The chair is moved farther away each night until it is out of the room and down the hall. The parent is instructed not to talk or interact with the child during this time. Children usually tolerate this routine well without crying; however, an occasional child will not stay in bed. The parent should be instructed to warn the child once, to leave the room and hold the door shut for 1 minute, and then return to the chair. This can be repeated, with a gradual increase in the time the door is held closed until the child stays in bed quietly. Before starting this routine, the plan should be explained to the child. For the child over 3 years of age, a sticker and praise can be given in the morning if they are cooperative. Besides teaching the child how to fall asleep alone and creating adaptive sleep associations, the chair-sitting routine can be used to gradually decrease parental contact during the NA.

Decreasing night-time feeding.   Night-time feeding is a common positive reinforcer for NA and is not required for nutrition in healthy children past the age of 4 months. If night-time feeding is present, it should be eliminated first before other issues are addressed. Changes in feeding should be made gradually over 1 to 2 weeks. For the child who is bottle fed, the parents should be instructed to put one ounce less in the bottle each night. The amount in the bottle (or bottles) should be decreased by one ounce each night until the parent reaches zero. This method works better than watering down the feed, as the parent is not left trying to eliminate a bottle of water at the end of the routine.

For breast-fed children the same principle is applied, but in this case, the feeding time is decreased by 1 to 2 minutes each night. The length of time between feeds can also be lengthened by half an hour each night.

Praising "good" night-time behavior.   Parents should be encouraged to praise the child in the morning for "good" night-time behavior. For children in the preschool and early elementary grades, the use of stickers is recommended.

Prevention of night awakenings.   Parents should be encouraged at the four month "well-baby visit" to put their baby in the crib awake and to establish a structured bedtime routine. Night-time positive reinforcers can be reduced by keeping night-time encounters with the child boring and brief, eliminating night-time feeding by 6 months of age and changing diapers at night-time only if necessary.

Techniques for Difficulty Settling

The same techniques described above for night awakenings under structured bedtime routines, teaching the child how to fall asleep alone (chair-sitting routine), and positive reinforcement of "good" sleep behavior are also used for difficulty settling. Parents should be encouraged to help their child to shift to quiet activities an hour before bedtime.

Techniques for Delayed Sleep Phase Syndrome

Intervention techniques for DSPS involve resetting the circadian clock (chronotherapy) of the child/adolescent. For children who have moved the bedtime and awakening time forward 2 to 4 hours, the parent should be counseled to move the awakening time in the morning earlier by 15 minutes to half an hour each day until the desired rising time is reached. This can be followed in a few days' time by moving the bedtime earlier. Parents should be counseled that bedtime and morning rising time need to be consistently reinforced 7 days a week. For the adolescent, often the shift is much greater than 4 hours. Bedtime can occur at 4 or 5 o'clock in the morning and rising time in the early afternoon. For individuals with this much shift, it is recommended that the time clock be moved forward (usually by 3 hours each night) until the desired bedtime is reached. For example, if an adolescent falls asleep at 4 am, in the next 24-hour period, he should stay up until 7 am and continue to shift the bedtime forward by 3 hours until the desired bedtime (for example, 11 pm) is reached. This resetting needs to be rigidly maintained 7 days a week, or it becomes easy to slip back into delaying the bedtime. Prior to starting these behavioral interventions, the child/adolescent and family require education about DSPS and need to be in agreement about the management suggestions. The clinical features of DSPS and the use of chronotherapy are well outlined by Czeisler[16] and Thorpy.[17]

Review of the Evidence Evaluating Behavioral Management

Over the past 10 to 15 years, there have been numerous research studies, many of them randomized controlled trials, evaluating the use of behavioral management in the treatment of the common pediatric sleep disorders such as night awakenings, difficulty settling, and delayed sleep phase syndrome. Table 20–2 summarizes research involving children who are developing normally, and Table 20–3 reviews research in children with neurodevelopmental disorders. Where two or more articles are identified evaluating the same behavioral technique, the article with the strongest study design (usually a randomized trial) is summarized.

As outlined in Table 20–2, the quality of the evidence is strong with multiple randomized controlled trials supporting the use of behavioral management for night awakenings and difficulty settling, and behavioral management receives an "A" recommendation. The use of chronotherapy for DSPS has not been specifically researched in children/adolescents and receives a "C" recommendation.

Although there are not as many randomized controlled trials, there is still good evidence ("A" recommendation) to support behavioral management in the treatment of night awakenings and difficulty settling in children with mental retardation. The treatment of DSPS with chronotherapy has not been extensively evaluated and receives a "C" recommendation. Behavioral management for other diagnostic conditions (for example, autism, visual impairment, cerebral palsy, acquired brain injury, and attention deficit hyperactivity disorder) have not been well evaluated. Further research evidence in these areas is required.

USE OF MEDICATION

Medication is rarely used in children who are developing normally. It can be considered in children with neurodevelopmental disorders resistant to behavioral intervention. Medication is considered a second-line approach and should be used in conjunction with a behavioral intervention program. The use of barbiturates, benzodiazepines, and antihistamines have been documented for sedation purposes. There are concerns about side effects, including complications from the interaction of barbiturates and other medications, the development

Table 20-2 Summary of Research Evaluating Behavioral Management in Children/Adolescents Developing Normally

Research Study	Objective/Study Design/Subjects	Behavioral Intervention	Results/Quality of Evidence	Recommendation
Rickert VI, Johnson CM[18] Reducing nocturnal awakening and crying episodes in infants and young children: a comparison between scheduled awakenings and systematic ignoring	• Objective: to evaluate systematic ignoring vs. scheduled awakenings vs. no tx in NA • Study design: RCT: three groups • Subjects: 33 children ages 6 to 54 months waking at least once per night	• Systematic ignoring: parents instructed to check on child and then leave the room • Scheduled awakenings: parents to wake and soothe child 15 to 60 minutes prior to expected NA	Results: • Both tx groups improved compared with the third group of no tx • High drop-out rate of parents randomized to the systematic ignoring group Quality of evidence: I	A
Adams LA, Rickert VI[19] Reducing bedtime tantrums: comparison between positive routines and graduated extinction	• Objectives: to evaluate positive bedtime routines vs. graduated extinction vs. no tx in children with difficulty settling • Study design: RCT: three groups • Subjects: 36 children ages 18 to 48 months with difficulty settling	• Positive routine: structured bedtime routine with 4 to 7 activities, with praise after each activity • Graduated extinction: ignoring tantrum for progressively longer, parents allowed to intermittently comfort child for 15 seconds or less	Results: • Children in both tx groups significantly improved compared with minimal change in the no tx group Quality of evidence: I	A
Seymour FW, Brock P, During M, Poole G.[20] Reducing sleep disruptions in young children: evaluation of therapist-guided and written information approaches: a brief report	• Objective: to evaluate a behavior intervention program vs written information alone vs no tx in children with NA • Study design: RCT: three groups • Subjects: 45 children ages 9 months to 5 years with NA	• Structured bedtime routine • Graduated removal of parents during the NA • Positive reinforcement of good sleep behavior	Results: • NA significantly improved in both tx groups and remained the same in the no tx group Quality of evidence: I	A

(continued)

Table 20–2 Summary of Research Evaluating Behavioral Management in Children/Adolescents Developing Normally *(continued)*

Research Study	Objective/Study Design/Subjects	Behavioral Intervention	Results/Quality of Evidence	Recommendation
Adair R, Zuckerman B, Bauchner H, et al.[21] Reducing night waking in infancy: a primary-care intervention	• Objective: to evaluate a written handout on sleep associations, and decreasing night feeding to prevent NA • Study design: prospective cohort with a historical control • Subjects: parents of four-month-old infants attending a pediatric office for a well-child visit (164/222 in tx group, 128/172 in control group)	• Parents given a handout at the 4th-month visit outlining the importance of putting the child to bed awake, and the safety of decreasing night feeding	Results: • At the 9th-month visit, the parents reported 36 percent less NA in the tx group compared with the control group Quality of evidence: II-1	A-B
Billiard M, Verge M, Toucon J, et al.[22] Delayed sleep phase syndrome: subjective and objective data chronotherapy and follow-up	• Objective: to evaluate the use of chronotherapy to tx DSPS • Study design: prospective case series • Subjects: 25 adolescents/adults (age range 17 to 76 yrs) with DSPS	• Ten subjects received chronotherapy moving the clock forward 3 hours each day	Results: • Five subjects demonstrated response (it is noted by the authors that there was a higher success rate in psychologically normal individuals Quality of evidence: III	C

(continued)

Table 20-2 Summary of Research Evaluating Behavioral Management in Children/Adolescents Developing Normally *(continued)*

Research Study	Objective/Study Design/Subjects	Behavioral Intervention	Results/Quality of Evidence	Recommendation
Pinella T, Birch LL[23] Help me make it through the night: behavioral entrainment of breast-fed infants' sleep patterns	• Objective: to evaluate if breast-fed infants could be taught to sleep throughout the night by 8 weeks of age • Study design: RCT • Subjects: 13 well term infants in each group	• Mother instructed to feed infant between 10 pm and 12 am • Parents asked to gradually lengthen the interval between feeds during the night • Parents instructed to make day and night activities different	Results: • 100 percent of tx group sleeping through the night compared with 23 percent of controls with no impact on weight gain Quality of evidence: I	A
Kerr SM, Jowett SA, Smith LN[24] Preventing sleep problems in infants: a randomized controlled trial	• Objective: to evaluate a health education prevention program for pediatric sleep problems • Study design: RCT • Subjects: parents of 3-month-old infants (86 in tx group, 83 in control)	• Structured bedtime routine • "Settling methods," not described in further detail	Results: • Decreased prevalence of difficulty settling and night awakenings in the tx group compared with the control Quality of evidence: I	A

tx = therapy; NA = night awakenings; RCT = randomized controlled trials; DSPS = delayed sleep phase syndrome

Table 20–3 Summary of Research Evaluating Behavioral Management in Children with Neurodevelopmental Disorders

Research Study	Objectives/Study Design/Subjects	Behavioral Intervention	Results/Quality of Evidence	Recommendations
Milan MA, Mitchell ZP, Berger MI, Pierson DF[25] Positive Routines: a rapid alternative to extinction for elimination of bedtime tantrum behavior	• Objective: to evaluate positive bedtime routines to treat difficulty settling in children with neurologic impairments • Study design: case series (? retrospective) • Subjects: 3 children with cerebral palsy, or seizure disorder, or mental retardation	• Structured bedtime routine with praise	Results: • Improvement in all three children Quality of evidence: III	C
Quine L[26] Helping parents to manage children's sleep disturbance: an intervention trial using health professionals	• Objective: to evaluate behavioral intervention in children with mental retardation and sleep disturbance • Study design: non-randomized trial with a voluntary tx group and non-tx group • Subjects: preschool children with mental retardation	• Structured bedtime routine • Teaching children to fall asleep without their parent's presence • Decreased parental contact during NA • Chair-sitting routine • Positive reinforcement of good sleep behavior	Results: • Significant improvement in difficulty settling and NA in the tx group with no change in the non-tx control group Quality of evidence: II-1	B
Bramble D[27] Rapid-acting treatment for a common sleep problem	• Objective: to evaluate behavioral tx for children with severe mental retardation and NA or difficulty settling • Study design: prospective case series • Subjects: 15 children with severe mental retardation ages 3.5 to 12 years	• Structured bedtime routine • Regular morning awakening time • Ignoring and returning the child to bed at bedtime • Praise in the morning for good sleep behavior	Results: • Significant improvement in parents' reports of sleep behavior and improvement in maternal stress Quality of evidence: II-3	C

(continued)

Table 20-3 Summary of Research Evaluating Behavioral Management in Children with Neurodevelopmental Disorders *(continued)*

Research Study	Objectives/Study Design/Subjects	Behavioral Intervention	Results/Quality of Evidence	Recommendations
Wiggs L, Stores G[28] Behavioral treatment for sleep problems in children with severe learning disabilities and challenging daytime behavior: effect on sleep patterns of mother and child	• Objective: to evaluate behavioral tx for NA, difficulty settling and early morning awakenings in children with severe mental retardation and daytime challenging behavior • Study design: RCT • Subjects: 30 children (mean age of 8.2)	• Gradual ignoring • Positive reinforcement of good sleep behavior	Results: • Significant improvement on parent ratings of sleep, but no change on wrist actigraphy (movement monitor), improvement in parent sleep Quality of evidence: I	A
Piazza CC, Hagopian LP, Hughes CR, Fisher WW[29] Using chronotherapy to treat severe sleep problems: a case study	• Objective: to evaluate the use of chronotherapy in an 8-year-old child with autism and mental retardation with erratic bedtimes, short sleep times and NA • Study design: case study	• Chronotherapy (moved bedtime forward) • Maintain regular schedule during daytime	Results: • Achieved an age-appropriate bedtime in 11 days that was maintained at 4 months follow-up Quality of evidence: III	C

tx = therapy; NA = night awakenings; RCT = randomized controlled trial of tolerance, and an insomnia rebound effect.[30] The two most commonly used medications are chloral hydrate[31] and melatonin.[32–34]

Chloral Hydrate

The American Academy of Pediatrics policy recommendations on chloral hydrate[31] refer to short-term sedation use only and not sleep disorders specifically. A theoretical risk of carcinogenicity has been found in animal studies; however, it is insufficient to warrant an alternative selection. There are no studies associating carcinogenicity and chloral hydrate in humans. Chloral hydrate is generally given 30 minutes prior to the desired bedtime at 10 mg/kg/dose. The dosage may need to be gradually increased to 25 mg/kg/dose. After 4 weeks of improved sleep, the child should be weaned from chloral hydrate over three to five nights. For recurrrence of sleep difficulties, the medication can be maintained for an additional 1 to 2 months and then the child weaned. There is no research evaluating the efficacy of chloral hydrate for sleep disorders in children. It therefore receives a "C" recommendation.

Melatonin

Melatonin is a naturally occurring hormone produced by the pineal gland and is felt to be related to the resetting of a person's biologic clock. Few side effects have been documented.[33–35] Long-term studies of both the safety and efficacy of melatonin are lacking. Melatonin is available in fast- and slow-release forms. In Canada, melatonin is available under the emergency drug release program through the Health Protection Branch of Canada. In the United States, melatonin is available as a nonprescription hormone and can be purchased over the counter in many drug and health food stores. The preparation most readily available is the fast-release form. Melatonin is given 30 minutes prior to the desired bedtime. The dosage range is 1 to 10 mg. A starting dosage for a toddler (less than 25 kg) is 2.5 mg, and school-age children (greater than 25 kg) is 5 mg. If there are no improvements after three nights, the dosage can be increased. In our clinical setting, the maximum dosage has been 9 mg. Following successful treatment over 2 to 4 months, the child can be weaned from melatonin over 1 week. If sleep problems return, melatonin can be restarted and then the child weaned again in 1 to 2 months. If there is no response after 2 to 3 weeks, it should be discontinued.[35]

As outlined in Table 20–4, the level of evidence for the use of melatonin is primarily from case series with only one randomized trial supporting its use. It therefore receives a "C" recommendation. Further randomized controlled trials are required.

PARASOMNIAS

Parasomnia is a disorder of sleep arousal associated with behaviors occurring during sleep, such as night terrors and sleepwalking. The behaviors are secondary to central nervous system motor and autonomic arousal.[42] Parasomnias are divided into two disorders of arousal, determined by their occurrence during either rapid eye movement (REM) or non-REM sleep. Night terrors and sleepwalking are both non-REM sleep arousal disorders. Nightmares are REM sleep arousal disorders. Parasomnias occur more frequently in males than in females.[42] Individuals who have one type of parasomnia have a greater likelihood of having a second parasomnia. A family history of parasomnias is also common in these individuals.[42]

Night Terrors

Night terrors occur during the transition from non-REM to REM sleep[43] and generally in the first 1 to 4 hours of sleep. They are considered a normal developmental phenomenon. Night terrors generally begin after 18 months of age. The reported prevalence is 6 percent for healthy children.[30] They often occur in clusters and then will disappear for several months before recurring. Night terrors in children can be extremely frightening for their

Table 20–4 Summary of Research Evaluating Melatonin in Children with Sleep Disorders

Research Study	Objective/Study Design/Subjects	Intervention	Results/Quality of Evidence	Recommendations
McArthur A, Budden S[36] Sleep dysfunction in Rett syndrome: a trial of exogenous melatonin treatment	• Objective: to test the safety and efficacy of a 4-week melatonin trial • Study design: double-blind placebo-controlled, cross-over trial • Subjects: nine females (4 to 17 years) with Rett syndrome with NA, difficulty settling, shortened total sleep time	• Melatonin (range 2.5 to 7.5 mg daily) versus placebo for 4 weeks with 1 week wash-out period	Results: • Significant improvement in NA, sleep onset time and total sleep time Quality of evidence: I	A
Palm L, Blennow G, Wetterberg L[37] Long-term melatonin treatment in visually impaired children and young adults with circadian sleep-wake disturbances	• Objective: to study the long-term safety and efficacy of melatonin • Study design: descriptive case series • Subjects: eight children with visual impairments, ages 3 to 23 years with fragmented sleep over a 24-hour period	• Sleep diaries kept for several months • Melatonin given 30 to 60 minutes prior to bedtime • Dosage range from 0.5 to 4 mg	Results: • Circadian rhythm improved in all subjects • No side effects reported • Length of follow-up ranged from 1 to 6 years Quality of evidence: III	C
Pillar G, Etzionia A, Shahar E, Lavie P[38] Melatonin in an institutionalized child with psychomotor retardation	• Objective: to describe a case report • Study design: single case study • Subjects: 13-year-old female institutionalized with mental retardation and an irregular sleep-wake cycle	• Melatonin 3 mg given at 18:00 • Wrist actigraphy 7 days prior to and 1 month after treatment	Results: • Increased total night sleep • Increased sleep efficiency • Increased daytime sleep • No overall change in total sleep/24 h Quality of evidence: III	C

(continued)

Table 20–4 Summary of Research Evaluating Melatonin in Children with Sleep Disorders   *(continued)*

Research Study	Objective/Study Design/Subjects	Intervention	Results/Quality of Evidence	Recommendations
Espezel H, Jan J, O'Donnell M, Milner R[39] Use of melatonin to treat sleep-wake rhythm disorders in children who are visually impaired	• Objective: to evaluate the efficacy of melatonin in visually impaired children • Study design: descriptive clinical experience • Subjects: 30/100 visually impaired children 3 mo to 17 yrs received melatonin	• Melatonin (2.5 to 10 mg) given	Results: • Treatment failed in 5 (query succeeded in 25) Quality of evidence: III	C
Jan J, Espezel H, Appleton R[32] Treatment of sleep disorders with melatonin	• Objective: to assess the potential role for melatonin in sleep disorders • Design: descriptive case series • Subjects: 15 children with multiple neurological disorders and NA, and difficulty settling	• Melatonin 2 to 10 mg	• 2/15 minimal sleep improvement • 13/15 improved sleep Quality of evidence: III	C
Camfield P, Gordon K, Dooley J, Camfield C[40] Melatonin appears ineffective in children with intellectual deficits and fragmented sleep: six "N of 1" trials	• Objective: to evaluate the use of melatonin in mentally handicapped children with frequent NA • Design: six n of 1 trials • Subjects: 6 children (3 to 13 years) with mental handicap and NA	• Each child underwent 10 week double-blind trial • Melatonin or placebo given daily at 18:00 dosage range 0.5–1.0 mg • Parents recorded child awake or asleep	Results: • No reportable difference in sleep pattern or daytime behavior • Subsequent letter to editor by Jan J, et al (1996) suggested the dosage was given too early and dosage was insufficient Quality of evidence: I	D

(continued)

Table 20–4 Summary of Research Evaluating Melatonin in Children with Sleep Disorders *(continued)*

Research Study	Objective/Study Design/Subjects	Intervention	Results/Quality of Evidence	Recommendations
Zhdanova I, Lynch H, Wurtman R[33] Melatonin: a sleep promoting hormone	• Objective: to review existing literature and author's clinical research on melatonin use in children with Angelman's syndrome • Study design: retrospective case series • Subjects: 13 children with Angelman's syndrome and "disturbed sleep"	• Melatonin 0.3 mg given 30 minutes prior to bedtime	Results: • No significant difference in total sleep time but night time sleep became "regularized" and less interrupted Quality of evidence: III	C
Sheldon S[41] Proconvulsant effects of oral melatonin in neurologically disabled children	• Objective: to evaluate the use of melatonin in children with multiple neurologic disabilities and sleep-wake disturbance • Study design: case series • Subjects: six children consecutively recruited 9 months to 18 years with NA, difficulty settling, and decreased total sleep time	• Behavioral intervention and 5 mg melatonin given at bedtime • Wrist actigraphy 2 weeks before and 2 weeks after melatonin	Results: • Improved total sleep time and settling, and decreased NA • 4/6 patients had increased seizures during the study • Seizure activity returned to pretreatment levels when melatonin was discontinued Quality of evidence: II-3	B (for total sleep time) D (for increased seizures)

NA = night awakenings

caregivers. Night terrors include a range of behaviors such as the child suddenly sitting upright in bed, screaming, staring with glassy eyes, having an irregular breathing pattern, and diaphoresis. The child is often inconsolable and does not appear to recognize the parent. The child will suddenly calm down and return to sleep. The episode can last from 30 seconds to 10 minutes. The child has no recall of the episode in the morning.

The treatment of night terrors begins with parental education and reassurance. The majority of children outgrow these episodes by their teen years. The parent should stay in the room to ensure a safe environment to protect the child from injury should they thrash about. The parent should be discouraged from awakening the child as this may prolong the episode.[44] As the child has no recall in the morning, the parents should not discuss the episode, as this can further confuse or frighten the child. For more resistant night terrors, Lask[45] described a behavioral intervention entitled scheduled awakenings. Lask reported an 80 percent improvement in night terror frequency. This technique consists of the following:

- Recording the timing of the night terror onset for five or six nights
- Wakening the child 10 to 15 minutes before the terror is likely to occur and keeping the child awake for 5 minutes duration
- Maintaining the intervention for five to seven nights

Although pharmacotherapy is not generally recommended, short-term use of benzodiazipines and tricyclic antidepressants has been reported to decrease arousals between sleep stages and therefore decrease night terrors and sleepwalking.[30] Side effects may include the rapid development of tolerance, rebound effects, and hyperactivity, and therefore long-term use is discouraged.[44,30] The medications are reserved for short-term use in situations/environments where night terrors and sleepwalking are difficult for the family to handle. The use of behavioral interventions and short-term pharmacotherapy have not been extensively researched in children and receive a "C" recommendation.

Nightmares

Nightmares usually occur in the last third of the night during REM sleep. The age of onset of nightmares is between 3 and 6 years. The reported prevalence is 10 to 50 percent for nightmares that are brought to parental attention.[42] The child often cries out, is visibly upset, and can easily be comforted by the parent. The child can recall the episode with vivid detail and return to sleep may be delayed due to fear or anxiety. As outlined in Table 20–5, nightmares can be differentiated from night terrors by their time of onset, sleep stage, response, and memory of the episode.

Table 20–5 Parasomnia Comparison

	Night Terrors	Nightmares
Onset	1-4 hr of sleep	Last third of sleep
Affect	Confused/disoriented	Upset/scared
Response	Not consolable	Comforted
Memory	None	Recall of dream detail
Return to sleep	Rapid return	Delayed
Sleep stage	Transition from non-REM stage IV to REM sleep	REM sleep

REM = rapid eye movement

Table 20–6 Summary of Research Evaluating Interventions for Parasomnias

Research Study	Objective/Study Design/Subjects	Intervention	Results/Quality of Evidence	Recommendations
Lask B Novel and nontoxic treatment for night terrors	• Objective: to assess a new intervention for night terrors • Study design: case series • Subjects: 19 children, 5 to 13 years of age	• Scheduled night awakenings 10 to 15 min before expected night terror	Results: • Night terrors stopped in each case in 1 week. Recurred in 3/19 but resolved with repeat tx Quality of evidence: III	C
Frank N, Spirito A, Stark L, Owens-Stively J The use of scheduled awakenings to eliminate childhood sleepwalking	• Objective: to assess the usefulness of scheduled night awakenings for the treatment of sleepwalking • Study design: case series • Subjects: three children	• Scheduled night awakenings to decrease the frequency of sleepwalking episodes	Results: • Resolution of sleepwalking in all subjects, which was maintained at the 6-month follow-up Quality of evidence: III	C

tx = therapy

The treatment of nightmares begins with the parents comforting the child at the time of the episode. It is recommended that night-time discussion of the details be minimal, as it may increase the child's anxiety. If further discussion is warranted, it should occur during the following day. If a stress can be identified, for example, frightening movies, an attempt should be made to decrease the exposure to or remove the stimuli. A drug history should be obtained as some medications, such as beta-adrenergic blockers, have been documented to increase nightmares.[30]

Sleepwalking

Sleepwalking also occurs during the transition from non-REM to REM sleep during the first 1 to 4 hours of sleep. Sleepwalking in young children has not been linked to emotional disturbance. The reported prevalence rate is 15 to 30 percent of children having at least one episode of sleepwalking. Less than 1 percent of adults are affected.[46] Parents describe the child purposelessly walking about the house, with poorly coordinated movement. The child may appear calm or agitated. To date, there has been no specific etiology identified for sleepwalking. Extreme fatigue or sleep deprivation have been hypothesized as triggers. A family history may be elicited; however, it has not been studied at this time.

The treatment of sleepwalking begins by ensuring a safe environment for the child. To alert parents who sleep through the episodes, the placement of bells on the child's door is recommended. Behavioral interventions can be tried, such as the scheduled awakening technique described for night terrors. Frank and colleagues[47] evaluated the use of scheduled night awakenings in three subjects prior to the typical sleepwalking onset. The intervention was successful in all three subjects and was maintained at a 6-month follow-up. An alternative approach includes a 30 to 60-minute nap late in the afternoon to decrease the amount of night-time non-REM sleep.[42] These recommendations have not been well evaluated in research studies and therefore receive a "C" recommendation. Lastly, benzodiazepines have been used for intractable cases; however, as in night terrors, tolerance quickly develops, and rebound effects upon drug withdrawal are described. For a history of severe sleepwalking or the new onset of sleepwalking in an adolescent, the clinician should rule out a sleep-related seizure disorder.[42] A summary of research evaluating the interventions for parasomnias is given in Table 20–6.

REFERENCES

1. Bernal JF. Night waking in infants during the first 14 months. Dev Med Child Neurol 1973;15:760–9.

2. Carey WB. Night waking and temperament in infancy. J Pediatr 1974;84:756–8.

3. Richman N, Stevenson JE, Graham PJ. Prevalence of behaviour problems in 3-year-old children: an epidemiological study in a London borough. J Child Psychol Psychiatry Allied Disciplines 1975;16:277–87.

4. Earls F. The prevalence of behavior problems in 3-year-old children. J Am Acad Child Psychiatry 1980;19:439–52.

5. Richman N. A community survey of characteristics of 1-2 year-olds with sleep disruptions. J Am Acad Child Psychiatry 1981;20:281–91.

6. Jenkins S, Owen C, Bax M, Hart H. Continuities of common behavior problems in preschool children. J Child Psychol Psychiatry Allied Disciplines 1984;25:75–89.

7. Lozoff B, Wolf AW, Davis NS. Sleep problems seen in pediatric practice. Pediatrics 1985;75:477–83.

8. Zuckerman B, Stevenson J, Bailey V. Division of developmental and behavioral pediatrics. Pediatrics 1987;80(5):664–71.

9. Largo RH, Hunziker UA. A developmental approach to the management of children with sleep disturbances in the first three years of life. Euro J Pediatr 1984;142:170–3.

10. Sander LW, Stechler G, Burns P, Julia H. Early mother-infant interaction and 24-hour patterns of activity and sleep. J Am Acad Child Psychiatry 1970;9(1):103–23.

11. Ferber R. Solve your child's sleep problems. New York: Simon and Schuster; 1985.

12. Keener MA, Zeanah CH, Anders TF. Infant temperament, sleep organization and nighttime parental interventions. Pediatrics 1988;81:762–71.

13. Adair R, Bauchner H, Philipp B, et al. Night waking during infancy: role of parental presence at bedtime. Pediatrics 1991;87:500–4.

14. Blader JC, Koplewicz HS, Abikoff H, Foley C. Sleep problems of elementary school children: a community survey. Arch Pediatr Adolesc Med 1997;51:473–80.

15. Richman N, Douglas J, Hunt H, et al. Behavioural methods in the treatment of sleep disorders: a pilot study. Journal of Child Psychology and Psychiatry 1985;26:581–90.

16. Czeisler CA, Richardson GS, Coleman RM, et al. Chronotherapy: resetting the circadian clocks of patients with delayed sleep phase insomnia. Sleep 1981;4:1–21.

17. Thorpy M, Korman E, Spielman A, Glovinsky P. Delayed sleep phase syndrome in adolescents. J Adolesc Health Care 1988;9:22–7.

18. Rickert VI, Johnson CM. Reducing nocturnal awakening and crying episodes in infants and young children: a comparison between scheduled awakenings and systematic ignoring. Pediatrics 1988;81:203–12.

19. Adams LA, Rickert VI. Reducing bedtime tantrums: comparison between positive routines and graduated extinction. Pediatrics 1989;84:756–61.

20. Seymour FW, Brock P, During M, Poole G. Reducing sleep disruptions in young children: evaluation of therapist-guided and written information approaches: a brief report. J Child Psychol Psychiatry Allied Disciplines 1989;30(6):913–8.

21. Adair R, Zuckerman B, Bauchner H, et al. Reducing night waking in infancy: a primary care intervention. Pediatrics 1992;89:585–8.

22. Billiard M, Verge M, Touchon J, et al. Delayed sleep phase syndrome: subjective and objective data chronotherapy and follow-up. Sleep Research 1993;22:172.

23. Pinilla T, Birch LL. Help me make it through the night: behavioral entrainment of breast-fed infants' sleep patterns. Pediatrics 1993;91:436–44.

24. Kerr SM, Jowett SA, Smith LN. Preventing sleep problems in infants: a randomized controlled trial. J Adv Nursing 1996;24:938–42.

25. Milan MA, Mitchell ZP, Berger MI, Pierson DF. Positive routines: a rapid alternative to extinction for elimination of bedtime tantrum behavior. Child Behav Ther 1981;3:13–25.

26. Quine L. Helping parents to manage children's sleep disturbance: an intervention trial using health professionals. The Children's Act 1989 and Family Support. London: HMSO; 1992. p. 101–37.

27. Bramble D. Rapid-acting treatment for a common sleep problem. Develop Med Child Neurol 1997;39:543–7.

28. Wiggs L, Stores G. Behavioural treatment for sleep problems in children with severe learning disabilities and challenging daytime behaviour: effect on sleep patterns of mother and child. J Sleep Research 1998;7(2):119–26.

29. Piazza CC, Hagopian LP, Hughes CR, Fisher WW. Using chronotherapy to treat severe sleep problems: a case study. Am J Mental Retard 1998;102:358–66.

30. Blum N, Carey W. Sleep problems among infants and young children. Pediatr Rev 1996;17:87–92.

31. American Academy of Pediatrics. Use of chloral hydrate for sedation in children. Am Acad Pediatr 1993;92:471–3.

32. Jan J, Espezel H, Appleton R. The treatment of sleep disorders with melatonin. Develop Med Child Neurol 1994;36:97–107.

33. Zhdanova I, Lynch H, Wurtman R. Melatonin: a sleep-promoting hormone. Sleep, 1997;20(10):899–907.

34. Durand M. Sleep better. Toronto: Brookes Publishing Company; 1998.

35. Jan J, Espezel H, Goulden K. Melatonin in sleep disorders in children with neurodevelopmental disabilities. In: Melatonin in psychiatric and neoplastic disorders. American Psychiatric Press; 1998; p. 169–88.

36. McArthur A, Budden S. Sleep dysfunction in Rett's syndrome: a trial of exogenous melatonin. Develop Med Child Neurol 1998;40:186–92.

37. Palm L, Blennow G, Wetterberg L. Long-term melatonin treatment in blind children and young adults with circadian sleep-wake disturbances. Develop Med Child Neurol 1997;39:319–25.

38. Pillar G, Etzioni A, Shahar E, Lavie P. Melatonin treatment in an institutionalized child with psychomotor retardation and an irregular sleep-wake pattern. Arch Dis Child 1998;79:63–4.

39. Espezel H, Jan J, O'Donnell M, Milner R. The use of melatonin to treat sleep-wake disorders in children who are visually impaired. J Visual Impairment Blindness 1996;90:43–50.

40. Camfield P, Godon K, Dooley J, Camfield C. J Child Neurol 1996;11:341–3.

41. Sheldon S. Proconvulsant effects of melatonin in neurologically disabled children. Lancet 1998;351(9111):1254.

42. Anders T, Eiben L. Pediatric sleep disorders: a review of the past 10 years. J Am Acad Child Adolesc Psychiatry 1997;36:9–20.

43. Lask B. Sleep disorders. J Am Acad Child Adolesc Psychiatry 1997;36:1161.

44. Dahl R. The pharmacologic treatment of sleep disorders. Psychiatric Clin N Am 1992;15:161–78.

45. Lask B. A novel and non-toxic treatment for night terrors. Br Med J 1988;297:592.

46. Thorpy M, Glovinsky P. Parasomnias. Psychiatric Clin N Am 1987;10:623–39.

47. Frank N, Spirito A, Stark L, Owens-Stively J. The use of scheduled awakenings to eliminate childhood sleepwalking. J Pediatr Psychol 1997;22:345–53.

CHAPTER 21

Common Skin Disorders

Sheila Jacobson, MD, FRCPC

Infants, children, and adolescents often present to physicians because of dermatologic concerns. Their lesions may be due to isolated dermatologic diseases, but not infrequently they are manifestations of systemic disorders. It is beyond the scope of this chapter to explore the innumerable diseases associated with dermatologic abnormalities. The focus, therefore, is on the few most common primary skin disorders, which are seen relatively frequently by pediatric health-care providers.

ATOPIC DERMATITIS

Atopic dermatitis affects between 10 and 12 percent of children[1] and has been estimated to account for 1 percent of all pediatric visits.[2] The etiology is poorly understood but appears to have a genetic component and is associated with other "atopic" diseases, such as asthma and allergic rhinitis. Immunoglobulin E (IgE) levels have been shown to be elevated in patients with atopic dermatitis,[3] but there is little correlation between serum levels and severity of skin manifestations.

Usually, the initial manifestations of atopic dermatitis occur around 2 to 3 months of age. In infants, the face, scalp, and extensor surfaces of the limbs are most frequently involved, while in older children and adolescents, lesions most commonly occur in the flexural creases, often with lichenification.

Detailed diagnostic criteria have been described by Hanifin.[4] These include pruritus, the typical morphology and distribution of the rash, a tendency to chronicity, and several other associated factors.

The mainstay of treatment of atopic dermatitis is topical therapy with emollients and topical steroids. Systemic steroids are rarely indicated. Because the natural history of atopic dermatitis is one of remissions and exacerbations, treatment is difficult to study, and there are many conflicting reports in the literature.

There are many well-conducted published randomized trials of different topical steroids, which generally concur that milder steroids are effective for milder disease, and that stronger formulations are indicated for more severe disease. [5–8]

Although almost all texts on the subject of atopic dermatitis recommend the use of emollients, their use is based on experience rather than evidence. One very small study (25 patients) compared the use of topical 2.5 percent hydrocortisone cream twice a day with the use of hydrocortisone once daily and with an emollient once a day, for a total period of 3 weeks. No differences were noted by an investigator, who was blinded to treatment assignment.[9] Ainley-Walker and colleagues found 1 percent hydrocortisone to be more effective than an emollient in 10 of 17 children.[10]

Antibiotic therapy does not appear to have a role in uncomplicated atopic dermatitis. A well-conducted randomized controlled trial of a 4-week course of oral flucloxacillin did demonstrate that skin colonization with *Staphylococcus aureus* was significantly decreased, but the clinical manifestations of the disease were not affected.[11] In addition, some of the subjects subsequently became colonized with methicillin-resistant organisms.

An 8-week double-blind trial of cetirizine (a newer H_1- antagonist) in children aged 6 to 12 years suggested that this drug is useful in controlling the pruritus associated with atopic dermatitis.[12] No adverse effects were noted.

Systemic cyclosporin is effective for treatment of refractory atopic dermatitis in adults, as has been shown in several randomized trials.[13-15] There are two published open-label trials in children, which suggest that in severe disease, cyclosporin may be useful.[16-17] Adverse effects in these patients were minimal.

Little has been published in the medical literature about the use of alternative therapies for the treatment of atopic dermatitis, although it is very likely that many herbal or naturopathic substances are employed, especially in an attempt to diminish the use of steroids. There is one small double-blind randomized trial of oral Chinese medicinal herbs (Zemaphyte), for the treatment of refractory eczema in children,[18] which did show a significant improvement in the treatment group. This was a short-term study. A 1-year open trial was offered to the participants in the original study, and ongoing improvement was described in those who continued the medication.[19] Two children were noted to have elevated liver enzymes during therapy, which resolved on discontinuation of the herbs. Larger studies are clearly indicated.

A randomized, double-blind controlled trial of oral evening primrose oil (essential fatty acids) in children with atopic dermatitis showed evening primrose oil to be more effective than placebo.[20]

There are two double-blind randomized placebo-controlled trials of oral pyridoxine (vitamin B_6) for treatment of atopic dermatitis. The first, which studied 20 patients, showed a significant improvement in the patients receiving pyridoxine.[21] However, when this study was repeated in a larger group of children (n=48), clinical benefit was not demonstrated.[22]

In adults with refractory atopic dermatitis, subcutaneous gamma interferon has been shown to be more effective than placebo in a 12-week study.[23] An open-label, follow-up study of the same group of patients showed continued efficacy for a period of up to 2 years.[24] Pediatric studies have not looked at the use of gamma interferon.

Much attention has focused on the prevention of atopic dermatitis, especially with regard to foods that have been implicated as triggers of the disease. Allergy testing (skin prick tests and serum radioallergosorbent test [RAST]) is not useful to assess or predict offending agents because of the large numbers of false-positive and false-negative results.[25-27] Parental reports of their children's adverse reactions to various foods and additives have also not been proved to be reliable in double-blind food challenge studies;[28-29] when these children were challenged with oral substances that they had previously reacted to, the majority showed no adverse effects.

Dietary interventions have also not been shown conclusively to affect the occurrence and severity of atopic dermatitis.[30] Two small, double-blind, placebo-controlled studies that examined the effects of eliminating cow's milk and egg from atopic infants' diets showed opposite results.[31,32] Mabin and colleagues completed a randomized single-blind study in 85 children, who were assigned to one of three groups — the control group continued to receive their normal diet, the other two groups both received a few-foods diet (eliminating all but 5 to 8 foods), with either a whey or casein hydrolysate formula, for a 6-week period. There was significant improvement in all three groups, with no differences among the three groups.[33] It is interesting that almost one-half of the study group dropped out because of non compliance!

A large cohort study published in 1930 showed a lower incidence of atopic dermatitis in breast-fed infants compared with those fed cow's milk.[34] Many of the ensuing studies have been fraught with methodologic difficulties, but the majority seem to support the protective effects of breast-feeding. [35] In one trial of premature infants, the infants were randomized to receive either banked breast milk or cow's milk–based formula; a higher incidence of atopic dermatitis was seen in the formula-fed group, but only in those who had a strong family history of allergy.[36]

The incidence of atopic dermatitis does not appear to be lowered by use of soy formula versus cow's milk–based infant formulas. This has been clearly shown in at least two well-controlled randomized clinical trials.[37,38] Extensively hydrolysed casein formulas (Nutramigen®, Alumentum®) and partially hydrolysed whey formula (Goodstart®) have been shown in randomized controlled trials to be associated with a lower incidence of atopic dermatitis in infancy.[39,40] A randomized controlled trial of cow's milk, which involved giving newborn infants either cow's milk protein supplements or placebo for the first 3 days of life, did not show an increased incidence of atopy in the exposed group at 1 year of age.[41] There was a higher incidence of atopic disease in children with strong family histories of allergy, but even within this subgroup, no increase in the exposed group was described. The period of exposure to cow's milk protein in this study was very short; it does not rule out the possibility that more prolonged exposure to cow's milk may predispose to atopy.

Avoidance of allergenic foods, such as egg and cow's milk, during pregnancy has been shown in randomized trials not to affect the development of atopic disease in the offspring.[42-44] The presence of food allergens in breast milk has been implicated in the development of atopic disease in infants with strong family histories of allergies. Two prospective studies (one of which was randomized) evaluated whether maternal avoidance of allergens, such as egg, cow's milk, and fish, during the first 3 months of lactation affected the incidence of atopy in high-risk infants . Both showed some reduction in atopic dermatitis for at least the first 18 months of life.[45,46] At 10 years of age, the difference was no longer evident.[47,48]

Prevention by avoidance of skin irritants, such as scented soaps, creams, and detergents, has been recommended. Although it does seem logical to avoid such irritants, there are no randomized trials to support this recommendation.

Table 21–1 Treatment of Atopic Dermatitis

Condition	Intervention	Quality of Evidence	Recommendation
Atopic dermatitis	• Topical steroids	I	A
	• Emollients	III	B
	• Topical 2.5 percent hydrocortisone cream, once daily and emollient once daily	I	A
	• Flucloxacillin	I	E
Pruritus of atopic dermatitis	Cetirizine 5 to 10mg/kg	I	A
Atopic dermatitis	• Cyclosporin	adults I	A
		children II-3	B
	• Gamma interferon	III	C
	• Pyridoxine	I	E
	• Evening primrose oil	I	A
	• Dietary restrictions	I	E
	• Chinese herbs (Zemaphyte)	I	B

DIAPER DERMATITIS

Despite the high incidence of diaper dermatitis in infants, it has not been the subject of extensive research, most likely because it is a self-limited problem that resolves when children become toilet trained.

The term "diaper dermatitis" includes several rashes occurring in the diaper area. The most common rash is irritant contact dermatitis, secondary to a number of factors, including occlusion, moisture, high pH, urine, and fecal enzymes. More severe, erosive rashes have been shown to harbor increased growth of fungal and/or bacterial organisms such as *Candida albicans*, group A beta-hemolytic *Streptococcus* and *Staphylococcus aureus*. Fungal infections usually cause papular, scaly rashes, predominantly in intertriginous areas.

Diaper dermatitis may be prevented by keeping the skin as dry as possible, avoidance of irritants, and the use of barrier creams, such as petrolatum or zinc oxide pastes. Several randomized controlled trials have shown that the incidence and severity of diaper rashes are significantly lower in infants who wear disposable diapers (versus cloth).[49-51] While these studies have been rigorously and scientifically conducted, it should be borne in mind that they have all been sponsored by diaper manufacturing companies. In the use of cloth and disposable diapers, the consequences on the environment remain controversial.[52]

Topical antifungal therapy for fungal diaper rashes has been shown to be effective. A double-blind, placebo-controlled trial of mycostatin versus placebo showed clinical cure rates of 32 percent with placebo, compared with 84 percent cure rates with topical mycostatin.[53] Small studies of topical clotrimazole have suggested similar cure rates to mycostatin.[54] Addition of oral antifungal medications to topical formulations does not appear to improve resolution of fungal diaper dermatitis.[55] The use of topical antibacterial creams has not been well studied in the current literature. In addition, there is very little evidence to support or refute the use of combinations of topical steroids and antifungal creams; one sample of five patients showed good effect[56] (Table 21–2).

SEBORRHEIC DERMATITIS

Seborrheic dermatitis is another very common skin affliction of infants. The pathogenesis and etiology are poorly understood. It usually presents as greasy, scaly lesions on the scalp but may also involve the face, the area around the ears, and the flexural creases. Unlike atopic dermatitis, seborrheic dermatitis is not usually itchy. It frequently resolves during the first year of life but may recur in a small percentage of adolescents as "dandruff" or blepharitis. Mimouni and colleagues followed up 88 infants diagnosed with seborrheic dermatitis; after 10 years, 85 percent were free of skin disease, and 8 percent had persistent signs of seborrheic dermatitis.[57]

Treatment regimens include frequent shampooing, applying oil to the scalp and combing out the scaly lesions, and applying keratolytic shampoos or topical steroids. A small, open study has suggested that topical ketoconazole is effective.[58] A randomized trial comparing 2 percent

Table 21–2 Treatment of Diaper Dermatitis

Condition	Intervention	Quality of Evidence	Recommendation
Fungal diaper dermatitis	• Topical antifungal therapy	I	A
	• Oral antifungal therapy	I	E
	• Topical antibacterial creams	III	C
	• Topical steroids	III	C

Table 21-3 Treatment of Seborrheic Dermatitis

Condition	Intervention	Quality of Evidence	Recommendation
Seborrheic dermatitis	• Topical steroids	III	B
	• Topical ketoconazole	II-3	B

ketoconazole cream with 1 percent hydrocortisone cream showed similar clinical efficacy.[59] The published literature on treatment of seborrheic dermatitis in children is sparse, probably because of the benign nature of the disease and its generally good prognosis (Table 21–3).

HEMANGIOMAS AND CONGENITAL VASCULAR MALFORMATIONS

Vascular malformations are the result of aberrant embryologic development, resulting in abnormal structures. Infantile hemangiomas are benign vascular neoplasms. They may be difficult to distinguish clinically.

Nevus Flammeus

These are congenital vascular malformations that commonly involve the forehead, face, and neck of newborns. Most are small and tend to disappear during infancy or childhood, especially those that are located in the midline of the face.[60] Portwine stains are large facial nevus flammeus lesions, which are usually unilateral and persist to adulthood.[61,62] Laser therapy has been shown to be effective in treating portwine stains;[63-65] these were not randomized trials.

Cavernous Hemangiomas

These are usually not true hemangiomas but, more often, are actually venous malformations that involute. The lesions that do not involute are true hemangiomas. The clinical course and histopathology of these two lesions differ substantially, although they may be very difficult to differentiate clinically in infants. Since the majority of these lesions involute, treatment is generally not indicated, unless the lesions interfere with important functions (eg, lesions on the eyelid that obstruct vision) or cause persistent cosmetic problems.

TINEA INFECTIONS

The term "tinea" incorporates about 40 fungal species that cause superficial infections in humans. These organisms invade keratin and, thus, have a predilection for hair, nails, and skin. Infection of the skin (tinea corporis) and scalp (tinea capitis) are the most common forms in children; nail infestations are unusual.

Tinea corporis forms superficial red scaly papules and small plaques, which enlarge to form expanding rings. Clearing of previously affected areas results in the typical "ringworm"

Table 21-4 Treatment of Tinea Infections

Condition	Intervention	Quality of Evidence	Recommendation
Tinea corporis /capitis	• Griseofulvin	I	A
Tinea corporis	• Ketoconazole	I	A
	• Itraconazole	III	B
	• Terbinafine	III	B

appearance. The cardinal clinical appearance of tinea capitis is inflammation, with hair loss and surrounding edema. Tinea infections may cause mild itching. Diagnosis is usually clinical but can be confirmed by potassium hydroxide (KOH) staining of scales, nails, or hair.

Tinea corporis is treated with topical antifungal agents, such as clotrimazole, miconazole, or terbinafine. Systemic therapy is indicated for tinea capitis so that antifungal therapy can penetrate growing hairs. Oral griseofulvin 20 mg/kg, for 8 to 12 weeks, is the most frequently prescribed medication for tinea capitis. In healthy children who are treated for less than 6 months, routine laboratory evaluation prior to or during therapy is not indicated. The newer antifungal medications have not been extensively evaluated in children. Fluconazole, itraconazole and ketoconazole have been shown to be as effective as griseofulvin in randomized controlled trials in adults and adolescents.[66-68] In a randomized controlled trial in children, oral ketoconazole has also been demonstrated to be as effective as griseofulvin.[69] Itraconazole 5mg/kg and terbinafine 3 to 5 mg/kg appeared to be effective in small groups of children, in open-label studies.[70-71] Further studies are indicated (Table 21–4).

ACNE VULGARIS

Up to 85 percent of people have acne during their adolescent years; the incidence peaks at 18 years of age, but older and younger individuals may also be affected.[72] Facial acne may cause severe psychosocial difficulties, including embarrassment, poor self-esteem, and social withdrawal.[73]

The pathogenesis of acne appears to be complex and is poorly understood. Multiple factors have been implicated; these include sebum production, bacterial infection with *Propionibacterium acnes*, and inflammation. Acne occurs on parts of the body that have the largest and most abundant sebaceous glands, that is, the face, neck, chest, back, and upper arms. The lesions which are characteristic of acne are as follows:

1. Noninflammatory lesions
   - Closed comedones ("whiteheads") which are whitish papules with apparently closed overlying surfaces
   - Open comedones ("blackheads") which are flat or slightly raised black or brown plugs. The color is due to oxidization of melanin (not dirt!)
2. Inflammatory lesions
   These may appear as papules, pustules, nodules, and cysts. They are usually red and "angry-looking"
3. Scarring
   Scarring generally follows inflammatory acne; it may be hypertrophic (keloid) or atrophic (so-called "ice-pick" lesions)
4. Hyperpigmentation

Several topical and systemic pharmacologic preparations are available for the treatment of acne. Research in this area has been quite extensive, and there are many well-conducted randomized controlled trials.

Topical therapy is indicated for milder disease, that is, noninflammatory or mild inflammatory acne. Topical retinoids, such as tretinoin and isotretinoin, have been shown in prospective cohort and randomized trials to be the most effective topical agents.[74-76] Their mechanism of action is the reversing of the abnormal desquamation that causes micro-comedon formation as well as their anti-inflammatory effects. Topical retinoids are available in a number of different strengths and formulations, including creams, liquids, and gels. They are also manufactured in combination with sunscreens. Treatment should be commenced with lower strength preparations and gradually increased, since side effects such as skin irritation and photosensitivity are relatively common. Most people do develop tolerance with continued use. It is important to remember that maximal clinical improvement may take several months.

Some newer, theoretically better topical retinoids have been developed recently. Adapalene is a synthetic retinoid that is more stable and lipophilic than tretinoin. One randomized trial has shown it to be at least as effective as and less irritant than 0.025 percent tretinoin for the treatment of mild to moderate acne.[77]

Benzoyl peroxide is bacteriocidal against *Propionibacterium acnes*. It is available in various strengths and preparations. It has been demonstrated in randomized controlled trials to be as effective as topical 1 percent clindamycin,[78] erythromycin lotion,[79] and 0.05 percent isotretinoin[80] for moderately inflammatory acne.

Topical salicylic acid has also been shown in randomized trials to be effective against comedones and inflammatory lesions.[81]

Several topical antibiotics have been used in the treatment of acne; clindamycin, erythromycin, and tetracycline have all been shown to be effective therapeutic agents in randomized trials.[78,79,82,83]

Combination therapy for the treatment of acne is very commonly prescribed. There is little evidence to support or refute multiple therapies, although it may seem intuitive to presume that more may be additive. There is some evidence from randomized trials to suggest that benzoyl peroxide is synergistic with both topical and oral antibiotics[84-86] and tretinoin.[87]

Systemic therapy for acne is indicated for more severe manifestations of acne or that which is unresponsive to topical agents. Tetracyclines are the most commonly prescribed antibiotics for acne and have been shown to be effective. Minocycline appears to be more effective than tetracycline or doxycycline,[88] presumably because it is the most lipophilic of the three. It is also the most expensive. Erythromycin, cotrimoxazole, and clindamycin have all been demonstrated to be effective in blinded randomized trials[89-91] but are less commonly prescribed because of potential associated adverse effects. Oral antibiotic therapy for acne should generally be continued for a period of at least 4 to 6 months.

Oral isotretinoin is indicated for the most severe manifestations of acne, for which it is extremely effective; this has been demonstrated in randomized controlled trials,[92] although the majority of studies are prospective cohort studies including large numbers of subjects, followed up for long periods of time.[93-95] Several dose-ranging studies have shown that higher doses (ie, 0.5 to 1 mg/kg) are associated with lower relapse rates.[96-98] Systemic isotretinoin, if taken during pregnancy, is associated with a high incidence of severe congenital defects, that is, the so-called retinoic acid embryopathy.[99] Counseling and contraception are essen-

Table 21–5 Treatment of Acne

Condition	Intervention	Quality of Evidence	Recommendation
Acne	• Topical retinoids	I	A
	• Benzoyl peroxide	I	A
	• Topical antibiotics (clindamycin, erythromycin, tetracycline)	I	A
	• Benzoyl peroxide in combination with systemic antibiotics	I	A
	• Benzoyl peroxide in combination with topical retinoic acid	I	A
Acne (severe)	Oral isotretinoin	I	A

tial aspects of treatment for women of childbearing age who are prescribed systemic isotretinoin (Table 21–5).

Hormonal therapy for acne is only occasionally indicated, usually for patients who have acne associated with endocrine disorders. Such treatment may include spironolactone, estrogens, androgen-blockers, and corticosteroids. Randomized trials of these medications have not been performed.

CONCLUSION

Skin disorders are common in children, and different diseases are seen frequently in children of different ages. This chapter has attempted to focus on new and/or controversial areas, to highlight the evidence — or the lack of it — for current management of dermatologic diseases frequently seen by pediatric primary health-care providers.

REFERENCES

1. Tong AKF, Mihm MC. The pathology of atopic dermatitis. Clin Rev Allergy 1986;4:27-42.

2. Sampson HA. Atopic dermatitis. Ann Allergy 1992;69:469-77.

3. Stone SP. IgE levels in atopic dermatitis. Arch Dermatol 1973;109:806–11.

4. Hanifin JM, Rajka G. Diagnostic features of atopic dermatitis. Acta Derm Venereol (Stockh) 1980;(Suppl)92:44-7.

5. Olsen EA. A double-blind controlled comparison of generic and trade-name topical steroids using the vasoconstrictor assay. Arch Dermatol 1991;127:197-201.

6. Sears HW, Bailer JW, Yeadon A. Efficacy and safety of hydrocortisone buteprate 0.1% cream in patients with atopic dermatitis. Clin Therapeutics 1997;19(4):710-9.

7. Wolkerstrofer A, Strobos A, Glazenberg EJ, et al. Fluticasone propionate 0.05% cream once daily versus clobetasone butyrate 0.05% cream twice daily in children with atopic dermatitis. J Am Acad Dermatol 1998;39(2 Pt 1):226-31.

8. Jorizzo J, Levy M, Lucky A, et al. Multicenter trial for longterm safety and efficacy comparison of 0.05% desonide and 1% hydrocortisone ointments in the treatment of atopic dermatitis in pediatric patients. J Am Acad Dermatol 1995;33(1):74-7.

9. Lucky AW, Leach AD, Laskarazewski P, et al. Use of an emollient as a steroid-sparing agent in the treatment of mild to moderate atopic dermatitis in children. Pediatr Dermatol 1997;14(4):321-4.

10. Ainley-Walker PF, Patel L, David TJ. Side to side comparison of topical treatment in atopic dermatitis. Arch Dis Child 1998;79:149-52.

11. Ewing CI, Ashcroft C, Gibbs AC, et al. Flucloxacillin in the treatment of atopic dermatitis. Br J Dermatol 1998;138(6):1022-9.

12. La Rosa M, Ranno C, Musarra F, et al. Double-blind study of cetirizine in atopic eczema in children. Ann Allergy 1994;73:117-22.

13. Sowden JM, Berth-Jones J, Ross JS, et al. Double-blind controlled crossover study of cyclosporin in adults with severe refractory atopic dermatitis. Lancet 1991;338:137-40.

14. Van Joost T, Heule F, Korstanje M, et al. Cyclosporin in atopic dermatitis: a multicenter placebo-controlled study. Br J Dermatol 1994;130:634-40.

15. Salek MS, Finlay AY, Luscombe DK, et al. Cyclosporin greatly improves the quality of life of adults with severe atopic dermatitis: a randomized double-blind placebo-controlled trial. Br J Dermatol 1993;129:422-30.

16. Berth-Jones J, Finlay AY, Zaki I, et al. Cyclosporin in severe childhood atopic dermatitis: a multicenter study. J Am Acad Dermatol 1996;34:1016-21.

17. Zaki I, Emerson R, Allen BR. Treatment of severe atopic dermatitis in childhood with cyclosporin. Br J Dermatol 1996;135(Suppl) 48:21-4.

18. Sheehan MP, Atherton DJ. A controlled trial of traditional Chinese medicinal plants in widespread non-exudative atopic eczema. Br J Dermatol 1992;126:179-84.

19. Sheehan MP, Atherton DJ. One-year follow-up of children treated with Chinese medicinal herbs for atopic eczema. Br J Dermatol 1994;130:488-93.

20. Hederos CA, Berg A. Epogam evening primrose oil treatment in atopic dermatitis and asthma. Arch Dis Child 1996;75(6):494-7.

21. Koller DY, Pirker C, Jarisch R, et al. Pyridoxine HCl improves atopic dermatitis: changes of IL-1 beta, IL-2, ACTH and cortisol in plasma [abstract]. Clin Exp Allergy 1992;22:126.

22. Mabin DC, Hollis S, Lockwood J, et al. Pyridoxine in atopic dermatitis. Br J Dermatol 1995;133:764-7.

23. Hanifin JM, Schneider LC, Leung DYM, et al. Recombinant interferon gamma therapy for atopic dermatitis. J Am Acad Dermatol 1993;28:189-97.

24. Stevens SR, Hanifin JM, Hamilton T, et al. Long-term effectiveness and safety of recombinant human interferon gamma therapy for atopic dermatitis despite unchanged serum IgE levels. Arch Dermatol 1998;134:799-804.

25. Bock SA, Buckley J, Holst A, et al. Proper use of skin tests with food extracts in diagnosis of hypersensitivity to food in children. Clin Allergy 1997;7:375-83.

26. Aas K. The diagnosis of hypersensitivity to ingested foods. Reliability of skin prick testing and the radioallergosorbent test with different materials. Clin Allergy 1978;8:39-50.

27. Lessoff MH, Buisseret PD, Merret J, et al. Assessing the value of skin tests. Clin Allergy 1980;10:115-20.

28. David TJ. Reactions to dietary tartrazine. Arch Dis Child 1987;62:119-22.

29. Bock SA. Prospective appraisal of complaints of adverse reactions to foods in children during the first three years of life. Pediatrics 1987;79:683-8.

30. David TJ, Patel L, Ewing CI, et al. Dietary regimens for atopic dermatitis in childhood. JR Soc Med 1997;90(Suppl)30:9-14.

31. Atherton DJ, Sewell M, Soothill JF, et al. A double-blind controlled crossover trial of an antigen-avoidance diet in atopic eczema. Lancet 1978;1:401-3.

32. Neild VA, Marsden RA, Bales JA, et al. Egg and milk exclusion diets in atopic eczema. Br J Dermatol 1986;114:117-23.

33. Mabin DC, Sykes AE, David TJ. Controlled trial of few foods diet in severe atopic dermatitis. Arch Dis Child 1995;73:202-7.

34. Grulee CJ, Sanford HN. The influence of breast and artificial feeding on infantile eczema. J Pediatr 1930;9:223-5.

35. Kramer MA. Does breastfeeding help protect against atopic disease? Biology, methodology and a golden jubilee of controversy. J Pediatr 1989;112:181-90.

36. Lucas A, Brooke OG, Morley R, et al. Early diet of preterm infants and development of allergic or atopic disease: randomized prospective study. Br Med J 1990;300:837-40.

37. Chandra RK, Singh G, Stridhara B. Effect of feeding whey hydrolysate, soy and conventional cow's milk formula on the incidence of atopic disease in high risk infants. Ann Allergy 1989;63:102-6.

38. Kjellman NIM, Johansson SGO. Soy versus cow's milk in infants with a biparental history of atopic disease: development of atopic disease and immunoglobulins from birth to four years of age. Clin Allergy 1979;9:347-58.

39. Chandra RK, Hamed A. Cumulative incidence of atopic disorders in high-risk infants fed whey hydrolysate, soy and conventional cow milk formulas. Ann Allergy 1991;67:127-32.

40. Chandra RK, Shakuntla P, Hamed A. Influence of maternal diet on development of atopic eczema in high risk infants. Br Med J 1989;299:228-30.

41. De Jonge MH, Scharp-vander Linden PTM, Aalberse RC, et al. Randomized controlled trial of brief neonatal exposure to cow's milk on the development of atopy. Arch Dis Child 1998;78:126-130.

42. Falth-Magnusson K, Kjellman NIM. Development of atopic disease in babies whose mothers were receiving exclusion diets during pregnancy — a randomized study. J Allergy Clin Immunol 1987;80:868-75.

43. Falth-Magnusson K, Kjellman NIM. Allergy prevention by maternal elimination diet during pregnancy — a five-year follow-up of a randomized study. J Allergy Clin Immunol 1999;89:709-13.

44. Lilja G, Dannaeus A, Foucard T, et al. Effects of maternal diet during late pregnancy and lactation on the development of atopic diseases in infants up to 18 months of age — in vivo results. Clin Exp Allergy 1989;19:473-9.

45. Chandra RK, Shakuntla P, Hamed A. Influence of maternal diet during lactation and use of formula feeds on development of atopic eczema in high risk infants. Br Med J 1989; 299:228-33.

46. Hatterig G, Kjellman B, Sigurs N, et al. Effect of maternal avoidance of eggs, cow's milk and fish during lactation upon allergic manifestations in infants. Clin Exp Allergy 1989;19:27-32.

47. Hatterig G, Sigurs N, Kjellman B. Maternal food antigen avoidance during lactation and allergy during the first 10 years of life. J Allergy Clin Immunol 1996;97(Part 3):241.

48. Sigurs N, Hatterig G, Kjellman B. Maternal avoidance of eggs, cow's milk and fish during lactation: effect on allergic manifestations, skin prick tests and specific IgE antibodies in children at age 4 years. Pediatrics 1992;89:735-9.

49. Campbell RL, Seymour JL, Stone LC, Milligan MC. Clinical studies with disposable diapers containing absorbent gelling materials: evaluation of effects on infant skin condition. J Am Acad Dermatol 1987;17:978-87.

50. Davis JA, Leyden JJ, Grove GL, Raynor WJ. Comparison of disposable diapers with fluff absorbent and fluff plus absorbent polymers: effects on skin hydration, skin pH and diaper dermatitis. Pediatr Dermatol 1999;6:102-8.

51. Campbell RL, Bartlett AV, Saurbough FC, Picking LK. Effects of diaper types on diaper dermatitis associated with diarrhea and antibiotic use in children in daycare centers. Pediatr Dermatol 1988;5:83-7.

52. Sutton MB, Weitzman M, Howland J. Baby bottoms and environmental conundrums: disposable diapers and the pediatrician. Pediatrics 1991;85(2):386-8.

53. Alban J. Efficacy of nystatin topical cream in the management of cutaneous candidiasis in infants. Curr Ther Res 1959:910-3.

54. Sawyer PR, Brogden RN, Pinder RM, et al. Clotrimazole: a review of its antifungal activity and therapeutic efficacy. Drugs 1975;9:424-7.

55. Munz D, Powell KR, Pai CH. Treatment of candidal diaper dermatitis: a double-blind placebo-controlled comparison of topical nystatin with topical plus oral nystatin. J Pediatr 1982;101:1022-5.

56. Bowring ARW, McKay D, Taylor FR. The treatment of napkin dermatitis: a double-blind comparison of two steroid-antibiotic combinations. Pharmatheurapeutica 1984;3:613-7.

57. Mimouni K, Mukamel M, Zeharia A, Mimouni M. Prognosis of infantile seborrheic dermatitis. J Pediatr 1995;127(5):744-6.

58. Taieb A, Legrain V, Palmier C, et al. Topical ketoconazole for infantile seborrheic dermatitis. Dermatologica 1990;181(1):26-32.

59. Katsambas A, Antoniou C, Frangouli E, et al. A double-blind trial of treatment of seborrheic dermatitis with 2% ketoconazole cream compared with 1% hydrocortisone cream. Br J Dermatol 1989;121(3):353-7.

60. Leung AKC, Telmesani AMA. Salmon patches in Caucasian children. Pediatr Dermatol 1989;6:185-7.

61. Alper JG, Holmes LB. The incidence and significance of birthmarks in a cohort of 4641 newborns. Pediatr Dermatol 1983;1:58-66.

62. Jacobs AH, Walton RG. The incidence of birthmarks in the neonate. Pediatrics 1976;58:218-22.

63. Garden JM, Polla LL, Tan OT. The treatment of portwine stains by the pulsed dye laser. Arch Dermatol 1988;124:889-96.

64. Renfro L, Geronemus RG. Anatomical differences of portwine stains in response to treatment with the pulsed dye laser. Arch Dermatol 1993;129:182-8.

65. Dover JS, Geronemus RG, Stern RS, et al. Dye laser treatment of portwine stains: comparison of the continuous-wave dye laser with a robotized scanning device and the pulsed dye laser. J Am Acad Dermatol 1995;32:237-40.

66. Del Palacio, Hernandez A, Lopez Gomez S, et al. A comparative double-blind study of terbinafine (Lamisil) and griseofulvin in tinea corporis and tinea cruris. Clin Exp Dermatol 1990;15(3):210-6.

67. Jolly HW, Daily AD, Rex IH. A multicenter double-blind evaluation of ketoconazole in the treatment of dermatomycoses. Cutis 1983;31(2):208-10.

68. Stratigos I, Zissis NP, Katsambas A, et al. Ketoconazole compared with griseofulvin in dermatophytoses: a randomized double-blind trial. Dermatologia 1983;166(3):161-4.

69. Martinez-Roig A, Torres-Rodriguez JM, Bartlett-Coma A. Double-blind study of ketoconazole and griseofulvin in dermatophytoses. Pediatr Infect Dis J 1988;7(1):37-40.

70. Ginter G. Microsporum canis infections in children: results of a new oral antifungal therapy. Mycoses 1996; 39(7-8):265-9.

71. Bakos L, Brito AC, Castro LCM, et al. Open clinical study of the efficacy and safety of terbinafine cream 1% in children with tinea corporis and tinea cruris. Pediatr Infect Dis J 1997;16:545-8.

72. Cunliffe WJ, Gould DJ. Prevalence of facial acne in late adolescence and in adults. Br J Dermatol 1979;1:1109-10.

73. Koo J. The psychosocial impact of acne: patients' perceptions. J Am Acad Dermatol 1995;32:S26-30.

74. Cunliffe WJ, Layton A, Knaggs HE, et al. Isotretinoin and acne: a longterm study. In: Saurat JH, editor. Retinoids:10 years on. Basel: S Karger; 1991. p. 274-80.

75. Lehucher-Ceyrac D, Weber-Buisset MJ. Isotretinoin and acne in practice: a prospective analysis of 188 cases over 9 years. Dermatology 1993;186(2):123-8.

76. Chalker DK, Lesher JL, Smith JG, et al. Efficacy of topical isotretinoin 0.05% gel in acne vulgaris: results of a multicenter, double-blinded investigation. J Am Acad Dermatol 1987;17:251-4.

77. Shalita AR, Weiss JS, Chalker DK, et al. A comparison of the efficacy and safety of adapalene gel 0.1% and tretinoin gel 0.025% in the treatment of acne vulgaris: a multicenter trial. J Am Acad Dermatol 1996;34:482-5.

78. Tucker SB, Tausend R, Cochran R, Flannigan SA. Comparison of topical clindamycin phosphate, benzoyl peroxide and a combination of the two for the treatment of acne vulgaris. Br J Dermatol 1983;108:199-204.

79. Burke B, Eady EA, Cunliffe WJ. Benzoyl peroxide versus topical erythromycin in the treatment of acne vulgaris. Br J Dermatol 1983;108:199-204.

80. Hughes BR, Norris JF, Cunliffe WJ. A double-blind evaluation of topical isotretinoin 0.05%, benzoyl peroxide gel 5% and placebo in patients with acne. Clin Exp Dermatol 1992;17(3):165-8.

81. Shalita AR. Treatment of mild and moderate acne vulgaris with salicylic acid in an alcohol-detergent vehicle. Cutis 1981;28:566-1.

82. Blaney DJ, Cook CH. Topical use of tetracycline in the treatment of acne: a double-blind study comparing topical and oral tetracycline therapy and placebo. Arch Dermatol 1976;112:971-3.

83. Shalita AR, Smith EB, Bauer E. Topical erythromycin versus clindamycin therapy for acne: a multicenter double-blind comparison. Arch Dermatol 1984;120:351-5.

84. Chalker DK, Shalita AR, Smith JG, Swann RW. A double-blind study of the effectiveness of a 3% erythromycin and 5% benzoyl peroxide combination in the treatment of acne vulgaris. J Am Acad Dermatol 1983;9:933-6.

85. Packman AM, Brown RH, Dunlap FE, et al. Treatment of acne vulgaris: combination of 3% erythromycin and 5% benzoyl peroxide in a gel compared to clindamycin phosphate lotion. Int J Dermatol 1996;35(3):209-11.

86. Lookingbill DP, Chalker DK, Lindhorn JS, et al. Treatment of acne with a combination clindamycin/benzoyl peroxide gel compared with clindamycin gel, benzoyl peroxide gel and vehicle gel: combined results of two double-blind investigations. J Am Acad Dermatol 1997;37(4):590-5.

87. Hurwitz S. The combined effect of vitamin A acid and benzoyl peroxide in the treatment of acne. Cutis 1976;17:585-90.

88. Hubbell CG, Hobbs ER, Rist T, et al. Efficacy of minocycline compared with tetracycline in the treatment of acne vulgaris. Arch Dermatol 1982;118:989-92.

89. Gammon WR, Meyer C, Lantis S, et al. Comparative efficacy of oral erythromycin versus oral tetracycline in the treatment of acne vulgaris: a double-blind study. J Am Acad Dermatol 1986;14:183-6.

90. Hersle K. Trimethoprim-sulphamethoxazole in acne vulgaris: a double-blind study. Dermatologica 1972;145:187-91.

91. Poulos ET, Tedesco FJ. Acne vulgaris: double-blind trial comparing tetracycline and clindamycin. Arch Dermatol 1976;112:974-6.

92. King K, Jones DH, Daltrey DC, et al. A double-blind study of the effects of 13-cis retinoic acid on acne, sebum excretion rate and microbial population. Br J Dermatol 1982;107:583-90.

93. Pochi PE. 13-cis retinoic acid in severe acne. N Engl J Med 1979; 300:369-80.

94. Gantt GG. Reduced anxiety and depression in cystic acne patients after successful treatment with oral isotretinoin. J Am Acad Dermatol 1987;17:25-32.

95. Spear KL, Muller SA. Treatment of cystic acne with 13-cis retinoic acid. Mayo Clin Proc 1983;58:509-14.

96. Jones DH, King KH, Miller AJ, et al. Dose-response study of 13-cis retinoic acid in acne vulgaris. Br J Dermatol 1983;108:333-43.

97. Strauss JS, Repini RP, Shalita AR, et al. Isotretinoin therapy for acne: results of a multicenter dose response study. J Am Acad Dermatol 1984;10:490-6.

98. Jones DH, Cunliffe WJ. Remission rates in acne patients treated with various doses of 13-cis retinoic acid (isotretinoin). Br J Dermatol 1984;111:123-5.

99. Lammer EF, Chen DT, Hoar RM. Retinoic acid embryopathy. N Engl J Med 1985;313:837-41.

CHAPTER 22

Learning Disabilities and Attention Deficit Hyperactivity Disorder

Saul Greenberg, MD, FRCPC

LEARNING DISABILITIES

Definition

The term "learning disabilities" (LDS) describes a group of disorders manifested as significant difficulties in the acquisition and use of listening, speaking, reading, spelling, writing, reasoning, or mathematical abilities. These disorders are intrinsic to the individual and presumed to be due to central nervous system dysfunction. The term does not include children whose learning problems result primarily from visual, hearing, or motor handicaps, mental retardation, and emotional disturbance, or environmental, cultural, or economic disadvantages. Children with LDS find it difficult to learn in the traditional way at the accepted rate for their age group. Their channels for learning do not process stimuli in the usual manner and, as a result, both receptive and expressive abilities can be affected. Nonetheless, children with LDS have average or above average intelligence.

Traditionally, children were considered to have a learning disability when they underachieved in reading, evidenced in a disparity between their intelligence quotient (IQ) scores and reading levels on standard measures of achievement, such as the Wide Range Achievement Test and the Peabody Individual Achievement Tests. However, IQ scores may depend on a child's ability to read and concentrate while taking the IQ test. Many children with lower IQ scores do learn to read, and poor readers of all IQ levels show equivalent difficulties with reading, spelling, short-term memory, and syntax. Reading disability may be better defined on the basis of performance below a particular score on a reading test that is appropriate for the child's chronologic age.[1]

In the United States, the Interagency Committee on Learning Disabilities concluded in 1987 that 5 to 10 percent of the population had a learning disability,[2] and according to a 1991 report of the United States Department of Education, nearly half of all children receiving special education services were considered learning disabled.[3] Boys and girls are equally affected, although more boys are referred for help, perhaps because they are more disruptive to parents and teachers.

Types and Manifestations

Learning disabilities may represent a deficit in one aspect of learning but commonly affect several areas of academic skills. These may include basic reading skills, reading comprehension, oral expression, listening comprehension, written expression, mathematical calculation, and mathematical reasoning. The age of identification of LDS depends on the type and severity and the presence or absence of associated deficits. Learning problems can be divided into two main groups: (1) reading disorders (dyslexia) due to language-based learning problems, and (2) poor handwriting (dysgraphia), problems with mathematics (dyscalculia), and deficits in social skills.

Children with reading disability/decoding problems usually manifest them by the end of grade 1, whereas children whose reading disability mainly involves comprehension may escape detection until the latter part of elementary school. Learning disabilities involving written expression are often associated with lack of composition ability or poor handwriting. They may also show up as failure to complete written assignments, difficulty copying board work, and low grades in mathematics or spelling. Learning disabilities in mathematics are often seen in conjunction with deficits in either reading or written expression.

Dyslexia: Language-Based Learning Disabilities

Dyslexia is the most common learning disability and the one that causes most long-term problems. Children who have normal intelligence but encounter difficulties in reading are typically referred to as dyslexic, reading disabled, or specific reading retarded. To warrant a diagnosis of dyslexia, a child must be reading at a level that is two grades behind his or her expected grade level. Dyslexia is the result of impaired language-processing skills. Good readers are able to decode letters quickly and automatically to concentrate on the meaning of the words. In contrast, children with dyslexia have problems in decoding phonemes, the individual speech sounds in the alphabet, and in mastering phonics, the ability to articulate words.

Dyslexic children show a weakness in verbal short-term memory and therefore have trouble recalling letters, words, phrases, names, dates, phone numbers, addresses, and other rote facts. Besides having problems comprehending written material, many of these children find it hard to understand what they hear. They may find it confusing to follow oral directions at home and in school and to distinguish similar sounds in words such as dog and log, especially in a noisy environment.

Mathematics presents a problem for dyslexic children because they have difficulty memorizing basic mathematical facts and remembering sequences of steps in computation. Preschool children who are later diagnosed as dyslexic often have a history of delayed speech, poor articulation, and difficulty with learning the names of numbers and letters. They have trouble rhyming and learning to associate sounds with letters. Following multistep directions is hard for them, and because they often cannot express their frustration in words, they are prone to hitting and kicking.[4,5]

Nonverbal Learning Disabilities

Problems with arithmetic and handwriting, and deficits in social awareness and social judgment are associated with nonverbal learning disabilities (NLDS). These comprise 1 to 10 percent of learning disabilities.[6] The right side of the brain processes nonverbal information and deals with spatial awareness, recognition of visual patterns, and coordination of visual information with motor processes (visual-motor integration).

Children with NLDS can manifest psychomotor and tactile-perceptual deficits and poorly coordinated gross- and fine-motor skills. They have visual-perceptual-organizational deficits and weak eye-hand coordination, reflected in handwriting, drawing, and copying from the blackboard.[7]

These children have problems understanding fundamental concepts of mathematics and determining the approach required to solve a problem. They do, however, have strong psycholinguistic skills, such as rote verbal learning, word recognition, and spelling.

Children with NLDS may have significant deficits in social perception, judgment, and interaction skills. They are often described as socially isolated, with few close friends and limited social activity. The meaning of jokes, strategies of games, motives of others, and social conventions may escape them. They often lack insight into their strengths and weaknesses and their own future. Nonverbal learning disabilities have been shown to persist into adulthood and even to worsen over time. The abnormal language characteristics, for example, poor prosody (intonation, accentuation, temporal variation, and voice quality) and pragmatics (the appropriate use of language in diverse social, cultural, or developmental contexts), yet good vocabulary, and pronounced social difficulties of these children have led some investigators to question whether NLDS are part of a continuum with pervasive developmental disorders and Asperger's syndrome.[8]

Coexisting Conditions

Attention Deficit Hyperactivity Disorder

Hyperactivity occurs in 25 to 41 percent of children with learning disabilities.[9] Some investigators suggest that attention deficit hyperactivity disorder (ADHD) may be a consequence of learning disability, as children become inattentive, learn poorly, and perhaps tune out. Children with LDS experience frustration and may be unable to sustain attention because the academic demands are too heavy. Evidence exists, however, that learning disability and ADHD are distinct disorders that frequently occur together.[10] Both have strong genetic components but appear to be inherited independently.[11]

Psychological Disturbances

Depression and anxiety occur in one-third of learning-disabled children, especially in those with nonverbal disabilities.[12,13] This is not surprising since these children often have low self-esteem after years of failing at school and being labeled "dumb" by peers.[14] Children with LDS are not as socially competent as their peers and appear to have difficulty understanding others' affective states, especially in complex or ambiguous situations.[15]

Causes

Heredity is a primary factor in language-based learning disabilities. Some 35 to 40 percent of close relatives of dyslexic persons have similar difficulties.[16] Linkage studies implicate loci on chromosomes 6 and 15 in reading disability.[17] As with ADHD, some children with LDS have mothers who abused alcohol and cocaine during pregnancy. Dyslexia is associated with left-brain dysfunction, the side of the brain specialized for language. Researchers have found that an area in the posterior portion of the temporal lobe, known as the planum temporale, which is normally larger on the left side than the right, is either the same size or smaller in dyslexic patients.[18] In adults with LDS, studies have shown functional changes on magnetic resonance imaging (MRI)[19] and areas of focal dysplasia in the language regions,[20] suggesting the presence of differences in the brain's structural and functional characteristics. Learning disabilities have been found in children who have suffered severe head injuries, are hydrocephalic, or have undergone radiation treatment of the head. Since these conditions entail destruction of white matter in the right hemisphere, some researchers attribute LDS of some children to early damage in this area.

Differential Diagnosis of Learning Disability

A child's poor performance in school may be due to reasons other than learning disability. Table 22–1 lists some of the other causes of inferior school performance that physicians must differentiate from LDS.

Diagnosis

Early diagnosis is crucial to effective treatment of LDS. It is important that a diagnosis be made before a child's skill levels and self-esteem slip to dangerous lows. Learning disabilities

Table 22-1 Differential Diagnosis of Learning Disability

- Mild and moderate mental retardation
- Gifted children who are bored
- Poor motivation, for example, from a family that does not value academic success
- Psychiatric disorders such as anxiety and depression
- Inappropriate expectations, for example, comparing a child to a high-achieving sibling or parent
- Teacher-student mismatch
- Attention deficit hyperactivity disorder
- Family issues: separation and divorce, illness of family member, alcoholism and drugs, poverty, physical, emotional or sexual abuse
- Physical illness: chronic or recurrent, for example, asthma, after-effects of head injury, brain tumor, very low birth weight sequelae, iron deficiency anemia, chronic lead poisoning
- Medication effects: theophylline, anticonvulsants, antihistamines, ethanol and recreational drugs
- Seizure disorders: absence or temporal lobe seizures
- Fetal alcohol syndrome
- Chromosomal syndromes: fragile X, Turner's, Williams, Down's, and Noonan's syndromes
- Nonchromosomal syndromes: Prader-Willi, Angelman's
- Visual and auditory impairment

can generally be diagnosed on the basis of a careful and detailed history, physical examination, and, if necessary, a pyschological assessment.

History

The physician should take a history of developmental milestones to rule out mental retardation or autism and inquire about behavior and attention span. Medications such as antihistamines, anticonvulsants, tranquilizers, and asthma medications may affect attention and learning. Information about a child's performance in school should be obtained from teachers. One should look for a history of delayed language development and problems with the sounds of words, for example, trouble rhyming or confusion of homonyms, and problems with expressive language, such as mispronunciations, hesitations, and word-finding difficulties. Children may have difficulty learning the letters of the alphabet, numbers, and days of the week, associating sounds with letters, or following directions or routines. Children may have trouble reading unfamiliar words; their oral reading may be inaccurate, slow, or labored and their spelling poor. They may also be slow to learn new skills and recall facts, relying heavily on memorization. Family history is important; the physician should obtain a history of reading and spelling difficulties of parents and siblings.

Physical Examination

The physician should look for neurologic dysfunction and assess hearing and vision to rule out any sensory or neurologic problem affecting learning. Physicians will vary in the detail and depth with which they wish to assess the academic skills of children. Simple screening tools may be used to evaluate comprehension of written and spoken language, mathematical skills, auditory memory, reading, spelling, and writing skills.[21] Formal assessment, by a psychologist, of intelligence and educational achievement is occasionally necessary. Reports from teachers and/or IQ test results can provide information about cognitive strengths and weaknesses and help define how well a child processes information. Some of the more frequently used intelligence tests for school-aged children are the Wechsler Intelligence Scale for Children (WISC-III) and the Stanford Binet Intelligence Scale. Academic achievement can be assessed by tests such as the Peabody Individual Achievement Test-Revised (PIAT-R), Woodcock-Johnson Tests of Achievement-Revised (WJ-R) and the Wide Range Achievement Test-Revised (WRAT-R).

Treatment

Educational Therapy

The cornerstone of treatment of LDS is educational therapy. It must be tailored to individual needs and depends on the child's learning strengths and weaknesses. To learn to read successfully, the child needs to master three component skills: phoneme analysis, visual memory, and comprehension. All children must first discover that spoken words can be broken down into smaller units of sound (phonemes) and that these are linked to specific letters and letter patterns (phonics). Once letter-to-letter decoding is achieved, whole words are usually committed to visual memory. Building up a sight-word vocabulary allows a child to read with increasing speed and automaticity. Speed in naming familiar symbols such as numbers or letters is slower in dyslexic children.[22] Comprehension is directly related to decoding skills but may present problems for students who are inattentive, have poor language skills generally, or fail to link the verbal information in words with nonverbal images of what they portray.[23] Many programs are available to teach reading skills, including intensive phonetic teaching programs. Reading remediation that emphasizes phonetic decoding has been shown to improve reading skills[24] (level I, recommendation A). See Table 22–2 for levels of LDS treatment, ranked on the basis of quality of evidence and perceived effectiveness. No evidence has been found, however, that any one reading technique is better than another. A number of protocols differing in method, format, intensity, and duration of intervention are now being tested to determine the most effective.[25]

Several studies have investigated whether children with LDS should be mainstreamed (placed in regular classes and helped by teacher's aides or tutors) or segregated in special classes with other learning-disabled children and a specially trained teacher. The studies suggest that with highly motivated teachers and aides, mainstreaming can lead to improvements in academic achievement, behavior, and self-esteem (level I, recommendation B) (see Table 22–2). Studies to determine whether children with LDS should repeat a school year (enabling them to acquire academic skills they missed the first time) or be promoted (retaining self-esteem) have proved inconclusive (level III, recommendation C).[26]

Table 22–2 Summary of Treatments for Learning Disabilities

Intervention	Quality of Evidence	Recommendation
Reading remediation	I	A
Repeating school year	III	C
Teaching learning strategies (mnemonics, rhymes, visual images)	I	A
Computer-based reading instruction	II	B
Social skills training	I	B
Psychotherapy	III	C
Behavior management	I	C
Medication (Piracetam)	I	C
Orthomolecular therapies (diets, vitamins)	I	E
Neurophysiologic therapies (sensorimotor integration, tinted lenses, eye muscle exercises)	I	E

Besides using remedial reading techniques, educators have tried teaching general learning strategies to children with LDS. They have achieved some success in helping children improve the way they approach new tasks, memorize new information (eg, using mnemonics) (level I, recommendation A),[27] and organize information (eg, using rhymes or visual images to link specific bits of information) (level I, recommendation A).[28]

Computer-based reading instruction has advanced recently with the use of interactive talking storybooks that encourage children to persist in the reading task and provide help in reading (eg, a child may select an unknown word to hear it read aloud). This method has been shown to improve skills in word recognition and decoding but may be less effective in improving comprehension.[29] Adding speech to text is a valuable addition to reading software and has been shown to double the rate of acquisition of decoding skills.[30] Children may have problems with written work because of poor spelling, weak fine-motor skills, or expressive language delays. Use of word processors has been shown to lead to positive changes in writing quality and the quantity of text written[31] and increased accuracy in spelling and grammar,[32] but these changes are not always found in all students. Children with writing disorders may be helped by using a classmate's notes, taping lectures, being assigned "homework buddies," and being allowed to take examinations orally.

Thus, computer-based reading instruction has resulted in improvement in some aspects of reading and writing skills (level II, recommendation B).

Other Therapies

Social skills training. Many children with LDS are not well accepted by their peers, have social skill deficits, and do not make and keep friends easily. Various interventions have been tried to help solve these problems, and some of them have proven effective.[33] Interventions with students in special programs have been less effective than with those who are mainstreamed, perhaps because the latter have more opportunities to observe desirable social behavior. Longer interventions (4 to 25 weeks of training) were more successful than shorter ones (1 to 14 weeks). Small groups of students achieved better results than larger groups, and students chosen because of significant social difficulties responded better than those selected simply because they were in an LDS class. Many studies that used techniques such as coaching, modeling, role-play, feedback, and problem solving had positive effects, although behavior changes occurring in controlled settings often did not generalize to natural settings. Nor was there evidence that peer acceptance increased as a result of these social skills interventions.[33]

Social skills training has resulted in improvement in these skills in selected groups of students (level I, recommendation B).

Counseling. Individual, family, or group counseling sessions may be required to treat psychological disorders. However, there is no good evidence that learning-disabled children treated with psychotherapy experience long-term benefits (level III, recommendation C).[34] However, counseling may deal with issues of the child's self-esteem and help relieve guilt about his or her problems. Education and information about LDS is important. One of the most valuable supports for parents is the Association for Children with Learning Disabilities. It provides parents with information about local services and new discoveries and helps organize support groups in which parents can compare notes and provide mutual encouragement.

Behavior management. Behavior management is often used with children diagnosed with LDS or ADHD. Reinforcing on-task behavior in children with LDS has been shown to improve academic performance in the short term.[35] The essentials of a behavior modification program have been extensively described,[36] with the expectation that it may produce desired behaviors and a positive parent-child relationship (level I, recommendation C).

Medication. In the child with combined LDS and ADHD, stimulant medications have been shown to improve classroom performance, not only through greater attentiveness and concentration, but also in the way the central nervous system processes information. In reading tasks, this effect is seen in improved word-finding abilities and a resultant improvement in reading vocabulary.[37] A different class of drug, pyrrolidine acetamide (Piracetam), was found to produce a significant improvement in the reading and writing ability of dyslexic boys, taking both rate and accuracy into consideration, compared with a placebo group.[38] This medication is still considered experimental (level I, recommendation C).

Alternative therapies. Patients with LDS and their families often seek out unconventional approaches to improving reading difficulties and behavior. Various diets have been advocated: additive-free, oligoantigenic, low-sugar, allergy-free, megavitamin–added, and trace mineral–added. Other therapies purported to help include anti–motion sickness medication for vestibular dysfunction, patterning, optometric training, sensorimotor integration, chiropractic manipulation, discontinuing fluorescent light, Irlen (colored) lenses, and negative ions. Few credible data are available to support the claims made for these therapies.[39,40] They are not considered useful and cannot be recommended for the treatment of LDS (level I, recommendation E).

Prognosis

Many follow-up studies have shown that some features of reading disabilities persist into late adolescence and young adulthood.[41] Although reading comprehension and word recognition skills may improve, many adults continue to have difficulty with spelling, reading unfamiliar words, and reading with reasonable speed.[42] Adults with untreated LDS have higher rates of unemployment, and many have difficulties in at least one activity of daily living, such as banking, using maps, and time management. Their frequent lack of organizational skills is reflected in unpredictability, inefficiency, poor punctuality, untidiness, and procrastination.[43] The outcome in children with LDS is determined by the severity of their learning deficits, the extent to which these are counteracted by their areas of strength, and the supports available to them. On an optimistic note, many people with LDS, such as Winston Churchill and Thomas Edison, went on to achieve high levels of academic and professional success.

ATTENTION DEFICIT HYPERACTIVITY DISORDER

Attention deficit hyperactivity disorder (ADHD) is now recognized as the most common neurobehavioral disorder affecting children. It is characterized by inattentiveness, impulsiveness, and hyperactivity that significantly impairs a child's functioning at home, at school, and with peers.[44] The prevalence of ADHD has been estimated to be between 1.7 and 16 percent, depending on the population and diagnostic methods used.[45,46] Recent reports indicate that 3 to 5 percent of school-aged children have ADHD.[44,47] On average, then, about one child in every classroom is affected. Some 40 percent of the children who cause problems in school likely have ADHD. This disorder is 2 to 8 times more frequent in boys than in girls.[48] Its symptoms persist into adolescence in 70 percent and into adulthood in 10 percent of those diagnosed with ADHD in childhood.[49,50]

Symptoms

The current and most widely used criteria for ADHD have been defined by the American Psychiatric Association (Table 22–3).[44] The symptoms of ADHD may vary substantially between home and school, structured and nonstructured settings, and large and small groups as well as in situations that make high or low demands on the child's performance. Children with ADHD can pay attention in situations they find novel, fascinating, or scary, or in a one-to-one situation with an adult. For example, a child with ADHD has difficulty concentrating when faced with routine, monotonous activities but has no problem when engaged in certain activities of his or her choice, like watching television or playing Nintendo. Most chil-

---

Table 22–3 DSM-IV Criteria for Attention Deficit Hyperactivity Disorder

---

Either (1) or (2)

1. Six or more of the following symptoms of inattention have persisted for at least 6 months to a degree that is maladaptive and inconsistent with the developmental level.

Inattention

- Often fails to give close attention to details or makes careless mistakes in schoolwork, work, or other activities
- Often has difficulty sustaining attention in tasks or play activities
- Often does not seem to listen when spoken to directly
- Often does not follow through on instructions and fails to finish schoolwork, chores, or duties in the workplace (not due to oppositional behavior or failure of comprehension)
- Often has difficulty organizing tasks and activities
- Often avoids, dislikes, or is reluctant to engage in tasks that require sustained mental effort (such as schoolwork or homework)
- Often loses things necessary for tasks or activities at school or at home (eg, toys, pencils, books, assignments)
- Is often easily distracted by extraneous stimuli
- Is often forgetful in daily activities

2. Six or more of the following symptoms of hyperactivity-impulsivity have persisted for at least 6 months to a degree that is maladaptive and inconsistent with the developmental level.

Hyperactivity

- Often fidgets with hands or feet or squirms in seat
- Often leaves seat in classroom or in other situations where remaining seated is expected
- Often runs about or climbs excessively in situations where it is inappropriate (in adolescents or adults, may be limited to subjective feelings of restlessness)
- Often has difficulty playing or engaging in leisure activities quietly
- Often talks excessively
- Is often "on the go" or often acts as if "driven by a motor"

Impulsivity

- Often has difficulty awaiting turn in games or group situations
- Often blurts out answers to questions before they have been completed
- Often interrupts or intrudes on others, for example, butts into other children's games

Onset Before the Age of 7 Years

- Some impairment from the symptoms present in two or more settings (eg, at school or work or at home)
- Clear evidence of clinically significant impairment in social, academic, or occupational functioning

---

dren with ADHD have trouble concentrating on activities that other children enjoy, like coloring, pasting, and doing puzzles. They may also show signs of the free flight of ideas, difficulty feeling satisfied, social immaturity, inconsistent performance, and mood swings. As these children get older, they exhibit excessive fidgeting and restlessness rather than gross motor activity.

Attention deficit hyperactivity disorder forms part of a more comprehensive diagnosis called attention deficit disorder (ADD), which is classified by the Diagnostic and Statistical Manual, 4th edition (DSM-IV) into three categories:

- ADD with predominant hyperactivity and impulsivity with minimal inattentiveness
- ADD with combined hyperactivity and inattentiveness
- ADD with predominant inattentiveness and minimal hyperactivity (ADD-H)

The first two groups are nearly indistinguishable from each other and will be referred to as children with ADHD.[51] Children with ADD-H function at a slower cognitive speed, appear more confused, apathetic and lethargic, show increased social withdrawal, and are more likely to suffer from anxiety or depression than children who have ADHD.[52] Children with ADD-H tend to be female and are diagnosed in later grades of elementary school, when they begin to fall behind academically. This group of children is often underdiagnosed, since their behavior and conduct problems are not as common or conspicuous as those in the ADHD group. These children are disorganized, inattentive, distracted, forgetful, and often labeled lazy or underachieving. In contrast, children with ADHD are described as more noisy, aggressive, disruptive, messy, irresponsible, immature, and less successful in establishing relationships with peers.

The paragraphs that follow describe the coexisting conditions, diagnosis, causes, and treatment of ADHD, by far the most prevalent condition among children with ADD.

Coexisting Conditions

In addition to exhibiting the core symptoms of inattentiveness, impulsiveness, and hyperactivity, some children with ADHD have learning problems and delays in speech, language, and motor skills.[53] Behavior disorders, low self-esteem, and psychiatric conditions such as anxiety disorders and depression are also common.[54] The prevalence rates of these comorbid conditions vary according to whether the patients are seen primarily by psychiatrists or pediatricians: conduct and oppositional defiant disorders seem to be higher in psychiatric studies and learning disorders higher in pediatric studies.

Academic Problems and Learning Disabilities

From 25 to 30 percent of children with ADHD also have a learning disability,[55] and the frequency is even higher in those with ADD-H.[56] Despite having normal or even superior intelligence, the ADHD child is often a chronic underachiever. By adolescence, up to one-third of these children have failed at least one grade. Both ADHD and reading disabilities have strong genetic components but appear to be inherited independently.[57]

Psychiatric Disorders

As many as 50 to 65 percent of children with ADHD referred to psychiatrists have at least one additional psychiatric disorder.[43] Virtually all childhood psychiatric disorders are more common in children with ADHD than in those who are unaffected. Tics may also be seen in some school-aged children with ADHD.[58] Problems with poor self-esteem are common; depressive disorders occur in 9 to 38 percent of children with ADHD, especially after they reach about 10 years of age.[45,59] Bipolar disorders have also been associated with ADHD.[60] Anxiety disorders resulting in fears and worries occur in up to 25 percent of children with ADHD.[43] These disorders are unlikely to worsen school performance but do cause more social difficulties.[61] Children with anxiety disorder and ADHD also respond less favorably to stimulant medication than those without anxiety.[62]

Conduct Disorder

Conduct disorder, or antisocial behavior, is characterized by cruelty, violence, and disregard for the rights of others. Affected children are aggressive, destroy property, and frequently lie and steal. They often skip classes and run away from home regularly. Approximately 25 percent of children with ADHD seen by psychiatrists have a conduct disorder.[45] The disorder is manifested less often in children and adolescents with ADD-H than in those with more pronounced hyperactivity. Children with both ADHD and conduct disorder come from families of lower socioeconomic status than ADHD children without conduct disorder.[63] They also have higher rates of reading disorders[64] and show an increased incidence of adult antisocial personality and criminal convictions.[65]

Oppositional Defiant Disorder

Oppositional defiant disorder, a term often used for younger children, involves negativism and hostility but, unlike conduct disorder, does not involve the violation of societal norms. The disorder is characterized by stubbornness, tantrums, disobedience, and defiance of authority. If the disobedience becomes a way of life for a child, he or she has an oppositional or defiant disorder. About 65 percent of ADHD children in one psychiatric study had this disorder, but it did not necessarily develop into a conduct disorder later on.[66]

Causes

Most experts believe that ADHD is an inherited neurobiologic disorder. Heredity plays a role, since children with relatives with the disorder are at high risk for ADHD, comorbid psychiatric disorders, school failure, and learning disability. One in every four children with diagnosed ADHD has a biologic parent who is similarly affected.[66] Identical twins are more likely to share ADHD than fraternal twins or other siblings.[67] Recent studies suggest an association between the dopamine transporter gene and ADHD[68] and differences between control subjects and ADHD patients in the D4 dopamine receptor gene (associated with novelty seeking).[69]

The frontal lobes of the brain, which have long been known to play a critical role in regulating attention, activity, and emotional reactions, may have a role in ADHD. Positron emission tomographic (PET) scans have shown that adults with ADHD have lower brain glucose metabolism in the frontal lobes than non-ADHD subjects when told to concentrate on a task.[70] This pattern of underactivity is thought to be due to abnormalities in the neurotransmitters in the frontal areas. Stimulant medication is postulated to compensate for these abnormalities, since ADHD subjects show increased activity in the frontal areas when treated. High concentrations of dopamine metabolites in the cerebrospinal fluid have also been shown to correlate with high degrees of hyperactivity and with good response to treatment with stimulant drugs.[71] Magnetic resonance imaging (MRI) studies have revealed structural differences in the brain in patients with ADHD. Non-ADHD boys showed an asymmetry of the caudate, the right side being larger than the left, whereas boys with ADHD demonstrated no asymmetry; subjects with the least asymmetry performed worst on tests of response inhibition.[72] Also, MRI has shown abnormal frontal lobes[73] and reduced volume in the rostrum and rostral body of the corpus callosum in patients with ADHD.[74]

Birth injuries associated with fetal distress and difficult labor play a negligible role in ADHD, but damage before birth may be a factor. Mothers who abuse drugs or alcohol during pregnancy may have children who suffer from ADHD and learning disabilities.[75]

Some have blamed environmental toxins, including lead, and artificial flavors, dyes, preservatives, and other food additives for ADHD, while others have singled out sugar, food allergy, and food additives as the causes. Anecdotal evidence and testimonials have been used to support these claims; however, double-blind controlled studies have not substantiated them.[76]

Differential Diagnosis

Physicians must distinguish between ADHD and other disorders or conditions that mimic its symptoms. Fidgeting, distractibility, and impulsiveness have many causes, only one of which is ADHD. If these behavioral problems have only recently begun to show up or are related to a particular event, a child may not have ADHD. For instance, a child who becomes distractible in grade 4 may be suffering from emotional problems, such as those caused by a divorce. Or if a child starts having trouble in mathematics, a problem that affects 5 to 10 percent of school-aged children,[77] a learning disability could be the cause.

Many of the conditions that coexist with ADHD may, on their own, cause hyperactivity in a child. Table 22–4 lists some of the other causes of hyperactivity that physicians must differentiate from ADHD.

Diagnosis

Physicians who see children with ADHD differ in their opinions about how to diagnose ADHD. Some recommend a large battery of tests, whereas others simply have the parent complete a brief rating scale for the child, then make a quick diagnosis and prescribe treatment. Neither extreme is in the patient's best interest.

No single medical, laboratory, or psychological diagnostic test definitively identifies ADHD.[44] The diagnosis is a clinical one made on the basis of a picture that begins early in life, persists over time, pervades different settings of the child's life, and impairs functioning at home, at school, or in leisure-time activity. The diagnosis is made through interviews with people who know the child, a physical examination, use of rating scales, and a review of previous psychological test results, if available.

History

The history of a child's longstanding problems with attention, impulsivity, and hyperactivity is the best source of information for identifying ADHD. The physician should obtain separate accounts of the child's behavior from parents and teachers, as symptoms are specific to situations.

When interviewing parents, the physician should take a full developmental history to rule out developmental delays, learning and language disabilities, and pervasive developmental disorder. The physician should
- ask about the child's behavior in infancy, such as resistance to cuddling, high activity levels, and sleep and feeding disturbances. Behavior at this stage is sometimes correlated with future ADHD behavior;

Table 22–4 Differential Diagnosis of Hyperactivity

- Age-appropriate overactivity
- Anxiety disorder
- Conduct disorder
- Oppositional defiant disorder
- Learning disability
- Speech or language disability
- Tourette's syndrome
- Affective disorder: mania, depression
- Schizophrenia or psychosis
- Inadequate environment or parenting
- Mental retardation
- In-utero exposure to alcohol, cocaine, lead
- Neurologic disorders: post-traumatic, postencephalitic
- Iatrogenic effects of medication: theophylline, barbiturates, steroids
- Eczema and other irritating skin conditions
- Endocrine disorders: hyperthyroidism, pheochromocytoma, hypoglycemia
- Chromosomal disorders: Down's syndrome, fragile X syndrome, Klinefelter's syndrome (XYY), Turner's syndrome

- elicit information about what the child's behavior is like in various settings, for example, when alone, playing with other children, or while shopping;
- review the behavior-management techniques the parents have used to ensure that they are appropriate for the child's age and not overly punitive or indulgent; and
- ask about the child's academic performance and peer relationships.

A family history of hyperactive behavior or learning difficulties is important because of the role played by heredity in ADHD. The physician should evaluate the child's emotional status to rule out depression and anxiety disorders and to distinguish ADHD from other disruptive behaviors, such as conduct disorder and oppositional defiant disorder.

Reports from teachers about the child's ability to finish work, stay on task, and respect others form an important part of the evaluation. As well, because of the association of ADHD with learning difficulties, these reports may help assess the child's level of academic achievement and general intelligence. Since underachievement is a hallmark of the child with ADHD, his or her grades usually do not match estimated ability levels.

An in-depth clinical interview with the child is necessary to rule out more serious disorders such as psychosis and to determine his or her degree of maturity and verbal skills. The physician should ascertain the child's feelings about home, school, and social life and ask whether the child feels sad, anxious, or fearful. Because the symptoms of anxiety or depression overlap those of ADHD (agitation, impulsivity, decreased concentration), these comorbid conditions may go unrecognized. The most common mistake physicians make when taking a history is forgetting to ask about coexisting conditions. It is important to remember that to be diagnosed with ADHD, a child must fulfill the DSM-IV criteria (see Table 22–3). Symptoms must be present before the age of 7 years and cause impairment in two or more settings.

Rating Scales

Various rating scales have been used to assess children's behavior at home and in school. The Conners Teacher Rating Scale[78] rates children on several aspects of behavior, as does the ADD-H Comprehensive Teacher Rating Scale, which allows separate evaluation of four areas of child behavior: attention, hyperactivity, social skills, and oppositionality. These scales help in making an initial diagnosis of ADHD, estimating symptom severity, and monitoring a child's response to treatment. However, none of them can provide a diagnosis. There are also performance tests that assess a child's ability to sustain and focus attention and to refrain from responding impulsively. These include the Matching Familiar Figures Test and the Continuous Performance Test.[79] Although these tests provide useful information, their results are not infallible and should be interpreted in the context of all available information.[80]

Physical Examination

Observation of the child's behavior in the physician's office can be helpful; however, only about 20 percent of children with ADHD exhibit overt hyperactivity during an office visit.[45] A physical examination is done primarily to rule out visual and hearing problems, which may impair attention and memory. It should also exclude physical illness, medication effects, and major neurologic or developmental problems. The examination may reveal some dysmorphic features characteristic of syndromes associated with ADHD, such as fragile X (an inherited condition associated with mental retardation) or fetal alcohol syndrome. As well, the physician should look for evidence of motor or vocal tics, which may indicate the presence of Tourette's syndrome as well as ADHD and influence the choice of medication.

The physician may pick up soft neurologic signs, such as fine-motor coordination problems and choreiform and motor-overflow movements. However, these are not diagnostic of ADHD, since normal children may also have them.

The electroencephalograms (EEGs) of some children with ADHD may also show abnormalities, such as an increase in slow-wave activity. However, since many affected children have normal EEGs, the test is not definitive. An EEG should not form a routine part of the examination unless the physician suspects other problems, such as a seizure disorder.

At this point, the physician should know if the child needs further assessments. If all or many of the tests suggest ADHD, the physician may decide on behavioral therapies, school modifications, and a trial of medication. If these interventions do not greatly improve the child's behavior and school performance, the physician may have to refer the child to other specialists, such as psychologists or psychiatrists. A positive response to stimulant medication, such as methylphenidate (Ritalin), however, does not ensure that the diagnosis of ADHD is correct, as the attention or behavior of children without ADHD may also improve when taking the medication.

Psychological Testing

Some, though not all, children with suspected ADHD are sent to a psychologist or educational consultant for IQ testing to rule out a learning disability. The relationship between the definition of LDS and IQ testing remains controversial. Currently, most clinicians prefer to define LDS on the basis of a significant discrepancy between a child's potential for learning and his or her actual achievement. As stated earlier, reading disability may be better defined on the basis of performance below a particular score on a reading test appropriate for the child's chronologic age.[1] Speech and language assessment may also be necessary if the child has a suspected communication problem.

Psychiatric Evaluation

Some children with ADHD exhibit symptoms of anxiety, depression, and anger. When these are severe, the child may require a psychiatric evaluation to determine whether the symptoms are causing, or complicating, the behavioral difficulties or are factors coexisting with ADHD. A child psychiatrist should be consulted if the child's psychological problems are severe or complex, the family is experiencing significant conflict, or the child needs alternative medications for coexisting symptoms.

Treatment

The goal of treatment for ADHD is to improve the child's functioning at home, in school, and with peers through modification of his or her inattention, impulsivity, and hyperactivity. It entails maximizing cognitive functioning, improving social and behavioral skills, and raising self-esteem while keeping side effects to a minimum. Multimodal therapy, described below, involves a combination of education, medication, psychological treatments, and appropriate classroom intervention. While many researchers assert that multimodal therapy is superior to medication or psychosocial intervention alone,[81,82] others think that empirical evidence to support this view is inconclusive.[83] (See Table 22–5 for summary of treatments for ADHD.)

Education

The first step in treatment is for the family and child to obtain comprehensive, accurate information from their doctor about ADHD, associated problems, and treatments. Parental support groups such as Children with Attention Deficit Disorders (CHADD) and Attention Deficit Disorders Association (ADDA) provide important educational and support services. They offer a forum in which parents can discuss problems, provide mutual emotional support, and share effective ways to deal with schools, doctors, and service institutions.

Medication

Medication, used either alone or in combination with psychological therapies, is the most widely used modality in the management of ADHD. It has been estimated that between 2 and

Table 22–5 Summary of Treatments for ADHD

Intervention	Quality of Evidence	Recommendation
Stimulants	I	A
Tricyclic antidepressants	I	A
Clonidine	I	A
Combined pharmacotherapy	III	C
Parent training	I	C
Classroom management	III	C
Cognitive behavior training	I	C
Group social skills training	I	A
Orthomolecular therapies (diets, vitamins)	I	E
Neurophysiologic therapies (sensorimotor integration, tinted lenses, eye muscle exercises)	I	E

2.5 percent of all school-aged children in North America receive some pharmacologic treatment for hyperactivity,[84] more than 90 percent of whom are treated with methylphenidate.[85]

Stimulants. Stimulants are sympathomimetic drugs structurally similar to endogenous catecholamines (eg, dopamine and norepinephrine). They are believed to act as neurotransmitters in certain areas of the brain, correcting a biochemical condition that interferes with attention and impulse control. Stimulants such as methylphenidate (Ritalin, the most commonly used stimulant), amphetamine (Dexedrine), and pemoline (Cylert) are the first choices for children with ADHD. More than 170 studies have shown that these drugs are effective in over 70 percent of children with ADHD.[86] If a child fails to respond to one of these drugs, he or she will react favorably to a second one in 70 percent of cases.[87] Stimulant medications work as well in adolescents as in children, but their effects vary more widely in preschool children and adults with ADHD.[88] These drugs have been unequivocally shown (in double-blind, placebo-controlled studies) to reduce the core symptoms of hyperactivity, impulsivity, and inattentiveness.[89] They also improve classroom behavior and academic performance, diminish oppositional and aggressive behaviors, reduce irritability and anxiety,[90] and promote interaction with teachers and family. Although long-term studies of stimulant medications are few, amphetamine has been shown in one randomized control trial to exert positive effects on inattention, hyperactivity, and other disruptive behaviour at home and in school for 15 months after the start of treatment.[91]

The usual starting dosage of methylphenidate is 0.3 mg/kg, given one to three times per day. If there is no response after 1 week, as measured by feedback from teachers and parents, the dosage may be gradually increased to 0.6 to 0.8 mg/kg. Starting doses of amphetamines are usually one-half to two-thirds that of methylphenidate. Higher doses of stimulant medication may improve general activity levels but have been shown to affect memory tasks and attentional tests adversely.[92] Excessive doses may cause "zombie-like" behavior, in which the child seems spaced-out and overfocused, and anxiety-associated behavior, such as nail biting and picking at scabs. Rebound hyperactivity is a deterioration in behavior, lasting one half hour or more, that follows the wearing off of short-acting stimulants. It may be managed by use of longer-acting drugs, increased structure in after-school activities, a small dose of medication in the late afternoon, or the addition of clonidine.

An important issue is whether medication should be given daily or just on school days. Drug holidays have the advantage of limiting potential toxicity; however, on occasions, when a child's impulsivity and activity interfere with peer and family interaction, the medication may be continued on weekends and holidays.

Stimulant medications have been shown in many studies to be quite safe, with minimal and mild side effects. Those most commonly seen are insomnia, loss of appetite, and weight loss. Other, less common side effects include sadness, depression, fearfulness, social withdrawal, sleepiness, headaches, nail biting, and stomach aches. All these effects are short term, and most disappear with a lowering of the dose. Long-term studies have found that stimulant medication is not addictive and does not lead to illegal drug use in later years.[93] Studies have also shown that stimulants may suppress growth during the first year or two of treatment; this problem, however, is transient and its effects on adult height are minimal.[94] It has traditionally been accepted that stimulants exacerbate tics and are thus contraindicated in children with tic disorders. However, recent well-controlled trials have shown that methylphenidate has no statistically significant effect on the frequency or severity of tics in children compared with a placebo group.[95]

Pemoline has been associated with hepatic toxicity and should be used as a second-line agent in treating ADHD and only in conjunction with monitoring of hepatic enzymes.

Stimulants are effective and are recommended in the treatment of ADHD (see Table 22–2) (level I, recommendation A).

Tricyclic antidepressants. Tricyclic antidepressants, such as imipramine and desipramine, can produce improvement in over 70 percent of children with ADHD.[96] Improvements in behavior are usually more prominent than those in attention. Tricyclics are thought to act as neurotransmitters but work by improving mood, impulsivity, and tolerance of frustration. Common side effects include dry mouth, constipation, and drowsiness. In rare cases, heart arrhythmias have been reported in children taking tricyclics, so regular electrocardiography is recommended for these children. Generally, tricyclics are used as a second line of drug therapy for children with ADHD who do not benefit from methylphenidate or develop side effects when on stimulant medication. They are the drug of choice in those who have depression or anxiety associated with ADHD and may also be used in children with ADHD who have tics or Tourette's syndrome. Sudden cessation may result in a flu-like anticholinergic withdrawal syndrome with nausea, cramps, headaches, and muscle pains. Therefore, tricyclics should be tapered over a 2- to 3-week period.

Tricyclic antidepressants are effective and are recommended in the treatment of ADHD (level I, recommendation A).

Clonidine. Clonidine is an alpha 2-adrenergic agonist that has been found to lower overactivity, aggression, and impulsivity in about 50 percent of ADHD children.[97] It also benefits children who have ADHD and tic disorders. Clonidine does not improve distractibility but may be used in combination with methylphenidate. Clonidine takes about 2 weeks to produce improvement. Its most common side effect is drowsiness, which is usually short lived. As with tricyclics, clonidine should never be stopped abruptly; doses should be carefully tapered off.

Clonidine is effective and is recommended in the treatment of ADHD (level I, recommendation A).

Combined Pharmacotherapy. Combined treatments can be used in various situations, for example, antidepressants plus a stimulant for ADHD and comorbid depression.[98] Clonidine may be given in the evening to ameliorate stimulant-induced insomnia. Clonidine, haloperidol, or pimozide may help children who have ADHD along with a tic disorder aggravated by stimulants.

The literature on combined pharmacotherapy is so sparse that no clear therapeutic guidelines can be developed (level III, recommendation C).

Psychological and Behavioral Therapies

A variety of psychological and behavioral therapies, alone and in combination, have been used in treating ADHD, with varying degrees of success. The aim of these therapies is to modify the associated problems such as oppositional defiant behavior and conduct problems.

Parent training. This training provides a variety of management strategies for the behavioral problems seen in ADHD children. A behavior modification program addresses problems such as noncompliance, defiance, and aggression. Training can be offered for individuals or groups and involves direct instruction, modeling, role playing, and discussion. Parents are taught to employ contingency management techniques and, in cooperation with the school, to use a daily report card to monitor the child's progress in areas where improvement is needed. Behavior modification for children with ADHD is most effective when administered in conjunction with stimulant medication.[99] Some studies, however, have shown that there is no significant benefit from adding parent training to the administration of medication.[100,101]

Parent training or behavior modification has not been shown to be useful adjuncts to pharmacotherapy in the treatment of ADHD (level I, recommendation C).

Classroom management. The purpose of behavior modification in the classroom is to improve classroom behavior and academic productivity. The procedures used are similar to the strategies parents learn in parent training (eg, praise and reinforcement, aggression management). The ideal classroom for the child with ADHD is highly structured and well organized, with clear expectations and a predictable schedule. The child should be seated near the teacher and away from windows and other distractions. Because children with ADHD work slowly, they should be allowed extra time to complete tests and assignments. In addition, the amount of written work should be reduced until the child is better able to cope. A daily homework planner will help develop organizational and time management skills. Parents need to communicate with teachers regularly to monitor the child's academic progress.

Classroom management in addition to medication may be helpful in managing ADHD (level III, recommendation C).

Cognitive-behavior training. This kind of training includes problem-solving and anger management. The goal of problem-solving training is to help the child with ADHD deal with impulsive behavior. The child is taught to solve a problem by saying to himself, "Stop, decide possible plans of action, carry out the plan, evaluate the success of the plan." Both parents and teachers must help the child by modeling and encouraging the use of problem-solving techniques. Used alone, this type of training is not as effective as stimulant medication or behavior modification.[102] One major problem is the difficulty children have in applying a general method to situations in which specific training has not occurred. Moreover, children tend not to use the strategies they have learned unless prompted.

Anger management training includes instruction in recognizing anger signals and using techniques like relaxation methods and coping self-statements to cope with it.

Some studies suggest that cognitive-behavior therapy may be a useful adjunct to pharmacotherapy,[103] while other investigators have questioned whether it offers any advantage over medication alone.[102,104] One randomized control trial evaluated whether an intensive 8-week behavior reinforcement and cognitive modeling program at home and school normalized the behavior of 28 children with ADHD. The study found that the program improved aggressive behavior but not attention, activity, and impulsivity while at school.[105]

Cognitive-behavior therapy or behavior modification are not useful adjuncts to pharmacotherapy in the treatment of ADHD (level I, recommendation C).

Group social skills training. Training of children and parents is helpful for children who have poor social skills and experience difficulties in peer relationships. The child is taught practical skills, such as maintaining eye contact, initiating and keeping up conversation, and cooperating. Children with ADHD are best helped by a combination of social skills training for themselves and their parents and stimulant medication.[106,107]

Social skills training involving patients and parents has resulted in improvement in social skills and peer adjustment (level I, recommendation A).

Academic intervention.   Children who have learning disabilities will require individual remedial education to optimize their learning. Parents and educators will have to decide on the best classroom placement for these children. This process is generally carried out through an individual placement and review committee at the child's school.

Unproved therapies.   Many nonstandard therapies have been tried for both ADHD and LDS. A few of these treatments are harmful, and they have not been shown to have any benefit. Orthomolecular therapies include the use of megavitamins and essential fatty acids and various restrictive diets (allergy-free, yeast-free, sucrose-restricted, salicylate-free).[108] Neurophysiologic therapies include alpha-wave conditioning, patterning, sensory integration training, optometric training, eye muscle exercises, and tinted lenses. Other therapies include anti–motion sickness therapy and chiropractic manipulation. None of these therapies have been shown to be effective when subjected to double-blind controlled clinical trials.[109,110]

These therapies are not useful and cannot be recommended for the treatment of ADHD (level I, recommendation E).

Prognosis

The symptoms of ADHD persist throughout childhood. About 70 percent of affected children continue to have the disorder in adolescence,[109] and it is more likely to persist in those who exhibit aggression or conduct problems in childhood.[110] Long-term studies have shown that 10 to 60 percent of children who have ADHD still have symptoms during adulthood.[47,48] Untreated adults, compared with controls with no school behavior problems in childhood, show an increased incidence of aggressive behavior, antisocial personality disorder, conduct disorder, depression and bipolar disorders, divorce, early school-leaving, and alcohol and drug abuse.[111] Adult ADHD is now being recognized more frequently and treated with medications similar to those for children with ADHD.

REFERENCES

1.   Siegel LS. Why we do not need intelligence test scores in the definition and analyses of learning disabilities. J Learn Disabil 1989;22:514–8.

2.   Learning disabilities: a report to the U.S. Congress, Bethesda (MD): National Institutes of Health, Interagency Committee on learning disabilities; 1987; p. 107–18.

3.   U.S. Department of Education: Thirteenth Annual Report to Congress on the Implementation of the Education of the Handicapped Act. Washington, D.C.: U.S. Government Printing Office;1991.

4.   Capin D. Developmental learning disorders: clues to their diagnosis and management. Pediatr Rev 1996;17:284–90.

5.   Shaywitz S. Dyslexia—current concepts. N Engl J Med 1998;5:307–12.

6.   Denckla MB. Academic and extracurricular aspects of nonverbal learning disabilities. Psychiatr Ann 1991;21:717–24.

7.   Harnadek M, Rourke BP. Principal identifying features of the syndrome of nonverbal learning disabilities in children. J Learn Disabil 1994;27:144–54.

8.   Semrud-Clikeman M, Hynd GW. Right hemispheric dysfunction in nonverbal learning disabilities: social, academic, and adaptive functioning in adults and children. Psychol Bul 1990;107:196–209.

9. Holbrow PL, Berry PS. Hyperactivity and learning difficulties. J Learn Disabil 1986;19:426–31.

10. Shaywitz B, Fletcher J, Shaywitz S. Attention deficit hyperactive disorder. In: Barness L, Morrow G, Rudolf A, et al, editors. Advances in pediatrics. Mosby; 1997; p. 336–41.

11. Faraone SV, Biederman J, Lehman BK, et al. Evidence for the independent familial transmission of attention deficit hyperactive disorder and learning disabilities: results from a family genetic study. Am J Psychiatry 1993;150:891–5.

12. Right hemisphere, white-matter learning disabilities associated with depression in an adolescent and young adult psychiatric population. J Nerv Ment Dis 19998;186(9):561–5.

13. A childhood learning disability that predisposes those afflicted to adolescent and adult depression and suicide risk. J Learn Disabil 1989;22:169–75.

14. Gregory JF, Shanahan T, Walberg HJ. A profile of learning disabled twelfth-graders in regular classes. Learn Disabil Q; 9:33–42.

15. Bryan M. Social problems and learning disabilities. In: Wong BY, editor. Learning about learning disabilities. San Diego: Academic Press; p. 195–229.

16. Shepherd MJ, Uhry JK. Reading disorder. Child Adolesc Psychiatr Clin N Am 1993;2:193–208.

17. Grigorenko EI, Wood FB, Meyer MS, et al. Susceptibility loci for distinct components of developmental dyslexia on chromosomes 6 and 15. Am J Hum Genet 1997;60:27–39.

18. Hynd GW, Semrud-Clikeman M. Dyslexia and brain morphology. Psychol Bull 1989;106:447–82.

19. Shaywitz SE, Shaywitz BA, Pugh KR, et al. Functional disruption in the organization of the brain for reading in dyslexia. Proc Natol Acad Sci USA 1998;95(5):2636–41.

20. Galaburda AM, Sherman GF, Rosen GD, et al. Developmental dyslexia: four consecutive cases with cortical anomalies. Ann Neurol 1985;18:222–33.

21. Rosenfeld J. Sampling academic skills. In: Fox M, Mahoney W, editors. Children with school problems: a physician's manual. Ottawa: Canadian Pediatric Society: 1998; p. 93–132.

22. Wolf M, Bally H, Morris R. Automaticity, retrieval processes, and reading: a longitudinal study in average and impaired readers. Child Dev 1986;57:988–1000.

23. Andrews D. Educational interventions. In: Fox M, Mahoney W, editors. Children with school problems: a physician's manual. Ottawa: Canadian Pediatric Society: 1998; p. 145–54.

24. Gittelman R, Feingold I. Children with reading disorders-I. Efficacy of reading remediation. J Child Psychol Psychiat 1983;24:167–91.

25. Lyon GR, Moats LC. Critical, conceptual, and methodological considerations in reading intervention research. J Learn Disabil 1997;30:578–88.

26. Feldman W. Learning disabilities. A review of available treatments. Springfield, Ill: Charles C. Thomas; 1990.

27. Elliott JL, Gentile JR. The efficacy of a mnemonic technique for learning disabled and nondisabled adolescents. J Learn Disabil 1996;19:237–41.

28. Rose MC, Cundick BP, Higbee KL. Verbal rehearsal and visual imagery: mnemonic aids for learning-disabled children. J Learn Disabil 1983;16:352–4.

29. Higgins K, Boone R. Technology as a tutor, tool, and agent for reading. J Special Edu Tech 1993;12:29–37.

30. Wise BW, Olson RK. Computer speech and the remediation of reading and spelling problems. J Special Edu Tech 1994;12:207–20.

31. Graham S, MacArthur C. Improving, learning disabled students' skills at revising essays produced on a word processor: self-instructional strategy training. J Special Edu Tech 1988;22:133–52.

32. Outhred L. Word processing: its impact on children's writing. J Learn Disabil 1989;22:262–4.

33. McIntosh R, Vaughn S, Zaragoza N. A review of social interventions for students with learning disabilities. J Learn Disabil 1991;24:451–7.

34. Feldman W. Learning disabilities. A review of available treatments. Springfield, Ill: Charles C. Thomas; 1990; p. 40.

35. Bowers DS, Clement PW, Fantuzzo JW, Sorense DA. Effects of teacher-administered and self-administered reinforcers on learning disabled children. Behav Ther 1985;16:335–69.

36. Andrews D. Behavioural management. In: Fox M, Mahoney W, editors. Children with school problems: a physician's manual. Ottawa: Canadian Pediatric Society 1998; p. 155–61.

37. Richardson E, Kupietz SS, Winsberg BG, et al. Effects of methylphenidate dosage in hyperactive reading-disabled children—II: reading achievement. J Am Acad Child Adolesc Psychiatry 1988;27:78–87.

38. Chase C, Russell G, Schmitt RL. Evaluation of the efficacy of piracetam in treating information processing, reading and writing disorders in dyslexic children. Inter J Psychophysiol 1986;4(1):41–52.

39. Fox M, Mahoney W. Children with school problems: a physician's manual. Canadian Pediatric Society; p. 176–7.

40. Silver LB. Controversial therapies. J Child Neurol 1995;10(Suppl 1):296–100.

41. Maughan B. Annotation: long-term outcomes of developmental reading problems. J Child Psychol Psychiatry 1995;36:357–71.

42. Denckla MB. The child with developmental disabilities grown up: adult residual of childhood disorders. Behav Neurol 1993;11:105–25.

43. Malcolm CB, Polatajko HJ, Simons J. A descriptive study of adults with suspected learning disabilities. J Learn Disabil 1990;23:518–20.

44. American Psychiatric Association. Diagnostic and statistical manual of mental disorders, 4th edition. Washington D.C.: American Psychiatric Association; 1994.

45. Esser G, Schmidt MH, Woerner W. Epidemiology and course of psychiatric disorders in school-age children: results of a longitudinal study. J Child Psychol Psychiatry 1990;31:243–63.

46. Bird HR, Canino G, Rubio-Stipec M, et al. Estimates of childhood and maladjustment in a community survey in Puerto Rico. Arch Gen Psychiatry 1988;45:1120–6.

47. Reiff MI, Banez GA, Culbert TP. Children who have attentional disorders: diagnosis and evaluation. Pediatr Rev 1993;14:455–64.

48. Shekim WO, Kashani J, Beck N, et al. The prevalence of attention deficit disorders in a rural midwestern community sample of nine-year-old children. J Am Acad Child Adolesc Psychiatry 1985;24:765–70.

49. Klein RG, Mannuzza S. Long-term outcome of hyperactive children: a review. J Am Acad Child Adolesc Psychiatry 1991;30:383–7.

50. Mannuzza S, Klein RG, Bessler A, et al. Adult outcome of hyperactive boys: educational achievement, occupational rank and psychiatric status. Arch Gen Psychiatry 1993;50:565–76.

51. Paternite CE, Loney J, Roberts MA. A preliminary validation of subtypes of DSM-IV attention-deficit hyperactivity disorder. J Attention Dis 1996;1:70–86.

52. Cantwell DP, Baker L. Attention deficit disorder with and without hyperactivity: a review and comparison of matched groups. J Am Acad Child Adolesc Psychiatry 1992;31:432–8.

53. Biederman MD, Newcord J, Sprich S. Comorbidity of attention deficit hyperactivity disorder with conduct, depressive, anxiety and other disorders. Am J Psychiatry 1991;148:564–77.

54. Pliszka S. Comorbidity of attention deficit hyperactive disorder with psychiatric disorder: an overview. 1998;59(Suppl 17):50–8.

55. Barkley RA. Attention deficit hyperactivity disorder: a handbook for diagnosis and treatment. New York, NY: Guilford Press; 1990; p. 75–7.

56. Jensen PS, Martin D, Cantwell DP. Comorbidity in ADD: implications for research, practice, and DSM-IV. J Am Acad Child Adolesc Psychiatry 1997;36:1065–79.

57. Gilger JW, Pennington BF, DeFries JC. A twin study of the etiology of comorbidity: attention deficit hyperactive disorder and dyslexia. J Am Acad Child Adolesc Psychiatry 1992;31:343–8.

58. Barkley R, McMurray M, Edelbrock C, et al. Side effects of MPH in children with attention deficit hyperactive disorder: a systematic placebo-controlled evaluation. Pediatrics 1990;86:184–92.

59. Anderson JC, Williams S, McGee R, et al. DSM-III disorders in preadolescent children: prevalence in a large community sample. Arch Gen Psychiatry 1987;44:69–76.

60. Faraone SV, Biederman J, Mennin D, et al. Attention deficit hyperactive disorder with bipolar disorder: a familial subtype? J Am Acad Child Adolesc Psychiatry 1997;36:1378–87.

61. Biederman J, Faraone SV, Chen WJ. Social adjustment inventory for children and adolescents: concurrent validity in ADHD children. J Am Acad Child Adolesc Psychiatry 1993;32:1059–64.

62. Plizka SR. Effect of anxiety on cognition, behavior, and stimulant response in ADHD. J Am Acad Child Adolesc Psychiatry 1989;28:873–81 .

63. Reeves JC, Werry JS, Elking GS, et al. Attention deficit, conduct, oppositional, and anxiety disorders in children—II: clinical characteristics. J Am Acad Child Adolesc Psychiatry 1987;26:144–55.

64. McGee R, Williams S, Silva PA. Behavioural and developmental characteristics of aggressive, hyperactive, and aggressive-hyperactive boys. J Am Acad Child Adolesc Psychiatry 1984;23:270–9.

65. Mannuzza S, Klein RG, Konig PH, et al. Hyperactive boys almost grown up—IV: criminality and its relationship to psychiatric status. Arch Gen Psychiatry 1992;49:728–38.

66. Biederman J, Faraone SV, Keenan K, et al. Further evidence for family-genetic risk factors in attention deficit hyperactive disorder (ADHD): patterns of comorbidity in probands and relatives in psychiatrically and pediatrically referred samples. Arch Gen Psychiatry 1992;49:728–38.

67. Lopez RE. Hyperactivity in twins. Can Psychiatr Assoc J 1965;10:421–6.

68. Cook EH, Stein MA, Krasowski MD, et al. Association of attention deficit disorder and the dopamine transporter gene. Am J Hum Genet 1995;56:993–8.

69. LaHoste GJ, Swanson JM, Wigal SB, et al. Dopamine D4 receptor gene polymorphism is associated with attention deficit hyperactive disorder. Mol Psychiatry 1996;1:1–4.

70. Zametkin A, Nordahl T, Gross M, et al. Cerebral glucose metabolism in adults with hyperactivity of childhood onset. N Engl J Med 1990;323(20):1361–6.

71. Cerebrospinal fluid homovanillic acid predicts behavioral response to stimulants in 45 boys with attention deficit/hyperactivity disorder. Neuropsychopharmacology 1996;14(2):125–37.

72. Castellanos FX, Giedd JN, Marsh WL, et al. Quantitative brain magnetic resonance imaging in attention deficit hyperactive disorder. Arch Gen Psychiatry 1996;53:607–16.

73. Giedd JN, Castelanos FX, Korzuch P, et al. Quantitative morphology of the corpus callosum in attention deficit hyperactive disorder. Am J Psychiatry 1994;151:665–9.

74. Hynd GW, Semrud-Clikeman M, Lorys AR, et al. Brain morphology in developmental dyslexia and attention deficit hyperactive disorder. Arch Neurol 1990;919–26.

75. Attention deficits and autistic spectrum problems in children exposed to alcohol during gestation: a follow-up study. Develop Med Child Neurol 1997;39(9):583–7.

76. Wender EH, Solanto MV. Effects of sugar on aggressive and inattentive behavior in children with attention deficit disorder with hyperactivity and normal children. Pediatrics 1991;88:960–6.

77. Phelan TW. All about attention deficit disorder. In: Child management. Illinois: Glen Ellyn; 1993.

78. Conners CK. A teaching rating scale for use in drug studies with children. Am J Psychiatry 1969;126:884–888.

79. Bain LJ. A parent's guide to attention deficit disorders. New York, NY: Dell;1991.

80. DuPaul GJ, Anastopoulos AD, Shelson TL, et al. Multimethod assessment of attention deficit hyperactive disorder: the diagnostic utility of clinic-based tests. J Clin Child Psychol 1992;21:194–402.

81. Pelham WE, Murphy HA. Attention deficit and conduct disorders. In: Hersen M, editor. Pharmacological and behavioral treatments: an integrative approach. New York, NY: John Wiley & Sons Inc; 1986; p. 108–48.

82. Richters JE, Arnold LE, Jensen PS, et al. NIMH Collaborative multi-site multimodal treatment study of children with ADHD—I: background and rationale. J Am Acad Child Adolesc Psychiatry 1995;34:987–1000.

83. Swanson JM. Effect of stimulant medication on children with attention deficit disorder: a "review of reviews." Exceptional Child 1993;60:154–62.

84. Bosco J, Robin S. Hyperkinesis: prevalence and treatment. In: Whalen C, Henker B, editors. Hyperkinetic children: the social ecology of identification and treatment. New York, NY: Academic Press; 1980; p. 173–87.

85. Greenhill L. Attention deficit hyperactive disorder: the stimulants. Child Adolesc Psychiatric Clin N Am 1995;4:123–68.

86. Elia J. Drug treatment of hyperactive children: therapeutic guidelines. Drugs 1993;46:863–71.

87. Elia J, Borcherding BG, Rapoport JL, et al. Methylphenidate and dextroamphetamine treatments of hyperactivity: are there true nonresponders? Psychiatry Res 1991;36:141–55.

88. Cantwell DP. Therapeutic management of attention deficit hyperactive disorder: participant workbook. New York, NY: SCP Communications 1994; p. 4–20.

89. Kavale K. The efficiency of stimulant drug treatment for hyperactivity: a meta-analysis. J Learn Disabil 1982;15:280–9.

90. Ahmann PA, Waltonen SJ, Olson RA, et al. Placebo-controlled evaluation of Ritalin side effects. Pediatrics 1993;91:1101–6.

91. Gillberg C, Melander H, Von Knorrins AL, et al. Long-term stimulant treatment of children with attention deficit hyperactivity disorder symptoms. Arch Gen Psychiatry 1997;54:857–64.

92. Sprague RL, Sleator EK. Methylphenidate in hyperkinetic children: differences in dose effects on learning and social behavior. Science 1977;198:1274–6.

93. Greenhill LL, Setterberg S. Pharmacotherapy of disorders of adolescents. Psychiatr Clin North Am 1993;16:793–814.

94. Safer DJ, Allen RP, Barr E. Growth rebound after termination of stimulant drugs. J Pediatr 1975;86:113–6.

95. Gadow KD, Sverd J, Sprafkin J, et al. Efficacy of methylphenidate for attention deficit hyperactive disorder in children with tic disorder. Arch Gen Psychiatry 1995;52:444–55.

96. Biederman J, Baldessarini RJ, Wright V, et al. A double-blind placebo-controlled study of desipramine in the treatment of ADD: I. Efficacy. J Am Acad Child Adolesc Psychiatry 1989;28:777–84.

97. Hunt RD, Minderaa RB, Cohen DJ. Clonidine benefits children with attention deficit hyperactive disorder: report of a double-blind placebo-crossover therapeutic trial. J Am Acad Child Adolesc Psychiatry 1985;24:617–29.

98. Gammon GD, Brown TE. Fluoxetine augmentation of methylphenidate for attention deficit and comorbid disorders. J Child Adolesc Psychopharmacol 1993;3:1–10.

99. American Academy of Child and Adolescent Psychiatry: practice parameters for the assessment and treatment of children, adolescents and adults with attention deficit hyperactive disorder. J Am Acad Child Psychiatry 1997;36(Suppl):85–121.

100. Firestone P, Kelly MJ, Goodman T, Davey J. Differential effects of parent training and stimulant medication with hyperactives. J Amer Acad Child Psychiatry 1981;20:135–47.

101. Gittelman-Klein R, Klein D, Abikoff H, et al. Relative efficacy of methylphenidate and behavior modification in hyperkinetic children: an interim report. J Abnor Child Psychol 1976;4:361–79.

102. Brown RT, Wynne ME, Borden KA, et al. Methylphenidate and cognitive therapy in children with attention deficit disorder. A double-blind trial. Dev Behav Pediatr 1986;7:163–70.

103. Hinshaw SP, Henker B, Whalen CK. Cognitive-behavioral and pharmacologic interventions in hyperactive boys: comparative and combined effects. J Consult Clin Psychol 1984;52:739–49.

104. Abikoff H, Gittelman R. Hyperactive children treated with stimulants. Is cognitive training a useful adjunct? Arch Gen Psychiatry 1985;42(10):953–61.

105. Abikoff H, Gittelman R. Does behavior therapy normalize the classroom behavior of hyperactive children. Arch Gen Psychiatry 1984;41:449–54.

106. Frankel F, Myatt R, Cantwell DP, Feinberg DT. Parent-assisted transfer of children's social skills training: effects on children with and without attention-deficit hyperactivity disorder. J Am Acad Child Adolesc Psychiatry 1997;36(8):1056–64.

107. Pfiffner LJ, McBurnett K. Social skills training with parent generalization: treatment effects for children with attention deficit disorder. J Consult Clin Psychol 1997;65(5):749–57.

108. National Advisory Committee on Hyperkinesis and Food Additives. Final Report to the Nutrition Foundation, October 1980. New York, NY: Nutrition Foundation; 1980.

109. Barkley R, Fischer M, Edelbroch C, et al. The adolescent outcome of hyperactive children diagnosed by research criteria: an 8 year prospective follow-up. J Am Acad Child Adolesc Psychiatry 1990;29:546–57.

110. Gittelman R, Mannuzza S, Shenker R, et al. Hyperactive boys almost grown up—I: psychiatric status. Arch Gen Psychiatry 1985;42:937–47.

111. Mannuzza S, Klein RG, Bessler A, et al. Adult outcome of hyperactive boys. Educational achievement, occupational rank, and psychiatric status. Arch Gen Psychiatry 1993; 50:567–76.

CHAPTER 23

Challenges in Adolescent Health

Debra K. Katzman, MD, FRCPC
Katherine A. Leonard, MD, FRCPC
Eudice Goldberg, MD, FRCPC

In the typical adolescent medicine clinic, the clinician encounters young people with complex problems and situations. The clinician may discuss contraception preferences with a 12-year-old girl who has recently become sexually active, inform a homeless adolescent female that she has a positive pregnancy test and help her consider various options, determine that a 15-year-old girl with severe menorrhagia has a hemoglobin level of 6 mg/dL, or discuss safer sex with a 17-year-old gay adolescent male infected with the human immunodeficiency virus, to name but a few of the possibilities.

These clinical experiences pose challenging questions about prevention and screening, diagnoses, treatment, prognosis, cost-effectiveness, and a host of other health-related issues. The busy clinician is faced with the daunting task of solving unique clinical problems, keeping up with the expanding body of sound external clinical evidence, and ultimately providing optimal patient care. Although the field of adolescent medicine is relatively young, it is growing rapidly, in large part because of the increasing knowledge available from clinical-care research that involves young people. The direct application of this growing body of evidence from research on adolescents to everyday clinical decisions is an opportunity for health-care providers to practice evidence-based adolescent medicine.

Evidence-based adolescent medicine can help clinicians deal with diverse adolescent health issues and make successful clinical decisions by integrating three important components: (1) an understanding of the adolescent's unique circumstances, (2) the health-care provider's clinical expertise, and (3) the best available research evidence.[1] To care for adolescents, the clinician must understand their role in making clinical decisions about their own health care and their unique circumstances: their rights, personal values, cultural beliefs and preferences, experiences, and education about making clinical decisions about their health care. The clinician's expertise is the proficiency and judgment acquired through the actual care of adolescent patients, as well as the advanced knowledge provided by continuing medical education. Current best–evidence research must also form an integral part of clinical decisions. Clinicians must formulate clear clinical questions, efficiently review the relevant literature that may bear on these questions, and correctly interpret the literature as it applies to the clinical situation so that, ultimately, they can provide optimal patient care. It is only by combining these three important components in our clinical practice of adolescent medicine that we will be able to deal with complex adolescent health issues adequately and make successful clinical decisions.[2–3]

Unlike adult medicine,[4] however, the extent to which evidence-based medicine is practiced in adolescent medicine has not been studied. The same principles should apply to both: evidence-based adolescent medicine is necessary to guide our clinical decisions to ensure that we ultimately do more good than harm to our adolescent patients.[5] Yet researchers, clinicians, and other decision makers must temper their use of these principles with the realization that adolescents, as a group, are not a homogenous clinical population and that they have unique biologic factors that distinguish them from children and adults. Consequently, these factors call into question the validity of extrapolating the results of trials undertaken in younger children or adults to adolescents.

Adolescent medicine is an exciting and challenging area in which to undertake clinical research. A diverse, heterogenous group, like adults, adolescents may have different sexual orientations or come from different ethnic and cultural backgrounds or at-risk, disabled, or marginalized populations. Other challenges include recruiting and retaining the full spectrum of adolescents for clinical trials; for example, adolescents with chronic illnesses tend to be more complicated than healthy adolescents; homeless adolescents have no fixed address and are more difficult to track down than adolescents from more traditional homes; adolescents with sexually transmitted diseases may prefer to receive treatment from anonymous and easily accessible clinics than university-based hospitals where clinical trials often take place; and adolescents with disabilities often feel more comfortable in their own community with their familiar social networks and supports than in a university health-care center where they may be involved in research studies.

The integration of evidence-based medicine into the routine clinical practice of adolescent medicine is a work in progress and will continue to increase with the generation of high-quality, easily accessible evidence. In this chapter, we present some common clinical scenarios often encountered in the practice of adolescent medicine that illustrate the potential use and the limitations of evidence-based approaches based on the currently available literature.

EXAMPLES OF EVIDENCE-BASED APPROACHES IN ADOLESCENT MEDICINE

Confidentiality

Background

One of the most important barriers to adolescents' use of health care is the issue of maintaining confidentiality.[6] Confidentiality is a basic principle and an important part of good quality care of the adolescent.[7] Consensus among major medical associations such as the American Medical Association,[8,9] the Canadian Pediatric Society,[10,11] The Society for Adolescent Medicine,[12,13] and the American Academy of Pediatrics[15] emphasizes that adolescents should have access to confidential care. The Adolescent Medicine Committee of the Canadian Pediatric Society in its Statements on Sexuality Education[12] and Office Practice Guidelines for the Care of Adolescents[11] emphasizes the importance of the clinician discussing and maintaining the confidentiality of patients' information with their adolescent patients. The American Academy of Pediatrics Policy Statement on Confidentiality in Adolescent Health Care states that, generally, adolescents underuse health-care resources, partially because of a lack of confidentiality, which is a significant barrier to adolescents' access to health care.[14] The Society for Adolescent Medicine's Position Paper on Access to Health Care for Adolescents includes confidentiality as one of the seven criteria for improving the adolescent's access to health care.[12]

Despite these recommendations, providers caring for adolescents are regularly challenged to maintain confidentiality and promote an appropriate private exchange of sensitive information between the adolescent and the provider. An example of such a scenario is outlined below.

Sample Case

A 15-year-old sexually active girl comes to your clinic requesting the oral contraceptive pill for birth control. A brief menstrual and sexual history reveals that menarche and the onset of sexual activity occurred at 12 years of age. She reports regular menses and rare condom use. She has used no other methods of birth control and has had a total of four sexual partners. She has never had a complete gynecologic examination and has never been tested for a sexually transmitted disease. Her mother, who is waiting for her in the waiting room, thinks that the reason her daughter has come to your clinic is to get some help for menstrual cramps. The patient does not want her mother to know the real reason for her visit to your office today.

Discussion

An important question that arises from this scenario is whether providing confidential health care in this instance will encourage this young girl to seek medical attention later when her parent or parents are not involved. The health-care provider is faced with the dilemma of whether or not to provide this young girl with confidential health care.

Surveys of adolescents have shown that young people are more likely to seek health care if they believe that the health-care providers will keep the details of the visit confidential.[15] Adolescents report that they are less likely to communicate with a physician or may even forgo health care because of concerns of confidentiality around sensitive health issues such as sexual behaviors, substance use, and mental health.

To date, only one randomized controlled trial (RCT) has investigated the issue of adolescents' concerns about confidentiality and their effect on care-seeking behavior.[16] This RCT tested whether the influence of physician assurances of confidentiality had an impact on the adolescents' willingness to disclose information and seek future health care. Adolescents were randomly assigned to one of three tape-recorded scenarios depicting an office visit during which they heard a physician who assured unconditional confidentiality, a physician who assured conditional confidentiality, or a physician who did not mention confidentiality. Otherwise, the groups were treated equally. The adolescents' willingness to disclose general information and information about sensitive topics, intended honesty, and the likelihood of return visits to the physician depicted in the scenario were assessed with an anonymous written questionnaire. Of the 615 students present on the date of the collection of the data, 568 students were eligible for randomization, and 562 (mean age, 14.9 years ± 0.82 SD) completed the study. All researchers were blinded to the experimental manipulation. The three experimental groups were similar at the start of the trial; differences in the sociodemographic variables and past experiences among the groups were not significant. Analysis of the data supported the hypothesis that assurances of confidentiality from a physician would influence adolescents' stated intentions to disclose sensitive information about sexuality, substance use, and mental health and would increase the number willing to seek future health care.

It is easy to see how the results of this single RCT could be used to influence our clinical decision-making in this case about confidentiality in adolescent health care. The study, however, has some potential limitations. First, whether adolescents' responses to the simulated scenarios depicted in this study would actually take place in a real-life clinical situation remains unknown. Although there is much skepticism about what adolescents say on a questionnaire and what they actually do in real-life situations, there is evidence[17] that adolescents' reported intentions are at least partially predictive of their behaviors. The ability to generalize the results of this study is also unknown. Second, the study population was derived from a school population of primarily white students of middle-to-high socioeconomic status. We do not know whether the outcome would be different in another setting or with a different adolescent population. Finally, the authors of this clinical trial present a scripted scenario with unconditional guarantees of confidentiality. This is clearly unrealistic since professionals have both ethical and legal obligations that require them to notify parents or other adults when the adolescent's life or well-being is at risk or if the adolescent is at risk of hurting someone else. In this trial, the adolescents who heard a scripted explanation of conditional confidentiality were less willing to seek future health care for common health issues than the adolescents who were not told the legal limitation of confidentiality.[16] Surprisingly, these same authors report in another study[17] that most primary-care physicians who discuss confidentiality with adolescents assure them of unconditional confidentiality.

This RCT supports the fact that adolescents' stated intentions are to communicate with and seek health care from physicians who assure confidentiality. On the basis of RCT[16] and the recommendations of professional organizations,[8,14,19] clinicians should discuss issues of confidentiality with their adolescent patients and their parents and include in these discussions a description of the limitations of confidentiality. Clinicians providing health care to adolescents need to be familiar with the legal and ethical limitations of confidentiality that are specific to this age group as well as with the conditions inherent in their respective health-care systems that may hinder confidential adolescent care.

Anorexia Nervosa and Osteopenia

Background

Anorexia nervosa (AN) is a complex illness that affects adolescents: 0.5 percent of girls between 15 and 19 years develop the disorder.[20–23] Anorexia nervosa is characterized by self-imposed starvation. Adolescents may refuse to maintain an appropriate body weight for their age and height or may fail to gain weight as they grow. These young people have an intense fear of gaining weight or becoming fat and a disturbance in the way they experience their body shape, weight, and size. Another sign of the disorder is the absence of at least three consecutive menstrual cycles in postmenarchal females.[24] While the exact etiology of AN remains unknown, the consensus is that the origins of this illness are multidimensional.[25]

Clinicians caring for adolescents will likely encounter patients with AN and need to be aware of the serious medical complications that result from the effects of voluntary starvation.[26] Among the earliest and most serious complications is peak bone-mass reduction.[27] If the bone mass acquired is inadequate or the loss of bone mass is excessive, significant reduction in bone mass occurs. This reduction in bone mass for age and sex is called osteopenia.

Osteopenia, a major cause of morbidity in adolescents with AN,[28] was first demonstrated in a study by Bachrach and colleagues.[28] They compared the bone mass of adolescents with AN (12 to 20 years of age) with that of a healthy control group by means of dual-energy x-ray absorptiometry (DEXA). Adolescents with AN had significantly lower lumbar vertebral bone density and whole-body bone mass than the controls. The bone density of two-thirds of the young girls with AN was less than normal value for their age by more than 2 standard deviations. Half these girls had received a diagnosis of AN less than 1 year earlier. Bone mineral density (BMD) correlated significantly with body mass index (BMI) in both the control group and the adolescents with AN. In addition, age at onset and the duration of AN correlated significantly with BMD. This was the first study to conclude that important deficits of bone mass occur as a frequent and often early complication of AN in adolescence.

The extent to which osteopenia in AN is reversible remains uncertain. A prospective longitudinal follow-up study[29] (12 to 16 months) of the spine and whole body with DEXA was undertaken in 15 adolescent patients with AN who were being treated in a tertiary-care pediatric eating disorder program. Bone mineral density of the lumbar spine did not change significantly, whereas whole-body BMD increased. Despite gains in bone mineral, eight patients had osteopenia of the spine or whole body or both. Changes in weight, height, and BMI were significant predictors of changes in BMD. Increased bone mass occurred with weight gain before the return of menses; conversely, weight loss was associated with further decreases in bone density. In this same report, another group of nine women who had recovered from AN during adolescence were also studied. All nine had normal whole-body BMD for their age, but three had osteopenia of the lumbar spine.

Both the longitudinal follow-up study and the cohort study of weight-restored women suggest that osteopenia in adolescents with AN reflects bone loss, perhaps combined with decreased bone accretion. Weight rehabilitation results in increased BMD before the return of menses. The persistence of osteopenia after recovery indicates that deficits in BMD acquired during adolescence may not be completely reversible.

There is no question that young girls with AN are at particular risk for osteopenia and may require intervention to prevent the ongoing progression of bone loss. However, the management of osteopenia in adolescents with AN remains unknown. The following scenario outlines these issues.

Sample Case

Ellen is a 16-year old adolescent with an 18-month history of AN. She has been followed up in your office, and her weight has not changed over the past 1 year; she remains below the 3rd percentile for her weight and at the 25th percentile for her height. Ellen's menarche was at age 11 years. Her menstrual periods were every 28 days and lasted 4 or 5 days. Her last normal menstrual period was 2 years ago. She denies ever having been sexually active. She denies having been sexually or physically abused. She feels that she is currently at an adequate weight but would like to lose another 5 kg (11 lb). She feels that her hips and thighs are too fat. You recently did a DEXA study and found that her lumbar and whole-body BMD were reduced. She is wondering what she can do about her BMD status; she has heard from one of the people in her psychoeducation group that hormone replacement therapy (HRT) would help her bones.

Discussion

This scenario raises the clinical question about what types of therapy are efficacious in the treatment and prevention of osteopenia in adolescents with AN.

Ellen, like other young girls with AN, is at risk for osteopenia.[28] There are several reasons for this. First, AN most commonly occurs during adolescence, a period of life when the rate of bone-mass acquisition is higher than in adulthood. Anorexia nervosa interrupts normal bone-mineral accretion and thus influences peak bone mass, defined as the highest level of bone mass achieved as a result of normal growth. Peak bone mass is important because it provides the bone reserve needed later in life.[30] Second, the nutritional intake (both general nutrition and calcium intake) required to achieve peak bone mass is reduced in patients with AN. Third, all patients with AN have hypothalamic-pituitary hypogonadism. Estrogen deficiency is thought to be a major risk factor for young women with AN, just as it is for postmenopausal women. Bone is a sex steroid–dependent tissue. There is a rapid increase in bone mass during puberty and a corresponding decrease in bone mass during menopause. The role of estrogen in the pathogenesis of postmenopausal bone loss is well established, whereas the role of estrogen in bone-mass acquisition is not completely understood. Furthermore, patients with AN are known to have high levels of circulating glucocorticoids.[31-34] A complication of glucocorticoid excess in children and adults is osteoporosis.[35] Finally, low body weight can also lead to low bone mass.[29] All these proposed mechanisms probably contribute simultaneously to the bone deficits described in patients with AN.

Since improvement in nutrition, weight restoration, and the return of normal hypothalamic-pituitary-ovarian function are not immediately and easily accomplished in adolescents with AN, many have advocated the use of HRT to prevent and perhaps reverse the osteopenia. Hormone replacement therapy is the first-line pharmacologic therapy for the treatment of established osteoporosis in postmenopausal women. It is fundamental in preventing osteopenia because it slows osteoclastic activity, thus preventing bone resorption.[36] In postmenopausal women, oral and transdermal estrogen decreases bone loss, reduces the incidence of fracture, and prevents loss of height. Recent studies[37] of postmenopausal women have demonstrated that HRT decreases bone loss and is associated with the highest BMD of all other regimens. Together, these findings suggest that HRT may confer skeletal protection in young girls with AN.

In preliminary studies[38,39] of amenorrheic adolescents with AN, HRT did not effectively improve BMD. Kreipe and colleagues[39] found that bone biopsies in a small number of patients with AN suggested that the use of estrogen replacement therapy without an accompanying weight gain was unlikely to protect bone mass. Seeman and colleagues[40] reported that the lumbar BMD of women with AN taking oral contraceptives was significantly higher than that of patients not supplemented with estrogen, although the BMD in both groups remained below normal for age.

Currently, only one RCT[41] has looked at the effects of estrogen administration on women with AN. Forty-eight women (mean age 24.9 ± 6.9 years) were randomized to receive HRT (either estrogen [0.625 mg/day, days 1 to 25] and progestin replacement [5 mg, days 16 to 25]) or an oral contraceptive containing 35 μg ethinyl estradiol), or no replacement. Spinal trabecular bone density was measured every 6 months for a mean of 1.5 years. The estrogen-treated group had no significant change in BMD, compared with the control group. However, patients with a less than 70 percent initial ideal body weight who were treated with estrogen had a 4.0 percent increase in mean BMD; controls (with a comparable low initial body weight) had a 20.1 percent decrease in BMD. This study supports the benefits of HRT in a subset of very low-weight women with AN.

This study has some limitations, including its small sample size, short intervention period, dose of estrogen administered to these premenopausal women and lack of information about monitoring compliance. In addition, the mean age of the study population was 24.9 ± 6.9 years, which is substantially older than that of an adolescent population. Whether the outcome would be different for an adolescent population needs to be determined.

So far, no existing evidence suggests that HRT is effective for the treatment and prevention of osteopenia in adolescents with AN. Long-term follow-up RCTs in adolescents with AN are needed to gain more knowledge about osteopenia and its treatment and prevention with HRT.

There are no long-term studies that have investigated the effect of calcium supplementation in young people with AN. It is apparent that healthy adolescent females are consuming substantially less calcium than recommended by current dietary intake standards.[42] Several studies have indicated that adolescents may gain more bone mass if they increase their intake of calcium. A number of relatively short (12 months to 3 years) clinical trials[43–49] with calcium supplements in children and adolescents indicate that calcium increases bone mass in healthy young people. Calcium supplementation during skeletal formation may contribute to both an increase in peak bone-mass acquisition and prevention of fractures during growth.[30] Other studies[48,49] suggest that the gains noted during the trial of supplementation were no longer detectable once the calcium supplementation ceased. These gains may not persist after the intervention is discontinued.

The role of calcium intake on BMD in patients with AN is unknown. Calcium consumption by adolescents with AN is less than the recommended dietary allowance.[28,29] A number of studies[28,50,51] have found no correlation between BMD and daily calcium intake in patients with AN. Patient compliance with dietary therapy as well as the validity of dietary recall are issues of concern in these studies.[28,51,52]

Long-term intervention studies with calcium supplementation in patients with AN are required. Until that time, however, patient recommendations should be based on our current understanding of bone mineralization and calcium intake in healthy children and adolescents. Since adolescents with AN are at increased risk for the development of skeletal inadequacy, it may be reasonable to recommend a calcium intake of 1,500 mg/day, the current standard of the National Institute of Health for the period of adolescent growth and development.[53] The recommended calcium supplement is calcium carbonate because it is inexpensive, easily absorbed, and available in a variety of forms (including chewable tablets, capsules, and effervescent forms).[36] Adolescents with AN need to maintain a diet that is rich in calcium (eg, dairy products, vegetables such as broccoli and collard greens, and sardines) as well as having sufficient calories and other nutrients for growth and development.

Published reports on the contribution of physical activity to BMD in healthy young people and in patients with AN present conflicting results. Most cross-sectional and prospective studies[54–57] of children and adolescents show a positive correlation between activity level and BMD. There are, however, conflicting findings about whether regular physical activity during childhood and adolescence has long-term benefits on BMD in adulthood. In their longitudinal study of the relationships among childhood growth, lifestyle, and peak bone mass in 153 young women, Cooper and colleagues[58] examined BMD at the lumbar spine and femoral neck, using DEXA and answers to questionnaires about previous and actual physical exercise. The authors concluded that physical activity in childhood was the major lifestyle determinant of peak bone mass in women. In contrast, a cross-sectional twin study[59] that quantified the role of genetic and lifestyle factors on bone mass in adolescent and young adult women found that physical activity did not have an impact on bone mass.

There may be several reasons for the conflicting conclusions of these two studies. Differences in study population and research methods may account for the disparate findings. These studies differ in the type, amount, and duration of exercise studied, use of randomization, controls, subject compliance, and emphasis on the choice of measurement site in the protocol.

Although the literature generally suggests that regular physical activity improves the skeletal development of healthy children and adolescents, the role of exercise in the prevention of low bone mass in adolescents with AN has not been established. Some studies[51] have reported that exercise may help protect patients with AN against osteopenia, whereas others[28,52] report the contrary. Consequently, no definitive recommendations about exercise for adolescents with AN are currently possible.

The type, quantity, intensity, frequency, and duration of activity that best promotes bone density are also currently unknown. The exercise therapy most physicians prescribe to prevent bone loss has been weight-bearing exercises, such as walking, jogging, and dancing.[60] Recent evidence[61] suggests that the effect of different types of exercise may not have a homogenous effect on the skeleton but, rather, are specific to the skeletal region stimulated by the selected activity. Regardless, exercise for young people with AN requires close monitoring, since any positive effects of physical activity may be diminished or lost by a combination of slow weight gain or weight loss, dietary restrictions, and amenorrhea in young girls.[62–66]

Bone formation and remodeling are influenced by body weight. Bone mass correlates positively with body weight and BMI in healthy adolescents and in those with AN.[29] Weight rehabilitation is an effective means of increasing BMD in adolescents with AN.[29] Increases in BMI result in increased bone mineralization, even before the return of menses.[29] At present, nutritional rehabilitation and weight gain with the resumption of normal spontaneous menses are the treatments of choice for the restoration of bone mass in adolescents with AN.

Reduction of Risk for Human Immunodeficiency Virus Infection in Adolescents

Background

Over the past decade, physicians and other health-care providers concerned with adolescent health issues have grown increasingly alarmed about the AIDS epidemic and the impact of human immunodeficiency virus (HIV) infection on the adolescent population. On the basis of the information obtained from seroprevalence studies, coupled with a greater understanding of the epidemiology of HIV infection, it is clear that HIV infection poses a major health threat to adolescents. In 1995, Hein and colleagues,[67] writing about the large proportion of young people infected with HIV worldwide, reported that the World Health Organization (WHO) estimated that half the 14 million people with HIV worldwide were infected between the ages of 15 and 24 years. According to data compiled by the UNAIDS/WHO Working Group on Global HIV/AIDS and Sexually Transmitted Disease (STD) Surveillance,[68] as of December 1997, this estimate has climbed to more than 30 million people. The majority of these in most parts of the world are between 15 and 24 years old.

In Canada, although the total number of teenagers with AIDS is relatively low, approximately 20 percent of people with AIDS are between 20 and 29 years of age.[69] Given that the incubation period from the start of the infection to the development of clinical signs and symptoms of the disease is usually measured in years, many of those with disease in early adulthood were infected with the virus as teenagers. In the United States, although the overall incidence of HIV infection declined in the early 1990s compared with that of the mid-1980s, heterosexual transmission increased during this same time period.[70] Rosenberg and Biggar[70] assessed national trends in the incidence of HIV in young people in the United States, using a statistical method known as back-calculation. When they compared people in successive birth cohorts who have become adults since the onset of the HIV epidemic in 1978, they found that younger cohorts became infected with HIV more frequently as teenagers, that this higher incidence in the younger cohort occurred irrespective of sex, race, ethnicity, or exposure group, and that HIV infection in young people attributed to heterosexual contact increased during this time period. The adolescent population is clearly at high risk for HIV infection. Intensive interventions to modify high-risk behaviors are warranted. The following case scenarios illustrate these issues.

Sample Cases

Case 1.   James is a 15-year-old boy, who has been living on the street on and off for the past 1 year. He has come to a walk-in clinic because he heard that a girl he had had sexual intercourse with was recently told that she had tested positive for HIV; he was concerned that he might also be infected. James has been in and out of foster care since he was 8 years old, when he was removed from his biological family because of a history of abuse. At 14 years of age, he ran away from his foster home and has been on the streets or in various group homes or shelters ever since. He is unsure of the number of sexual partners he has had during this time—he thinks he has had at least 20. He denies having engaged in "survival sex" (a young person involved in prostitution activities to financially support himself/herself) but does admit to "getting high" before having sex on several occasions. He has tried using condoms but cannot afford to buy them regularly. He has had only heterosexual relationships that involved anal sex on occasion, as well as oral and vaginal sex. He admits to smoking marijuana and crack cocaine and also to taking LSD when he has the opportunity. He does not like to drink alcohol because he says it makes him sick. He denies any intravenous drug use. He has no knowledge of the drug and sexual practices of his partners.

Case 2.   Jennifer is a 16-year-old girl, who has been monitored by her pediatrician all her life and has never had any major health problems. She is a good student, lives at home with her parents and two siblings, and has aspirations to go to university and become a veterinarian. Over the past 1 year, she started seeing a boy in her class. They have been having vaginal intercourse for the past few months. She has been reluctant to approach her pediatrician before now to discuss birth control because she has been worried that he might be upset with her. She has not used condoms, other than on one occasion, because her boyfriend says they make intercourse less pleasurable for him. She has never used any drugs and does not think that her boyfriend has either, although she has never really discussed the matter with him. She does not know if he has ever had any other sexual partners. She is very worried that she might be pregnant because her period is 1 week late. She is also concerned about sexually transmitted infections (STIs), especially HIV.

Discussion

Both these case scenarios raise important clinical questions about the risk of HIV infection, as well as about the potential of interventional strategies to reduce this risk. There is a vast and growing literature in the area of HIV prevention and risk-reduction interventions for adolescents. Assuming that neither of these teenagers is yet HIV positive, the question of whether anything can be done to reduce their risk for HIV infection in the future should be of the highest priority. Although the two cases are very different, they both illustrate risk factors for HIV infection. The identified high-risk activities include unprotected intercourse, multiple sexual partners, concurrent drug use, and lack of knowledge of the partners' sexual and drug histories.

Although risk-taking is a normal developmental feature of adolescence, certain high-risk behaviors can have devastating long-term consequences, such as infection with the AIDS virus. Teenagers are developmentally inclined to experimentation, which includes health-risk behaviors such as early sexual activity and drug use.[71] High-risk sexual activities and drug use contribute to increase the risk of HIV infection.[67,72–80] Because of these risk factors, many adolescent populations have been the target of intervention strategies[79,81–104] that attempt to increase adolescents' knowledge about HIV infection, change their attitudes, and reduce their risk-taking behaviors. These have ranged from AIDS education and counseling interventions in physicians' offices to implementing intervention strategies in outreach settings and evaluating their effectiveness. Specific high-risk adolescent populations have been targeted, including runaways, inner-city teenagers, incarcerated youth, and substance-using adolescents.

Informative work has been done in the school system. For example, Kirby and colleagues[85] reviewed the effectiveness of 23 school-based intervention strategies that met the inclusion criteria of having (1) been implemented in the schools, (2) been published in peer-reviewed journals, and (3) reported sexual or contraceptive behaviors or their outcomes. Both experimental and quasiexperimental studies were reviewed by a panel of experts. In some, subjects were randomly assigned to an intervention or interventions; in others, they were not. The authors concluded that the interventions that were most effective in changing HIV knowledge, attitudes, and behavior were those with "(1) theoretical grounding in social learning or social influence theories, (2) a narrow focus on reducing specific sexual risk-taking behaviors, (3) experiential activities to convey the information on the risk of unprotected sex and how to avoid those risks and to personalize that information, (4) instruction on social influences and pressures, (5) reinforcement of individual values and group norms against unprotected sex that are age and experience appropriate, and (6) activities to increase relevant skills and confidence in those skills."

In 1996, the meta-analysis of the HIV-prevention literature based on social learning theory done by Kalichman and colleagues[92] discerned four requirements for behavioral change: (1) accurate information to increase awareness and knowledge of the risks associated with specific behaviors, (2) social and self-management skills, (3) enhancement of skills and development of self-efficacy, and (4) social supports and reinforcements for behavior changes.

Although these reviews by Kirby and colleagues[85] and Kalichman and colleagues[92] attempted to sort out what intervention strategies have been effective for HIV risk reduction, not many of the studies they reviewed were well-designed prospective RCTs, which calls into question the ability of these reviews to guide future work in HIV prevention and intervention.

However, since the mid-1990s, several RCTs[96,100–105] have been published. Orr and colleagues[100] tried to determine whether condom use among high-risk female adolescents could be increased through a brief behavioral intervention. Infection with *Chlamydia trachomatis* as a biomarker of condom practices was used when subjects returned for follow-up assessment 5 to 7 months after the intervention. As compared with those receiving a standard (control) intervention, subjects receiving the behavioral intervention reported a three-fold greater condom use at follow-up. However, incident infection with *C. trachomatis* did not differ between groups. The authors suggested that condom use, although increased, remained inconsistent. As they pointed out, interpretation of this biomarker data has to include such factors as the prevalence of the infection in the population and the transmissibility of the organism. Important limitations of the study included a very high attrition rate. Dropouts were significantly younger, more likely to have enrolled from a family planning clinic, and more likely to have been sexually active for a shorter period of time than those who returned for follow-up. As well, the ability to generalize these results was limited because all subjects had had an STI, and the majority were African Americans and had had more than one sexual partner. In spite of these limitations, the study suggests that brief behavioral interventions may increase condom use amongst high-risk adolescents.

Unlike Orr and colleagues, Kamb and colleagues[104] found significant decreases in STIs as well as increased condom use in their large (about 6,000 participants) multicenter RCT, even at 12 months after the intervention. Not only did they find that their interventions were effective but also that even their brief interactive intervention (two client-centered counseling sessions) achieved these results. The researchers found that the greatest impact of their interventions was amongst subjects under 20 years of age.

Stanton and colleagues,[96] in a longitudinal RCT of about 400 African American youth aged 9 to 15 years, tried to evaluate the effects of an AIDS risk-reduction intervention on the use of condoms and other prescription and nonprescription birth-control methods. They obtained self-reported data at baseline, 6, 12, and 18 months after the intervention. They found that those who received the intervention used more effective contraceptive practices; more than 80 percent of the youth who used oral contraceptives also used condoms. These findings were stable over time. Although the study was limited by its sample size, the use of convenience sampling, and possible problems with self-reported data, the results are extremely encouraging.

Jemmott and colleagues[102] reported a well-designed rigorous RCT that evaluated the relative efficacy of two intensive interventions, abstinence and safer sex, and compared these with a control intervention on health matters unrelated to sexual behavior. The study answered these clinical and research questions: Are HIV risk-reduction interventions effective? Are there differences in effect on the basis of whether the intervention is derived from abstinence or a safer-sex model? Are the effects of the intervention or interventions long lasting? Is there a difference in effectiveness on the basis of implementation by adult or peer cofacilitators? The editorial in the same issue of the *Journal of the American Medical Association*[106] praised this study in these words: "This methodologically rigorous study provides much needed data for evaluating the relative efficacy of these two intervention approaches." The trial involved 659 African American youth, who were randomly assigned to one of three interventions. Follow-up assessments occurred at 3, 6, and 12 months after the intervention. Either adults or peer facilitators delivered the interventions. Although the abstinence intervention group reported less likelihood of sexual intercourse at 3 months after the intervention, this significant finding was no longer present at the 6- and 12-month follow-up assessments. The safer-sex group, however, did show sustained decreases in sexual intercourse at the 6- and 12-month follow-up assessment, as well as less unprotected intercourse at all the follow-up assessments, compared with the other two groups. Although the adolescents in the peer-facilitator groups gave more favorable evaluations to the program and their facilitators than did those in the adult-led groups, this factor had no bearing on the effectiveness of the interventions. Because no biomarker data were reported in this paper, a possible limitation of this study was its complete reliance on self-report. This may be of relevance in interpreting the behavioral outcomes of the study. However, Kamb and colleagues[104] did demonstrate significant behavioral changes with counseling interventions, using biomarker outcomes in addition to self-report.

From these and other studies, the literature supports the important, clinically relevant concept that theory-based HIV interventions are useful, not only in increasing knowledge and changing attitudes about HIV infection, but also in altering high-risk behaviors. Although the findings in the study by Jemmott and colleagues[102] should be replicated in other clinical trials aimed at different high-risk adolescent populations, there is fairly strong evidence that a risk-reduction model is more effective in altering behavior over time than an abstinence model. However, other authors[98] have warned that with certain subgroups of adolescents, such as incarcerated youth, additional work must be done on the motivation for change so that the interventions will be effective. Troubled youth who cannot see beyond today need convincing that changing behavior will benefit them in the long run.

Applying all this to the two case scenarios, health-care providers can be confident that their attempts to intervene to reduce the risk for HIV infection in these young people may be successful. They should consider both the similarities and differences between these patients and modify their interventions accordingly, taking into account the important evidence derived through a critical appraisal of the literature.

Suicide

Background

Suicide is a leading cause of death in adolescents. In Canada, it is second only to motor vehicle injuries as a cause of death in 15 to 19-year-olds.[107] Males comprise the majority of suicide completers; 81 percent of 15 to 19-year-old suicide victims were males in 1994. The suicide rate for males in this age group was 20.39 per 100,000, and suicides accounted for 24 percent of all 15 to 19-year-old male deaths that year.

In the United States, suicide ranks third as a cause of death, after motor vehicle injuries and homicides.[108] According to this report, firearms were the leading method for those 15 to 19-year-olds who successfully committed suicide, accounting for 71 percent of suicides.[109] Firearms were more frequently chosen as the method of suicide in males (73 percent) compared with females (38 percent). In Canada, after many years of being the leading method of suicide in adolescents, firearms fell to second place in the early 1990s, being used in 38 percent of male suicides and 6 percent of female suicides in 15 to 19-year-olds. The rate of home ownership of firearms in Canada is 23 percent,[109] whereas that in the United States has been estimated to be 50 percent.[110]

Although males complete suicide more frequently than do females, females attempt suicide up to four times more frequently than do males.[111] In an Oregon[112] study of fatal and nonfatal suicide attempts, ingestions accounted for 75 percent of nonfatal attempts, while firearms were used in 64 percent of fatal attempts. Suicidal ideation is common in adolescents. Smith and Crawford[113] studied a midwestern high school and reported that 62.2 percent of students had had suicidal ideation and 8.4 percent had made an attempt. Adolescents who have attempted suicide are at a higher risk of successfully committing suicide than the general population.[114]

There are certain racial differences in adolescent suicide rates that merit mentioning. In the United States, suicide rates are markedly different between African American and Caucasian youth.[115] In 1995, the suicide rates for 10 to 19-year-old Caucasians were 42 percent higher than those for African Americans. Nonetheless, the suicide rates for African American youth has been increasing faster than that of Caucasian youth. In addition, aboriginal populations in both Canada and the United States have youth suicide rates much higher than the general population.[116,117]

The best evidence about suicide risk factors in adolescents comes from psychological autopsy studies. These involve extensive study of the psychiatric status of the person completing suicide through interviews with family members and friends. Mounting evidence from these psychological autopsy studies indicates that as many as 80 to 90 percent of persons completing suicide have a diagnosable psychiatric illness. When Shaffer and colleagues[118] studied the psychological autopsies of 120 persons under the age of 20 years completing suicide and those of 147 control subjects, matched for age, sex, and ethnicity, they found that 93 percent of persons completing suicide had a probable Axis I disorder (various clinical disorders or conditions that may be a focus of clinical attention except for personality disorders and mental retardation), as defined by the DSM-III.[119] In this study, 61 percent of those completing suicide had a mood disorder. Adjustment disorder, conduct disorder, and anxiety disorder; substance and alcohol abuse were also frequently implicated.

Suicide prevention has been a much discussed initiative. Unfortunately, many initiatives are based on incorrect assumptions and ideas about adolescent suicide. The following case scenario provides the groundwork to illustrate the evidence for effectiveness of three interventions.

Sample Case

Robert is a 16-year-old Caucasian male brought to an adolescent medicine clinic by his parents because of deteriorating school performance. His parents wonder if he has attention deficit disorder because lately he seems unable to complete his homework. During your psychosocial interview, you elicit a history of 3 months of increasing sleep disturbances, fatigue, and difficulty concentrating during the day, loss of appetite, social withdrawal, and intense feelings of sadness. For the past 3 weeks, Robert has thought almost daily about wanting to die, though he has not made an attempt or formulated a plan. A hunting rifle, owned by Robert's grandfather, who died 3 years ago, is still kept in the home. With the patient's consent, you call the school to get a further history. The school principal is very concerned about the subject of adolescent suicide and asks you to develop and present a suicide prevention program for the school as a whole.

Your diagnosis of Robert's condition is depression with suicidal ideation. The following questions outline three of the many decisions you must now make:

1. Should you initiate pharmacologic antidepressant therapy?
2. What should you recommend the parents do about the firearm?
3. What should you tell the principal about the subject of the school-based education program he wishes you to initiate?

Pharmacologic Therapy

Effective pharmacologic treatment of adolescents with depression has been hampered by a lack of adolescent-specific studies evaluating the effectiveness of antidepressant medication. However, emerging evidence indicates that tricyclic antidepressant medication, though effective in adults, is not superior to a placebo in adolescents and children.[120–122] In light of its toxicity and the risk of overdosing, this class of medication cannot be recommended for treatment of adolescent depression. In recent years, attention has turned to the selective serotonin reuptake inhibitor (SSRI) class of medication, which seems to have a superior side-effect profile and reduced toxicity, compared with tricyclic antidepressants.[123] Although most studies on SSRIs have not focused on adolescents, a randomized double-blinded placebo-controlled study[124] has evaluated the use of fluoxetine in children and adolescents. Emslie and colleagues[124] studied 96 outpatients between the ages of 7 and 17 years with nonpsychotic major depressive disorder. The patients were randomized to receive either 20 mg of fluoxetine or placebo and followed up for a period of 8 weeks. Improvement was assessed with the Clinical Global Impressions Scale and the Children's Depression Rating Scale. Significant differences were noted between the fluoxetine and placebo groups: 56 percent of the patients in the fluoxetine group were rated as much or very much improved at the end of the study, as opposed to 33 percent of the placebo group. When the results were broken down by age, the response was similar for patients who were 7 to 12 years old and those 12 to 17 years old.

Although there is little evidence about the efficacy of pharmacotherapy for the reduction of suicidal behaviors in adolescents, Greenhill and Waslick[125] did an open study in which depressed adolescent suicide attempters and depressed nonattempters were treated with fluoxetine; both groups had a significant reduction in their suicide assessment scales after 8 weeks of treatment with fluoxetine. Since there was no placebo group, it cannot be determined definitively whether the improvement in suicidality was caused by the treatment with fluoxetine. When Beasley and colleagues[126] did a meta-analysis of controlled studies that compared treatment with fluoxetine with that of a placebo or tricyclic antidepressants, they found a significant reduction in the incidence of substantial suicidal ideation with fluoxetine, compared with the placebo. However, of the 17 studies in the meta-analysis, only one included adolescents.

In summary, a double-blinded RCT of the use of fluoxetine in the treatment of adolescent depression showed the medication's effectiveness. An open pilot study of adolescents on fluoxetine showed a significant reduction in suicidal ideation, and a meta-analysis of controlled, predominantly adult studies showed a significant reduction in the suicidal ideation in patients on fluoxetine compared with that of controls. Therefore, there is good evidence to support the use of fluoxetine in adolescents with depression and fair evidence to suggest that this will result in a reduction of suicidal ideation and behaviors.

Firearms and Suicide

Several well-designed case–control studies have shown that the presence of a firearm in the home increases the risk for completed suicide.[127–129] Brent and colleagues[128] compared a group of 47 adolescent suicide completers, aged 19 years or younger, with 47 psychiatric inpatients who had attempted suicide and with a control group of 47 psychiatric inpatients who were never suicidal. The attempters and the controls were matched with the suicide completers for age, county of origin (western Pennsylvania), and sex. The authors found that firearms were twice as likely to be present in the homes of the suicide completers as in those of the attempters (odds ratio 2.1, 95 percent confidence interval) and the psychiatric control group (odds ratio 2.2, 95 percent confidence interval). The majority of suicide completers who had firearms in their homes used the firearms in their suicide; none of the suicide attempters used guns. Suicide by firearm was rare when the suicide completers did not have firearms in their homes. The method of storage of firearms in the home did not differ among the three groups. Although the trend was towards less safe storage of the guns (ie, guns stored loaded or unlocked) in the homes of suicide completers, this was not statistically significant: of the 5 suicide completers who lived in a home where the gun was locked up, 3 killed themselves with that gun. Kellermann and colleagues[129] studied 438 suicide completers of all ages who had committed suicide at home and matched them with control subjects in the same neighborhood. After controlling for subjects living alone, taking psychotropic medication, abusing alcohol or drugs, or not graduating from high school, the authors found that the presence of a firearm in the home was associated with a significantly increased risk of suicide (adjusted odds ratio, 4.8; 95 percent confidence interval).

Teenagers who have reduced access to firearms seem not to compensate fully for this by committing suicide in other ways. Sloan and colleagues[130] did a comparative study of suicide rates and relative risks of suicide in Vancouver and Seattle. Vancouver has stricter gun control laws and lower firearm ownership rates than Seattle; the two cities are otherwise very similar demographically. For the 15- to 24-year-olds in the study, the non-firearm suicide rate in both cities was similar. However, the total suicide rate in Seattle was significantly higher (Seattle 15.72 versus Vancouver 11.43 deaths per 100,000, relative risk, 1.38) because Seattle had a three-fold increased risk of suicide by firearms that was not offset by an increase in suicides by other methods in Vancouver. Interestingly, the study found that in the older age groups in Vancouver, the rate of suicides by methods other than with a firearm *did* increase and offset the decreased rate of suicide by firearms. This suggests that measures aimed at reducing the availability of firearms could particularly benefit young people.

The presence of a firearm in the home, therefore, should be seen as an important risk factor for suicide in adolescents. This information should be included in general pediatric safety counseling. Questioning about the presence of a firearm in the home should be an automatic part of the assessment of suicide risk for every suicidal adolescent. Lastly, every effort should be made to remove all firearms from the homes of suicidal adolescents. Safe storage of firearms does not appear to be an adequate safeguard against teenage suicide by firearms.

School-Based Suicide Prevention Programs for Adolescents

The purpose of most school-based curricula programs for the prevention of adolescent suicide is to heighten awareness of the problem of adolescent suicide and to encourage teenagers to recognize when they or their friends are at risk for suicide and to get help. The rationale for these programs is that suicidal teenagers are more likely to discuss their concerns with a peer than with an adult. The teenagers who have had school-based education will be more likely to seek help for their troubled friend. It is hoped that students exposed to the intervention will be more likely to seek help for themselves as well.

In 1996, Ploeg and colleagues[131] did a systematic overview of this popular type of program. They found 187 articles relevant to suicide prevention curricula programs for adolescents. Of these, only 11 met the following relevance criteria:

- Evaluation of an intervention
- Provision of information on client-focused outcomes or cost or both
- Description of a prospective study
- Use of a control group

The validity of the 11 articles was assessed on such criteria as methods of allocation to study groups and data collection, level of agreement to participate, control for confounding variables, and percentage of participants available for follow-up. The design of the studies was judged to be weak by the authors (as opposed to moderate or strong) because at least one of the validity criteria was not met. Eight of the 11 studies were done in the United States, 2 in Israel, and 1 in Australia. Ten of the studies evaluated a program of teaching a suicide prevention curriculum, and one evaluated a "postvention" (an intervention in a school after a suicide) program consisting of counseling.

Although the majority of the studies showed increased knowledge among participants about suicide, the programs had a more mixed effect on students' attitudes about suicide. Five studies showed an improvement in attitudes, two showed no change. One study showed that after the program, *more* students (mostly males) thought that suicide was a possible solution to their problems. Evaluation of hopelessness was another area of concern. In two studies, there was an improvement in the students exposed to the intervention; however, in one study, there was a decrease in hopelessness for girls but an increase for boys. Of the 11 studies, most studied only attitudes. Only one (the "postvention" study) evaluated changes in actual behavior; there was no significant difference between exposed and nonexposed groups in the rate of hospitalization for suicide attempts. On the basis of these findings and the limitations of the studies, the authors concluded that there was insufficient evidence to support the use of the methods of these programs.

In summary, before school-based programs to prevent suicide can be recommended, research must determine which approaches will positively affect suicide risk factors *and* behaviors in both male and female adolescents. Health-care providers should be wary of involvement in programs that, though well-intentioned, may do harm as well as good.

CONCLUSION

Adolescent medicine is a rapidly advancing field. It is our responsibility to develop the field in such a way that we ensure careful and critical use of our clinical experience, together with the best available published information. From the case scenarios highlighting evidence-based approaches in adolescent medicine that we have presented here, it is clear that there is much work to be done and many questions to be answered. As advocates for our adolescent patients, we want to provide optimal patient care by integrating our clinical expertise with sound evidence and the active participation of our patients in their health-care decisions. A summary of the interventions for various issues in adolescence is provided in Table 23–1.

Table 23–1 Summary of Recommendations for the Prevention and Management of Selected Adolescent Issues

Condition	Intervention	Level of Evidence	Recommendations
Confidentiality and the adolescent's intentions to disclose sensitive information and modify their willingness to seek future health care	Assuring confidentiality	I	A
Osteopenia in anorexia nervosa	• Hormone replacement therapy	II	C
	• Calcium supplementation	III	B
	• Increased physical activity	III	C
Adolescent HIV risk reduction	Safer sex and risk reduction interventions	I	A
Adolescent depression	SSRI	I	A
Suicidal ideation in adolescent depression	SSRI	II-2	B
Adolescent suicide	• Remove firearm from home	II-2	B
	• School-based suicide prevention program	II-2	C

SSRI = selective serotonin reuptake inhibitor

REFERENCES

1. Haynes RB, Sackett DL, Gray JMA, et al. Transferring evidence from research into practice: 1. The role of clinical care research evidence in clinical decisions. ACP J Club 1996;November/December:A14–6.

2. Mulrow CD, Cook DJ, Davidoff F. Systematic reviews: critical links in the great chain of evidence. Ann Intern Med 1997;126:389–91.

3. Sackett DL, Rosenberg WMC, Gray JAM, et al. Evidence-based medicine: what it is and what it isn't. Br Med J 1996;312:71–2.

4. Ellis J, Mulligan I, Rowe J, Sackett DL. Inpatient general medicine is evidence-based. Lancet 1995;346:407–10.

5. Feldman W. Evidence-based pediatrics. Evidence-Based Med 1998;September/October:134–5.

6. Ginsburg KR, Slap GB, Cnaan A, et al. Adolescents' perceptions of factors affecting their decisions to seek health care. JAMA 1995;273:1913–8.

7. Wibblesman CJ. Confidentiality in an age of managed care: can it exist? Adolescent Medicine State-of-the-art Reviews. 1997;8:427–32.

8. American Medical Association National Coalition on Adolescent Health: Policy Compendium on Confidential Health Services for Adolescents. Chicago: American Medical Association; 1993.

9. Rationale and recommendations: delivery of health services to adolescents. In: Elster A, editor. AMA guidelines for adolescent preventive services: recommendations and rationale. Baltimore, Maryland: Williams and Wilkins; 1994; p. 191.

10. Adolescent Medicine Committee CPS. Office practice guidelines for the care of adolescents. Can Med Assoc J 1994;1:121–3.

11. Adolescent Medicine Committee and Bioethics Committee CPS. Sexuality education: counselling guidelines for the primary care physician. Paediatr Child Health 1997;2:45–8.

12. Klein JD, Slap GB, Elster AB, Schonberg SK. Access to health care for adolescents: a position paper of the Society for Adolescent Medicine. J Adolesc Health 1992;13:162–70.

13. Emans SJ, Brown RT, Davis A, et al. Society for Adolescent Medicine. Position paper on reproductive health care for adolescents. J Adolesc Health 1991;12:649–61.

14. Policy reference guide: a comprehensive guide of American Academy of Pediatrics policy statements published through December 1991. Elk Grove Village, IL: American Academy of Pediatrics; 1991.

15. Cheng TL, Savageau JA, Sattler AL, De Witt TG. Confidentiality in health care. A survey of knowledge, perceptions and attitudes among high school students. JAMA 1993;269:1420–4.

16. Ford CA, Millstein SG, Halpern-Felsher BL, Irwin CE. Influence of physician confidentiality assurances on adolescents' willingness to disclose information and seek future health care. A randomized controlled trial. JAMA 1997;278:1029–34.

17. Adler NE, Kegeles SM, Irwin CE, Wibbelsman C. Adolescent contraceptive behavior: an assessment of decision processes. J Pediatr 1990;116:463–71.

18. Ford CA, Millstein SG. Delivery of confidentiality assurances to adolescents by primary care physicians. Arch Pediatr Adolesc Med 1997;151:505–9.

19. Council on Scientific Affairs, American Medical Association. Confidential health services for adolescents. JAMA 1993;269:1420–4.

20. Rooney B, McClelland L, Crisp AH, Sedgwick PM. The incidence and prevalence of anorexia nervosa in three suburban health districts in South West London, U.K. Inter J Eating Disorders 1995;18:299–307.

21. Eagles JM, Johnston MI, Hunter D, et al. Increasing incidence of anorexia nervosa in the female population of Northeast Scotland. Am J Psychiatry 1995;152:1266–71.

22. Lucas AR, Beard CM, O'Fallon WM, Kurland LT. 50 Year trend in the incidence of anorexia nervosa in Rochester, Minn.: a population based study. Am J Psychiatry 1991;148:917–22.

23. Hsu LK. Epidemiology of the eating disorders. Psychiatr Clin N Am 1996;18:681–700.

24. American Psychiatric Association. Diagnostic and statistical manual of mental disorders, 4th ed. Washington, D.C.: American Psychiatric Association; 1994.

25. Garfinkel PE, Garner DM. Anorexia nervosa: a multidimensional perspective. New York, NY: Brunner/Mazel; 1982.

26. Palla B, Litt IF. Medical complications of eating disorders in adolescents. Pediatrics 1988;81:613–23.

27. Katzman DK, Zipursky RB. Adolescents with anorexia nervosa: the impact of the disorder on bones and brains. Ann NY Acad Sci 1997;817:127–37.

28. Bachrach LK, Guido D, Katzman DK, et al. Decreased bone density in adolescent girls with anorexia nervosa. Pediatrics 1990;86:440–7.

29. Bachrach L, Katzman D, Litt I, et al. Recovery from osteopenia in adolescent girls with anorexia nervosa. J Clin Endocrinol Metab 1991;72:602–6.

30. Matkovic V, Kostia lK, Simonovic I, et al. Bone status and fracture rates in two regions of Yugoslavia. Am J Clin Nutr 1979;32:540–9.

31. Ferrari E, Franschini F, Brambilla F. Hormonal circadian rhythms in eating disorders. Biol Psychiatry 1990;27:1007–20.

32. Gold PW, Gwirtsman H, Avgerinos PC, et al. Abnormal hypothalamic-pituitary-adrenal function in anorexia nervosa. Pathophysiologic mechanisms in underweight and weight-corrected patients. N Engl J Med 1986;314:1335–42.

33. Kaye W, Gwirtsman H, George D, et al. Elevated cerebrospinal fluid levels of immunoreactive corticotropin-releasing hormone in anorexia nervosa: relation to state of nutrition, adrenal function, and intensity of depression. J Clin Endocrinol Metab 1987;64:203–8.

34. Kling M, Demitrack M, Whitfield H, et al. Effects of the glucocorticoid antagonist RU 486 on pituitary-adrenal function in patients with anorexia nervosa and healthy volunteers: ement of plasma ACTH and cortisol secretion in underweight patients. Neuroendocrinology 1993;57:1082–91.

35. Lukert BP, Raisz LG. Glucocorticoid-induced osteoporosis: pathogenesis and management. Ann Intern Med 1990;112:352–65.

36. Canadian Consensus Conference on Menopause and Osteoporosis. Osteoporosis. J Soc Obstet Gynaecol Can 1998;20:1264–72.

37. Barrett-Connor E. Risks and benefits of replacement estrogen. Annu Rev Med 1992;43:239–51.

38. Kreipe RE, Hicks DG, Rosier RN, Puzas JE. Preliminary findings on the effects of sex hormones on bone metabolism in anorexia nervosa. J Adolesc Health 1993;14:319–24.

39. Hergenroeder AC. Bone mineralization, hypothalamic amenorrhea, and sex steroid therapy in female adolescents and young adults. J Pediatr 1995;126:683–9.

40. Seeman E, Szmukler GI, Formica C, et al. Osteoporosis in anorexia nervosa: the influence of peak bone density, bone loss, oral contraceptive use, and exercise. J Bone Miner Res 1992;7:1467–74.

41. Klibanski A, Biller BMK, Schoenfeld DA, et al. The effects of estrogen administration on trabecular bone loss in young women with anorexia nervosa. J Clin Endocrinol Metab 1994;80:898–904.

42. Fleming KH, Heimbach JT. Consumption of calcium in the U.S.: food sources and intake levels. J Nutr 1994;124(8 Suppl):1426–30S.

43. Johnston CC, Miller JZ, Slemenda CW, et al. Calcium supplementation and increases in bone mineral density in children. N Engl J Med 1992;327:82–7.

44. Lloyd T, Andon MB, Rollings N, et al. Calcium supplementation and bone mineral density in adolescent girls. JAMA 1993;270:841–4.

45. Lee TWK, Leung SSF, Wang SF, et al. Double-blind, controlled calcium supplementation and bone mineral accretion in children accustomed to a low-calcium diet. Am J Clin Nutr 1994;60:744–50.

46. Bonjour JP, Carrie AL, Ferrarri S, et al. Calcium-enriched foods and bone mass growth in prepubertal girls: a randomized, double-blind, placebo-controlled trial. J Clin Invest 1997;99:1287–94.

47. Cadogan J, Eastell R, Jones N, Barker ME. Milk intake and bone mineral acquisition in adolescent girls: randomised, controlled intervention trial. Br Med J 1997;315:1255–60.

48. Lee WTK, Leung SSF, Leung DMY, Cheng JCY. A follow-up study on the effects of calcium-supplement withdrawal and puberty on bone acquisition of children. Am J Clin Nutr 1996;64:71–7.

49. Slemenda CW, Peacock M, Hui S, et al. Reduced rates of skeletal remodeling are associated with increased bone mineral density during the development of peak skeletal mass. J Bone Mineral Res 1997;12:676–82.

50. Hay PJ, Delahunt JW, Hall A, et al. Predictors of osteopenia in premenopausal women with anorexia nervosa. Calcified Tissue International 1992;50:498–501.

51. Rigotti NA, Nussbaum SR, Herzog DB, Neer RM. Osteoporosis in women with anorexia nervosa. N Engl J Med 1984;311:601–6.

52. Biller BMK, Saxe V, Herzog DB, et al. Mechanisms of osteoporosis in adult and adolescent women with anorexia nervosa. J Clin Endocrinol Metab 1989;68:548–54.

53. NIH Consensus Conference. Optimal calcium intake. NIH Consensus Development Panel on Optimal Calcium Intake. JAMA 1994;272:1942–8.

54. vandenBergh MF, DeMan SA, Witteman JC, et al. Physical activity, calcium intake, and bone mineral content in children in the Netherlands. J Epidemiol Comm Health 1995;49:299–304.

55. Nordstrom P, Thorsen K, Nordstrom G, et al. Bone mass, muscle strength and different body constitutional parameters in adolescent boys with a low or moderate exercise level. Bone 1995;17:351–6.

56. Gunnes M, Lehmann EH. Physical activity and dietary constituents as predictors of forearm cortical and trabecular bone gain in healthy children and adolescents: a prospective study. Acta Paediatrica 1996;85:19–25.

57. Boot AM, de Ridder MA, Pols HA, et al. Bone mineral density in children and adolescents: relation to puberty, calcium intake and physical activity. J Clin Endocrinol Metab 1997;82:57–62.

58. Cooper C, Cawley M, Bhalla A, et al. Childhood growth, physical activity, and peak bone mass in women. J Bone Mineral Res 1995;10(6):940–7.

59. Young D, Hopper JL, Nowson CA, et al. Determinants of bone mass in 10- to 26-year-old females: a twin study. J Bone Mineral Res 1995;105:558–67.

60. Marcus R, Drinkwater B, Dalsky G, et al. Osteoporosis and exercise in women. Med Sci Sports Exercise 1992;24:S301–7.

61. Snow-Harter CM. Bone health and prevention of osteoporosis in active and athletic women. Clin Sports Med 1994;13:389–404.

62. Kannus P, Haapasalo H, Sankelo M, et al. Effect of starting age of physical activity on bone mass in the dominant arm of tennis and squash players. Ann Intern Med 1995;123(1):27–31.

63. Heinonen A, Oja P, Kannus P, et al. Bone mineral density in female athletes representing sports with different loading characteristics of the skeleton. Bone 1995;17:197–203.

64. Fehling PC, Alekel L, Clasey J, et al. A comparison of bone mineral densities among female athletes in impact loading and active loading sports. Bone 1995;17:205–10.

65. Guglielmini C, Cavallini R, Mazzoni G, et al. Relationship between physical activity level and bone mineral density in two groups of female athletes. Quart J Nuclear Med 1995;39:280–4.

66. Okano H, Mizumuma H, Soda M, et al. Effects of exercise and amenorrhea on bone mineral density in teenage runners. Endocrine J 1995;42:271–6.

67. Hein K, Dell R, Futterman D, et al. Comparison of HIV+ and HIV- adolescents: risk factors and psychosocial determinants. Pediatrics 1995;95:96–104.

68. UNAIDS/WHO Working Group on Global HIV/AIDS and STD Surveillance. Report on the global HIV/AIDS epidemic: estimates as of December 1997. Geneva: World Health Organization; 1998.

69. Lab Centre for Disease Control. Ottawa, Ontario: Health Canada; 1995.

70. Rosenberg PS, Biggar RJ. Trends in HIV incidence among young adults in the United States. JAMA 1998;279:1894–9.

71. Chassin L, Presson CC, Sherman SJ, Edwards DA. The natural history of cigarette smoking: predicting youth adult smoking outcomes from adolescent smoking patterns. Health Psychol 1990;9:701–16.

72. Wendell DA, Onorato IM, McCray E, et al. Youth at risk. Sex, drugs and human immunodeficiency virus. Am J Dis Child 1992;146:76–81.

73. Battjes RJ, Leukefeld CG, Pickens RW. Age at first injection and HIV risk among intravenous drug users. Am J Drug Alcohol Abuse 1992;18:263–73.

74. DeMatteo D, Major C, Bock B, et al. Toronto street youth and HIV/AIDS: prevalence, demographics and risks. J Adolesc Health 1998. [In press]

75. Fortenberry JMD. Adolescent substance use and sexually transmitted diseases risk: a review. J Adolesc Health 1995;16:304–8.

76. Friedman LMD, Strunin LP, Hingson RS. A survey of attitudes, knowledge, behavior related to HIV testing of adolescents and young adults enrolled in alcohol and drug treatment. J Adolesc Health 1993;14:442–5.

77. Kipke M, O'Connor S, Palmer R, MacKenzie RG. Street youth in Los Angeles. Profile of a group at high risk for human immunodeficiency virus infection. Arch Pediatr Adolesc Med 1995;149:513–9.

78. McDonald C, Loxley W, Marsh A. A bridge too near? Injecting drug users' sexual behaviour. AIDS Care 1994;6:317–26.

79. St. Lawrence J, Jefferson K, Alleyne E, Brasfield T. Comparison of education versus behavioral skills training interventions in lowering sexual HIV-risk behavior of substance-dependent adolescents. J Consult Clin Psychol 1995;63:154–7.

80. MacDonald N, Fisher W, Wells G, et al. Canadian street youth: correlates of sexual risk-taking activity. Pediatr Infect Dis J 1994;13:690–7.

81. Magura S, Kang S, Shapiro M. Outcomes of intensive AIDS education for male adolescent drug users in jail. J Adolesc Health Care 1994;15:457–63.

82. Graham CA. AIDS and the adolescent. Inter J STD AIDS 1994;5:305–9.

83. Kipke MD, Boyer CP, Hein KMD. An evaluation of an AIDS risk reduction education and skills training (ARREST) program. J Adolesc Health 1993;14:533–9.

84. Kelly JA. Sexually transmitted disease prevention approaches the work. Interventions to reduce risk behavior among individuals, groups and communities. Sex Trans Dis 1994;21:73–5.

85. Kirby DP, Short LP, Collins JP, et al. School-based programs to reduce sexual risk behaviors: a review of effectiveness. Public Health Records 1994;3:339–60.

86. Caceres CF, Rosasco AM, Mandel JS, Hearst N. Evaluating a school-based intervention for STD/AIDS prevention in Peru. J Adolesc Health 1994;15:582–91.

87. Mansfield C, Conroy M, Emans S, Woods ER. A pilot study of AIDS education and counseling of high-risk adolescents in an office setting. J Adolesc Health 1993;14:115–9.

88. Jemmott L, Jemmott J. Increasing condom-use intentions among sexually active black adolescent women. Nursing Res 1992;41:273–9.

89. Rotheram-Borus MJ, Koopman C, Haignere C, Davies M. Reducing HIV sexual risk behaviors among runaway adolescents. JAMA 1991;266:1237–41.

90. Walter H, Vaughan MS. AIDS risk reduction among a multiethnic sample of urban high school students. JAMA 1993;270:725–30.

91. St. Lawrence J, Brasfield T, Jefferson K, et al. Cognitive-behavioral intervention to reduce African American adolescents' risk for HIV infection. J Consult Clin Psychol 1995;63:221–37.

92. Kalichman S, Carey M, Johnson B. Prevention of sexually transmitted HIV infection: a meta-analytic review of the behavioral outcome literature. Ann Behav Med 1996;18:6–15.

93. Quirk M, Godkin M, Schwenzfeier E. Evaluation of two AIDS prevention interventions for inner-city adolescent and young adult women. Am J Prevent Med 1993;9:21–6.

94. Morton M, Nelson L, Walsh C, et al. Evaluation of an HIV/AIDS education program for adolescents. J Comm Health 1996;21:23–8.

95. O'Hara P, Messick B, Fichtner R, Parris D. A peer-led AIDS prevention program for students in an alternative school. J School Health 1996;66:176–83.

96. Stanton B, Li X, Ricardo I, et al. A randomized, controlled effectiveness trial of an AIDS prevention program for low-income African-American youth. Arch Pediatr Adolesc Med 1996;150:363–72.

97. Main D, Iverson D, McGloin J, et al. Preventing HIV infection among adolescents: evaluation of a school-based education program. Prevent Med 1994;23:409–17.

98. Slonim-Nevo V, Auslander W, Ozawa M, Jung K. The long-term impact of AIDS-preventive interventions for delinquent and abused adolescents. Adolescence 1996;31:409–21.

99. Wren P, Janz N, Carovano K, et al. Preventing the spread of AIDS in youth: principles of practice from 11 diverse projects. J Adolesc Health 1997;21:309–17.

100. Orr DP, Langefeld CD, Katz BP, Caine VA. Behavioral intervention to increase condom use among high-risk female adolescents. J Pediatr 1996;128:288–95.

101. Thomas BH, DiCenso A, Griffith L. Adolescent sexual behaviour: results from an Ontario sample. Part II: Adolescent use of protection. Can J Public Health 1998;89:94–7.

102. Jemmott JB, Jemmott LS, Fong GT. Abstinence and safer sex HIV risk-reduction interventions for African American adolescents. A randomized controlled trial. JAMA 1998;279:1529–36.

103. DiClemente RJ, Wingood GM. A randomized controlled trial of an HIV sexual risk-reduction intervention for young African-American women. JAMA 1995;274:1271–6.

104. Kamb JL, Fishbein M, Douglas JM, et al. Efficacy of risk-reduction counseling to prevent human immunodeficiency virus and sexually transmitted diseases. JAMA 1998;280:1161–7.

105. Rusakaniko S, Mbizvo MT, Kasule J, et al. Trends in reproductive health knowledge following a health education intervention among adolescents in Zimbabwe. Central Afr J Med 1997;43:1–6.

106. DiClemente RJ. Preventing sexually transmitted infections among adolescents. JAMA 1998;279:1574–5.

107. Statistics Canada. Mortality, Summary List of Causes, 1994. Statistics Canada; 1996. Catalogue No. 84-209.

108. National Center for Health Statistics, Vital Statistics, U.S. National Summary of Injury Mortality Data. Department of Health and Human Services, Public Health Service, Centers for Disease Control and Prevention; 1998.

109. Angus Reid Group. Firearm ownership in Canada. Angus Reid Group; 1991.

110. The Gallup Organization. Handgun ownership in America. Los Angeles Times Syndicate; May 29, 1991.

111. Suicide among children, adolescents, and young adults—United States, 1980-1992. JAMA 1995;274:451–2.

112. MMWR. Fatal and nonfatal suicide attempts among adolescents. Gregon, 1988–1993. MMWR 1995;44:312–315.

113. Smith K, Crawford S. Suicidal behavior among "normal" high school students. Suicide Life Threat Behav 1986;16:313–325.

114. Shaffer D, Garland A, Gould M, et al. Preventing teenage suicide: a critical review. J Am Acad Child Adolesc Psychiatry 1988;27:675–87.

115. Suicide among black youths—United States, 1980-1995. JAMA 1996;279:1431.

116. Berlin IN. Suicide among American Indian adolescents: an overview. Suicide and life-threatening behavior 1987;17:218–32.

117. Moffatt ME. Adolescence and health in Canada's aboriginal people. In: Westwood M, editor. Report of the Eighth Canadian ROSS Conference in Paediatrics. Montreal: Ross Laboratories; 1991.

118. Shaffer D, Gould MS, Fisher P, et al. Psychiatric diagnosis in child and adolescent suicide. Arch Gen Psychiatry 1996;53:339–48.

119. American Psychiatric Association. Diagnostic and statistical manual of mental disorders, 3rd ed. Washington, D.C.: American Psychiatric Association; 1987.

120. Kutcher S, Boulos C, Ward B, et al. Response to desipramine treatment in adolescent depression: a fixed-dose, placebo-controlled trial. J Am Acad Child Adolesc Psychiatry 1994;33:686–94.

121. Kye CH, Waterman GS, Ryan ND, et al. A randomized, controlled trial of amitriptyline in the acute treatment of adolescent major depression. J Am Acad Child Adolesc Psychiatry 1996;35:1139–44.

122. Geller B, Cooper TB, Graham DL, et al. Double-blind placebo-controlled study of nortriptyline in depressed adolescents using a "fixed plasma level" design. Psychopharmacol Bull 1990;26:85–90.

123. Leonard HL, March J, Rickler KC, Allen AJ. Pharmacology of the selective serotonin reuptake inhibitors in children and adolescents. J Am Acad Child Adolesc Psychiatry 1997;36:725–36.

124. Emslie GJ, Rush AJ, Weinberg WA, et al. A double-blind, randomized, placebo-controlled trial of fluoxetine in children and adolescents with depression. Arch Gen Psychiatry 1997;54:1031–7.

125. Greenhill L, Waslick B. Management of suicidal behavior in children and adolescents. Psychiatr Clin N Am 1997;20:641–6.

126. Beasley CM Jr, Dornseif BE, Bosomworth JC, et al. Fluoxetine and suicide: a meta-analysis of controlled trials of treatment for depression. Br Med J 1991;303:685–9.

127. Brent DA, Perper JA, Goldstein CE, et al. Risk factors for adolescent suicide. A comparison of adolescent suicide victims with suicidal inpatients. Arch Gen Psychiatry 1988;45:581–8.

128. Brent DA, Perper JA, Allman CJ, et al. The presence and accessibility of firearms in the homes of adolescent suicides. A case-control study. JAMA 1991;266:2989–95.

129. Kellermann AL, Rivara FP, Somes G, et al. Suicide in the home in relation to gun ownership. N Engl J Med 1992;327:467–72.

130. Sloan JH, Rivara FP, Reay DT, et al. Firearm regulations and rates of suicide. A comparison of two metropolitan areas. N Engl J Med 1990;322:369–73.

131. Ploeg J, Ciliska D, Dobbins M, et al. A systematic overview of adolescent suicide prevention programs. Can J Public Health 1996;87:319–24.

Index

Please note: italicized page numbers refer to tables or figures.